LEADING
and MANAGING
in NURSING

SIXTH EDITION

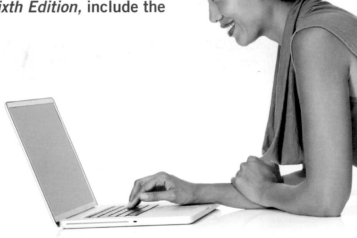

LEADING
and MANAGING
in NURSING

SIXTH EDITION

Patricia S. Yoder-Wise
Texas Tech University Health Sciences Center
Lubbock, Texas

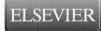

MOSBY

3251 Riverport Lane
St. Louis, Missouri 63043

LEADING AND MANAGING IN NURSING
SIXTH EDITION   978-0-323-18577-6

Notices

Knowledge and best practice in this field are constantly changing. As new research and experience broaden our understanding, changes in research methods, professional practices, or medical treatment may become necessary.

Practitioners and researchers must always rely on their own experience and knowledge in evaluating and using any information, methods, compounds, or experiments described herein. In using such information or methods they should be mindful of their own safety and the safety of others, including parties for whom they have a professional responsibility.

With respect to any drug or pharmaceutical products identified, readers are advised to check the most current information provided (i) on procedures featured or (ii) by the manufacturer of each product to be administered, to verify the recommended dose or formula, the method and duration of administration, and contraindications. It is the responsibility of practitioners, relying on their own experience and knowledge of their patients, to make diagnoses, to determine dosages and the best treatment for each individual patient, and to take all appropriate safety precautions.

To the fullest extent of the law, neither the Publisher nor the authors, contributors, or editors, assume any liability for any injury and/or damage to persons or property as a matter of products liability, negligence or otherwise, or from any use or operation of any methods, products, instructions, or ideas contained in the material herein.

Library of Congress Cataloging-in-Publication Data

Leading and managing in nursing / [edited by] Patricia S. Yoder-Wise. – Sixth edition.
     p. ; cm.
  Includes bibliographical references and index.
  ISBN 978-0-323-18577-6 (pbk. : alk. paper)
  I. Yoder-Wise, Patricia S., 1941- editor of compilation.
  [DNLM: 1. Nurse Administrators–organization & administration. 2. Leadership. WY 105]
  RT89
  362.17'3–dc23
                                                    2014001017

Senior Content Strategist: Yvonne Alexopoulos
Content Development Manager: Jean Sims Fornango
Senior Content Development Specialist: Danielle Frazier
Publishing Services Manager: Jeff Patterson
Senior Project Manager: Tracey Schriefer
Design Direction: Ashley Miner

Printed in China.
Last digit is the print number: 10 9 8 7 6 5 4 3

Working together
to grow libraries in
developing countries

www.elsevier.com • www.bookaid.org

This book is dedicated to the families and friends who supported us as we created it; to the faculty who are dedicated to producing the nursing service leaders for the ever changing healthcare services; to the learners who have committed to an exciting career in nursing administration; and to the nurse leaders who face the incredible issues of health care every day, who do their best in leading important changes in practice, and who remain committed to the glory of nursing: the care we deliver to patients.

Lead on! ¡Adelante!

CONTRIBUTORS

Michael R. Bleich, PhD, RN, NEA-BC, FAAN

President and Maxine Clark and Bob Fox Dean and Professor Goldfarb School of Nursing at Barnes-Jewish College
St. Louis, Missouri
Chapter 1: Leading, Managing, and Following

Mary Ellen Clyne, MSN, RN, NEA-BC

President and Chief Executive Officer
Clara Maass Medical Center
Belleville, New Jersey
Chapter 16: Strategic Planning, Goal-Setting, and Marketing

Jeannette T. Crenshaw, DNP, RN, LCCE, IBCLC, NEA-BC, FAAN

Doctor of Nursing Practice
Executive Leadership in Nursing Specialization
Assistant Professor
Texas Tech University Health Sciences Center
Lubbock, Texas
Chapter 6: Making Decisions and Problem Solving
Chapter 28: Self-Management: Stress and Time

Richard G. Cuming, RN, MSN, EdD, NEA-BC

Nurse Executive – Operations Management
Performance Management & Innovation
Tenet Healthcare Corporation
Dallas, Texas
Chapter 19: Workforce Engagement and Collective Action

Mary Ann T. Donohue, PhD, RN, APN, PMH-CNS, NEA-BC

Vice President and Chief Nursing Executive
Jersey Shore University Medical Center
Meridian Health System
Neptune, New Jersey
Chapter 28: Self-Management: Stress and Time

Karen A. Esquibel, PhD, RN, CPNP-PC

Associate Professor of Nursing
Pediatric Nurse Practitioner
Texas Tech University Health Sciences Center School of Nursing
Lubbock, Texas
Chapter 9: Cultural Diversity in Health Care

Michael L. Evans, PhD, RN, NEA-BC, FACHE, FAAN

Dean and Professor
Texas Tech University Health Sciences Center School of Nursing
Lubbock, Texas
Chapter 3: Developing the Role of Leader

Victoria N. Folse, PhD, APN, PMHCNS-BC, LCPC

Director and Associate Professor, School of Nursing
Illinois Wesleyan University
Bloomington, Illinois
Chapter 20: Managing Quality and Risk
Chapter 23: Conflict: The Cutting Edge of Change

Jacqueline Gonzalez, DNP, ARNP, MBA, NEA-BC, FAAN

Senior Vice President & Chief Nursing Officer and Patient Safety Officer
Miami Children's Hospital
Miami, Florida
Chapter 4: Developing the Role of Manager

Ginny Wacker Guido, JD, MSN, RN, FAAN

Regional Director for Nursing and Assistant Dean, College of Nursing
Washington State University Vancouver
Vancouver, Washington
Chapter 5: Legal and Ethical Issues

Debra Hagler, PhD, RN, ACNS-BC, CNE, ANEF, FAAN
Clinical Professor
College of Nursing & Health Innovation
Arizona State University
Phoenix, Arizona
Chapter 29: Managing Your Career

Karen Kelly, EdD, RN, NEA-BC
Associate Professor & Director, Continuing
Education
Southern Illinois University Edwardsville School of
Nursing
Edwardsville, Illinois
Chapter 10: Power, Politics, and Influence

Shari Kist, PhD, RN
Assistant Professor
Goldfarb School of Nursing at
Barnes-Jewish College
St. Louis, Missouri
Chapter 1: Leading, Managing, and Following

Karren Kowalski, PhD, RN, NEA-BC, FAAN
Professor
Texas Tech University Health Sciences Center
Lubbock, Texas;
President and CEO
Colorado Center for Nursing Excellence
Denver, Colorado
Chapter 18: Building Teams Through
  Communication and Partnerships
Chapter 24: Managing Personal/Personnel
  Problems

Mary E. Mancini, PhD, RN, NE-BC, FAHA, FAAN
Professor and Associate Dean of Undergraduate
Nursing Programs
The University of Texas—Arlington
College of Nursing
Arlington, Texas
Chapter 7: Healthcare Organizations
Chapter 8: Understanding and Designing
  Organizational Structures

Maureen Murphy-Ruocco, ANP, C, MSN, EdM, DPNAP, FNAP
Professor and Associate Dean School of Nursing and
Health Education Graduate Program
Felician College School of Education
Rutherford, New Jersey
Chapter 26: Delegation: An Art of Professional
  Nursing Practice

Dorothy A. Otto, EdD, MSN, RN, ANEF
Associate Professor
University of Texas Health Science Center-Houston
School of Nursing
Houston, Texas
Chapter 9: Cultural Diversity in Health Care

Elaine S. Scott, PhD, RN, NE-BC
Associate Professor
Director, East Carolina Center for Nursing
Leadership
College of Nursing
East Carolina University
Greenville, North Carolina
Chapter 17: Leading Change

Ashley Sediqzad
Clinical Informatics Manager
Children's Mercy Hospitals and Clinics
Kansas City, Missouri
Chapter 11: Caring, Communicating,
  and Managing with Technology

Janis B. Smith, RN, DNP
Director, Clinical Informatics and Professional
Practice
Children's Mercy Hospitals and Clinics
Kansas City, Missouri
Chapter 11: Caring, Communicating,
  and Managing with Technology

Susan Sportsman, PhD, RN, ANEF, FAAN
Director, Academic Consulting Group
Nursing and Health Professions
Elsevier, Inc.
St. Louis, Missouri
Chapter 13: Care Delivery Strategies
Chapter 14: Staffing and Scheduling

Sylvain Trepanier, DNP, RN, CENP

Senior Director, Patient Care Services
Tenet Healthcare Corporation
Dallas, Texas
Chapter 6: Making Decisions and Problem
  Solving
Chapter 12: Managing Costs and Budgets

Diane M. Twedell, DNP, RN, CENP

Chief Nursing Officer, Southeast
Minnesota Region
Mayo Clinic Health System
Austin, Minnesota
Chapter 15: Selecting, Developing, and
Evaluating Staff
Chapter 27: Role Transition

Jana Wheeler, RN, MSN, CPN

Manager, Clinical Informatics
Children's Mercy Hospitals & Clinics
Kansas City, Missouri
Chapter 11: Caring, Communicating,
  and Managing with Technology

**Crystal J. Wilkinson, DNP, RN,
CNS-CH, CPHQ**

Assistant Professor
Texas Tech University Health Sciences Center
School of Nursing
Lubbock, Texas
Chapter 25: Workplace Violence
and Incivility

**Patricia S. Yoder-Wise, RN, EdD, NEA-BC,
ANEF, FAAN**

Professor and Dean Emerita
Texas Tech University Health Sciences Center
Lubbock, Texas
Chapter 2: Safe Care: The Core of Leading and
  Managing
Chapter 30: Thriving for the Future

Margarete Lieb Zalon, PhD, RN, ACNS-BC, FAAN

Professor
Department of Nursing
University of Scranton
Scranton, Pennsylvania
Chapter 21: Translating Research into Practice
Chapter 22: Consumer Relationships

David Zambrana, DNP, MBA, RN

Chief Operating Officer
University of Miami Hospital
Miami, Florida
Chapter 19: Workforce Engagement and Collective
  Action

EVOLVE RESOURCES
Test Bank

Joyce Engel, PhD, RN, BEd, MEd

Associate Professor
Department of Nursing
Brock University
St. Catharines, Ontario

Peer review is a critical aspect of most publications. Peers tell us what is strong and what is missing. They direct the content of a publication from their area of knowledge and experience. These individuals provide insightful comments and suggestions to hone the information presented in a text or article, and we are indebted to them. The end result of their efforts, as in any peer review process, is a stronger presentation of information for the readership. We are grateful to the masked reviewers of this publication. Thank you!

Mary T. Boylston, RN, MSN, EdD, AHN-BC

Professor of Nursing
Eastern University
St. Davids, Pennsylvania

Elizabeth P. Crusse, MS, MA, RN, CNE

Clinical Assistant Professor
Towson University
Department of Nursing
Towson, Maryland

Dee Ernesti, RN, MSN, CENP

Instructor
University of Nebraska Medical Center College of Nursing
Omaha, Nebraska

Mary L. Fisher, PhD, RN

Professor of Nursing
Associate Vice Chancellor for Academic Affairs
Indiana University-Purdue University Indianapolis
Indianapolis, Indiana

Shirley Garick, PhD, RN

Interim Director of Nursing
Professor of Nursing
Texas A&M University-Texarkana
Texarkana, Texas

Beth Bates Gaul, PhD, RN

Professor of Nursing
Grand View University
Des Moines, Iowa

Evalyn J. Gossett, MSN, RN

Clinical Assistant Professor
Indiana University Northwest
College of Health and Human Services
School of Nursing
Gary, Indiana

Judy Gregg, MS, RN

Nursing Instructor
Mount Vernon Nazarene University
Mount Vernon, Ohio

Nancy Grove, PhD, RN

Associate Professor (Retired)
University of Pittsburgh
School of Nursing
Johnstown, Pennsylvania

Emma Kientz, MS, APRN-CNS, CNE

Assistant Professor
The University of Oklahoma
Tulsa, Oklahoma

Mary B. Killeen, PhD, RN, NEA-BC

Adjunct Associate Professor
Department of Nursing
University of Michigan-Flint
Flint, Michigan

Dimitra Loukissa, PhD, RN

Associate Professor
North Park University
School of Nursing
Chicago, Illinois

Catherine Poillon Lovecchio, PhD, RN

Assistant Professor of Nursing
The University of Scranton
Scranton, Pennsylvania

Anne Boulter Lucero, MSN, RN

Assistant Director
Nursing Instructor
Cabrillo College
Aptos, California

Dorothea E. McDowell, PhD, RN
Professor of Nursing
Henson School of Science and Technology
Salisbury University
Salisbury, Maryland

Lynn A. Menzel, RN, BSN, MA
Case Management
Martin Health System
Stuart, Florida

Bettie G. Miller, MSN, MS, BSE, BSN, RN-BC
Instructor of Nursing
Eleanor Mann School of Nursing
PhD (Candidate)
Public Policy Program-Policy Studies in Aging
University of Arkansas
Fayetteville, Arkansas

Juleann H. Miller, PhD, RN
Associate Professor
Assistant Director of the Nursing Program
St. Ambrose University
Davenport, Iowa

Jack E. Rydell, DNP, RN
Assistant Professor
Concordia College
Moorhead, Minnesota

Charlotte Silvers, RN, MSN, CPHQ
Assistant Professor
Texas Tech University Health Sciences Center School
of Nursing
Lubbock, Texas

Darlene Sredl, PhD, RN
Professor of Nursing
College of Nursing
University of Missouri-St. Louis
St. Louis, Missouri

Charlotte A. Wisnewski, PhD, RN, CDE, CNE
BSN Program Director
University of Texas Medical Branch School of
Nursing at Galveston
Galveston, Texas

Joyce Wright, PhD, RN, CNE, CNL
Associate Professor
Coordinator of the RN to BSN Program
New Jersey City University
Jersey City, New Jersey

Judith Young, DNP, CCRN
Clinical Assistant Professor
Indiana University School of Nursing
Indianapolis, Indiana

ACKNOWLEDGMENTS

From the beginning of the precedent setting first edition leadership/management text to this sixth edition, many people had a part in making this publication possible. Perhaps the group that is often overlooked is, in a sense, the most important—the graduates who tell me how valuable information was in this text and how it prepared them for the evolving role of nurses as they take on new roles and responsibilities in their careers. Thank you for sharing your wisdom with us!

Special acknowledgment goes to the team at Elsevier—the "behind the scenes" people who turn Word documents into a graphically appealing and colorful presentation. To our content strategist, Yvonne Alexopoulos; to our content development specialist, Danielle Frazier; and to our project manager, Tracey Schriefer: THANKS!

To the authors who made this edition possible: thank you for helping the next generation of nurses be well prepared to enter the profession of nursing and to exercise both leadership and management in responsible and artistic ways. To the educators who have used this textbook and provided feedback, we listened and, as with the comments of the reviewers, incorporated suggestions as needed.

Most of all, for me personally, I have to thank my husband and best friend, Robert Thomas Wise. He has lived through six editions of this text and knows by now that when the deadlines tighten, his humor and creativity need to increase. And they do! His willingness to take on more of the things that might be deemed mutual tasks is a small example of his ongoing support. You are the best!

As has been true since the beginning of *Leading and Managing in Nursing,* we who created and revised this edition learned more about a particular area and the impact of each area on the whole of leadership and management. Our learning reflects the condition of nursing today: there is no room for stagnation on any topic. The context in which nurses lead and manage is constantly changing—so the key to success is to learn continuously. Keep learning, keep caring, and maintain our passion for nursing and the patients we serve. That message, if nothing else, must be instilled in our leaders of tomorrow.

Lead on! ¡Adelante!

Patricia S. Yoder-Wise
RN, EdD, NEA-BC, ANEF, FAAN
Texas Tech University Health Sciences Center
Lubbock, Texas

Leading and managing are two essential expectations of all professional nurses and become increasingly important throughout one's career. To lead, manage, and follow successfully, nurses must possess not only knowledge and skills but also a caring and compassionate attitude.

This book results from our continued strong belief in the need for a text that focuses in a distinctive way on the nursing leadership and management issues of today and tomorrow. We continue to find that we are not alone in this belief. This edition incorporates reviewers from both service and education to be sure that the text conveys important and timely information to users as they focus on the critical roles of leading, managing, and following. Additionally, we took seriously the various comments by educators and learners offered as I met them in person or heard from them by email.

CONCEPT AND PRACTICE COMBINED

Innovative in both content and presentation, *Leading and Managing in Nursing* merges theory, research, and practical application in key leadership and management areas. Our overriding concern in this edition remains to create a text that, while well grounded in theory and concept, presents the content in a way that is real. Wherever possible, we use real-world examples from the continuum of today's healthcare settings to illustrate the concepts. Because each chapter contributor synthesizes the designated focus, you will find no lengthy quotations in these chapters. We have made every effort to make the content as engaging, inviting, and interesting as possible. Reflecting our view of the real world of nursing leadership and management today, the following themes pervade the text:

- Every role within nursing has the basic concern for safe, effective care for the people for whom we exist—our clients and patients.
- The focus of health care continues to shift from the hospital to the community at a rapid rate.
- Healthcare consumers and the healthcare workforce are increasingly culturally diverse.

- Today virtually every professional nurse leads, manages, and follows, regardless of title or position.
- Consumer relationships play a central role in the delivery of nursing and health care.
- Communication, collaboration, team-building, and other interpersonal skills form the foundation of effective nursing leadership and management.
- Change continues at a rapid pace in health care and society in general.
- Change must derive from evidence-based practices wherever possible and from thoughtful innovation when no or limited evidence exists.
- Healthcare delivery is highly dependent on the effectiveness of nurses across roles and settings.

DIVERSITY OF PERSPECTIVES

Contributors are recruited from diverse settings, roles, and geographic areas, enabling them to offer a broad perspective on the critical elements of nursing leadership and management roles. To help bridge the gap often found between nursing education and nursing practice, some contributors were recruited from academia and others from practice settings. This blend not only contributes to the richness of this text but also conveys a sense of oneness in nursing. The historical "gap" between education and service must become a sense of a continuum and not a chasm.

AUDIENCE

This book is designed for undergraduate learners in nursing leadership and management courses, including those in BSN-completion courses and second-degree programs. In addition, we know that nurses in practice, who had not anticipated formal leadership and management roles in their careers, use this text to capitalize on their own real-life experiences as a way to develop greater understanding about leading and managing and the important role of following. Numerous examples and The Challenge/Solution in each chapter provide relevance to the real world of nursing.

ORGANIZATION

We have organized this text around issues that are key to the success of professional nurses in today's constantly changing healthcare environment. So the content flows from the core concepts (leading, managing, and following; patient safety; and role development as a leader and manager) to the context in which leading and managing occur (legal considerations, organizational aspects, culture, and power) to managing resources (technology, costs, staffing, change, building teams, quality, and applying research) to personal and professional skills (consumer relationships, conflicts, delegation, personal role transition, self and career management and preparing for the future).

Because repetition plays a crucial role in how well learners learn and retain new content, some topics appear in more than one chapter and in more than one section. For example, because disruptive behavior is so disruptive, it is addressed in several chapters that focus on conflict, personal/personnel problems, incivility, and self management. Rather than referring learners to another portion of the text, the key information is provided within the specific chapter, but perhaps in less depth.

We also made an effort to express a variety of different views on some topics, as is true in the real world of nursing. This diversity of views in the real world presents a constant challenge to leaders, managers, and followers, who address the critical tasks of creating positive workplaces so that those who provide direct care thrive and continuously improve the patient experience.

DESIGN

The functional full-color design, still distinctive to this text, is used to emphasize and identify the text's many learning strategies, which are featured to enhance learning. Full-color photographs not only add visual interest but also provide visual reinforcement of concepts, such as body language and the changes occurring in contemporary healthcare settings. Figures expand and clarify concepts and activities described in the text graphically.

LEARNING STRATEGIES

The numerous strategies featured in this text are designed both to stimulate learners' interest and to provide constant reinforcement throughout the learning process. Color is used consistently throughout the text to help the reader identify the various chapter elements described in the following sections.

CHAPTER OPENER ELEMENTS

- The introductory paragraph briefly describes the purpose and scope of the chapter. It is a preview of what the chapter contains.
- Objectives articulate the chapter's learning intent, typically at the application level or higher.
- *Terms to know are listed and* appear in color type in each chapter. Definitions appear alphabetically in the Glossary at the end of the text.
- The Challenge presents a contemporary nurse's real-world concern related to the chapter's focus. It is designed to allow us to "hear" a real-life situation. The Challenge ends with a question about what you might do in such a situation.

ELEMENTS WITHIN THE CHAPTERS

Exercises stimulate learners to reason critically about how to apply concepts to the workplace and other real-world situations. They provide experiential reinforcement of key leading, managing, and following skills. Exercises are highlighted within a full-color box and are numbered sequentially within each chapter to facilitate using them as assignments or activities. Each chapter is numbered separately so that learners can focus on the concepts inherent in a specific area and educators can readily use chapters to fit their own sequence of presenting information.

Research Perspectives and *Literature Perspectives* illustrate the relevance and applicability of current scholarship to practice. Perspectives always appear in boxes with a "book" icon in the upper left corner. These remain the same in the edition of the text and additional research and literature perspectives are updated on a scheduled basis so that newer information is available should educators wish to substitute any perspectives.

Theory Boxes provide a brief description of relevant theory and key concepts.

Numbered boxes contain lists, tools such as forms and work sheets, and other information relevant to the chapter.

The vivid full-color chapter opener *photographs* and other photographs throughout the text help convey each chapter's key message. Figures and tables also expand concepts presented to facilitate a greater grasp of important materials.

END OF CHAPTER ELEMENTS

The Solution provides an effective method to handle the real-life situations set forth in *The Challenge*. It reflects the response the author of The Challenge took and ends with a question about how that solution would fit for you.

The Evidence contains one example of evidence related to the chapter's content or it contains a summary of what the literature shows to be evidence related to the topic.

What New Graduates Say is a new feature that illustrates comments recent graduates have made related to the concepts discussed in the chapter.

The *Chapter Checklist* summarizes the main point in a brief paragraph and an itemized list of the major headings from the chapter.

Tips offer practical guidelines for learners to follow in applying some aspect of the information presented in each chapter.

References and *Suggested Readings* provide the learner with a list of key sources for further reading on topics found in the chapter.

OTHER TEACHING/ LEARNING STRATEGIES

The *Glossary* contains a comprehensive list of definitions of all boldfaced terms used in the chapters.

COMPLETE TEACHING AND LEARNING PACKAGE

In addition to the text *Leading and Managing in Nursing*, Educator Resources are provided online through Evolve (http://evolve.elsevier.com/Yoder-Wise/). These resources are designed to help educators present the material in this text and include the following assets:

- UPDATED! PowerPoint Slides for each chapter with lecture notes where applicable
- UPDATED! ExamView Test Bank. Answers and a rationale are also provided.
- NEW! TEACH for Nurses

Learning Resources can also be found online through Evolve (http://evolve.elsevier.com/Yoder-Wise/). These resources provide learners with additional tools for learning and include the following assets:

- NCLEX-Style Questions
- Sample Resumes

CONTENTS

PART 1

Core Concepts

Leading, Managing, and Following

Michael R. Bleich, Shari Kist

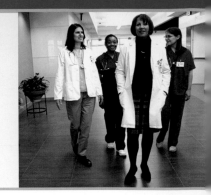

The hallmark Institute of Medicine report, The Future of Nursing: Leading Change, Advancing Health, *calls for all nurses to lead change, to manage care within interprofessional teams, and to follow in the spirit of collaboration. As health reform expands the scope of nursing practice and opportunities for nurses, the concepts of leading, managing, and following are essential to nursing practice at the point-of-care, to influence new settings and models of care delivery used, and to advocate for individuals, families, and communities.*

LEARNING OUTCOMES

- Relate leadership and other organizational theories to behaviors that serve the role(s) and functions of professional nursing.
- Link self-knowledge and emotional intelligence to the constructive use of power and influence, and the exercise of authority and responsibility needed for professional practice.
- Develop strength in bringing a professional nursing lens to the interprofessional team while advocating for quality and safety.
- Improve decision making when acting as a leader, manager, or follower by enlarging the view of the individual, family, or community being cared for to include the social network and organizational context for outcomes achievement.

KEY TERMS

Advanced Practice Registered
  Nurses (APRN)
clinical processes
complexity theory
emotional intelligence
evidence-based organizational
  practice
followership

leadership
Magnet Recognition Program®
management
management theory
motivation
Patient Protection and Affordable
  Care Act

process of care
social networking
triple aim
values
vision

THE CHALLENGE

Barbara Primm, BSN, RN-BC
Assistant Administrator and former Nursing Director Loch
Haven Senior Living Community, Macon, Missouri

Leading Culture Change in Long-Term Care: Where to Begin?

Administrators of our long-term care facility desired to be increasingly responsive to the needs of our stakeholders. With 180 skilled-care beds, we cared for individuals with dementia and those who required complex skilled care. Additionally, we had residents in 24 licensed residential care apartments. Fifteen semiprivate rooms had been converted to private rooms, but we still had a waiting list of individuals and their families who requested private rooms. The leadership team also felt the need to use the private room concept to increase our focus on resident-centered care. We recognized this national trend of resident-centered care to be in tune with our mission.

Where does one start when undertaking something as dramatic as a change in culture and processes of care? What role do staff, residents, and community members play in the implementation of resident-centered care?

What do you think you would do if you were this nurse?

INTRODUCTION

The nursing profession constitutes the backbone of the healthcare system, both in numbers and its span of influence across the clinical spectrum. Two major developments reveal the central nature of nursing to the health and well-being of citizens: the public acknowledgement of nursing in the landmark Institute of Medicine report (IOM) entitled, *The Future of Nursing: Leading Change, Advancing Health* (IOM, 2011) and the passage of the Patient Protection and Affordable Care Act (PPACA). After close analysis of the IOM report and the summary of the PPACA, one can conclude that no substantial health reform can unfold without active nursing engagement (Focus on Health Reform). Each document emphasizes that nurses must lead, manage, and collaboratively follow—not in the traditional sense of following orders or clinical protocols for care—but as active collaborators with other members of the health team and with those being served.

Beyond the expectation to lead, manage, and follow, nurses are also expected to help fulfill health care's triple aim. Coined by the Institute for Healthcare Improvement (IHI), the triple aim relates to access, quality, and cost of care (Berwick, Nolan, & Whittington, 2008). Nurses who practice in expanded roles help solve access to care in practice settings beyond traditional hospital and ambulatory centers. Increasingly, all nurses practice in the widest array of settings of any healthcare worker, including school clinics; public health; palliative, hospice, and home care; urgent care; and more. Many states allow advanced practice registered nurses (APRNs) the freedom to practice independently.

As access increases, nurses are also vigilant in delivering care that is scientific, state of the art, and sensitive to patients' needs, collectively creating a quality experience. Beyond respectful treatment, patients want their values and beliefs accommodated in partnership with the care team. Further, nurses must bring health literacy into the quality equation, ensuring the patient's ability to comprehend health-related information so that appropriate health decisions and informed post-treatment follow-up is ensured (Koh et al., 2012). Patients also demand a safe clinical experience, free from medical error and catastrophic events, including death.

Lastly, the triple aim includes impacting the cost of health care, as costs have mounted and even destabilized economies worldwide. Technology, institutional care, supplies, and human resource requirements place a staggering cost burden on individuals and businesses. At the individual level, a single major health event could drive a family into bankruptcy. The cost of insurance, insurance company profits tied to limits placed on coverage, and high deductibles are active public conversations—even with passage of the PPACA, which is designed to begin correcting many of these issues. The new terminology references accountable care organizations (ACOs), health insurance exchanges, and mandated coverage, all which challenge the public and health professionals to acquire common meaning from these and other terms.

This introduction should signal to all that point-of-care service is but one, albeit a very significant dimension of what it takes to be a high performing nurse in today's health system. As a discipline, we are called upon to develop expanded roles congruent with societal needs. We influence policy development within and beyond institutional settings. We design care processes to ensure patient- and family-centered experiences that are safe and reflect quality.

Nursing education, focused on individual, family, and community-based needs and how each intersects, adds to care coordination with health professionals who share a restricted view of care. Exercising these added functions requires self-confidence, knowledge of organizations and health systems, and an inner desire to lead, manage, and follow. This chapter starts to frame that journey, and the chapters that follow add to professional formation. In the end, nurses with leadership, management, and followership abilities will make better clinical decisions, consider the organizational and societal context of decisions, and act as advocates and stewards of resources for individuals receiving care and the impact of these decisions on families and the environment.

DIFFERENTIATING LEADING, MANAGING, AND FOLLOWING

Too often, nurses new to the profession believe their ability to perform clinical procedures is what makes them appear professional to those receiving care, to their peers, or to the public. Often, a view that leadership is isolated to those holding managerial positions prevails; and so does the view that a direct care nurse is subject to following by adhering to the direction of others. Such views fail to incorporate the fact that to be a nurse requires each licensed individual to lead, manage, and follow when practicing at the point-of-care and beyond. To appreciate why this is the case requires understanding operational definitions and appreciating leadership and organizational theories.

Leadership has been defined by individuals who have represented many different disciplines over time—it is not unique to health care. Early practitioners in organizational science noted the differences in the ways some organizations or units within those organizations operated. Morale was different, more uplifted in some areas over others. Work output was more generative. Relationships were more congenial. The traits of individuals were studied, leading to awareness that some individuals possessed traits that

seemed to produce better organizational outcomes. From these studies, trait theory was developed and is still examined as a leadership factor today.

Closely tied to this appreciation of traits as one leadership ingredient were observations that a leader could be successful in one environment yet not necessarily in another. The situation at hand and the work environment itself were variables, beyond traits, that mattered. Activities being performed were yet another variable that was studied. When the setting required reproducible and repetitive tasks, a charismatic leader may be less effective than in an unpredictable or unstructured situation where the tasks required on-the-spot innovation. These variables advanced knowledge about leading, managing, and following and promoted the development of other theories that are presented later. These include situational/contingency theory, which examines variables in the external and internal environment, including the nature of the work itself, worker behaviors (individually or in groups), the predictability or unpredictability of work, and the risk associated with work. Management theories, which require planning, organizing, and directing, and controlling aspects of the design of work are also included.

These theories, originating from the mid-1950s, are still relevant today. They continue to evolve and often are combined with other theories to guide professionals into evidence-based organizational practices, including those in health care.

From this early work, leadership can be defined as the use of individual traits and abilities, in relationship with others, and the ability to (often rapidly) interpret the environment/context where a situation is emerging, and enter that situation in the absence of a script or defined plan that could have been projected. Leadership is required when the unknown presents itself, necessitates the use of principles to improvise solutions, and helps others to cope, thrive, and function at a high capacity based on the situation. Key traits that leaders possess include articulating a vision for the desired future state; seeing possibilities in this midst of challenging, often complex, uncharted, or even dire circumstances; communicating effectively, sometimes powerfully, with others; adapting to new situations and environments; and using experience and knowledge to judge reasonable risks.

Nurses face the unknown every day. New diseases emerge. Clinical procedures have to be adapted to a patient's physical challenges. Natural disasters, such as hurricanes or tornadoes, create havoc, which leaves many people in need of immediate health care. Each of these requires stepping into the unknown, using principles, showing a commanding presence, and taking risks.

Management is the ability to plan, direct, control, and evaluate others in situations where the outcomes are known or preestablished, where one of more ways of performing have been agreed upon based upon evidence, where feedback and communication is shared to improve clinical processes and outcomes, and where sustained relationships advance consistency of purpose. Traits needed for effective managers include (1) the ability to identify recurring problems that exist where the design of evidence-based routines create structure and improved work efficiency, (2) persistent and vigilant behavior in self and others, and (3) communication that maintains esprit de corps in the face of repetitive work tasks.

Considerable time is spent on developing both leadership and management abilities. Courses, such as Advanced Cardiac Life Support (ACLS), that emphasize procedures or clinical algorithms teach management: if "A" happens, then "B" follows; if "C" emerges from "B", then "D" is performed. Less emphasis has been given to leadership development, which deals with relationships and movement toward an aim. Clinical simulation and experiences provide some opportunities for increasing these skills. Both leadership and management are needed to deal with complexity, relationship dynamics, new information, and new organizational systems and structures.

Management is needed to provide organization in the workplace, a sense of purpose, and safety. The complexities of blood or chemotherapy administration are examples of highly complex management routines. Even basic care routines, such as oral care and skin hygiene, if neglected, have serious clinical outcomes for patients. Nursing and scientific knowledge supports what we know to be best practice, yet without persistence and vigilance, efforts shift to monitoring basics such as hand hygiene and lift practices.

These examples support the idea that leadership and management is not an either/or scenario. Care routines must be managed. Nurses are on the front line when dealing with new and unknown experiences, which demands leadership. A professional nurse must have abilities to both lead and manage.

Either role, leader or manager, requires engagement with others; one does not lead or manage in isolation. Similarly one cannot follow if no direction is indicated. Unfortunately, the terms *following* and *followership* fail to get credit for what actually transpires within a healthy leader-follower or manager-follower transaction. Following sounds passive, non-directed, or unable to perform. In the health team today, collaboration requires that all team members bring knowledge, skills, abilities, and experience to deal with many complex clinical issues. A healthy definition of *followership* is that each member contributes optimally, but acquiesces to a peer who is leading or managing in a setting where a team has gathered to ensure the best clinical decision-making and actions are taken to achieve clinical or organizational outcomes. When in the following role, teamwork is palpable, where each person acts together in purpose and in a rhythm that addresses the aim at hand. Traits that great followers possess include acting synergistically with others, relieving others and stepping into leading and managing situations to prevent fatigue, speaking and acting with principle and integrity, adding value to the work being accomplished, and questioning decisions and directions when they are unclear or fail to be patient-focused. Box 1-1 is a composite of the traits needed to lead, manage, and follow.

BOX 1-1   DESIRED ATTRIBUTES OF LEADERS, MANAGERS, AND FOLLOWERS

- Use focused energy and stamina to accomplish a vision
- Use critical-thinking skills in decision making
- Trust personal intuition and then back up intuition with facts
- Accept responsibility willingly and follow up on the consequences of actions taken
- Identify the needs of others
- Deal with people skillfully: coach, communicate, counsel
- Demonstrate ease in standard/boundary setting
- Examine multiple options to accomplish the objective at hand flexibly
- Be trustworthy and handle information from various sources with respect for the source
- Motivate others assertively toward the objective at hand
- Demonstrate competence or be capable of rapid learning in the arena in which change is desired

TRADITIONAL AND EMERGING LEADERSHIP AND MANAGEMENT ROLES

The way nurses lead, manage, and follow has changed over time. Formerly, nurses took direction from physicians or senior nurses exclusively, such as "head" or "charge" nurses. These formal roles still exist in title and responsibility today, but the expectation has shifted from top-down, order-giving tied to an expectation of unquestioned following to a model in which shared decision making with collaborative action is the norm. As knowledge expands and the array of treatment interventions available to patients has grown, care delivery today is far beyond what a command-and-control top-down structure can accommodate in a traditional hierarchically-led organization. Especially in acute care settings, acuity requires immediate and autonomous responses separate from those that can be predicted and pre-assigned. Health care is now delivered in a collaborative and interprofessional manner, such as that reflected in the movement toward primary care/medical homes. In this model of care, care is delivered by providers who ensure comprehensive, patient-centered, coordinated, accessible care and quality and safety. With a team-driven approach, the model is morphing to consider the needs of populations of patients with similar care needs, focused on outcomes and true cost, aligning payment models with value-based improvement, and integrating with specialty providers, as needed (Porter, Pabo, & Lee, 2013). This holistic approach to care delivery suggests that holistic leadership is equally important. The literature perspective on p. 8 relates how communication, mentoring, and professional development can advance the function of a team.

New theories will emerge to capture the complexity and globalization of health care and other organizations. Complexity science recognizes that organizations developed under the bureaucratic model during the industrial age, where the parts in an assembly-line approach contributed to the whole, flexibility in an environment was absent, knowledge was contained, the Internet and social media were absent, and specialized knowledge-workers created webs of relationships with little regard to organizational boundaries or structures. Health care today is an amalgamation of both traditional and dynamic structures. It is unpredictable and focused on deterministic problem solving.

Professional nurses will need to practice within a system that is both predictable and unpredictable.

In this chapter and in Chapters 3 and 4, various perspectives on the concepts of leading (leadership), managing (management), and following (followership) are presented. These concepts are integrated, meaning that nurses can lead, manage, and follow concurrently. Leading, managing, and following are not institutionally role-bound concepts—the nurse must lead, manage, and follow within *any* nursing role, from direct care nurse to chief executive nurse. For organizations to thrive, each person has to assume personal responsibility by becoming the CEO of his/her own roles. We need to "lead where we are planted and shine where we find ourselves" (Sharma, 2010, p. 17). We do not have to have a "title" to be a leader; we just have to be a living human being. In other words, the synchrony of leading, managing, and following is within each of us.

The collective behaviors that reflect leading, managing, and following enhance each other. All interdisciplinary healthcare providers, including professional nurses, experience situations each day in which they must lead, manage, and follow. Some institutional formal positions, such as a nurse manager or charge nurse, require an advanced set of attributes and know-how to establish organizational goals and objectives, oversee human resources, provide staff with performance feedback, facilitate change, and manage conflict to meet patient care and organizational requirements. In other positions, the nursing role demands shifting between leading, managing and following on a moment-by-moment basis. A nurse who discovers a patient in cardiac arrest may initiate leading (dealing with the unknown), use clinical management/ACLS protocols to resuscitate the patient, and acquiesce to a follower role when the code team arrives.

EXERCISE 1-1

Using the definitions for leading, managing, and following noted previously, observe how work is organized on a clinical unit. What situations occurred that could not be predicted at the onset of the shift? What work followed a routine nature or was driven by protocol? Identify an activity that was driven by principles rather than by formal evidence. Identify an activity that was driven by evidence-based practice or evidence-based organizational practice. Then, notice team functioning. Who led? Who managed? Who followed? Did this happen seamlessly, or were there times when there was tension in efforts?

EMOTIONAL INTELLIGENCE DEVELOPMENT FOR PROFESSIONAL PRACTICE

Leading, managing, and following require different skills from those associated with the technical skills-based aspects of nursing. Goleman (2000) and others refer to emotional intelligence, characterized by social skills, interpersonal competence, psychological maturity, and emotional awareness that help people harmonize to increase their value in the workplace. Nurses have countless interactions throughout the workday in the face of emotionally-laden challenges that involve life and death. A professional nurse's portfolio contains five domains that are necessary for leading, managing, and following:

- Deepening self-awareness and encouraging others to do the same (stepping outside oneself to envision the context of what is happening while recognizing and owning feelings associated with an event)
- Managing emotions in self and others (owning feelings such as fear, anxiety, anger, and sadness and acting on those feelings in a healthy manner; avoiding passive-aggressive and victim responses)
- Motivating self and others (focusing on a goal, often with delayed gratification, such that emotional self-control is achieved and impulses are stifled)
- Being empathetic (valuing differences in perspective and showing sensitivity to the experiences of others in ways that demonstrate an ability to reveal another's perspective on a situation)
- Fostering and handling relationships (exhibiting socially appropriate behavior, expanding social networks, and using social skills to help others manage emotions).

Emotionally intelligent nurses are credible as leaders, managers, and followers because they possess awareness of the individual, family, or community that is the locus of caregiving, have enhanced organizational skills because they have invested in relationships, and are able to collaborate, show insight into others, and commit to self-growth. When coupled with performing clinical tasks tied to critical thinking and action, the emotionally intelligent nurse demonstrates the capacity to be a high-performing professional. The synergy associated with credibility and capability fuse to become makers of success. Without self-reflective skills, growth in emotional intelligence is stymied, work becomes routine, and asynchrony with others results.

Being empathetic and showing sensitivity to the experiences of others helps nurse leaders develop their emotional intelligence.

EXERCISE 1-2

Reflect on the world view of how family, friends, and others see you. Think about the historical markers that influenced your life perspective. Think about your religious or other belief systems. Review the extent to which others with diverse ideas and beliefs were a part of your life experience. As you journal these thoughts, how do they impact your emotional intelligence? Are there ways for you to expand your life experience and build your emotional capacity? What role can a mentor and continuing education play in advancing your life perspective? Most of all, do you comprehend that professional nursing demands emotional intelligence in the five domains noted earlier? For you, which domain is the most developed and which is the least developed?

THEORY DEVELOPMENT IN LEADING, MANAGING, AND FOLLOWING

Theory has several important functions for the nursing profession. First, theory can help address important questions that have yet to be answered. Second, theory (and the expanding array of research methods available to research) adds to evidence-based care and management practices (Goode, 2004). Third, theory directs and sharpens the ability to predict or guide clinical and organizational problem solving and outcomes. Nurses often have less exposure to organizational theories than to clinical theories. Leadership, management, and organizational theories are still evolving as the complexity of healthcare organizations grow, and the variables that influence care delivery increase and become more apparent. Unfortunately, a single universal theory to guide all organizational and human interactions does not exist.

Theory development associated with leading, managing, and following concepts has been a process of testing, discarding, expanding, creating, and applying. These theories overlap and have ties to the development of business and industry in the United States, as

 LITERATURE PERSPECTIVE

Resource: Hubbard, L.A. (2012). Advancing holistic nursing leadership. *Beginnings, 32*(6), 4-7.

All nurses need to be holistic leaders in the profession. Because of the nature of many nursing positions, nurses are inherently expected to lead, something that is often either forgotten or ignored. Three critical domains for leading are: communication, mentoring, and professional development. Communication and mentoring go hand in hand. Maintaining open and appropriate communication channels are essential in most aspects of nursing practice, especially when working with other members of the healthcare team. Effective mentoring of the team provides social support that improves cohesiveness; builds confidence and trust in the knowledge, skills, and abilities of the new member; decreases burnout; and improves teamwork.

Professional development in three interrelated areas is needed to advance leadership performance: evidence-based practice, quality improvement, and informatics. Evidence-based practice can be viewed as holistic care because it considers the needs and preferences of the patient, along with research-based scientific evidence. Skills in evidence-based practice and technological applications are used as part of quality improvement processes to enhance patient safety and outcomes. Collectively, these three domains foster holistic leadership, with individuals possessing a repertoire of skills.

Implications for Practice

It is just as important for a nurse to have a holistic perspective on leading, managing, and following as providing holistic care to patients. Whether in a leadership role or caring for patients, maintaining a holistic focus can be challenging, particularly during times of change and high stress. Holistic approaches to leadership require basic and ongoing skill development in the areas of communication, mentorship, and professional development. None of these areas has an endpoint in terms of opportunities to improve; novice to seasoned nurses can improve their approaches with patients and other members of the healthcare team through ongoing leadership development.

noted earlier in the chapter. Terms such as leadership theory, transformational leadership, servant leadership, management theory, and motivational theory and even attempts at followership theories are interrelated and cannot be categorized in any mutually exclusive manner. Developing theories in leading, managing, and following is a complicated task. Furthermore, the theories that leaders, managers, and follower use are drawn from yet another set of theories, many addressed within the later chapters of this book. These include theories related to change, conflict, economic, clinical, individual and group interactions, communication and social networking, and many more. The Theory Box on pp. 9–11 is organized as an overview to highlight sets of theoretical work that are commonly referenced for the purpose of demonstrating the variety, approach, and constant evolution of theory development in organizational studies. The complex factors associated with clinical care and organizational functioning explain why no single theory fully addresses the totality of leading, managing, and following.

COMPLEXITY SCIENCE TAKES HOLD

Too often, theories are believed to have been developed in the distant past, but this idea was dispelled earlier in this chapter. Complexity theory is important because it is a nontraditional theory, emerging from the work of physical sciences and, more recently, social sciences. It is addressed here because healthcare organizations are going through major transformation during a time of health systems reform.

Classic physical and, now, organizational sciences developed theory based on assumptions that by reducing something into its component parts it could be better understood. Think of the learning that took place in biology through the process of dissection. Organizations are sometime referenced as silos; like dissection, each has been organized by functional clusters (radiology, laboratory, nutrition, nursing, and medical services, for instance). Complexity science promotes the idea that the world is full of patterns that interact and adapt through relationships. These interactive patterns can be missed when one focuses solely on the part, so complexity scientists pay keen attention to what naturally occurs as patterns in the universe and how these patterns create adaptive change rather than planned or forced change. Stated

THEORY BOX

Leadership Theories

THEORY/CONTRIBUTOR	KEY IDEA	APPLICATION TO PRACTICE
Trait Theories Trait theories were first studied from 1900 to 1950. These theories are sometimes referred to as the *Great Man* theory, from Aristotle's philosophy extolling the virtue of being "born" with leadership traits. Stogdill (1948) is usually credited as the pioneer in this school of thought.	Leaders have a certain set of physical and emotional characteristics that are crucial for inspiring others toward a common goal. Some theorists believe that traits are innate and cannot be learned; others believe that leadership traits can be developed in each individual.	Self-awareness of traits is useful in self-development (e.g., developing assertiveness) and in seeking employment that matches traits (drive, motivation, integrity, confidence, cognitive ability, and task knowledge).
Style Theories Sometimes referred to as *group and exchange* theories of leadership, style theories were derived in the mid-1950s because of the limitations of trait theory. The key contributors to this renowned research were Shartle (1956), Stogdill (1963), and Likert (1987).	Style theories focus on what leaders do in relational and contextual terms. The achievement of satisfactory performance measures requires supervisors to pursue effective relationships with their subordinates while comprehending the factors in the work environment that influence outcomes.	To understand "style," leaders need to obtain feedback from followers, superiors, and peers, such as through the Managerial Grid Instrument developed by Blake and Mouton (1985). Employee-centered leaders tend to be the leaders most able to achieve effective work environments and productivity.
Situational-Contingency Theories The situational-contingency theorists emerged in the 1960s and early 1970s to mid-1970s. These theorists believed that leadership effectiveness depends on the relationship among (1) the leader's task at hand, (2) his or her interpersonal skills, and (3) the favorableness of the work situation. Examples of theory development with this expanded perspective include Fiedler's (1967) Contingency Model, Vroom and Yetton's (1973) Normative Decision-Making Model, and House and Mitchell's (1974) Path-Goal theory.	Three factors are critical: (1) the degree of trust and respect between leaders and followers, (2) the task structure denoting the clarity of goals and the complexity of problems faced, and (3) the position power in terms of where the leader was able to reward followers and exert influence. Consequently, leaders were viewed as able to adapt their style according to the presenting situation. The Vroom-Yetton model was a problem-solving approach to leadership. Path-Goal theory recognized two contingent variables: (1) the personal characteristics of followers and (2) environmental demands. On the basis of these factors, the leader sets forth clear expectations, eliminates obstacles to goal achievements, motivates and rewards staff, and increases opportunities for follower satisfaction based on effective job performance.	The most important implications for leaders are that these theories consider the challenge of a situation and encourage an adaptive leadership style to complement the issue being faced. In other words, nurses must assess each situation and determine appropriate action based on the people involved.

Continued

THEORY BOX—cont'd

Leadership Theories

THEORY/CONTRIBUTOR	KEY IDEA	APPLICATION TO PRACTICE
Transformational Theories Transformational theories arose late in the past millennium when globalization and other factors caused organizations to fundamentally re-establish themselves. Many of these attempts were failures, but great attention was given to those leaders who effectively transformed structures, human resources, and profitability balanced with quality. Bass (1990), Bennis and Nanus (2007), and Tichy and Devanna (1997) are commonly associated with the study of transformational theory.	Transformational leadership refers to a process whereby the leader attends to the needs and motives of followers so that the interaction raises each to high levels of motivation and morality. The leader is a role model who inspires followers through displayed optimism, provides intellectual stimulation, and encourages follower creativity.	Transformed organizations are responsive to customer needs, are morally and ethically intact, promote employee development, and encourage self-management. Nurse leaders with transformational characteristics experiment with systems redesign, empower staff, create enthusiasm for practice, and promote scholarship of practice at the patient-side.
Hierarchy of Needs Maslow is credited with developing a theory of motivation, first published in 1943.	People are motivated by a hierarchy of human needs, beginning with physiologic needs and then progressing to safety, social, esteem, and self-actualizing needs. In this theory, when the need for food, water, air, and other life-sustaining elements is met, the human spirit reaches out to achieve affiliation with others, which promotes the development of self-esteem, competence, achievement, and creativity. Lower-level needs will always drive behavior before higher-level needs will be addressed.	When this theory is applied to staff, leaders must be aware that the need for safety and security will override the opportunity to be creative and inventive, such as in promoting job change.
Two-Factor Theory Herzberg (1991) is credited with developing a two-factor theory of motivation, first published in 1968.	Hygiene factors, such as working conditions, salary, status, and security, motivate workers by meeting safety and security needs and avoiding job dissatisfaction. Motivator factors, such as achievement, recognition, and the satisfaction of the work itself, promote job enrichment by creating job satisfaction.	Organizations need both hygiene and motivator factors to recruit and retain staff. Hygiene factors do not create job satisfaction; they simply must be in place for work to be accomplished. If not, these factors will only serve to dissatisfy staff. Transformational leaders use motivator factors liberally to inspire work performance.
Expectancy Theory Vroom (1994) is credited with developing the expectancy theory of motivation.	Individuals' perceived needs influence their behavior. In the work setting, this motivated behavior is increased if a person perceives a positive relationship between effort and performance. Motivated behavior is further increased if a positive relationship exists between good performance and outcomes or rewards, particularly when these are valued.	Expectancy is the perceived probability of satisfying a particular need based on experience. Therefore nurses in leadership roles need to provide specific feedback about positive performance.

Leadership Theories

THEORY/CONTRIBUTOR	KEY IDEA	APPLICATION TO PRACTICE
OB Modification Luthans (2011) is credited with establishing the foundation for Organizational Behavior Modification (OB Mod), based on Skinner's work on operant conditioning.	OB Mod is an operant approach to organizational behavior. OB Mod Performance Analysis follows a three-step *ABC* Model: *A*, antecedent analysis of clear expectations and baseline data collection; *B*, behavioral analysis and determination; and *C*, consequence analysis, including reinforcement strategies.	The leader uses positive reinforcement to motivate followers to repeat constructive behaviors in the workplace. Negative events that de-motivate staff are negatively reinforced, and the staff is motivated to avoid certain situations that cause discomfort. Extinction is the purposeful non-reinforcement (ignoring) of negative behaviors. Punishment is used sparingly because the results are unpredictable in supporting the desired behavioral outcome.

in nursing terms, professional nurses can care for individual patients repeatedly, whereas each patient is a unique challenge. But with time and perspective, patterns emerge and nurses learn that these patterns lead to ways to control pain, engage family members in care at the end-of-life, and address a host of other issues. As healthcare providers are very focused on problems and predictable solutions, it is possible that reframing care to build on an individual, family, or community strengths presents quite a different perspective that unleashes solutions to complex problems and shifts human energy toward a positive outcome. Therefore complexity science expands the repertoire of nursing actions to include strategies that are multidimensional and with a different patient or organizational view.

In adaptive leadership, consistent with the definition of leadership provided earlier, the goal in responding to patient and organizational problems is to examine a problem through a different lens. This view might examine the "whole" that includes potential threats, exposes conflict, or challenges norms as part of the art of improvising change. An adaptive leader understands that systems are ecological—they restore themselves—and that change can happen equally from the bottom up or from the top down. One leads by entering the stream, not observing it and sitting off to the side to critique it. Questioning, observing patterns, and generating new patterns through being involved is how change unfolds. Imagine the power of social networking where no top-down leader exists.

Rather, a series of powerful interactions and messages constantly shift to first re-create reality and then major social change. Adaptive leaders appreciate that they have influence and can help shape direction, with no sense that absolute control is either necessary or possible.

In complexity theory, traditional organizational hierarchy plays a less significant role as the "keeper of high-level knowledge." It is replaced with decision making distributed among the human assets within an organization without regard to hierarchy. Less time is spent trying to control the future (which is not predictable anyway), and more time is spent moving toward and into energy while influencing, innovating, and responding to the many factors that are influencing health care. In complexity science, every voice counts and every encounter with patients and families emerge to co-create a desired outcome.

Change is an important dimension of leadership. Eoyang and Holladay (2013) contrast three kinds of change, using performance appraisal as an example. The same example is used here, as each professional nurse is subject to an appraisal of performance. The first example is static change. A performance appraisal in this model is one where an annual overview of performance is described, with comparison to the performance of the previous year, against a set of defined goals and objectives. The second model is the dynamic change model. It is illustrated in the Research Perspective on p. 12. Contrary to the static model, this approach yields periodic feedback, enough that

RESEARCH PERSPECTIVE

Resource: Hauck, S., Winsett, R.P., & Kuric, J. (2012). Leadership facilitation strategies to establish evidence-based practice in an acute care hospital. *Journal of Advanced Nursing, 69*(3), 664-674.

A prospective comparative design was used to assess the effect of leadership facilitation strategies on beliefs regarding change, and use of evidence-based practice (EBP) as well as organizational readiness for change. A strategic plan to implement EBP in an acute care hospital was designed. All currently employed registered nurses (RNs) were surveyed at baseline and 2 years later following implementation. Three measures were used to assess beliefs, use, and organizational culture regarding EBP in their hospital. Baseline results demonstrated that direct care RNs perceived limited support from their unit directors. In response, an educational program was developed specifically for those in formal nurse leader roles. The follow-up measures demonstrated statistically significant improvement from baseline on beliefs and readiness regarding EBP, as well as meeting performance goals that were established in the strategic plan. The overall use of EBP in nursing practice improved but was not statistically significant. Evidence-based practice use was significantly lower in direct care nurses than those nurses in non-direct care who were not considered part of the management team.

Implications for Practice

This is an example of dynamic change, requiring individual attributes consistent with leading, managing, and following behaviors as new processes are designed and implemented in practice. The use of a well-developed plan with specific target measures and engagement of all RNs enhanced the effectiveness of this study. This study demonstrates how important it is for nurses in leadership roles to be well versed in EBP in order to facilitate EBP use by direct care nurses. Though the results of this study cannot be generalized to all facilities implementing EBP, they do demonstrate the importance of a well-designed plan with measurable outcomes.

much is dynamic (aimed at projects that interject incremental improvement), and some is dynamical (unpredictable and interactive). Adaptive leaders are driven by complexity science by nature of the shifting environment.

Historically, Marion and Uhl-Bien (2001) identified five ways in which complexity science encourages individuals to lead, manage, and follow. Those who use complexity principles:

Develop Networks. A network is any related group with common involvement in an area of focus or concern. Social networks are found within organizations but also beyond organizational boundaries. For example, a nursing program is not considered a part of the hospital or agency setting where clinical experiences take place; however, common interests (supply and preparation of a qualified workforce and demand for clinical services) make this network critically important for both organizations.

Encourage Non-hierarchical, "Bottom-up" Interaction Among Workers. As noted earlier, those who lead, manage, and follow may have responsibilities that are not served within the traditional hierarchy. Shared governance is an example of a decision-making structure in which staff at any level in the hierarchy are engaged in shaping policy and practices that affect patient care. In this model, each nurse is a valued human resource with rich perspective and possesses a voice in shaping direction.

Become a Leadership "Tag". The term *tag* references the philosophic, patient-centered, and values-driven characteristics that give an organization its personality, the "energy" that it has; a tag is sometimes called an *attractor* or a *hallmark of culture*, similar to values. Although clinical organizations often perform similar procedures and functions, an intangible sense that this particular organization has a "caring" or "good energy" attractor differs from one where the sense is the focus on efficiency and cost only. The term *tag* refers to these distinctions.

Focus on Emergence. The concept of emergence addresses how individuals in positions of responsibility engage with and discover, through active organizational involvement, those networks that are best suited to respond to problems in creative, surprising, and artful ways—those who think "outside the box." Emergence is tied to unleashing constructive energy rather than constraining energy.

it functions as a kind of thermostat and with work assignments that are marked with milestones, especially when meeting project deadlines or other work targets. The third change model is quite different. The dynamical model focuses on the interrelationship of the leader with feedback that is both regular (even daily) and summative (annually). The appraisal provides feedback relative to systems and interactions, and autonomy is given to move with opportunities that emerge, not just projects to be completed. These three change models represent that challenge in health care today: some work is static (predictable),

Think Systematically. The principles of systems thinking theory have been characterized classically by Anderson and Johnson (1997) as:

* *Thinking of the "Big Picture"* The nurse who looks past an individual assignment and comprehends the needs of all units of the hospital, or who can focus on the needs of all the residents in a long-term care facility, or who can think through the complications of emergency department overcrowding in an urban setting is seeing the big picture. These nurses have the ability to envision the context of their work beyond the immediate tasks.
* *Balancing Short-Term and Long-Term Objectives* The nurse who recognizes the consequences of actions taken today on the long-term effect of the organization or patient care, such as the decision of a patient to terminate clinical treatment, can guide thinking about how to balance decision making for quality outcomes.
* *Recognizing the Dynamic, Complex, and Interdependent Nature of Systems* All things are connected. Patients are connected to families and friends. Together, they are connected to communities and cultures. Communities and cultures make up the fabric of society. The cost of health care is linked to local economies, and local businesses are connected to global industries. Identifying and understanding these relationships helps solve problems with full recognition that small decisions can have a large impact.
* *Using Measurable versus Nonmeasurable Data Systems* This thinking triggers a "tendency to 'see' only what we measure." If we focus our measuring on morale, working relationships, and teamwork, we might miss the important signals that only

---

EXERCISE 1-3

Identify a clinical scenario in which a complex problem needs to be addressed. Who would you include in a network to engage in creative problem solving? How would you go about linking to other social networks if the problem was "bigger than" your immediate contacts? Identify one member of the network and map the potential connections of that individual that could influence problem resolution. Concentrate on the power of these influencing individuals. The patient/family is part of the network. What role would they play in co-creating the resolution strategies? How would you encourage non-hierarchical interaction among workers? Cite instances (personally or professionally) in which a small change in a system has had a big effect.

---

objective statistics can show us. On the other hand, if we consider only numbers, (e.g., number of patients seen), we might miss a big perspective, such as lack of engagement in the workplace.

TASKS OF LEADING, MANAGING, AND FOLLOWING

When dealing with theory and concepts, we can lose sight of the practical behaviors that are needed to put these ideas into practice. Gardner (1990) was the first to recognize this. He described tasks of leadership in his seminal book, *On Leadership*. The purpose of describing tangible behaviors associated with leading, managing, and following is to facilitate an understanding of the distinctions between the tasks and the definitions of leadership, management, and followership presented earlier in the chapter.

Gardner's Tasks of Leadership

Gardner's leadership tasks are presented in Table 1-1 to demonstrate that leading, managing, and following are relevant for nurses who hold clinical positions, formal management positions, and executive positions. Note that each role represents the interests of the organization, although the locus of attention is different.

Envisioning Goals

Leading requires envisioning goals in partnership with others. At the point of care, leading helps patients envision their life journey when health outcomes are unknown. It might help a patient envision walking again, participating in family events, or changing a lifestyle pattern. In the case of leading peers (not dissimilar to working with patients and family members), leader competence, trustworthiness, self-assuredness, decision-making ability, and prioritization skills envision crafting solutions to care delivery problems. Imagine leading a change to an electronic health record from a traditional paper record: the leader uses the aforementioned abilities to engage with, convince, or persuade colleagues about the relevance of this change and proceeds with setting direction. Envisioning goals is contingent upon trustful relationships, shared information, and agreement on mutual expectations.

Establishing a shared **vision** is an important leadership concept. "Visioning" requires the leader to

TABLE 1-1   GARDNER'S TASKS OF LEADING/MANAGING APPLIED TO PRACTICE, MANAGEMENT, AND EXECUTIVE POSITIONS

GARDNER'S TASK	BEHAVIORS		
	CLINICAL POSITION	MANAGEMENT POSITION	EXECUTIVE POSITION
Envisioning goals	Visioning patient outcomes for single patient/families; assisting patients in formulating their vision of future well-being	Visioning patient outcomes for aggregates of patient populations and creating a vision of how systems support patient care objectives; assisting staff in formulating their vision of enhanced clinical and organizational performance	Visioning community health and organizational outcomes for aggregates of patient populations to which the organization can respond
Affirming values	Assisting the patient/family to sort out and articulate personal values in relation to health problems and the effect of these problems on lifestyle adjustments	Assisting the staff in interpreting organizational values and strengthening staff members' personal values to more closely align with those of the organization; interpreting values during organizational change	Assisting other organizational leaders in the expression of community and organizational values; interpreting values to the community and staff
Motivating	Relating to and inspiring patients/families to achieve their vision	Relating to and inspiring staff to achieve the mission of the organization and the vision associated with organizational enhancement	Relating to and inspiring management, staff, and community leaders to achieve desired levels of health and well-being and appropriate use of clinical services
Managing	Assisting the patient/family with planning, priority setting, and decision making; ensuring that organizational systems work in the patient's behalf	Assisting the staff with planning, priority setting, and decision making; ensuring that systems work to enhance the staff's ability to meet patient care needs and the objectives of the organization	Assisting other executives and corporate leaders with planning, priority setting, and decision making; ensuring that human and material resources are available to meet health needs
Achieving workable unity	Assisting patients/families to achieve optimal functioning to benefit the transition to enhanced health functions	Assisting staff to achieve optimal functioning to benefit transition to enhanced organizational functions	Assisting multidisciplinary leaders to achieve optimal functioning to benefit patient care delivery and collaborative care
Developing trust	Keeping promises to patients and families; being honest in role performance	Sharing organizational information openly; being honest in role performance	Representing nursing and executive views openly and honestly; being honest in role performance
Explaining	Teaching and interpreting information to promote patient/family functioning and well-being	Teaching and interpreting information to promote organizational functioning and enhanced services	Teaching and interpreting organizational and community-based health information to promote organizational functioning and service development

TABLE 1-1   GARDNER'S TASKS OF LEADING/MANAGING APPLIED TO PRACTICE, MANAGEMENT, AND EXECUTIVE POSITIONS—cont'd

GARDNER'S TASK	BEHAVIORS		
	CLINICAL POSITION	MANAGEMENT POSITION	EXECUTIVE POSITION
Serving as symbol	Representing the nursing profession and the values and beliefs of the organization to patients/families and other community groups	Representing the nursing unit service and the values and beliefs of the organization to staff, other departments, professional disciplines, and the community at large	Representing the values and beliefs of the organization and patient care services to internal and external constituents
Representing the group	Representing nursing and the unit in task forces, total quality initiatives, shared governance councils, and other groups	Representing nursing and the organization on assigned boards, councils, committees, and task forces, both internal and external to the organization	Representing the organization and patient care services on assigned boards, councils, committees, and task forces, both internal and external to the organization
Renewing	Providing self-care to enhance the ability to care for staff, patients, families, and the organization served	Providing self-care to enhance the ability to care for staff, patients, families, and the organization served	Providing self-care to enhance the ability to care for patients, families, staff, and the organization served

engage with others to assess the current reality, determine and specify a desired end-point state, and then strategize to reduce the difference. When this is done well, the nurse and the patient or nurses within an organization experience creative tension. Creative tension inspires the patient and others to work in concert to achieve a desired goal. Shared visioning gives direction to accelerate change.

Affirming Values

Values are the connecting thoughts and inner driving forces that give purpose, direction, and precedence to life priorities. An organization, through its members, shares collective values that are expressed through its mission, philosophy, and practices. Leaders influence decision making and priority setting as an expression of their values. People (either patients or peers being influenced by the leader) also use their values to achieve their goals, which are then manifested through behavior.

The word *value* connotes something of worth; intentional actions reflect our values. A leader continuously clarifies and acknowledges the values that draw attention to a problem and the resources in human and material terms to solve it. Values are powerful forces that promote acceptance of change and drive achievement toward a goal.

Motivating

When values drive our actions, they become a source of motivation. Motivation energizes what we value, personally and professionally, and stimulates growth and movement toward the vision. Motivators are the reinforcers that keep positive actions alive and sustained, fueling the desire to engage in change. Theories of motivation identify and describe the forces that motivate people. Examples of motivation theory are presented in the Theory Box on Motivation on pp. 9–11.

Managing

The ability to manage is an important aspect of organizational functioning, because management requires determining routines and practices that offer structure and stability to others. This is especially true in certain positions of influence within a clinical setting, such as a nurse manager, clinical nurse specialist, or clinical nurse leader, all of whom share responsibility for creating effective structures that support clinical and organizational outcomes. Being effective as a manager requires behaviors different from those associated with effective leadership, and vice versa. Ideally, those charged with managing are good leaders and followers, because no organizational position is limited to one exclusive set of behaviors over another. Good leaders need management skills and abilities, and good managers need leading skills and abilities, and good followers need both skills too. The tasks of management are discussed on p. 18.

Achieving Workable Unity

Another leadership challenge is to achieve workable unity between and among the parties being affected by change and to avoid, diminish, or resolve conflict so that vision can be achieved (see Chapters 17 and 23). Conflict resolution skills are essential for leaders. When a dispute occurs as a result of conflicting values or interests, following a defined set of principles to guide conflict resolution is an excellent aid. In their classic work, Ury, Brett, and Goldberg (1988) described a highly effective approach for restoring unity and movement toward positive change through conflict management, as shown in Box 1-2.

BOX 1-2 PRINCIPLES OF CONFLICT RESOLUTION

1. Put the focus on interests:
   - Examine the real issues of all parties.
   - Be expedient in responding to the issues.
   - Use negotiation procedures and processes such as ethics committees and other neutral sources.
2. Build in "loop-backs" to negotiation:
   - Allow for a "cooling off" period before reconvening if resolution fails.
   - Review with all parties the likely consequences of not proceeding so that they understand the full consequences of failure to resolve the issue.
3. Build in consultation before and feedback after the negotiations:
   - Build consensus and use political skills to facilitate communication before confrontation, if anticipated, occurs.
   - Work with staff or patients after the conflict to learn from the situation and to prevent a similar conflict in the future.
   - Provide a forum for open discussion.
4. Provide necessary motivation, skills, and resources:
   - Make sure that the parties involved in conflict are motivated to use procedures and resources that have been developed; this requires ease of access and a nonthreatening mechanism.
   - Ensure that those working in the dispute have skills in problem solving and dispute resolution.
   - Provide the necessary resources to those involved to offer support, information, and other technical assistance.

Modified from Ury, W., Brett, J., & Goldberg, S. (1988). *Getting disputes resolved: Designing systems to cut the costs of conflict.* San Francisco: Jossey-Bass.

Developing Trust

A hallmark task of leadership is to behave with consistency so that others believe in and can count on the leader's intentions and direction. Trust develops when leaders are clear with others about this direction, and the way to achieve high performance is through building on strengths and mitigating poor performance. Inherent in this concept is the behavior of truth telling. Although leaders cannot always share all information, it is unwise to misdirect others in their thinking and actions. Trust, according to Lencioni's (2002) classic work, is the key component of a team. Without it, the team is dysfunctional. Trustworthiness is reflected in actions and communications.

Explaining

Leading and managing require a willingness to communicate and explain—again and again. The art of communication requires the leader to do the following:

1. Determine what information needs to be shared.
2. Know the parties who will receive the information. Ask, "What will they 'hear' in the process of the communication?" Information that addresses the listener's self-interest must be presented.
3. Provide the opportunity for dialogue and feedback. Face-to-face communication is preferred when the situation requires immediate feedback because it offers the opportunity to clarify information. Written communication through the use of e-mail and text messages increasingly are used as primary communication mechanisms. Although expedient, these mechanisms have limitations that must be acknowledged.
4. Plan the message. Giving too much information can temporarily paralyze the listener and divert energy away from key responsibilities.
5. Be willing to repeat information in different ways, at different times. The more diverse the group being addressed, the more important it is to avoid complex terms, concepts, or ideas. Information should be kept simple. Remember, a message is heard when a person is ready to hear it, not before.
6. Always explain why something is being asked or is changing. The values behind the change should be reinforced.
7. Acknowledge loss and provide the opportunity for honest communication about what will be missed, especially if change is involved.

8. Be sensitive to nonverbal communication. It may be necessary in complex situations to have someone re-interpret key points and provide feedback about the clarity of the message after the meeting. Leaders must use every opportunity for explaining as a vehicle to fine-tune communication skills. (See Chapter 18 for additional discussion of communication.)

Serving as a Symbol

Every leader has the opportunity to be an ambassa-dor for those he or she represents. Nurses may be symbolically present for patients and families, rep-resent their department at an organizational event, or be involved in community public relations events. Serving as a symbol reflects unity and collective identity.

Representing the Group

More than being present symbolically, many opportu-nities exist for leaders to represent the group through active participation. Progressive organizations create opportunities for employees to participate in and foster organizational innovation (e.g., organizations seeking Magnet Recognition Program® designation). Nurses may participate on human resource committees, pa-tient safety task forces, improvement committees, and departmental initiatives. When nurses offer their "voice" in each of these leadership opportunities, they are thinking beyond personal needs and staying clear on group outcomes. When decision making is decen-tralized and layers of management are compressed, nurses have more leadership accountability. A leader treats these newfound opportunities with respect and represents the group's interests with openness and in-tegrity. Ultimately, leaders must understand the orga-nization's objectives and contribute to its mission and purpose.

Renewing

Leaders can generate energy within and among others. A true leader attends to the group's energy and does not allow it to lose focus. In organizations and nursing practice, constantly balancing prob-lem solving (energy-expending) with vision setting (energy-producing) is important. When changes are made based on a shared vision, they can be made with renewed spirit and purpose. Taking time to cel-ebrate individual accomplishments or creating a "Hall of Honor" to post photos, letters, and other forms of positive feedback renews the spirit of workers.

Furthermore, leaders must be proponents of self-care—eat a balanced diet, get adequate sleep and exercise, and participate in other wellness-oriented activities—to maintain their own perspective and neces-sary energy level. Likewise, they must ensure that their constituents are given similar opportunities for physical and mental renewal. Gardner (1990) states, "The consid-eration leaders must never forget is that the key for re-newal is the release of human energy and talent" (p. 136). This requires focused energy and personal well-being.

Bleich's Tasks of Management

The ability to manage is very much aligned with how an organization structures its key systems and pro-cesses to deliver service.

A care delivery system is composed of multiple processes to achieve all of the requisite components required by patients. Some of the key processes relate to medication procurement, ordering, and admin-istration; patient safety practices; patient education; and discharge planning and care coordination. A pro-cess of care specifies the desired sequence of steps to achieve clinical standardization, safety, and outcomes. Effective management depends on knowing, adhering to, and improving processes for efficiency and effec-tiveness. Each person must respect and act on his or her prescribed role in a process of care. Data-driven outcome measurements add to good management and support feedback, coaching, and mentoring opportu-nities. Rewards for individual and team effectiveness reinforce desired behaviors.

Box 1-3 lists tasks of management that are essential to effective functioning.

Followers complement leaders and managers with their skills. Followers and leaders fill gaps that exist to build on each other's cognitive, technical, interpersonal, and emotional strengths. Followers, showing sensitivity to leaders, offer respite in times of stress. Followers need and respond to feedback from leaders to stay on course. The follower must acquiesce to the skills and abilities of the leader or manager to promote teamwork. This does not mean that the follower does not have the skills and abilities of the leader or manager, because the follower may be thrust into one of those roles when circumstances demand.

BOX 1-3   BLEICH'S TASKS OF MANAGEMENT

1. Identify systems and processes that require responsibility and accountability, and specify who owns the process.
2. Verify minimum and optimum standards/specifications, and identify roles and individuals responsible to adhere to them.
3. Validate the knowledge, skills, and abilities of available staff engaged in the process; capitalize on strengths; and strengthen areas in need of development.
4. Devise and communicate a comprehensive big picture plan for the division of work, honoring the complexity and variety of assignments made at an individual level.
5. Eliminate barriers/obstacles to work effectiveness.
6. Measure the equity of workload, and use data to support judgments about efficiency and effectiveness.
7. Offer rewards and recognition to individuals and teams.
8. Recommend ways to improve systems and processes.
9. Use a social network to engage others in decision making and for feedback, when appropriate or relevant.

BOX 1-4   BLEICH'S TASKS OF FOLLOWERSHIP

1. Demonstrate individual accountability while working within the context of organizational systems and processes; do not alter the process for personal gain or shortcuts.
2. Honor and implement care to the standards and specifications required for safe and acceptable care/service.
3. Offer knowledge, skills, and abilities to accomplish the task at hand.
4. Collaborate with leaders and managers; avoid passive-aggressive or nonassertive responses to work assignment.
5. Include evidence-based feedback as part of daily work activities as a self-guide to efficiency and effectiveness and to contribute to outcome measurement.
6. Demonstrate accountability to the team effort.
7. Take reasonable risks as an antidote for fearing change or unknown circumstances.
8. Evaluate the efficiency and effectiveness of systems and processes that affect outcomes of care/service; advocate for well-designed work.
9. Give and receive feedback to others to promote a nurturing and generative culture.

EXERCISE 1-4

Examine one structured process in the delivery of patient care from start to finish (e.g., food ordering, preparation, and delivery). How is the process organized? How many steps does the process take? Who is responsible for each step in the process? Who has the responsibility and authority for managing the process? What data are available in the organization to measure how well the process is working?

Images associated with followers portray workers who are passive, uninspired, not intellectual, and waiting for direction. In reality, the effective follower is willing to be led, to share time and talents, to create and innovate solutions to problems synergistically, and to take direction from the manager. Simultaneously, followers must perform their assigned structured duties. These duties are not devoid of critical thinking or decision making (see Box 1-4).

The relationship between followers and leaders or managers is complex. The key to building a competent team requires transformational leaders, who can envision a desired future (Hutchinson & Jackson, 2013), or patient quality will suffer. Equally, peers need to invest in each other in terms of time, knowledge, and resources if leadership skills are to be enhanced (Perkins, 2013). "Transformational leaders recognize a clear consistent focus on the vision by the team and an ability to keep the dream bigger than any fears are a key ingredient to success" (Marshall, 2011, p. ix).

At times the leader is the follower and vice versa. In any given work shift, a charge nurse may hold a leading/managing role. During a shift, the charge nurse assesses resources needed, sees the unit as a complete entity, notes when patients may be admitted or discharged, and delegates according to this big picture view. Throughout the shift, critical clinical events arise that are better led by one of the senior direct care nurses. Ideally, the charge nurse and senior direct care nurse shift their relationship so that the functioning of the unit is balanced. Assignments are temporarily adjusted and talents and skills of individual nurses are deployed to patients and families in need, all with little or no fanfare. But, examine the complexity, respect, and team achievement factors at play as the system adapts!

LEADING, MANAGING, AND FOLLOWING IN A DIVERSE ORGANIZATION

The healthcare industry is spiraling through unparalleled change, often away from the traditional industrial models that reigned throughout the twentieth century. The culture in most healthcare organizations today is more ethnically diverse; has an expansive educational chasm (from non–high school graduates to doctorally-prepared clinicians); has multiple generations of workers with varying values and expectations of the workplace; involves the increased use of technology to support all aspects of service functioning; and challenges workers, patients, families, and communities environmentally with medical waste, antibiotic-resistant strains of microorganisms, and other risks.

The complexity of the healthcare system is marred with chronic problems, information imbalance (sometimes too much, sometimes not enough), an abundance of job roles that challenge resource allocation, intense work that makes examining patterns of practice difficult, increased consumer and regulatory demands, and fatigue from too many cues and reminders! Reforms will exacerbate this problem.

These and other variables make leading, managing, and following increasingly challenging. A leader must address the needs of the diverse community of those seeking care. Language and cultural barriers create the opportunity for misunderstanding. Those who manage the systems and processes of care may find a temporary workforce—individuals unfamiliar with organizational standards of care and practice—as their primary resource. Followers may have leaders of other generations with values different from their own, and therefore the opportunity for conflict is omnipresent.

CONCLUSION

Developing the leading, managing, and following skills and abilities noted throughout this chapter will sustain professional nurses to adapt to and accept differences as a positive rather than a negative force in daily work life. Building on gender strengths; generational values, gifts, and talents; cultural diversity; varying educational and experiential perspectives; and a mobile and flexible workforce is rewarding. It is also rewarding to be led in different ways, to experience the strength of a good manager, and to achieve positive outcomes as a follower, knowing that the team approach generated a successful work experience.

THE SOLUTION

Engaging stakeholders in the shared development of a vision for the care model, thinking through the triple aim (access, quality and cost), and creating a plan together that would change the culture was a conscious strategy by those who held formal leadership roles. Based in a small town in northeast Missouri, we did not have the fiscal resources that some organizations do to bring in consultants, but nonetheless, we self-educated ourselves. Two videos, *Tale of Transformation* and *Green House Project*, exemplified how culture change in long-term care could be implemented and we studied these references. In addition, a member of the leadership team visited two facilities in other parts of the United States that were using the cottage model to provide care to 10 to 14 residents in a more home-like environment. Seeing the positive results at those facilities developed a sense of urgency in getting our project underway. In small group sessions, staff at all levels, residents, nursing home board of directors, and community members helped envision what the living and care delivery experience would look like. As is typical of change, early adopters were excited about the planning, others less so. With a long history of recognizing and satisfying resident needs, we discussed change—what was and was not changing—with staff in groups large and small, helping naysayers move to a more positive place. What was actually changed is that some residents receive care in a cottage-like environment, and all residents receive more personal, more intimate, and more dignified care. Most recognized that this focus had been key to the success of our organization's 40 years in operation.

Using change theory as a basis for our work, Kotter's eight-step change model was the organizing framework for the project (Kotter & Cohen, 2002). Stakeholder sessions developed a sense of urgency that change was needed to meet consumer preferences. Building something that was tangible—two cottage-style buildings with 12 private rooms each—allowed us to share that our vision was taking a physical reality and that the physical design would help modify how we delivered personalized services.

To mitigate naysayers, a sustaining strategy was ongoing education of staff and community members with the intent of gaining buy-in. Extensive staff education was provided to those who would be resident caregivers in the cottages. An important second strategy was to not forget the value of service for caregivers who would not be going over to the cottage model. The concept of resident-centered care that was not limited by physical structures was reinforced for those in the traditional parts of our facilities. And throughout, we made presentations to about every community group possible and those that asked about the changes we were making. In the end, we created a new model of care, everyone adhered to a new resident-sensitive care delivery model, and the community held us to a level of accountability tied to those new standards.

Evaluating change in the short and long term is a critical aspect of change management. Both staff and community members have had overwhelmingly positive responses. Projects such as this are never really complete. They must be monitored and adjustments made on an ongoing basis.

—*Barbara Primm*

Would this be a suitable approach for you? Why?

THE EVIDENCE

The roles of leader, manager, and follower are different, and each is needed in a successful organization. Leaders are known by their actions, not by their titles, so top-down only organizational structures are no longer sustainable in creating change. Change can originate at any point and is effective when supported by webs of interested and committed individuals.

Collaboration requires a set of special conditions between leaders and followers. Among these conditions is the idea that each voice will be valued in an equitable manner, that power is evenly distributed among all of the stakeholders, and that conditions exist for innovation to occur.

Organizations often function with effective leaders and managers who preside over work groups with common, short-term goals. When true team work is required the work is longer to allow for team relationships to build.

Complexity science does not refer to the complexity of the decision to be made or to the work environment but, rather, to examining how systems adapt and function—where co-creation of ideas and actions unfold in a non-prescriptive manner. The goal of leadership and management should be to reduce the complexity of the work itself. Only in simplicity does compliance and useful "fit for practice" occur.

Social networking is being recognized as a web of relationships that can be tapped and used for communication, problem solving, support, and real-time information, critical to decision making. It is a real tool for individuals to use when leading, managing, or following.

WHAT NEW GRADUATES SAY

- I learned in school all nurses are leaders ... not sure I really understood that. However, it is true.
- I feel like I am a leader especially when I work with nursing students, nursing techs, and families.
- I now better understand the difference between management and leadership ... not all managers are leaders.

CHAPTER CHECKLIST

This chapter provided an overview of leading and managing and how following relates to both. Understanding the theoretical basis for these role elements in nursing provides the basis for nurses moving health care ahead and making the best care possible for many people.

- Differentiating leading, managing, and following
- Traditional and emerging leadership and management roles
- Emotional intelligence development for professional practice
- Theory development in leading, managing, and following
- Complexity science takes hold
  - Develop networks
  - Encourage non-hierarchical, bottom-up interaction among workers
  - Become a leadership tag
  - Focus on emergence
  - Think systematically
- Tasks of leading, managing, and following
  - Gardner's tasks of leadership
    - Envisioning goals
    - Affirming values
    - Motivating
    - Managing
    - Achieving workable unity
    - Developing trust
    - Explaining
    - Serving as a symbol
    - Representing the group
    - Renewing
  - Bleich's tasks of management
- Leading, managing, and following in a diverse organization

TIPS FOR LEADING, MANAGING, AND FOLLOWING

- Recall that leading and managing require making decisions and taking collective action. If the situation is mostly known, refer to the tasks of management. If the situation is mostly unknown, refer to the tasks of leadership.
- To be effective in clinical care, nurses must be able to lead, manage, and follow. It is about the actions, not the titles.
- Examine how decisions get made. Some decisions are made through a formal hierarchy; others are autonomous. Knowing when and how to make clinical and organizational decisions adds to credibility early in one's career.

- Remember that both contingency theory and complexity science approaches require knowledge about the context of care. Use this knowledge to examine the individual patient in the context of family and community.
- Leadership, management, and organizational theories provide useful frameworks when faced with complex decisions. Select relevant theories to guide thoughtful reflection and to aid in advancing clinical and organizational outcomes.

REFERENCES

Anderson, V., & Johnson, L. (1997). *Systems thinking basics: From concepts to causal loops.* Waltham, MA: Pegasus Communications.

Bass, B. M. (1990). From transactional to transformational leadership: Learning to share the vision. *Organizational Dynamics, 18,* 19–31.

Bennis, W. G., & Nanus, B. (2007). *Leaders: The strategies for taking charge* (2nd ed.). New York: Harper Business.

Berwick, D. M., Nolan, T. W., & Whittington, J. (2008). The triple aim: Care, health and cost. *Health Affairs, 27*(3), 759–769.

Blake, R. R., & Mouton, J. S. (1985). *The managerial grid III.* Houston: Gulf Publishing.

Eoyang, G. H., & Holladay, R. J. (2013). *Adaptive action: Leveraging uncertainty in your organization.* Stanford, CA: Stanford Business Books.

Fiedler, F. A. (1967). *A theory of leadership effectiveness.* New York: McGraw-Hill.

Focus on health reform: Summary of the affordable care act (retrieved July, 2013). http://kaiserfamilyfoundation.files.wordpress.com/2011/04/8061–021.pdf.

Gardner, J. W. (1990). *On leadership.* New York: Free Press.

Goleman, D. P. (2000). *Working with emotional intelligence.* New York: Bantam Books.

Goode, C. J. (2004, April). *Using evidence to transform your work environment.* Presented at the meeting of Nursing Leadership: Rising on the Wings of Change, Phoenix, AZ.

Hauck, S., Winsett, R. P., & Kuric, J. (2012). Leadership facilitation strategies to establish evidence-based practice in an acute care hospital. *Journal of Advanced Nursing, 69*(3), 664–674.

Herzberg, F. (1991). One more time: How do you motivate employees? In M. J. Ward & S. A. Price (Eds.), *Issues in nursing administration: Selected readings.* St. Louis: Mosby.

House, R. J., & Mitchell, T. R. (1974, Autumn). Path-goal theory of leadership. *Journal of Contemporary Business, 3,* 81–97.

Hubbard, L. A. (2012). Advancing holistic nursing leadership. *Beginnings, 32*(6), 4–7.

Hutchinson, M., & Jackson, D. (2013). Transformational leadership in nursing: Towards a more critical interpretation. *Nursing Inquiry, 26*(1), 11–22.

Institute of Medicine (IOM), *The future of nursing: Leading change, advancing health.* (2011). Washington, DC: The National Academies Press.

Koh, H. K., Berwick, D. M., Clancy, C. M., Baur, C., Brach, C., Harris, L. M., et al. (2012). New federal policy initiatives boost health literacy can help the nation move beyond the cycle of costly crisis care. *Health Affairs, 31*(2), 434–443.

Kotter, J., & Cohen, D. (2002). *The heart of change: Real life stories of how people change their organization.* Boston: Harvard Business School Press.

Lencioni, P. M. (2002). *The five dysfunctions of a team: A leadership fable.* San Francisco: Jossey-Bass.

Likert, R. (1987). *New patterns of management.* New York: Garland.

Luthans, F. (2011). *Organizational behavior* (12th ed.). Burr Ridge, IL: McGraw-Hill.

Marion, R., & Uhl-Bien, M. (2001). Leadership in complex organizations. *The Leadership Quarterly, 12,* 389–418.

Marshall, E. S. (2011). *Transformational leadership in nursing: From expert clinician to influential leader.* New York, NY: Springer.

Maslow, A. (1943). A theory of human motivation. *Psychological Review, 50,* 370–396.

Patient Protection and Affordable Care Act (PPACA). (March 11, 2013). HHS notice of benefit and payment parameters for 2012, 78 Fed. Reg. 15410. (to be codified at 45 C.F.R. pts. 153, 155,156, 157, & 158).

Perkins, K. M. (2013). "Investation" … an original leadership concept. *Nursing Management, 44*(4), 35–39.

Porter, M. E., Pabo, E. A., & Lee, T. H. (2013). Redesigning primary care: A strategic vision to improve value by organizing around patient needs. *Health Affairs, 32*(3), 516–525.

Sharma, R. (2010). *The leader who had no title.* New York: Free Press.

Shartle, C. L. (1956). *Executive performance and leadership.* Englewood Cliffs, NJ: Prentice Hall.

Stogdill, R. M. (1948). Personal factors associated with leadership: A survey of the literature. *Journal of Psychology*, *25*, 35–71.

Stogdill, R. M. (1963). *Manual for the leader behavior description questionnaire, form XII*. Columbus: The Ohio State University, Bureau of Business Research.

Tichy, N. M., & Devanna, M. A. (1997). *The transformational leader*. New York: John Wiley & Sons.

Ury, W., Brett, J., & Goldberg, S. (1988). *Getting disputes resolved: Designing systems to cut the costs of conflict*. San Francisco: Jossey-Bass.

Vroom, V. H. (1994). *Work and motivation*. New York: John Wiley & Sons.

Vroom, V. H., & Yetton, P. (1973). *Leadership and decision-making*. Pittsburgh, PA: University of Pittsburgh Press.

SUGGESTED READINGS

Anklam, P. (2007). *Network: A practical guide to creating and sustaining networks at work and in the world*. Burlington, MA: Butterworth-Heinemann.

Bass, B. M., & Avolio, B. J. (1994). *Improving organizational effectiveness through transformational leadership*. Thousand Oaks, CA: Sage Publications.

Birute, R., & Lewin, R. (2003). Third possibility leaders: The invisible edge women have in complex organizations. Retrieved September 23, 2009, from http://plexusinstitute.org/services/stories/show.cfm?id=28.

Brafman, O., & Beckstrom, R. (2006). *The starfish and the spider: The unstoppable power of leaderless organizations*. New York: Penguin Group.

Brafman, O., & Brafman, R. (2008). *Sway: The irresistible pull of irrational behavior*. New York: Doubleday.

Bridges, W. (1991). *Managing transitions: Making the most of change*. Reading, MA: Addison-Wesley.

Covey, S. (1991). *Principle-centered leadership*. New York: Summit.

Gerzon, M. (2006). *Leading through conflict: How successful leaders transform differences into opportunities*. Boston: Harvard Business School Press.

Gladwell, M. (2000). *The tipping point*. Boston: Little, Brown.

Grossman, R. J. (2000). Emotions at work: Health care organizations are just beginning to recognize the importance of developing a manager's emotional quotient, or interpersonal skills. *Health Forum Journal*, *43*, 18–22.

Heifetz, R., Grashow, A., & Linsky, M. (2009). *The practice of adaptive leadership: Tools and tactic for changing your organization and the world*. Boston: Harvard Business Press.

Katzenbach, J. R., & Smith, D. K. (1993). *The wisdom of teams: Creating the high-performance organization*. New York: Harper Business.

Kellerman, B. (Fall, 2012). What every leader needs to know about followers. *Harvard Business Review*, 96–103.

Lentz, S. (1999). The well-rounded leader: Knowing when to use consensus and when to make a decision is crucial in today's competitive health care market. *Health Forum Journal*, *42*, 38–40.

Maeda, J. (2006). *The laws of simplicity*. Cambridge, MA: The MIT Press.

McDaniel, R. R. (1997). Strategic leadership: A view from quantum and chaos theories. *Health Care Management Review*, *22*, 21–37.

Noll, D. C. (1997). Complexity theory 101. *Medical Group Management Journal*, *44*(3), 22, 24–26, 76.

Northouse, P. G. (2013). *Leadership theory and practice* (6th ed.). Thousand Oaks, CA: Sage Publications.

Plsek, P. E., & Wilson, T. (2001). Complexity, leadership, and management in healthcare organisations. *BMJ*, *323*, 746–749.

Runde, C., & Flanagan, T. (2007). *Becoming a conflict competent leader: How you and your organization can manage conflict effectively*. San Francisco: Jossey-Bass.

Trott, M. C., & Windsor, K. (1999). Leadership effectiveness: How do you measure up? *Nursing Economic$*, *17*, 127–130.

Useem, M. (1998). *The leadership moment*. New York: Three Rivers Press.

Wakeman, C. (2010). *Reality-based leadership*. San Francisco: Jossey-Bass.

Weeks, D. (1994). *The eight essential steps to conflict resolution*. New York: G. Putney Sons.

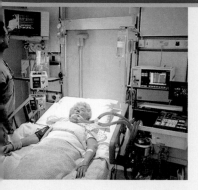

Safe Care: The Core of Leading and Managing

Patricia S. Yoder-Wise

In any discipline, most practitioners think of a leader as someone with positional authority. Terms such as manager, director, chief, *and* leader *convey positional authority. Realistically, however, every registered nurse is legally a leader—someone who has the opportunity and authority to make changes for his or her patients. Although Florence Nightingale was concerned with safety, it wasn't until the end of the twentieth century that major efforts became intense. This shift to being consumed with a passion for patient safety is a hallmark of today's healthcare delivery and the target for the care of tomorrow. This chapter provides an overview of some major patient safety efforts as the basis for all aspects of leading and managing in nursing. Patient safety, and subsequently quality of care, is why the public entrusts us with licensure and why we use our passion for caring.*

LEARNING OUTCOMES

- Differentiate the key organizations leading patient safety movements in the United States.
- Value the need for leaders and managers to focus on patient safety.
- Apply the concepts of today's expectations for how patient safety is implemented.

KEY TERMS

Agency for Healthcare Research and Quality (AHRQ)

American Board of Quality Assurance and Utilization Review Physicians (ABQAURP)

Det Norske Veritas (DNV)

Institute for Healthcare Improvement (IHI)

Institute of Medicine (IOM)

Magnet Recognition Program®

National Integrated Accreditation for Healthcare Organizations℠ (NIAHO)

National Quality Forum (NQF)

Quality and Safety Education for Nurses (QSEN)

TeamSTEPPS (an AHRQ strategy to promote patient safety)

The Joint Commission

THE CHALLENGE

Vickie S. Simpson, BA, BSN, RN, CCRN, CPN
Dell Children's Medical Center of Central Texas, Austin, Texas

Over the years, our hospital has focused on pressure ulcers. In 2002, for example, we reviewed literature on pediatric pressure ulcer risk assessment scales and prevention interventions. Later, as we were doing our pediatric pressure ulcer risk policy, we realized that pressure ulcers were not tracked. So it was impossible to determine the true incidence. Thus we instituted a tracking system. We also developed a pediatric SKIN bundle. SKIN stands for **S**urface selection, **K**eep turning, **I**ncontinence management, and **N**utrition.

Many of these efforts included broad interdisciplinary teams. For example, after moving to our new facility we noticed a trend of pressure ulcer development in nasally intubated patients. When a root cause analysis was completed with members of the anesthesia and respiratory therapy departments, staff in the critical care unit, and the cardiovascular surgeon, numerous issues were identified. These issues included not purchasing arms for the new ventilators and identifying the need for a different taping process for nasally intubated children, which was developed by our respiratory therapists. Our outcome is that now we have no pressure ulcers on nasally intubated children in our facility.

Then we identified a trend in our patient population: more overweight teenagers. We had to decide what to do.

What do you think you would do if you were this nurse?

INTRODUCTION

This book focuses on the concepts of leading and managing. The question is, however, leading and managing for what? No issue is more prominent in the literature or in healthcare organizations than the concern for patient safety, and that is at the core of leading and managing in nursing. Many factors and individuals have influenced the nursing profession's and the public's concern about patient safety, but the seminal work was *To Err is Human: Building a Safer Health System* (2000), produced by the Institute of Medicine (IOM). From that report through the numerous additional publications, the IOM has focused its work on multiple issues surrounding patient safety. This focus fits well with the basic patient advocacy role that nurses have supported over decades and that makes us so valued by patients.

Because the core of concern in any healthcare organization is safety, it also is the core for leaders and managers in nursing. Safety, and subsequently quality, should drive such aspects of leading and managing as staffing and budgeting decisions, personnel policies and change, and information technology and delegation decisions. Three major driving forces are behind the current emphasis on quality: the IOM, the Agency for Healthcare Research and Quality (AHRQ), and the National Quality Forum (NQF). Other groups such as The Joint Commission, the Det Norske Veritas (DNV), and the Magnet Recognition Program® have incorporated specific standards and expectations about safety and quality into their respective work. Additionally, specifically focused efforts such as those of the Quality and Safety Education for Nurses (QSEN) and TeamSTEPPS initiatives, have addressed patient safety issues. The American Board of Quality Assurance and Utilization Review Physicians provides a certification program for physicians, nurses, and other healthcare professionals. No nurse can function today without a focus on patient safety, nor can any nurse leader or manager.

THE CLASSIC REPORTS AND EMERGING SUPPORTS

Several reports are reflective of the efforts to refocus health care to quality. Many other reports also support these efforts. Table 2-1 highlights the key groups.

THE INSTITUTE OF MEDICINE REPORTS ON QUALITY

Of the eight reports from the IOM cited in Table 2-1, two focus specifically on nursing, whereas the others include nursing in a broader context. For example, *To Err is Human* spelled out six major aims in providing health care, as shown in Box 2-1. Those aims apply equally to all professions.

TABLE 2-1   MAJOR FORCES INFLUENCING PATIENT SAFETY

ELEMENT	CORE RELEVANCE	IMPLICATIONS FOR LEADERS AND MANAGERS
Institute of Medicine Reports	*To Err is Human* (2000): Defined the number of deaths attributed to patient safety issues	Moved safety issues from the incident report level to an integrated patient safety report for the organization
	Crossing the Quality Chasm (2001): Identified the six major aims in providing health care (see Box 2-1)	Moved care from discipline-centric foci to patient-centered foci
		Reinforced the disparities that occur within health care, which, in turn, led to a focus on best practices (and reinforced the need to be patient centered)
		Addressed issues such as healing environments, evidence-based care and transparency, which led to a more holistic environment that was built on evidence and that was transparent
	Health Professions Education: A Bridge to Quality (2003): Addressed the issue of silo education among the health professions in basic and continuing education (see Box 2-2)	Attempted to shrink the chasm between education and practice so that interprofessional teams would work more effectively together
		Increased expectation for participation in lifelong learning
	Keeping Patients Safe: Transforming the Work Environment of Nurses (2004): Identified many past practices that had a negative impact on nurses and thus on patients	Focused on direct care nurses, supporting their involvement in decision making related to their practice
		Supported the concept of shared governance
		Provided a framework for considering how nurses could determine staffing requirements
		Moved the Chief Nursing Officer into the boardroom as a key spokesperson on safety and quality issues
	Improving the Quality of Health Care for Mental and Substance-Use Conditions (2005): Addressed issues related to this patient population, including those who can be found among a general care population	Provided a focus on mental health needs of patients who were not admitted for the primary reason of mental health issues
	Preventing Medication Errors (2006): Addressed many of the issues surrounding the use of medications	Validated the complexity of providing medications to patients
	Future of Nursing: Leading Change, Advancing Health (2010): Identified 8 recommendations based on evidence that the profession must attend to (See Box 2-3)	Created state coalitions focused on improving nursing
		Created nursing/community/business coalitions to accomplish the work
		Moved the issue of nurses as leaders to a more visible level
Agency for Healthcare Research and Quality	Federal agency devoted to improving quality, safety, efficiency, and effectiveness (2008) www.ahrq.gov	Outcomes research sections provide resources for nurses.
		Source of Five Steps to Safer Health Care (www.ahrq.gov/consumer/5step.htm) (see Box 2-4)
		Source of Stay Healthy checklists for men and women
		Source of TeamSTEPPS
National Quality Forum	Membership-based organization related to quality measurement and reporting www.nqf.org	Source for Centers for Medicare & Medicaid's never events
		Resource for Healthcare Facilities Accreditation Program (a CMS-deemed authority) (uses NQF's Safe Practices)
		Source of nurse-sensitive care standards
The Joint Commission	Not-for-profit organization that accredits healthcare organizations internationally www.jointcommission.org	Focused on outcomes redirected accreditation processes and thus nurses' roles with the process
		Changed to unannounced visits and thus changed the way organizations prepared for accreditation
		Issues annual patient safety goals
		Issues sentinel event announcements

Continued

TABLE 2-1	MAJOR FORCES INFLUENCING PATIENT SAFETY—cont'd	
ELEMENT	**CORE RELEVANCE**	**IMPLICATIONS FOR LEADERS AND MANAGERS**
Det Norske Veritas/ National Integrated Accreditation for Healthcare Organizations	Internationally based organization that accredits many fields, including health care www.dnvaccreditation.com	Based on an internationally understood set of standards known as ISO (International Organization for Standardization) Visits annually and thus changed the way accreditation is viewed
Magnet Recognition Program®	A designation built on and evolving through research Emphasizes outcomes www.nursecredentialing.org/Magnet/ ProgramOverview.aspx	Created unified approaches to seek this designation Redirected focus to outcomes, including data and efforts related to patient safety
Institute for Healthcare Improvement	Independent, not-for-profit Source of TCAB (Transforming Care at the Bedside)	Provides rapid cycle change projects designed to improve care rapidly (see Theory Box on p. 29)
Quality and Safety Education for Nurses	Comprehensive resource, including references and video modules www.qsen.org	Created knowledge, skills, and attitudes for students and graduates related to safety

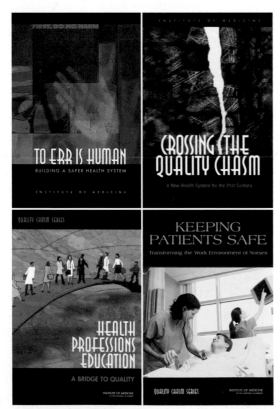

Knowing the relevant literature about safe patient care guides nursing practice.

BOX 2-1   THE AIMS OF PROVIDING HEALTH CARE

- Safe
- Effective
- Patient-centered
- Timely
- Efficient
- Equitable

From Institute of Medicine (IOM). (2001). *Crossing the quality chasm: A new health system for the 21st century.* Washington, DC: National Academy Press.

For the first time, the concern about education in silos was identified in *Health Professions Education* (IOM, 2003), which exposed publicly one of the major concerns about safety, namely that we educate disciplines in silos and then expect them to function as an integrated whole. Box 2-2 emphasizes five competencies this report endorsed.

One final report of importance, even though it is not focused directly on patient safety, is *The Future of Nursing: Leading Change, Advancing Health* (IOM, 2011). The numerous citations of evidence related to education, scope of practice, and leadership clearly indicate that if the eight recommendations (see Box 2-3) were fully implemented, the quality of care, including safety, would be enhanced.

EXERCISE 2-1

The Institute of Medicine, through its report, *The Future of Nursing: Leading Change, Advancing Health* (2010), advocated for having at least 80% of the registered nurse population prepared at the baccalaureate level. This recommendation is based on research indicating that lower morbidity and mortality rates are correlated with a better educated nursing workforce. Conduct a brief online search regarding the rationale behind this recommendation. Assume that you work in a facility that does not require an all baccalaureate-prepared nursing staff and does not provide support (time off, tuition reimbursement, recognition of educational achievement). How could you use the information you found to change workplace policies and practices to benefit patients and nurses who do not hold the baccalaureate degree in nursing?

BOX 2-2   COMPETENCIES OF HEALTH PROFESSIONALS

- Provide patient-centered care
- Work in interdisciplinary teams
- Employ evidence-based practice
- Apply quality improvement
- Utilize informatics

From Institute of Medicine (IOM). (2003). *Health professions education: A bridge to quality.* Washington, DC: National Academy Press.

BOX 2-3   THE FUTURE OF NURSING RECOMMENDATIONS

1. Remove scope-of-practice barriers.
2. Expand opportunities for nurses to lead and diffuse collaborative improvement efforts.
3. Implement nurse residency programs.
4. Increase the proportion of nurses with a baccalaureate degree to 80% by 2020.
5. Double the number of nurses with a doctorate by 2020.
6. Ensure that nurses engage in lifelong learning.
7. Prepare and enable nurses to lead change to advance health.
8. Build an infrastructure for the collection and analysis of inter-professional healthcare workforce data.

From Institute of Medicine (IOM). (2011). *The future of nursing: Leading change, advancing health.* Washington, DC: National Academies Press.

AGENCY FOR HEALTHCARE RESEARCH AND QUALITY

The **Agency for Healthcare Research and Quality (AHRQ)** is the primary federal agency devoted to improving quality, safety, efficiency, and effectiveness of

health care (AHRQ, 2013). An example of AHRQ's work is the fairly well known, "Five Steps to Safer Health Care," which is available at *http://www.ahrq.gov/patients-consumers/care-planning/errors/5steps/index.html*. Nurses who work in clinics find these steps especially helpful in working with patients. This list identifies ways in which nurses can support people in assuming a more influential role in their own care. Further, supporting people in assuming a larger role in their care helps them receive care that is patient-centered. Box 2-4 lists the five steps.

AHRQ is also the source for the *stay healthy* checklists for men and women. These checklists can be useful in any clinical setting in helping people assume a greater understanding of their own care.

EXERCISE 2-2

Go to *www.ahrq.gov/legacy/consumer* and review what sources of information are available to people for whom you may provide care. Click on "Staying Healthy," and then scroll to "Preventing Disease & Improving Your Health" and click on "Men: Stay Healthy at 50+." Review the information there, and then use the back button to return to the prior page and click on "Women: Stay Healthy at 50+." What are the differences in the checklists based on gender?

AHRQ also provides TeamSTEPPS: a well-used resource in nursing practice. TeamSTEPPS is an evidence-based system designed to improve various skills, especially communication. The curriculum includes special foci on patients with limited English skills, those in long-term care, and those who receive primary care. This site also provides a rapid response team curriculum.

More recently, the AHRQ issued a report on evidence-based practices, *Making Health Care Safer II*

BOX 2-4   FIVE STEPS TO SAFER HEALTH CARE

1. Ask questions if you have doubts or concerns.
2. Keep and bring a list of ALL medications you take.
3. Get the results of any test or procedure.
4. Talk to your doctor about which hospital is best for your health needs.
5. Make sure you understand what will happen if you need surgery.

From www.ahrq.gov/consumer/5steps.htm. Retrieved March 10, 2013.

(AHRQ, 2013). The outcome was the identification of 22 practices that were either strongly encouraged (n = 10) or encouraged (n = 12). Among the strongly encouraged practices were preoperative checklists, bundles to prevent central line–associated bloodstream infections, interventions to reduce urinary catheter care, hand hygiene, "do not use" abbreviations, and barrier precautions to prevent healthcare-associated bloodstream infections. Among the encouraged practices were multicomponent interventions to reduce falls, documentation of patient preferences for life-sustaining treatment, team training, rapid response systems, and simulation exercises in patient safety efforts. Examples of these practices are cited in the evidence section at the end of the chapter (see p. 32).

EXERCISE 2-3

Refer to Gardner's Tasks of Leadership in Chapter 1 (pp. 14-15). Create a 3 × 10 grid. Enter Gardner's tasks in the left vertical column. Go to the AHRQ Website and find the report on *Making Health Care Safer II*. Select one of the encouraged or strongly encouraged practices. Using your selected practice, enter one behavior expected of a leader in column two to illustrate each of Gardner's tasks. Then in the third column, enter one behavior expected of a manager to illustrate each task. Finally reflect on your latest day in the clinical setting. Did you see evidence of the best practices being employed? What leadership and management behaviors were observable?

THE NATIONAL QUALITY FORUM

The National Quality Forum (NQF) is a membership-based organization designed to develop and implement a national strategy for healthcare quality measurement and reporting. As a result, the Centers for Medicare & Medicaid Services (CMS) formed its no-pay policy based on NQF's identification of "never-events." In other words, CMS will no longer pay for certain conditions that result from what might be termed *poor practice* or events that should never have occurred while a patient was under the care of a healthcare professional. The Healthcare Facilities Accreditation Program, a CMS-deemed authority, has adopted the NQF's 34 Safe Practices.

NQF refers to nurses as "the principal caregivers in any healthcare system" (National Quality Forum [NQF], 2008). This acknowledgment, while welcome, is also a challenge for nurses to perform in the best manner possible to lead organizations in their quests for quality and safety. Examples of measures related directly to nurses are pressure ulcer prevalence, ventilator-associated pneumonia, skill mix, voluntary turnover, and nursing care hours per patient day.

THE JOINT COMMISSION

The Joint Commission (TJC), formerly known as the *Joint Commission on Accreditation of Healthcare Organizations (JCAHO)*, is a not-for-profit organization that accredits healthcare organizations. It has "deemed" status from the CMS, which means that an organization that meets TJC standards is deemed to have met the standard that CMS sets.

When TJC changed its focus from process to outcomes, it also emphasized patient safety. As a result, TJC issues, with input from hospitals and healthcare professionals, annual patient safety goals that are setting specific; a list of "do-not-use" terms, symbols, and abbreviations; and sentinel events. All of these efforts are directed toward improving patient safety. In addition, with the NQF, TJC sponsors the Eisenberg Award for patient safety to highlight exemplars of quality.

THE DET NORSKE VERITAS/NATIONAL INTEGRATED ACCREDITATION FOR HEALTHCARE ORGANIZATIONS^SM

More recently, an internationally based organization that provides accreditation in a variety of fields entered healthcare accreditation. The Det Norske Veritas (DNV), or National Integrated Accreditation for Healthcare Organizations^SM (NIAHO^SM), is a direct competitor of TJC, and is also concerned with quality of care. The DNV/NIAHO work is based on a set of international standards known as *International Organization for Standardization (ISO)*.

The main difference between TJC and the DNV/NIAHO is that the latter surveys accredited organizations annually rather than the every three years of the TJC so that an organization has considerably more information to work with. Also, the DNV/NIAHO employs in health care the same

THEORY BOX

Diffusion Theory

THEORY/CONTRIBUTOR	KEY IDEA	APPLICATION TO PRACTICE
Rogers (2003)	• A process of communication about innovation to share information over time and among a group of people. • Allows for nonlinear change. • More complex change is less likely to be adopted. • Early adopters serve as role models	• Engage key leaders in a change to infuse the energy from early adopters. • Using Twitter in the hospital culture to engage employees communicates changes quickly.

approaches it has used in other fields where safety and quality are concerns.

MAGNET RECOGNITION PROGRAM®

The Magnet Recognition Program® is the only national designation built on and evolving through research that is designed to recognize nursing excellence of healthcare organizations through a self-nominating, appraisal process. Through the Magnet Recognition Program® Model *(www.nursecredentialing.org/Magnet/ProgramOverview/New-Magnet-Model)*, organizations must demonstrate how they provide excellence. Five elements comprise the model: transformational leadership; structural empowerment; exemplary professional practice; new knowledge, innovation, and improvements; and empirical quality results. From initial designation to redesignation, greater emphasis is placed on empirical quality results. Magnet™, like other organizations mentioned here, focuses on quality care.

INSTITUTE FOR HEALTHCARE IMPROVEMENT

The Institute for Healthcare Improvement (IHI) is dedicated to rapidly improving care through a variety of mechanisms including rapid cycle change projects. (See the Theory Box for the classic view of rapid cycle change.) IHI's work, *Transforming Care at the Bedside* (TCAB), has created numerous clinical practice changes for nursing. The common core of most projects is patient safety. The Open School *(www.ihi.org/offerings/IHIOpenSchool/Pages/default.aspx)* provides numerous resources for individuals to enhance their skills that relate to improving care.

QUALITY AND SAFETY EDUCATION FOR NURSES

Equally important for actual safe practice is the education students receive about safety. As a result, a project known as Quality and Safety Education for Nurses (QSEN) serves as a repository for resources related to the knowledge, skills and attitudes that learners need to develop to serve as safe practitioners. Competencies are identified for both prelicensure and graduate students, and numerous resources are available. In the prelicensure competencies, for example, one element relates directly to leading and managing: teamwork and collaboration. An example of what is expected in communication is this:

Analyze differences in communication style preferences among patients and families, nurses and other members of the health team Describe impact of own communication style on others Discuss effective strategies for communicating and resolving conflict	Communicate with team members, adapting own style of communicating to needs of the team and situation Demonstrate commitment to team goals Solicit input from other team members to improve individual, as well as team, performance Initiate actions to resolve conflict	Value teamwork and the relationships upon which it is based Value different styles of communication used by patients, families and health care providers Contribute to resolution of conflict and disagreement

Source: http://qsen.org/competencies/pre-licensure-ksas/#teamwork_collaboration.

MEANING FOR LEADING AND MANAGING IN NURSING

Many of the approaches to patient safety, and before that, aviation and nuclear energy safety, consist of strategies to alert us to safety issues. For example, the use of SBAR (Situation, Background, Assessment, and Recommendation) and checklists are designed to decrease omission of important information and practices. These practices are not designed to limit a professional's distinctive contributions. Rather they are designed to increase the likelihood of safe practice. Related issues of worker safety, such as the work environment itself and safe patient handling, also impinge on basic safe care of patients.

This concern for patient safety is not limited solely to hospitals or to the United States. For example, Accreditation Canada International *(www.internationalaccreditation.ca/accreditation/patientsafety.aspx)* identifies nine required organizational practices related to safety. The World Health Organization provides information on patient safety in five languages *(www.jointcommissioninternational.org/WHO-Collaborating-Centre-for-Patient-Safety-Solutions)*. Practices that were once mostly studied in hospital settings are now scrutinized in other settings. For example, outpatient clinics (KuKanich, Kaur, Freeman, & Powell, 2013), nursing homes (Castle, Wagner, Ferguson, & Handler, 2011), and rural settings (MacKinnon, 2011) report work related to patient safety.

To think that manager and leader decisions do not affect patient safety is erroneous. Creating a positive environment, assuring appropriate staffing, intervening and supporting others in doing so in cases of incivility, and supporting the use of the best evidence in practice all create a safer patient environment.

Often managerial and leadership tasks, like many others we perform, are squeezed into a hectic day. By stopping to concentrate on the work before us, we increase our chances of understanding the complexity of the situation and the ramifications of various decisions. By thinking through various scenarios, we are likely to eliminate strategies and methods that would not meet our needs and be more likely to narrow our choices of best actions to take. Then, if after an action, we took time to reflect on how well some decision was enacted, we would increase our knowledge about particular types of problems and enhance our skill at making decisions.

One of the challenges for nurses in any position, and especially for leaders and managers, is the obligation to have the greatest influence for patient safety. For example, Hendrich et al. (2012) identifies how nurse executives maximize their influence in advancing quality and safety. (See the following Literature Perspective.) Malloch and Melnyk (2013) refer to the nurse executive as having "evidence-driven consciousness" (p. 62). Many frontline nurses are unaware of the work that happens at this level on behalf of patient safety. Yet this work is equally critical to the organization's overall success in addressing patient safety issues.

The challenge for competent practice today is to stay well-informed about the best evidence or best

LITERATURE PERSPECTIVE

Resource: Hendrich, A.L., Batcheller, J., Ellison, D.A., Janik, A.M., Jeffords, N.B., Miller, L. Perlich, G.L., Staffileno, G., Strom, M., & Williams, C. (2012). The Ascension health experience: Maximizing the chief nursing officer role in a large, multihospital system to advance patient care quality and safety. *Nursing Administration Quarterly, 36*(4), 277-288.

Because of the magnitude of this healthcare system, the chief nursing officers (CNOs) created an advisory council to achieve multiple purposes, one of which was the identification and dissemination of best practices throughout the various hospitals and health ministries. The original focus was to align the work of nursing with the patient safety goals identified by The Joint Commission. The work then turned to other objectives including promoting interdisciplinary practice, involving the CNO with shared governance and considering major system issues to build consensus.

Six clinical examples were presented along with the identified issue and the impact and performance related to the example. For hand hygiene, as an example, the advisory council wanted to develop a standardized process and monitoring tool. The CNOs knew variation in handwashing procedures existed and wanted to unify all of the hospitals and ministries around best practices. A more dramatic example related to an expenditure of $60 million on new beds and surfaces to prevent pressure ulcers. The rate of decubiti across the system reduced by 43.4%.

Implications for Practice

A focus on patient safety is required of everyone in an organization. Nurses in administrative positions have the opportunity to influence patient safety in very different ways from frontline nurses. Maximizing everyone's potential advances the cause of patient safety.

practices that exist in any practice situation, including that of management and leadership. Eliminating barriers to integrating best practices is the role of leaders and managers. When they fail to support an environment that embraces evidence-based practice work, frontline nurses recognize that as a stumbling block for doing their best for patients. (See the following Research Perspective.)

RESEARCH PERSPECTIVE

Resource: Melnyk, B.M., Fineout-Overholt, E., Gallagher-Ford, L., & Kaplan, L. (2013). The state of evidence-based practice in US nurses: Critical implications for nurse leaders and educators. *The Journal of Nursing Administration, 42*(9), 410-417.

This descriptive study, involving a sample of 20,000 nurse members of the American Nurses Association and conducted by an email link to SurveyMonkey, included a demographic questionnaire, an 18-item Likert-scale survey about clinician's perspectives and needs related to evidence-based practices (EBP), and open-ended questions. Only 1105 nurses responded, which is a 5% response rate. One of the demographic questions allowed the researchers to compare Magnet™-designated hospitals from those without such designation. Nurses in Magnet™ organizations reported more consistency in implementing EBP, greater availability of experts, a supportive culture, and routine education and recognition about EBP.

One of the open-ended questions asked what barriers existed for implementing EBP. In addition to the culture and lack of skills and access to knowledge, leader/manager resistance was identified by 51 of the respondents as an issue. When asked about what would help them implement EBP routinely, manager support was identified by 55 of the respondents.

Implications for Practice
Although the number of nurses identifying that "leaders/managers" was an area to be addressed was small, the finding is still a concern. Coupling the number of responses for manager/leader resistance (n = 51) with the organizational culture (an area of accountability for the leader/manager) (n = 123), concerns should arise related to how to develop effective leaders and managers for today's healthcare practice.

CONCLUSION

Creating a culture of safety is everybody's business; and nurses, who are so integral to care, are key players in this important work. Every nurse has the accountability to challenge any act that appears unsafe and to stop actions that are not in the patient's best interest. Being proactive is insufficient in itself; examining practices and conditions that support errors is critical, as is sharing knowledge that can redirect care. In this challenging context, nurses continue to provide care and provide the organizational "glue" that supports patient care being accomplished in a safe, effective, and efficient manner. Nurses who serve as leaders and managers have additional opportunities to create conditions where ideas are heard, problems are solved, and the best evidence is employed.

THE SOLUTION

A multidisciplinary group was formed to address the problem. Our facility did not have some of the necessary equipment such as lift equipment, adult-sized positioning devices, and beds large enough to accommodate larger patients. We purchased the necessary equipment, and we also implemented a safe patient-handling program. The facility "skin champions "also developed an incontinence protocol and a friction/shear protocol.

Participation by our hospital in a multisite research study on pressure ulcer development in critically ill children has shown that our pressure ulcer incidence is significantly lower than that of other participating children's hospitals.

Success of the pediatric pressure ulcer prevention program is the result of extensive multidisciplinary collaboration—support from hospital administration, physicians, and frontline nurses. Use of evidence-based practice and research has also driven successful changes in our program. The desire to continually improve pressure ulcer prevention strategies has become the culture within our hospital.

—*Vickie S. Simpson*

Would this be a suitable approach for you? Why?

THE EVIDENCE

Making Health Care Safer II: An Updated Critical Analysis of the Evidence for Patient Safety Practices (AHRQ, 2013) identified 10 strongly encouraged practices and 12 encouraged practices, both sets of which are based on evidence. (The full listings are available at *http://archive.ahrq.gov/clinic/ptsafety.*)

Sample evidence

Strongly Encouraged
1. Preoperative checklists
2. Bundles that include checklists to prevent central line–associated bloodstream infections
5. Hand hygiene
6. "Do Not Use" list for hazardous abbreviations

Encouraged
1. Multicomponent interventions to reduce falls
3. Documentation of patient preferences for life-sustaining treatment
5. Team training
9. Rapid response systems
12. Use of simulation exercises in patient safety efforts

WHAT NEW GRADUATES SAY

- Know how to retrieve literature related to best practice and evidence in your area of practice.
- Wash your hands so patients see you do this.
- Practice what to say to stop an unsafe practice.
- Observe and listen to what nurses say about patient safety on your unit.
- Act on behalf of patients.

CHAPTER CHECKLIST

This chapter focused on the core of leading and managing in nursing, namely an intense passion for patients and their safety. To lead and manage effectively, a nurse must be passionate about quality and patient safety. The nurse leader and manager, as well as followers, must be able to identify potential safety issues, intervene quickly when a safety issue exists, and think skillfully after a safety violation so that all may learn.
- The classic reports and emerging supports

- The Institute of Medicine reports on quality
- Agency for Healthcare Research and Quality
- The National Quality Forum
- The Joint Commission
- The DNV/NIAHO℠
- Magnet Recognition Program®
- Institute for Healthcare Improvement
- Quality and Safety Education for Nurses
- Meaning for leading and managing in nursing

TIPS FOR PATIENT SAFETY

- Use the IOM competencies to frame your actions.
- Keep current with the evidence and best practices.
- Use only quality sources, especially Websites.
- Read general nursing literature regarding other organizations' work related to safety.

REFERENCES

Accreditation Canada International. *Required organizational practices.* Retrieved March 14, 2013 from www.internationalaccreditation.ca/accreditation/patientsafety.aspx.

Agency for Healthcare Research and Quality (AHRQ). *AHRQ mission.* Retrieved March 10, 2013, from www.ahrq.gov.

Agency for Healthcare Research and Quality (AHRQ). *Making health care safer II: An updated critical analysis of the evidence for patient safety practices.* Retrieved March 6, 2013 from www.ahrq.gov/research/findings/evidence-based-reports/ptsafetyuptp.html.

Castle, N. G., Wagner, L. M., Ferguson, J. C., & Handler, S. M. (2011). Safety culture of nursing homes: Opinions of top managers. *Health Care Management Review, 36*(2), 175–187. http://dx.doi.org/10.1097/HMR.0b013e3182080d5f.

Det Norske Veritas (DNV). *Managing risk to improve patient safety.* Retrieved March 14, 2013, from www.dnv.com/industry/healthcare/index.asp.

Hendrich, A. L., Batcheller, J., Ellison, D. A., Janik, A. M., Jeffords, N. B., Miller, L., et al. (2012). The ascension health experience: Maximizing the chief nursing officer role in a large, multihospital system to advance patient care quality and safety. *Nursing Administration Quarterly, 36*(4), 277–288. http://dx.doi.org/10.1097/NAQ.0b013e31826692a6.

Institute of Medicine (IOM), *To err is human: Building a safer health system.* (2000). Washington, DC: National Academy Press.

Institute of Medicine (IOM), *Crossing the quality chasm: A new health system for the 21st century.* (2001). Washington, DC: National Academy Press.

Institute of Medicine (IOM), *Health professions education: A bridge to quality.* (2003). Washington, DC: National Academy Press.

Institute of Medicine (IOM), *Keeping patients safe: Transforming the work environment of nurses.* (2004). Washington, DC: National Academy Press.

Institute of Medicine (IOM), *Improving the quality of health care for mental and substance-use conditions: Quality Chasm Series.* (2005). Washington, DC: National Academy Press.

Institute of Medicine (IOM), *Preventing medication errors: Quality Chasm Series.* (2006). Washington, DC: National Academy Press.

Institute of Medicine (IOM), *The future of nursing: Leading change, advancing health.* (2011). Washington, DC: National Academy Press.

KuKanich, K. S., Kaur, R., Freeman, L. C., & Powell, D. A. (2013). Evaluation of a hand hygiene campaign in outpatient health care clinics. *American Journal of Nursing, 113*(3), 36–42.

MacKinnon, K. (2011). Rural nurses' safeguarding work: Reembodying patient safety. *Advances in Nursing Science, 34*(2), 199–29. http://dx.doi.org/10.1097/ANS.0b013e3182186b86.

Malloch, K., & Melnyk, B. M. (2013). Developing high-level change and innovation agents: Competencies and challenges for executive leadership. *Nursing Administration Quarterly, 37*(1), 60–66. http://dx.doi.org/10.1097/NAQ.0b013e318275174a.

Melnyk, B. M., Fineout-Overholt, E., Gallagher-Ford, L., & Kaplan, L. (2013). The state of evidence-based practice in US nurses: Critical implications for nurse leaders and educators. *The Journal of Nursing Administration, 42*(9), 410–417. http://dx.doi.org/10.1097/NNA.0b013e3182664e0a.

National Quality Forum. (2008), *Nursing care quality at NQF.* Retrieved Mary 15, 2013, from, www.qualityforum.org/nursing.

Quality and Safety Education for Nurses. *Competencies: Prelicensure KSAs.* Retrieved March 14, 2013, from http://qsen.org/competencies/pre-licensure-ksas.

Rogers, E. M. (2003). *Diffusion of innovations* (5th ed.). New York: The Free Press.

World Health Organization. *Patient safety solutions.* Retrieved March 14, 2013, from www.jointcommissioninternational.org/WHO-Collaborating-Centre-for-Patient-Safety-Solutions.

SUGGESTED READINGS

Agency for Healthcare Research and Quality. www.ahrq.gov.

Ashe, P. A., & Weeks, S. K. (2012). Positive changes, positive outcomes: The DNV/ISO/NPPM connection. *Nurse Leader, 10*(4), 20–23.

Institute for Healthcare Improvement. www.ihi.org.

Institute of Medicine. www.iom.org.

McHugh, M. D., & Stimpfel, A. W. (2012). Nurse reported quality of care: A measure of hospital quality. *Research in Nursing and Health, 35*(6), 566–575. http://dx.doi.org/10.1002/nur.21503.

Petersen, M. A., Blackmer, M., McNeal, J., & Hill, P. D. (2013, January). What makes handover communication effective? *Nursing Management,* 15–18. http://dx.doi.org/10:1097/01.NUMA.0000424026.21411.65.

West, G., Patrician, P. A., & Loan, L. (2012). Staffing matters—Every shift. *American Journal of Nursing, 112*(12), 22–27.

3

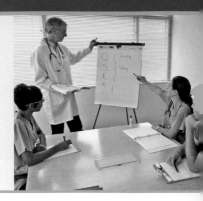

Developing the Role of Leader

Michael L. Evans

This chapter focuses on leadership and its value in advancing the profession of nursing. Leadership development is explained with examples of how to survive and thrive in a leadership position. The differences between the emerging and entrenched workforce generations are explored, and the desired characteristics of a leader for the emerging workforce are described. Leadership in a variety of situations, such as clinical settings, community venues, organizations, and political situations, is described. This chapter provides an introduction to the opportunities, challenges, and satisfaction of leadership.

LEARNING OUTCOMES

- Analyze the role of leadership in creating a satisfying working environment for nurses.
- Evaluate transactional and transformational leadership techniques for effectiveness and potential for positive outcomes.
- Value the leadership challenges in dealing with generational differences.
- Compare and contrast leadership and management roles and responsibilities.
- Describe leadership development strategies and how they can promote leadership skills acquisition.
- Analyze leadership opportunities and responsibilities in a variety of venues.
- Explore strategies for making the leadership opportunity positive for both the leader and the followers.

KEY TERMS

emerging workforce	management	transactional leadership
entrenched workforce	mentor	transformational leadership
leadership		

THE CHALLENGE

Katheren Koehn, MA, RN
Executive Director
Minnesota Organization of Registered Nurses, Minneapolis MN

Leadership is occasionally about the heroic moment. More often, it is about the day-to-day efforts to keep your team headed generally the same way, guiding them and making sure they have what they need to do their best work. As a leader, I have found that one of the most important things I can do is to make sure that all members of the team know where we are headed by having a common definition of the terms we are using.

Why would we worry about a common definition for the terms we use? They are all in English, aren't they? They are common and easily understood, aren't they? Maybe yes, but then, maybe no ...

The first time I became aware that standard definitions could be a problem is when I was president of a state nurses association. As our board of directors was reviewing the previous board's strategic plan, we saw that one of the main goals was to increase the diversity of our membership. Our board noted that we had failed this one miserably; our members were no more ethnically or racially diverse than they had been before the creation of this goal. We talked about steps we might take to try to achieve this goal, never considering what the word "diversity" meant. Everyone knows, we thought, that diversity is ethnic and racial. No question.

It was more than a year later, when we were still unable to achieve that goal that we finally talked to some people who had helped write it in the first place. Much to our surprise, their definition of diversity was not based on race or ethnicity. It was based on education and practice setting! The state nurses' association membership was primarily made up of direct care nurses, and the former board's goal was to add educators, managers, and others to the demographics of the membership. Without knowing the definition of diversity, our board was unable to create strategies that could help us achieve that goal. We failed before we started.

This experience was put to even greater use a couple of years later. The hospital where I worked had a newly formed patient care delivery committee made up of direct care nurses, managers, and directors, plus human resources representatives. The Vice President of Nursing and I, as a direct care nurse, were co-chairs of the committee. Practice changes were to come to our committee for deliberation before implementation. This was shared decision making at a higher level than we had tried before and making it work was going to take a lot of growing pains.

At one meeting, a discussion about a proposed change turned into a disagreement, then an argument. The meeting ended abruptly, no solution available. As co-chairs, we decided to stop meeting for a while. We needed a "cooling-off" period. This had been a really big disagreement!

What do you think you would do if you were this nurse?

INTRODUCTION

Leadership is a complex, highly important, and challenging skill expected of all nurses. Leader refers to performance, not a formal position. We lead when we intervene with courage for a patient. We lead when we organize a group of colleagues to address an organizational problem. We lead when we are formally placed in charge of a project or when we are promoted to a specific management position.

WHAT IS A LEADER?

A leader is an individual who works with others to develop a clear vision of the preferred future and to make that vision happen. Historically, Oakley and Krug (1994) called that type of **leadership** *enlightened leadership,* or the ability to elicit a vision from people and to inspire and empower those people to do what it takes to bring the vision into reality. Leaders bring out the best in people. McBride (2011) states that "leaders develop over time rather than being born with 'the right stuff'" (p. 16).

Leadership is a very important concept in life. Great leaders have been responsible for helping society move forward and for articulating and accomplishing one vision after another throughout time. Dr. Martin Luther King, Jr., called his vision a *dream,* and it was developed because of the input and lived experiences of countless others. Mother Teresa called her vision a *calling,* and it was developed because of the suffering of others. Steven Spielberg calls his vision a *finished motion picture,* and it is developed with the collaboration and inspiration of many other people. Florence Nightingale called her vision *nursing,* and it was developed because people were experiencing a void that was a barrier to their ability to regain or establish health.

Leaders have followers. An individual can have an impressive title, but that title does not make that person a leader. No matter what the person with that title does, he or she can never be successful without having the ability to inspire others to follow. The leader must be able to inspire the commitment of followers.

McBride (2011) sees leadership as much larger than simply inspiring followers. It is about "moving a profession, or institution, or some aspect of health care down a new path with different expectations, structures, and ways of conceptualizing how to achieve the mission in light of changing conditions" (p. 165).

Covey (1992), in his classic work, identified eight characteristics of effective leaders (Box 3-1). Effective leaders are continually engaging themselves in lifelong learning. They are service-oriented and concerned with the common good. They radiate positive energy. For people to be inspired and motivated, they must have a positive leader. Effective leaders believe in other people. They lead balanced lives and see life as an adventure. Effective leaders are synergistic; that is, they see things as greater than the sum of the parts and they engage themselves in self-renewal.

EXERCISE 3-1

List Covey's eight characteristics of effective leaders on the left side of a piece of paper or a word document. Next to each characteristic, list any examples of your activities or attributes that reflect the characteristic. Some areas may be blank; others will be full. Think about what this means for you personally.

Healthcare organizations are complex. In fact, health care is complex. Continual learning is essential to stay abreast of new knowledge, to keep the organization moving forward, and to continue delivering the best possible care. An emphasis must be present

---

BOX 3-1   COVEY'S EIGHT CHARACTERISTICS OF EFFECTIVE LEADERS

1. Engage in lifelong learning
2. Are service-oriented
3. Are concerned with the common good
4. Radiate positive energy
5. Believe in other people
6. Lead balanced lives and see life as an adventure
7. Are synergistic; that is, they see things as greater than the sum of the parts
8. Engage themselves in self-renewal

---

on organizations becoming learning organizations, to provide opportunities and incentives for individuals and groups of individuals to learn continuously over time. A learning organization is one that is continually expanding its capacity to create its future (Senge, 2006). Leaders are responsible for building organizations in which people continually expand their ability to understand complexity and to clarify and improve a shared vision of the future—"that is, they are responsible for learning" (Senge, 2006, p. 340).

The roles of manager and leader are often considered interchangeable, but they are actually quite different. The manager may also be a leader, but the manager is not required to have leadership skills within the context of moving a group of people toward a vision. The term *manager* is a designated leadership position. *Leadership* is an abilities role, and it is most effective if the manager is also a leader. **Management** can be taught and learned using traditional teaching techniques. Leadership can also be taught, but it is usually a reflection of rich personal experiences.

Management and leadership are both important in the healthcare environment. Leaders are developed over time and through experience. Thus we must value, support, and provide our leaders with the one thing vital for good leadership—good followership. Leadership is a social process involving leaders and followers interacting. Followers need three qualities from their leaders: direction, trust, and hope (Bennis, 2009). The trust is reciprocal. Leaders who trust their followers are, in turn, trusted by them. Leaders have learned to be effective leaders from their experience of being effective followers. Followers learn the skills involved in leadership from the follower vantage point. Effective leaders support and nurture their followers in part because they are creating the next generation of leaders.

The manager is concerned with doing things correctly in the present. The role of manager is very important in work organizations because managers ensure that operations run smoothly and that well-developed formulas are applied to staffing situations, economic decisions, and other daily operations. The manager is not as concerned with developing creative solutions to problems as with using known strategies to address today's issues. A well-managed entity may be proceeding correctly but, without leadership, may be proceeding in the wrong direction (Covey, 1992).

Wakeman (2010, p. 50) states, "the difference between management and leadership is that management is working on your business, and leadership is working on your people."

Leadership as an Important Concept for Nurses

Nurses must have leadership to move forward in harmony with changes in society and in health care. Within work organizations, certain nurses are designated as managers. These individuals are important to ensuring that care is delivered in a safe, efficient manner. Nurse leaders are also vital in the workplace to elicit input from others and to formulate a vision for the preferred future.

Moreover, leadership is key for nursing as a profession. The public depends on nurses to advocate for the public's needs and interests. Nurses must step forward into leadership roles in their workplace, in their professional associations, and in legislative and policy-making arenas. Fortunately, as McBride (2011) points out, nurses have many leader abilities such as "integrity, practical intelligence, and systems thinking" (p. 16). Nurses depend on their leaders to set goals for the future and the pace for achieving them. The public depends on nurse leaders to move the consumer advocacy agenda forward.

Leadership as a Primary Determinant of Workplace Satisfaction

Nurse satisfaction within the workplace is an important construct in nursing administration and healthcare administration. Turnover is extremely costly to any work organization in terms of money, expertise, and knowledge, as well as care quality. Thus, being mindful of nurse satisfaction is both an economic and a professional concern.

Followers expect their leaders to provide them with:
- Respect
- A future-focused direction
- Control of the decisions that affect them
- Rewards and recognition
- Balance of life and work
- Professional development guidance

The effective leader in healthcare settings needs to be aware of these important facets of work life that influence followers. The leader should also work with followers to find a way to actualize these important aspects of work life.

A study by Moneke and Umeh (2013), which examines the factors influencing critical care nurses' job satisfaction, found a statistically significant relationship between perceived leadership and job satisfaction. They found that "organizational success and an employee's ability to thrive are influenced by a leader's ability to inspire outstanding performance" (p. 206).

The leader, not the manager, inspires others to work at their highest level. The presence of strong leadership sets the tone for achievement in the work environment. Effective leadership is the basis for an effective workplace, and therefore creating leadership succession is an important consideration. This means that, in addition to supporting current leaders in their roles, new leaders must be encouraged and developed.

EXERCISE 3-2

Follower behavior nurtures and supports—or deteriorates—leader behavior. Identify the behavior you exhibited during your most recent clinical experience. What was supportive? What did not support the leader?

THE PRACTICE OF LEADERSHIP

Leadership Approaches

How one approaches leadership depends on experience and expectations. Many leadership theories and styles have been described. Two of the most popular theory-based approaches are transactional leadership and transformational leadership. (See the Theory Box on p. 38.)

Transactional Leadership

A transactional leader is the traditional "boss" image. In a **transactional leadership** environment, employees understand that a superior makes the decisions with little or no input from subordinates. Transactional leadership relies on the power of organizational position and formal authority to reward and punish performance. Followers are fairly secure about what will happen next and how to "play the game" to get where they want to be. A transactional leader uses a *quid pro quo* style to accomplish work (e.g., I'll do x in exchange for you doing y). Transactional leaders reward employees for high performance and penalize them for poor performance. The leader motivates

THEORY BOX

A Comparison of Outcomes in Transactional and Transformational Leadership

TRANSACTIONAL LEADERSHIP	TRANSFORMATIONAL LEADERSHIP
Leader Behaviors	**Leader Behaviors**
• Contingent reward *(quid pro quo)* • Punitive • Management by exception (active)—monitors performance and takes action to correct • Management by exception (passive)—intervenes only when problems exist	• Charismatic • Inspirational and motivational • Intellectual stimulation • Individualized consideration
Effect on Follower	**Effect on Follower**
• Fulfills the contract or gets punished • Does the work and gets paid • Errors are corrected in a reactive manner	• A shared vision • Increased self-worth • Challenging and meaningful work • Coaching and mentoring happens • A sense of being valued
Organizational Outcomes	**Organizational Outcomes**
• Work is supervised and completed according to the rules • Deadlines are met • Limited job satisfaction • Low to stable levels of commitment	• Increased loyalty • Increased commitment • Increased job satisfaction • Increased morale • Increased performance

Modified from McGuire, E., & Kennerly, S.M. (2006). Nurse managers as transformational and transactional leaders. *Nursing Economic$, 24*(4), 179-185.

the self-interest of the employee by offering external rewards that generate conformity with expectations.

Transformational Leadership

Transformational leadership is based on an inspiring vision that changes the framework of the organization for employees. Employees are encouraged to transcend their own self-interest. This style of leadership involves communication that connects with employees' ideals in a way that causes emotional engagement. The transformational leader can motivate employees by articulation of an inspirational vision; by encouragement of novel, innovative thinking; and by individualized consideration of each employee, thus accounting for individual needs and abilities. Drenkard (2013) describes true transformational leadership as occurring when leaders and followers have a relationship in which the leader does not hold all of the power and authority, but the leader "created an environment that brought leaders and followers together to solve problems, create new ways of doing work, and manage change together" (p. 57). This synergy of bringing people together around an inspiring vision and yet valuing individuals as distinct beings

suggests a finely tuned, mindful approach to the role of leader.

Covey (1992) states, "The goal of transformational leadership is to transform people and organizations in a literal sense, to change them in mind and heart; enlarge vision, insight, and understanding; clarify purposes; make behavior congruent with beliefs, principles, or values; and bring about changes that are permanent, self-perpetuating, and momentum-building" (p. 287).

Kouzes and Posner (2012) identify five key practices in transformational leadership, as follows:

1. Challenging the process, which involves questioning the way things have been done in the past and thinking creatively about new solutions to old problems
2. Inspiring shared vision or bringing everyone together to move toward a goal that all accept as desirable and achievable
3. Enabling others to act, which includes empowering people to believe that their extra effort will have rewards and will make a difference
4. Modeling the way, meaning that the leader must take an active role in the work of change

5. Encouraging the heart by giving attention to those personal things that are important to people, such as saying "thank you" for a job well-done and offering praise after a long day

A transformative leader style seems particularly suited to the nursing environment. For example, the Magnet Recognition Program® places great emphasis on this type of leadership to move an organization to high levels of quality. A transformative leader creates a vision of what quality could look like and then provides specific actions that create a sense of community, which supports satisfaction, retention, communication, and interprofessional work. This type of leader listens to the views of others, finds ways to remove barriers, and serves as an advocate for those who care for patients.

The role of the Chief Nursing Officer (CNO) is key to truly transformational leadership in a healthcare organization (Clavelle, Drenkard, Tullai-McGuinness, & Fitzpatrick, 2012). In fact, "the Chief Nursing Officer's effectiveness as a change agent is dependent upon effective transformational leadership practices, such as creating a shared vision, inspiring others, and empowering others to lead" (p. 195).

Murphy (2012) describes a different construct of leadership involving the CNO. Authentic leadership is the CNO being oneself, and "has been identified as the single most important quality of leadership" (p. 507). Authentic leaders understand their values, convictions, and the purpose of their leadership, and they develop this understanding by constructing a life story. "Through ongoing reflection on the significant people and experiences influencing them, these leaders frame and reframe their stories, giving them new meaning with each iteration. In constructing their life stories, authentic leaders discover the true purpose of their leadership" (p. 507). Positive outcomes are derived from effective leadership in organizations. Boev (2012) found that direct care nurse perceptions of the nurse manager's leadership and ability was significantly related to patient satisfaction and the role of the nurse manager is pivotal in both nurse and patient satisfaction. In addition, leadership has the potential to influence nurses' use of clinical guidelines, a vital tool for making evidence-based practice decisions (Gifford et al., 2013).

Transformational leadership is hard work; investment of time and energy is required to bring out the best in people. And a leader does not have to be good at everything. A good leader seeks to create a whole from the various members of a team. Transformational leadership is not unique to nursing as the following Research Perspective illustrates.

 RESEARCH PERSPECTIVE

Resource: Bulmer, J. (2013). Leadership aspirations of registered nurses: Who wants to follow us? *Journal of Nursing Administration*, 43(3), 130-134.

This descriptive, correlational study measures relationships among perceived support, career stage, educational preparation, and leadership aspiration in registered nurses. The predictors of leadership aspiration were years of experience, educational preparation, and perceived available support.

Overall, fewer than 12.5% of registered nurses aspire to leadership roles. Those newly entering nursing have higher percentages of interest, but the interest wanes over time as nurses become disillusioned with those whom they see as ineffective in leadership roles and with the obstacles they face. Nurses with higher degrees tend to have higher interest in leadership roles. Nurses who perceive that they have support from colleagues, from direct supervisors, and from non-workplace individuals are more likely to be interested in such formal leadership roles.

Implications for Practice

The estimate is that 75% of current formal nurse leaders plan to leave the workforce by 2020. Therefore more attention must be given to the identification and development of nurse leaders for the future. Because early career nurses and those with higher education are the ones most interested in progressing to formal leadership positions, they should not be overlooked. Past practices of targeting nurses with several years of experience for development should be questioned.

More nurses are graduating from second degree accelerated BSN programs and many of those already have a wealth of experience outside of health care. Those nurses who are interested in a leadership role should be carefully assessed and formally developed early in their careers while the interest is still high. Nurses who have achieved higher levels of education should also be actively assessed for possible leadership development. Support from the nurse's nurse manager and from having a career coach external to the direct work environment are also correlated with inspiring interest in a formal leadership role.

Because baccalaureate and higher degree programs are expected to provide exposure to content dealing with leadership, these individuals may be ready for career advancement earlier in their careers than has been the case in the past. Actively identifying and developing registered nurses for formal leadership roles is essential in all workplace organizations.

Barriers to Leadership

Leadership demands a commitment of effort and time. Many barriers exist to both leading and following. Good leadership and good followership go hand in hand, and both strengthen the mission of the organization.

False Assumptions

Some people have false assumptions about leaders and leadership. For example, some believe that position and title are equivalent to leadership. Having the title of Chief Executive Officer or Chief Nursing Officer does not guarantee that a person will be a good leader. Consequently, a good executive is not necessarily a good leader. Furthermore, assuming a management or administrative role does not automatically confer the title of leader on an individual. Inspired and forward-moving organizations often select these executives specifically because of their ability to forge a vision and lead others toward it. Leadership is an earned honor and an action-oriented responsibility.

Others believe that workers who do not hold official management positions cannot be leaders. Some nursing units are managed by the nurse manager but led by the unit clerk. Leaders are those who do the best job of sharing their vision of where the followers want to be and how to get there. Many new nurse managers make the mistake of assuming that along with their new job comes the mantle of leadership. Leadership is an earned right and privilege.

Time Constraints

Leadership requires a time commitment; it does not just happen. The leader must fully comprehend the situation at hand, investigate and research options for action, assume the responsibility to communicate the vision to others, and continually reevaluate the organization or the team to ensure that the vision remains relevant and attainable. All of these activities take time. The twenty-first century has been described as the period of doing more with less. Everyone is busy. Finding time to lead is, therefore, a barrier for many who have inspirational ideas but lack time to develop the skills needed to lead effectively.

LEADERSHIP DEVELOPMENT

Leadership effectiveness depends on mastering the art of persuasion and communication. Success depends on persuading followers to accept a vision by using convincing communication techniques and making it possible for the followers to achieve the shared goals. Several important leadership tasks, when used effectively, will help ensure success (Box 3-2). These are discussed in the following sections.

Select a Mentor

A **mentor** is someone who models behavior, offers advice and criticism, and coaches the novice to develop a personal leadership style. A mentor is a confidante and coach, as well as a cheerleader and teacher. In other words, a mentor is knowledgeable and skilled. Where do you find a mentor? Usually, a mentor is someone who has experience and some success in the leadership realm of interest, such as in a clinical setting or in an organization. A respected faculty member; a nurse manager, director, or clinician; or an organizational officer or active member may be a mentor. Mentorship is a two-way street. The mentor must agree to work with the novice leader and must have some interest in the novice's future development. A mentor can be close enough geographically to allow both observation and practice of leadership

---

EXERCISE 3-3

Define a clinical or management issue that sparks your passion. Assume you have 6 weeks to make a difference. Create a plan identifying your leadership tasks, the support required from others, and the time frame to move the issue toward resolution. Think about what your message is and how and when you will deliver it. Think about what you would do if no one were responsive to your issue. Think about why the issue may be important for you but not for others.

BOX 3-2 LEADERSHIP DEVELOPMENT TASKS

1. Select a mentor.
2. Lead by example.
3. Accept responsibility.
4. Share the rewards.
5. Have a clear vision.
6. Be willing to grow.

behaviors, as well as timely feedback. A mentor may also be geographically remote and yet well-connected to the mentee. A mentor should provide advice, feedback, and role-modeling. In addition, the mentor has a right to expect assistance with projects, respect, loyalty, and confidentiality. In a mentoring relationship, aspiring leaders soak up knowledge and experience and should expect to return it by serving as a mentor to a young, aspiring leader in the future.

Lead by Example

An effective leader knows that the most effective and visible way to influence people is to lead by example. Desired behavior can be modeled. For example, if an organization has a vision of becoming a political player in the state or community, the leader should be seen engaging in political activities. If the goal is to have improved relationships among followers, the leader must exhibit respect and patience with followers. A key skill to develop is the ability to understand that the leader serves the followers. The effective

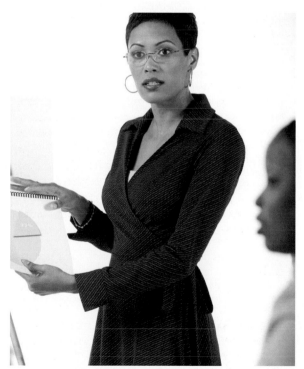

Leading by example helps developing leaders see the mission in action.

leader does not send members to do a job but, rather, leads them toward a mutual goal as a team.

Accept Responsibility

Even when the outcome is below expectations, the leader is ultimately responsible for the organization or activity. Effective leaders sometimes react in strange ways when negative outcomes occur. Sometimes these leaders seek to blame others or to make excuses for undesirable or unintended outcomes. Some refuse to accept any responsibility at all. In accepting responsibility, the leader needs to know that there is reward in victory and growth in failure. No one plans to fail, but an effective leader sees failures as opportunities to learn and grow so that previous failures are never repeated. This is called *experience.*

Share the Rewards

An effective leader is as eager to share the glory as to receive it. The more that respect and trust are shared with others, the more they are returned to the leader. Followers who believe their major task is to make the leader look good will soon tire of the task. Empowerment, the act of sharing power with others, is a dynamic process. In essence, sharing power has a synergistic effect that increases power overall. Followers who think the leader is working to make them look good will follow eagerly. Followers form a network and a support base for the leader.

Have a Clear Vision

Leaders see beyond where they are and see where they are going. Strong leaders are proactive and futuristic. The effective leader knows why the journey is necessary and takes the time and energy to inspire others to go along. The ability to communicate and promote the vision is a vital part of achieving it. Effective leaders share their vision and empower followers to come along to achieve it. They also share their leadership skills and successes toward achievement of a goal.

Be Willing to Grow

Thinking that growth for the person or organization is automatic is a misconception. Complacency leads to stagnation. Leaders must continually read about new ideas and approaches, experiment with new concepts, capitalize on a changing world, and seek or create continuing education opportunities to enhance their abilities to lead. Growth takes risk, planning, investment, and work. Setting goals that complement the vision will help the aspiring leader know where to invest time and energy to grow into the desired role.

Leadership development is a lifetime endeavor. Effective leaders are constantly striving to improve their leadership skills. The good news is that leadership skills can be learned and improved. A commitment to improvement strengthens the leader's ability to lead effectively and raises the bar for followers to achieve. As organizations and health care change, the leader is better able to work effectively with an increasingly diverse workforce. The best leaders bring out the best in their followers, as seen in the following Literature Perspective.

DEVELOPING LEADERS IN THE EMERGING WORKFORCE

Generational differences have always created challenges in the workplace. At the dawn of the twenty-first century, the workplace found an **emerging workforce** with goals, priorities, and work preferences that were vastly different from those of their Baby Boomer parents. Helping each generation understand and tolerate others is often a delicate orchestration of needs and wants, incentives and motives. Transgenerational leadership must focus on building an understanding and acceptance of each other.

Nurse leaders need to understand generational differences in order to enhance performance. Multiple dimensions of diversity exist in the workplace, including religion, gender, culture, and race, but a nurse leader must also think about generation (not age) differences. A nurse leader must be able to become a

 LITERATURE PERSPECTIVE

Resource: Covey, S.M.R. (2012). *Smart trust*. New York: Free Press.

The role of leader includes building trust between the leader and followers and between followers and leaders.

Stephen M.R. Covey, the son of the late Stephen Covey, describes a method for instilling trust in organizations. He describes the dilemma of not knowing whom to trust in an untrusting world. We are born to be very trusting, but the older we get and after learning many life lessons about trust, we grow less willing to trust.

Smart trust is all about judgment. It enables us to have high trust in a low-trust world. It is how to trust in a low-trust world. It combines the human propensity to want to trust with analysis.

Analysis in smart trust involves assessment of three very important variables:

1. The opportunity or the situation and what you are trusting someone with.
2. Risk or the level of risk involved in the situation.
3. Credibility or the character and competence of the people who are involved.

In the absence of analysis, low propensity to trust produces no trust or indecision, and high propensity to trust produces blind trust or gullibility. In the absence of propensity to trust, low analysis produces distrust or suspicion, and high analysis produces smart trust or judgment. So, Covey posits that application of both propensity to trust and analysis will produce the most positive leadership results.

Smart trust is based on five smart trust actions for leaders to master:

1. Choose to believe in trust. Leaders must create the foundational paradigm out of which all the other trust-building behaviors follow.
2. Start with self. Leaders must focus first on developing character and competence, which is their credibility. This enables leaders to trust themselves and to also give others someone or something in which they can trust.
3. Leaders declare their intent and assume positive intent in others. They signal the goals and intended actions in advance and assume that others also have good intent and want to be trustworthy.
4. Leaders then do what they say they are going to do. They follow through in carrying out the declared intent.
5. They lead out in extending trust to others. These leaders are the first to extend trust to others, which initiates the cycle of mutual trust.

Covey describes the outcome of high levels of mutual trust between leaders and followers. He calls it a performance multiplier that can translate directly into greatly improved outcomes, both interpersonally and for productivity of leadership interactions.

Implications for Practice

People notice differences in various workplaces and they tend to choose the workplace where there is a high level of trust demonstrated between leaders and followers. The culture of the workplace reflects the effectiveness of the leader's ability to create, nurture, and develop relationships based on trust.

generationally fluent translator, able to communicate among the different generations (Clipper, 2013).

The Emerging Workforce: The 1965 to 1995 Generation

Part of this cohort, born between 1965 and 1976, represents the smallest workforce entry pool since 1930, with just 44 million, compared with the 77 million Baby Boomers preceding them and the 70 million Generation Ys following them. They have a mindset and work ethic that Baby Boomers do not understand. They are hard workers, but unlike the Baby Boomers, they do not have confidence in leaders and institutions. They tend to change jobs more frequently. Their focus is on work-life balance and they seek feedback about their performance

Their younger siblings, the Generation Ys (also known as *Generation Net, Nexter,* or the *Millennium Generation*), who were born between 1977 and 1995, share many of the same approaches to work but bring their own challenges with no brand loyalty and a blatant disregard for status symbols. They are highly skilled in technology and seek to "figure out" how something works rather than read a manual. They tend to believe in themselves and are generally optimistic.

Successfully leading the emerging workforce means the leader must shape a vision and win the 20-somethings to it. The vision must be one that excites them, because fun and balance are an important part of their lives. A vision that is powerful enough can transform the workplace.

The successful leader must mobilize followers to act. The required actions must provide value to the followers (e.g., learning a new skill or attaining certification or recognition). The younger generations are happy to follow as long as they can retain balance in their lives, have information about and input into the decisions that affect them, and see some benefit in the activity. It is the leader's challenge to provide the type of environment in which younger-generation followers want to follow.

The Entrenched Workforce: The 1946 to 1965 Generation

Baby Boomers, born after World War II, see work life very differently compared with the emerging workforce. Boomer workers are much more likely to believe in the power of collective action, based on

their successes with social movements in their formative years in the 1960s. They tend to mistrust authority and are very comfortable with the process of getting to a goal. They find the journey of getting to the goal almost as important as reaching the goal. They are tolerant of, even depend on, meetings and ongoing discussions that the younger generation finds tedious and wasteful.

The preferred leader of the entrenched workforce shares some of the characteristics of the younger generation's leader, such as being motivational, honest, approachable, competent, and knowledgeable. However, Baby Boomers also expect their leaders to be professional and supportive and have high integrity.

Challenges for the entrenched workforce are sharing leadership with the younger generation, empowering them to lead in their own model rather than trying to make them into second-generation Baby Boomers, and retaining the younger leaders in leadership ranks. Many younger employees are opting out of traditional work roles to become entrepreneurs. They take their leadership potential with them where there are few older role models for them to follow. A risk for aging Boomers is that the best and the brightest potential leaders will lose interest in leading and will opt for personal satisfaction and wealth accumulation rather than leadership and service roles.

The challenges of generational acceptance are some of many facing twenty-first century leaders. Attention to the needs of both the leader and the follower will create an environment in which everyone thrives.

> **EXERCISE 3-4**
> List the names of the people with whom you work most frequently. Determine to which workforce (emerging or entrenched) each belongs. Describe known benefits of the workplace that support each generation's view. (One list may be longer than the other.) What elements of benefits are present in the personnel policies and workplace practices that benefit each? What elements are absent?

SURVIVING AND THRIVING AS A LEADER

The keys to leadership are to believe in the vision and to enjoy the journey. The leader has a responsibility to self and to followers to stay healthy and enthusiastic for the mission of the group. Surviving and thriving as a leader are based on the rules in Box 3-3. Each element is discussed in the following sections.

The Leader Must Maintain Balance

Time management is essential for an effective leader. Many new leaders, in their zeal to be accessible to their constituents, lose control of their lives. A good strategy for retaining or regaining control is to get control of communication. Good leaders use the simplest and fastest method of communication that makes them accessible but does not tie them down. The keys to success are setting priorities and keeping in control. Effective leaders also maintain work-life balance in their own lives as well as providing time for balance for followers.

The Leader Must Generate Self-Motivation

Leaders who expect their followers to provide them with motivation, to be grateful for the time spent on followers' needs, and to offer frequent and lavish praise are in for a painful awakening. Followers in organizations, work situations, and elected constituencies feel they have earned the right to criticize the leader by being followers. Followers will have an opinion about everything. Sometimes the comments are favorable, and sometimes they are not. The reason that self-motivation is so essential is because the leader can expect very little external motivation. Most leaders are risk takers and self-starters who are enthused by and believe in the vision they have created. Enthusiasm leads to an energized base, which is a hallmark of a vibrant, healthy organization.

The Leader Must Work to Build Self-Confidence

An effective leader must have self-confidence. This confidence comes from an acceptance of self, despite imperfections. Self-confidence is a self-perpetuating virtue. Effective leaders perform an honest self-appraisal on a

regular basis and work to feel good about the job they are doing. A leader who is surrounded by people who enhance the leader's own characteristics makes a formidable leader and strengthens self-confidence in the ability to lead.

The more confident a leader feels, the more likely that success will follow. Success builds self-confidence. Two important factors are related to developing self-confidence. One is avoiding the tendency to become arrogant. The other is maintaining self-confidence despite setbacks.

The Leader Must Listen to His or Her Constituents

Followers always have something to say. Leaders must listen to their constituents and determine whether action is indicated. Active listening, which in the U.S. culture includes looking the person in the eye and offering questioning probes, shows an interest in what a person is saying. However, listening does not obligate the leader to any course of action. Clear boundaries must be communicated. A smart leader listens to all sides and makes decisions based on the vision and direction that is best for the group.

The Leader Must Have a Positive Attitude

Positive attitude is vital to leadership success. No one wants to follow a pessimist anywhere. People expect the leader to have the answers, to know where the organization is going, and to take the initiative to get the group to its goal. A positive attitude can be a great ally in sharing and maintaining the vision. Attitude is a choice, not a foregone conclusion. The effective leader uses positive thinking and positive messages to create an environment in which followers believe in the organization, the leader, and themselves. The problems and challenges in health care demand that nurses seek and fill leadership positions in a positive and future-oriented manner.

EXERCISE 3-5

Using the five rules for leaders, create a personal description of how you maintain balance, generate self-motivation, build self-confidence, listen to constituents, and maintain a positive attitude.

THE NURSE AS LEADER

Nurses in numerous positions and various organizations serve as leaders. Because every nurse has the opportunity to serve as a leader, every nurse can exercise the right to lead.

Leadership Within the Workplace

Nurse Executive as Leader

Leader is a term often used interchangeably with the term nurse executive. Although that statement is true, it is also limiting because many others in any organization can be and are seen as leaders. A primary goal of the nurse executive is leadership within the workplace. The nurse executive has an outstanding opportunity to shape the future of professional practice within a working environment by creating opportunities for direct care nurses and managers to have optimal input into organizational decision making related to the future. The nurse executive thus helps create a shared vision of the preferred future.

The concept of empowerment is important to the role of leadership for the nurse executive in a work organization. Empowerment theory suggests that power must be given away or shared with others in the organization. Direct care nurses may be encouraged to have input into decisions, or they may be given considerable information about how decisions are made. The ability to make or influence changes in the organization is a powerful tool. Nurses must believe that their input and ideas are considered when change occurs. Having input in decisions, having some control over the environment, and receiving feedback about actions taken or not taken all contribute to a feeling of being empowered to have control over one's practice and one's life.

Nurse executives need to be aware of the importance of succession planning (Patrician, Oliver, Miltner, Dawson, & Ladner, 2012). "The critical need for succession planning in nursing leadership has been demonstrated, yet two-thirds of CNOs reported they do not have succession plans in place. Proactive planning is clearly needed to prepare the next generation of nursing leaders" (p. 461). Effective nurse executives have a plan for identification of charge nurses and nurse managers who have great potential for development as nurse leaders.

The importance of managers and executives being leaders rather than managers is a recurring theme in the nursing literature. The fact is that both management and leadership skills in the nurse executive are essential. The ability to balance the day-to-day operating knowledge with the ability to lead a nursing service organization into the future is a winning combination.

Nurse Manager as Leader

Management and leadership, although different constructs, can be a strong combination for success. The nurse in the role of manager ensures that the day-to-day elements of the workplace are done correctly. Just as the effective manager pays attention to employee selection, hiring, orientation, continuing employee development, and financial accountability, in the role of leader, the manager raises the level of expectations and helps employees reach their highest level of potential excellence. A primary role of the leader is to inspire. The nurse manager may be seen as the embodiment of leadership in nursing. That person is the "face of leadership" to those in direct care.

Developing with direct care nurses a shared vision of the preferred future is a goal of the nurse manager in the role of leader. Everyone tends to resist change that is thrust upon them. When nurses are active participants in change from its inception, they are far more likely to be invested in outcomes.

An essential element of success for the nurse manager as a leader is the inclusion of direct care nurses in decision making. This contribution can enhance their organizational commitment and create a sense of pride in successful outcomes. The nurse manager inspires staff by involving them in changing the workplace to make it more satisfying. In so doing, the nurse manager also develops personal leadership skills.

Direct Care Nurse as Leader

Workplace leaders create an environment in which others can experience satisfaction and have ideas for increasing the level of workplace satisfaction for nurses on the team. Leaders are those who creatively pose solutions to problems and capitalize on opportunities in the workplace. Furthermore, they support others, who offer numerous ideas about various issues, including patient safety. Nurses who believe that they have good ideas for future improvements should volunteer for opportunities to lead. These opportunities might include practice councils, clinical unit standards committees, or legislative committees to pose new solutions. They also might include opportunities to be a group spokesperson or team advocate. If the hospital or other workplace has no formalized mechanism for nurse input into organizational decision making, nurses find informal avenues for influence. Those strategies might include asking thought-provoking questions, filing official complaints, creating unit campaigns, or holding informal discussions.

Developing leadership skills for direct care nurses can happen in several ways. Some of these may be employment opportunities (e.g., practice councils), others may be professional opportunities (e.g., a local professional association), and still others may be clinically focused opportunities (e.g., the heart association). Leadership can be developed, and direct care nurse leaders can help establish workplaces that are satisfying and rewarding. Magnet™ facilities, for example, depend on direct care nurse leadership to create the intensity of quality work.

Novice leadership skills that contribute to future leadership success involve learning how to work in groups, deal with difficult people, resolve conflict, reach consensus on an action, and evaluate actions and outcomes objectively (Figure 3-1). These opportunities create skills that can lead to some expertise that could transfer to subsequent practice.

Fagin (2000) describes a 10- to 15-year leadership development plan for neophyte nurses that build on their leadership skills from their beginning nurse-patient experiences. The reality of development toward true leadership expertise takes place over a long period and should not be expected during the first year or two of nursing practice. Nevertheless, every leader started somewhere. Movement toward an increasingly complex leadership experience allows the new nurse to move from leading and planning with an individual to working with groups, such as families or communities. Further leadership development occurs during interactions with larger groups and through instituting changes in research and application of new techniques and moving toward health policy and political activities. With increasing educational achievement and career experience comes increasing complexity of leadership capabilities.

Leadership Within Professional Organizations

In the United States, the best and most important step to take in becoming a leader within the nursing profession is to join a professional organization. Many nurses today take part in several organizations. These associations may be general and broad (e.g., the American Nurses Association), role-based (e.g., the American Organization of Nurse Executives), or clinically focused (e.g., the American Association of Critical-Care Nurses). Volunteering for local or committee memberships is a valued and useful way to learn and to grow within the association.

Many of the professional specialty organizations maintain a national or regional presence rather than having state or local chapters. Some of them have local chapters (e.g., Association of periOperative Registered Nurses), especially in the larger, more populated areas across the country. The major impact of the professional specialty organization is sharing and dissemination of information, discussion of mutual clinical or role concerns, and education regarding the latest innovations in the field. Leadership opportunities are available to present posters or papers at local, regional, or national conferences, as well as to serve on committees and boards.

After becoming established and known in a local association, running for elected office in the local district or chapter association is a way many leaders within professional associations start their leadership careers. It is not unusual to be unsuccessful in the first attempt at running for an elective office in a

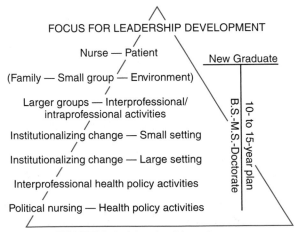

FIGURE 3-1 A leadership trajectory.

professional association, but persistence can do two things: (1) it can help with name recognition, and (2) it can let members know that you are serious about being an association leader.

Leaders, often from local levels, later hold office at the state level. Volunteering for committee assignments and running for elected office in a state level association establish leadership interest within a professional association. Leadership efforts at the national level are usually more successful after establishing a record of successful leadership at the state level.

This pathway of professional involvement and leadership may seem like a linear progression to more global opportunities for leadership in the profession. However, many successful nursing leaders conceptualize the progression as circular rather than linear. Many well-known leaders who have held high offices at the national or state level take their experience and expertise to return to offices and committee appointments at another level.

Leadership in the Community
Nurses as Community Opinion Leaders

Nurses are valued and respected members of their communities. As trusted professionals, nurses have an opportunity to serve as catalysts in leadership opportunities in the community. In partnership with others in the community, nurses can help build a more just, more peaceful, and more healthful society.

Many avenues are available for nurses to serve as community opinion leaders. Attendance at civic gatherings, such as city commission and school board meetings, is an excellent way to be aware of what is happening and to offer input from a nursing perspective. For instance, when the school board begins deliberating whether the budget will accommodate a registered nurse for every school or whether to replace a registered nurse with a trained clerk who can record vaccinations, a nursing voice in the audience could clarify the importance of school nurses to a school population. Writing letters to the editor of a newspaper and participating in public forums give the nurse an avenue to share expertise and mold community opinion.

Nurses as Community Volunteers

Many opportunities exist for volunteer participation in the community. Nurses bring a unique leadership skill set to community activities. The ability to understand complex systems, as well as to understand interpersonal dynamics and communication techniques, constitutes knowledge that is valuable in community volunteer opportunities.

Leadership in mobilizing volunteers for health fairs, screening activities, and educational events is a community need that nurses can and do fill. Such activities promote health and advance the health of the community in important ways. Nurses can also lead efforts to engage others in the community in volunteer activities. In addition, nurses can organize individuals in the community to help develop a vision for the future of the community's health, healthcare opportunities, and healthcare delivery.

From the perspective of the nurse as a community leader, a unique opportunity exists to work with schools, city or county governments, and other community entities to formulate a vision for improving the health of the community through disease prevention and health promotion. The nurse can be a catalyst for a community to recognize present problems and to develop a plan to reach a preferred future.

Leadership Through Appointed and Elected Office

Nurses are valuable leaders in elected and appointed offices at the local, state, and national levels. Because of the trustworthiness of nurses in general, nurses should be able to mobilize resources to raise monies, develop support, and get elected to offices. The numbers of nurses in offices at all three levels of government are continually growing. However, the number is small in relation to the percentage of the population nursing represents. In addition to typical sources of campaign support, various healthcare-related political action committees provide assistance to nurses who want to run for office. Nurses who are elected members of governmental bodies can exert their leadership to shape the vision of the government to help meet the health and societal needs of citizens.

Local government opportunities include school boards, city councils, and community boards dealing with various community initiatives.

At the state level, opportunities include serving in the state legislatures, being appointed to state boards, such as the state board of nursing or the state board of health, or serving on special task forces such as those created by the legislature, a state board, or the governor. At the national level, opportunities include being elected as a U.S. representative (nurses are few, but present), being elected as a U.S. senator (no nurse has served in this capacity), being appointed to a federal commission or board, or serving as an expert for a legislator or legislative body.

CONCLUSION

The nurse is in a trusted role as nurturer and provider of care to the most vulnerable in our society. Nurses who choose leadership roles have many of the needed talents to serve their followers and their profession. Visionary and responsible leadership is vital to the future success of nursing as an art and a science. Professional nursing has been blessed with excellent leaders in the past and will continue to be led by the visionary nurse leaders of tomorrow.

THE SOLUTION

After a couple of weeks, we needed to find a way to bring the committee back together. I sat with the Vice President of Nursing (VPN), in her office, considering what our options were. We couldn't just start meeting again without dealing with the issue that had divided us. We had to acknowledge it and work through it before we could move on to other things.

As we were trying to come up with a strategy to bring people together, I remembered the strategic plan definition problem and suggested that we might be having the same sort of problem. We might be fighting over words without a common definition.

It was kind of a funny thing to consider. The words were things like "skill mix," "patient acuity," "hours per patient day," and "assistive personnel." These are common terms; surely we all knew what the words meant. Even so, we decided to test our assumption and see if we had been using the terms differently from each other. It was risky for both of us. The VPN had to deal with the managers and directors. I had to make it okay for the rest of the nurses.

We brought the committee back together for a meeting in subgroups, making sure that each table had at least one direct care nurse, one manager, one director, and a human resources representative. No one liked the assigned seating, but we were firm that they had to comply with it. Then we gave table assignments to come up with

a common definition for certain terms—the ones we were sure they could define. The groups began their assignments and found that they had trouble completing them. It was hard to develop a common definition of these terms that "everyone knows what they mean." After discussion, some groups were able to come up with a definition all could agree to; other groups could not. We discovered that we had actually been fighting different fights. It had been like parallel conversations. We couldn't come to consensus on practice changes if we were talking about different things, even though we were using the same terms.

Understanding that we had been disagreeing about different things ended the impasse. The practice committee could continue its work. As leaders, we learned that our first job was to make sure everyone understood what was being talked about, that we were all talking the "same language." The practice committee continued meeting for several years. Debates about practice change were robust—sometimes "spirited." But, we always made sure that we were using our words in the same way so that a lack of definition was never the issue.

—Katheren Koehn

Would this be a suitable approach for you? Why?

THE EVIDENCE

Leadership requires effective communication, responsibility, empowerment, job clarity, continuing of care, and interprofessional collaboration. Enhancing any of those strategies promotes more effective leadership.

In recent years, great emphasis has been placed on transformational leadership. It is closely associated with followers' working conditions—namely involvement, influence and meaningfulness. Leaders create the workplace environment.

Nurse managers with effective leadership skills are an essential component to addressing the nursing shortage. The manager is the "face" of formal leadership and influences the local workplace environment. When positive places are present, staff turnover is lower.

The presence of a supportive culture in which learning is valued is a key factor in implementing and sustaining best practice guidelines. Transformational leadership creates the supportive culture.

Emerging workforce members have different views of what they seek in their managers/leaders. They want a leader who is receptive to people, who serves as a team player, who is honest, approachable, knowledgeable, motivating, and competent. That person must also be a good communicator and have a positive attitude and good people skills.

WHAT NEW GRADUATES SAY

- I was surprised that I was expected to lead, even though others were very supportive. At least I didn't have to take on formal management work!
- I was a leader in the student association. I was very surprised how few of the nurses I work with belong to any professional group.
- Leadership sounds important but like a lot of hard work! I am constantly thinking about what to do that is best for my patients and my team.

CHAPTER CHECKLIST

The role of the nurse leader is to share a vision and provide the means for followers to reach it. When the group succeeds, the leader succeeds. Members of different generations have expectations and needs that are different from those of a leader. Various leadership opportunities are available; it is up to the nurse to take advantage and contribute to the progress of the nursing profession.
- What is a leader?
  - Leadership as an important concept for nurses
  - Leadership as a primary determinant of workplace satisfaction
- The practice of leadership
  - Leadership approaches
    - Transactional leadership
    - Transformational leadership
  - Barriers to leadership
    - False assumptions
    - Time constraints
- Leadership development
  - Select a mentor
  - Lead by example
  - Accept responsibility
  - Share the rewards

- Have a clear vision
- Be willing to grow
- Developing leaders in the emerging workforce
  - The emerging workforce: The 1965 to 1995 generation
  - The entrenched workforce: The 1946 to 1965 generation
- Surviving and thriving as a leader
  - The leader must maintain balance
  - The leader must generate self-motivation
  - The leader must work to build self-confidence
  - The leader must listen to his or her constituents
  - The leader must have a positive attitude
- The nurse as leader
  - Leadership within the workplace
    - Nurse executive as leader
    - Nurse manager as leader
    - Direct care nurse as leader
  - Leadership within professional organizations
  - Leadership in the community
    - Nurses as community opinion leaders
    - Nurses as community volunteers
  - Leadership through appointed and elected office

TIPS FOR BECOMING A LEADER

- Take advantage of leadership opportunities, and practice your leadership skills.
- Expect to stumble occasionally, but learn from your mistakes and continue. Every leader has made mistakes. The truly inspired leaders have learned from them and moved forward.
- Get some help—having a caring mentor is the best way to develop leadership ability. The mentor can give you the benefit of experience and will serve as a resource to get feedback on actions and to explore options.
- Take risks. A person does not become a leader by maintaining the status quo. Leaders forge a vision and bring followers forward. However, change involves risks. Do not be foolhardy, but do not be complacent either.

REFERENCES

Bennis, W. (2009). *On becoming a leader*. New York: Basic Books.

Boev, C. (2012). The relationship between nurses' perception of work environment and patient satisfaction in adult critical care. *The Journal of Nursing Scholarship*, 44(4), 368–375.

Bulmer, J. (2013). Leadership aspirations of registered nurses: Who wants to follow us? *Journal of Nursing Administration*, 43(3), 130–134.

Clavelle, J. T., Drenkard, K., Tullai-McGuinness, S., & Fitzpatrick, J. J. (2012). Transformational leadership practices of chief nursing officers in magnet organizations. *Journal of Nursing Administration*, 42(4), 195–201.

Clipper, B. (2013). *The nurse manager's guide to an inter-generational workforce*. Indianapolis: Sigma Theta Tau International Honor Society of Nursing.

Covey, S. M. R. (2012). *Smart trust*. New York, NY: Free Press.

Covey, S. R. (1992). *Principle-centered leadership*. New York: Simon & Schuster.

Drenkard, K. (2013). Transformational leadership; Unleashing the potential. *Journal of Nursing Administration*, 43(2), 57–58.

Fagin, C. (2000). *Essays on nursing leadership*. New York: Springer Publishing.

Gifford, W. A., Davies, B. L., Graham, I. D., Tourangeau, A., Woodend, A. K., & Lefebre, N. (2013). Developing leadership capacity for guideline use: A pilot cluster randomized control trial. *Worldviews on Evidence-Based Nursing*, 10(1), 51–65.

Kouzes, J., & Posner, B. (2012). *The leadership challenge: How to make extraordinary things happen in organizations*. San Francisco: Jossey-Bass.

McBride, A. B. (2011). *The growth and development of nurse leaders*. New York: Springer Publishing Company.

Moneke, N., & Umeh, O. (2013). Factors influencing critical care nurses' perception of their overall job satisfaction. *Journal of Nursing Administration*, 43(4), 201–207.

Murphy, L. (2012). Becoming and remaining an authentic nurse leader. *Journal of Nursing Administration*, 42(11), 507–512.

Oakley, E., & Krug, D. (1994). *Enlightened leadership*. New York: Simon & Schuster.

Patrician, P. A., Oliver, D., Miltner, R. S., Dawson, M., & Ladner, K. A. (2012). Nurturing charge nurses for future leadership roles. *Journal of Nursing Administration*, 42(10), 461–466.

Senge, P. M. (2006). *The fifth discipline: The art and practice of the learning organization*. New York: Doubleday.

Wakeman, C. (2010). *Reality-based leadership*. San Francisco: Jossey-Bass.

SUGGESTED READINGS

Atchison, T. A. (2004). *Followership: A practical guide to aligning leaders and followers*. Chicago: Health Administration Press.

Dierckx de Casterle, B., Willemse, A., Verschueren, M., & Milisen, K. (2008). Impact of clinical leadership development on the clinical leader, nursing team and care-giving process: A case study. *Journal of Nursing Management*, 16(3), 266–274.

Lencioni, P. (2012). *The advantage: Why organizational health trumps everything else in business*. San Francisco, CA: Jossey-Bass.

Raup, G. H. (2008). The impact of ED nurse manager leadership style on staff nurse turnover and patient satisfaction in academic health center hospitals. *Journal of Emergency Nursing*, 34(5), 403–409.

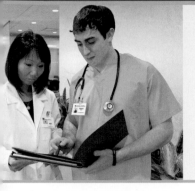

Developing the Role of Manager

Jacqueline Gonzalez

This chapter identifies key concepts related to the role of the nurse manager. It describes basic manager functions, illustrates management principles that are inherent in the role of professional practice, and identifies descriptive competencies for the nurse manager that are integral in creating a positive and healthy work environment. Role development is crucial to forming the right questions to ask in a management or clinical situation that will help the practitioner identify problems and anticipate needs. This chapter provides an overview for the further development of practical skills.

LEARNING OUTCOMES

- Analyze roles and functions of a nurse manager.
- Analyze the relationship of the nurse manager with others.
- Describe the role of the nurse manager in creating a healthy work environment.
- Analyze management of healthcare settings.
- Evaluate management resource allocation/distribution.
- Evaluate behaviors of professionalism of the nurse manager.

KEY TERMS

case management	managed care	quantum theory
change agent	manager	role
follower	organizational culture	role theory
leader	quality indicators	

THE CHALLENGE

Erika Vila, DNP, MSN, RN, NE-BC
Nursing Director, The Heart Program, Miami Children's Hospital

In today's customer service–oriented healthcare system, service excellence has been a challenge for healthcare providers, but it is expected by patients and their families. Coordination of care has been one of the biggest challenges for nurse managers in leading teams within a facility to help in reducing waiting times, improving patient flow processes, and positively increasing the patient's experience. In the pediatric cardiovascular surgery department, one of the biggest challenges faced by the professional and medical team is the total length of time of the preoperative process the day before surgery. The preoperative process consists of a series of diagnostic procedures, such as chest x-ray, EKG, and echocardiogram, and consultations with the cardiologist or anesthesiologist. A meeting with a specialized pediatric surgical APRN (advanced practice registered nurse) focuses on patient and family education, including the preoperative and postoperative processes. The preoperative process was estimated to take about 6 hours, and because most of the patients were infants and toddlers, parents and caregivers often felt a huge sense of frustration and dissatisfaction at the end of the day because their child required NPO status for several of the diagnostic procedures. This dissatisfaction was clearly reflected in this department's overall admission process and negatively affected overall patient satisfaction scores. The nurse manager's new goal is to improve the overall coordination of care across departments and providers to decrease the preoperative process time.

What do you think you would do if you were this nurse?

INTRODUCTION

Chapter 1 provided a general overview of leading and managing. Chapter 4 looks at management from different perspectives. The core of role theory began with management theory, a science that has undergone numerous changes in the past century. In the early 1900s, the theory of scientific management, introduced by Frederick Taylor (Thornton, 2013), was embraced. This theory is based on the idea that one best way exists to accomplish a task. This view equates the production of work with financial reward. Practice in the 1930s through the 1970s was dominated by participative, humanistic management theories. Although changes in healthcare delivery no doubt are affecting the roles of nurse managers, the relevance of role theory remains a constant. Conway's (1978) historic definition, "**role theory** represents a collection of concepts and a variety of hypothetical formulations that predict how actors will perform in a given role, or under what circumstances certain types of behaviors can be expected" (p. 17), is still appropriate. Role theory explains that there are socially desired behavioral norms, and there are three central components that are modeled after certain social behaviors. These include role expectations, the assumption of social roles, and the subsequent enactment of those roles (Newman & Newman, 2012).

Role expectations are the behavioral expectations that are shared or related to each person's role. When a nurse manager enters or enacts his or her new role, behaviors are associated with attaining that role. In this case, the nurse manager has assumed the social role, and the enactment of this role includes the predictable qualities of social behavior of the role, such as demonstrating leadership, managing financial resources, and creating a positive work environment.

The evolutionary process of management theories has affected how managers address workers' concerns and needs. The beginning management theories discounted concern for workers' psychological needs and focused on productivity and efficiency. When theories relating to human relations evolved from the Hawthorne Corporation's studies of working conditions, workers' social needs and motivations became focal points for the nurse manager. Perhaps often used in nursing, Maslow's original (1954) hierarchy of needs reflects on the needs of human beings that must be satisfied at their most basic level (physiologic, safety) before reaching higher levels (love and self-esteem) in order to achieve self-actualization. Conversely, situational theories, such as the Path-Goal theory, focused on the environment, clarifying the relationship between the pathway employees take and the outcome or goal they wish to attain. As seen in the Theory Box, McGregor's (1960) Theory X and Theory Y made two basic opposing assumptions about employees and how the manager should interact with them.

THEORY BOX

Mcgregor's Theory X and Theory Y

MCGREGOR'S THEORY	ASSUMPTIONS	IMPLICATIONS
Theory X	People basically do not like their work and must be coerced to perform.	Lower level basic needs are important, e.g., safety, security.
Theory Y	People are more content when they have self-discipline and autonomy at work.	People aim to satisfy through higher level accomplishments to achieve self-actualization.

McGregor, D. (1960). The human side of enterprise. New York: McGraw-Hill.

What do all of these theories mean to a manager? One might ask in a self-appraisal, just what do I have to do to prepare to synthesize this information and prepare for all of the challenges I may face as a nurse manager? Is being a clinically expert nurse a prerequisite for becoming a nurse manager? What kind of educational preparation and experience do I need to prepare myself for this new role? Have I identified my current and future career goals and mapped out a path to achieve them? What specific knowledge, skills, and personal qualities do I need to develop to be most effective in practice? Which mentors will guide me in this direction? Will my organization that I work for have succession planning, including development opportunities such as tuition reimbursement and advanced educational offerings? Today's fast-paced and changing environment of health care calls for leaders who cannot only lead, manage, and successfully communicate the change but also participate in and drive reform. The opportunities that present themselves for nurse leaders will be plentiful as the Patient Protection and Affordable Care Act (2010) is implemented. Innovative solutions are needed from nurse managers (and staff) during this exciting and somewhat turbulent time of reform. The nurse manager must operate and navigate within healthcare agencies and also within the larger social system, including the community they serve. A nurse manager must recognize the need for growth within, which then translates into improving one's practice and serving as a mentor to others. A prerequisite for self-actualization is a bond between the nurse and the community, because the community includes a nurse manager's patients and staff.

Nurse managers have many roles in leading their unit or department. Stefancyk, Hancock, and Meadows (2013) pose the question as to whether the role of the nurse manager is a change agent or a change coach. Nurse managers have the responsibility of day-to-day decisions for their units, and they must manage change and also lead change initiatives that have positive impact on patient outcomes in the interest of patient quality and safety. In order to lead change the nurse manager must identify and develop skill sets that enable them to facilitate others, provide guidance, and inspire those around them. These tools allow the nurse managers to not only coach their staff and colleagues but also encourage their leaders in leading by example. These collaborative efforts to bring about change require active listening to understand the viewpoints of others and demonstrating integrity by communicating directly and fairly with their teams. The complexity of management is this and much more.

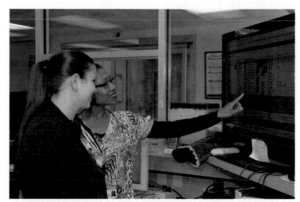

Nurse manager as coach. (From Miami Children's Hospital with permission.)

THE DEFINITION OF MANAGEMENT

Management is a generic function that includes focusing on completing the work that must be done.

Thus almost every nurse has a vested interest in management. Nurses must self-manage and manage others for whom they are accountable, even when their titles do not reflect a formal management role. Drucker (1974), one of the world's most studied authors of management, describes seven foundational concepts of management today:

- Management of personnel, including their salaries and wages, job descriptions, and evaluations
- Decentralization, as much as possible
- Productivity as linked to scientific management
- Manager development to ensure professional growth
- Use of information and data analysis in decision-making
- Marketing of services
- Long-range planning for future needs

Though Drucker (1974) described these concepts as the basis for management, he went on to say that a manager must not only work within these concepts, but also rise to new demands in order to excel. For example, although managers must manage personnel, they must also lead people and view them as resources in accomplishing today's work. Another example of the role of the manager is in understanding and leveraging the work of people as knowledge workers who use concepts, theories, and thoughts rather than merely relying on everyday skills to complete a task.

Drucker (1974) described the five operational roles of the manager as being essential to driving results in work performance.

1. Establishes objectives and goals for each area and communicates them to the persons who are responsible for attaining them
2. Organizes and analyzes the activities, decisions, and relations needed and divides them into manageable tasks
3. Motivates and communicates with the people responsible for various jobs through teamwork
4. Analyzes, appraises, and interprets performance and communicates the meaning of measurement tools and their results to staff and superiors
5. Develops people, including self

The American Organization of Nurse Executives (AONE) (2006) offers a framework with three separate domains for the learning framework of the nurse manager. These domains are reviewed in Figure 4-1 and include:
- The science: Managing the business
- The art: Leading the people
- The leader within: Creating the leader in yourself

The nurse manager is responsible for fostering and managing relationships with those above themselves, their peers, and staff for whom they are accountable; maintaining the highest level of professionalism; and managing resources.

Fennimore and Wolf (2011) describe what is needed for the development of the nurse leader in establishing a culture of high performance and excellent patient outcomes. Managers are described as "chief culture builders" (p. 204) who are able to establish a positive work environment and culture, where staff are able to work at their best in delivering outstanding patient care. Duffield, Roche, Blay, and Stasa (2011) studied 2488 nurses across Australia, and results also confirmed that staff job satisfaction and satisfaction with nursing was integrally related to their perception of their nurse manager. Common behavioral characteristics included high visibility, consultation with staff, recognition, praise, and overall perception of the manager as a good leader.

Managers are able to focus on both the individual and the larger goals of the department and organization. Their aim is to enable people to develop their abilities and strengths to the fullest and to achieve excellence, thus contributing to the department's overall success. The manager must help people develop realistic, attainable goals that provide an avenue of individual growth. Active participation, encouragement, and guidance from the manager and from the organization are needed for the individual's developmental efforts to be fully actualized. Nurse managers who are successful in motivating staff often provide an inclusive environment that facilitates clearly set, achievable goals that can result in both team and personal satisfaction.

The nurse manager must possess qualities similar to those of a good leader: knowledge, integrity, ambition, good judgment, courage, stamina, enthusiasm, communication skills, planning skills, and administrative abilities. The arena of management versus leadership has been addressed by numerous authors, and although points of view differ,

Nurse Manager Leadership Partnership Learning Domain Framework

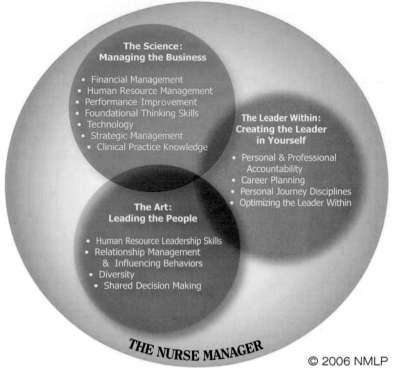

The Science: Managing the Business
- Financial Management
- Human Resource Management
- Performance Improvement
- Foundational Thinking Skills
- Technology
- Strategic Management
- Clinical Practice Knowledge

The Leader Within: Creating the Leader in Yourself
- Personal & Professional Accountability
- Career Planning
- Personal Journey Disciplines
- Optimizing the Leader Within

The Art: Leading the People
- Human Resource Leadership Skills
- Relationship Management & Influencing Behaviors
- Diversity
- Shared Decision Making

THE NURSE MANAGER

© 2006 NMLP

FIGURE 4-1 Nurse Manager Leadership Partnership Learning Domain Framework. (Reprinted with permission from the publisher. NMLP Learning Domain Framework. (2011). American Organization of Nurse Executives. All rights reserved.)

some similarities exist between managers and leaders. Many nurses would concur that these same skills, applied differently, are equally important for followers.

Managers address complex issues by organizing, planning, budgeting, and setting target goals. They meet their goals by organizing, staffing, controlling, and solving problems. By contrast, leaders build a culture of teamwork, set a direction, develop a vision, and communicate that direction to staff; and followers collaborate and communicate to translate that direction into action and share perceptions about facilitators and barriers to achieving the vision. Managers address complexity *and* change, whereas leaders primarily address change. Followers implement patient care change and provide input into organizational change. Successful organizations embrace manager, leader, and follower traits that are relationship based, thus driving change and positive outcomes, and providing and ensuring a healthy and effective work environment. Table 4-1 shows the traits of leaders, managers, and followers.

EXERCISE 4-1

In a small group, discuss the staffing needs of a very busy intensive care unit for a particular night shift. The patient care staffing needs of this unit are very high, and today the unit has extra staff on duty. The last few days have been very busy and the staff have worked very hard. Leaving extra staff on duty today, however, may drive the unit over its budget at a time when hospital resources are scarce. How does the manager handle the conversation with the staff while also contributing to cost-effectiveness? How would you want to hear this conversation? What messages suggest insincerity in addressing concerns for staff?

TABLE 4-1   LEADER, MANAGER, AND FOLLOWER TRAITS

LEADER TRAITS	MANAGER TRAITS	FOLLOWER TRAITS
Values commitments, relationships with others, and esprit de corps in the organization	Emphasizes organizing, coordinating, and controlling resources (e.g., space, supplies, equipment, people)	Perceives the needs of both the leader and other staff
Provides a vision that can be communicated and has a long-term effect on the organization that moves it in new directions	Attends to short-term objectives/goals	Demonstrates cooperative and collaborative behaviors
Communicates the rationale for changing paths; charts new paths that lead to progress	Maximizes results from existing resources	Exerts the power to communicate through various channels
Endorses and thrives on taking risks that bring about change	Interprets established policy, procedures, and mandates	Remains fully accountable for actions while relinquishing some autonomy and conceding certain authority to the leader
Demonstrates a positive feeling in the workplace and relates the importance of workers	Moves cautiously; dislikes uncertainty	Exhibits willingness to both lead and follow peers, as the situation warrants, allowing for competency-based leadership
	Enforces policy mandates, contracts, etc. (acts as a gatekeeper)	Assumes responsibility to understand what risks are acceptable for the organization and what risks are unacceptable

American Association of Critical-Care Nurses. (2005). AACN standards for establishing and sustaining healthy work environments: A Journey to excellence. Retrieved April 20, 2013, from www.aacn.org/WD/HWE/Docs/HWEStandards.pdf.

American Organization of Nurse Executives (AONE). (2004). Principles & elements of a healthful practice/work environment. Retrieved September 23, 2009, from www.aone.org/aone/pdf/PrinciplesandElementsHealthfulWorkPractice.pdf.

AORN position statement. (2009). Key components of a healthy perioperative work environment. Retrieved March 31, 2013, from www.aorn.org/WorkArea/DownloadAsset.aspx?id=21934.

NURSE MANAGER ROLE AND THE INTERGENERATIONAL WORKFORCE

The literature abounds with complexities that the nurse manager faces in the everyday roles they encounter when leading their staff. One of those challenges is managing an intergenerational nurse workforce while continuing to ensure the establishment and maintenance of the positive workplace environment. In one study (Wieck, Dois, & Landrum, 2010) of perceptions of intergenerational nursing staff regarding their nurse manager and their work environment, generational perceptions were compared as to what staff valued as nurse manager characteristics. Study cohorts included Millenials (18 to 26 years old), Generation X (27 to 40 years old) and Baby Boomers (older than 40 years). Commonly, all generations desired a supportive manager who was a communicator and worked well with people. Generation X-ers and Baby Boomers most valued a "supportive manager," whereas Millenials preferred a "dependable manager." Stanley (2010) cites the following implications for nurse leaders in managing different generations: maintaining an open-door policy for employees (especially younger generations who desire to be heard), focusing on each individual, being mindful of including everyone, promoting individual goals/advancement, encouraging work/life balance, providing benefits, recognizing and respecting skills and achievements, promoting opportunities for growth and development, and providing motivational opportunities for all generational groups.

Warshawsky, Havens, and Knafl (2012) describe the importance and influence of strong interpersonal relationships in improving nurse engagement and in more proactive performance in the workplace. The nurse manager's work engagement was most influenced by their interpersonal relationships with nurse administrators. Authentic leadership along with empowerment of new graduate nurses promotes a practice environment of interprofessional collaboration and must be a focus for the nurse manager to build and create a workforce that is engaged and effective (Laschinger & Marie, 2013). Sherman and Pross (2010) discuss the importance of developing nurse managers who can build desirable unit-level work environments. The nurse manager's continued growth and development has a direct correlation to one's continued effectiveness. The younger generation of staff will enjoy working in teams and in taking advantage of developmental opportunities. The nurse manager can create winning situations by engaging these teams in establishing and working toward accomplishing departmental goals and objectives.

The manager is always assessing the context in which a practice and work environment that is positive and healthy can affect people's performance. Paris and Terhaar (2011) describe the stress of the work environment for nurses as having the most

influence on direct care nurse intent to leave and job satisfaction. In this study, empowerment of staff, making practice decisions in their workplace environment, along with communication and teamwork, were key elements for staff retention. The nurse manager has a critical role in ensuring that the environment is balanced, and staff have the tools they need to practice safely and at their best, especially in terms of staffing and workload. Table 4-2 demonstrates the necessary domains of a healthy work environment as defined by professional nursing organizations.

Quantum theory's foundation was based on a rapidly changing dynamic environment; it does not represent one event and at its very foundation is connectedness. Porter-O'Grady and Malloch (2011) identified qualities for nurse leaders such as self-awareness, vision, and empathy that are grounded in the complexity of quantum theory leadership. These authors suggest that a team player knows that the greatest outcome is achieved from the sum of small acts or parts and uses an analytical approach to view problems as opportunities. Flexibility is key for the leader in striving for win-win solutions. Nurse

TABLE 4-2 STANDARDS FOR CREATING AND MAINTAINING HEALTHY WORK ENVIRONMENTS

DOMAINS OF A HEALTHY WORK ENVIRONMENT	AONE (2004)	AACN (2005)	AORN (2009)
Collaboration	A culture that promotes collaboration through trust, diversity, and team orientation	True collaboration: ongoing and multidisciplinary	Collaborative practice culture: all team members are acknowledged and treated respectfully
Communication	A culture with clear, respectful, open, and trusting communication	Skilled communication: communication skills must be equal to clinical skills	Communication-rich culture: communication is clear, respectful, open, and trusting
Decision making	A structure for participation in shared decision making	Effective decision making: nurses must feel valued in policy development and in directing and leading	Shared decision making: nurses participate in decision making and policy development; responsible for their practice
Staffing	Adequate numbers of qualified staff to meet patient expectations and provide balance to the work and home life of staff	Appropriate staffing: effectively meeting patient needs with matched nurse competencies	Presence of adequate numbers of qualified perioperative registered nurses: work and on-call schedules promote positive work-life balance; quality care provided by adequate staffing

Continued

TABLE 4-2	STANDARDS FOR CREATING AND MAINTAINING HEALTHY WORK ENVIRONMENTS—cont'd		
DOMAINS OF A HEALTHY WORK ENVIRONMENT	**AONE (2004)**	**AACN (2005)**	**AORN (2009)**
Recognition	Recognition of contributions of nursing staff and recognition by nurses of the contributions they provide to practice	Meaningful recognition: recognize value that each nurse brings to workplace	Recognition of value of contributions from nursing: recognized by peers and team members for performance; growth options available. Recognition by nurses for meaningful contribution to practice: formal recognition of perioperative practice excellence
Leadership	Presence of a leader who serves as an advocate for nursing, supports empowerment of nurses, and ensures availability of resources	Authentic leadership: authentically embrace healthy work environment and engage team in achieving	Presence of expert, visible, and credible nursing leadership: leadership skills are at every level; nurses are advocates and share decision making; resources support profession
Accountability	A culture in which everyone is accountable and knows what is expected		A culture of accountability: role expectations and definitions are clear
Self-actualization	Ongoing education and professional development		Encouragement of professional practice, growth/development: ongoing education, certification and development encouraged and promoted

leaders today must serve as quantum leaders embracing uncertainty and seeking to understand behaviors and relationships before attempting to change them. Now, when new nurses enter the workforce with enormous technologic demands for their knowledge and skills, it is up to the nurse leader to help foster their growth and their comfort with flexibility and the unknown. Quantum leaders are change catalysts and innovators. They are also transformational, and as such they must be courageous. Developing courage has never been more needed in health care than it is today. Having the courage and ability to own one's opinions and to stand up when it is more popular not to is a hallmark of great leadership and a trait of a quantum leader.

CONSUMING RESEARCH

Nurse managers' responsibilities are twofold: they must participate in research, and they must be an advocate for and interpreter of research. Nursing literature, especially in nursing administration journals, reflects that nurse managers are contributing to research either by conducting unit research or participating in large-scale agency research projects. (See the Research Perspectives on p. 59.) Likewise, nurse managers interpret published research findings that have implications for the staff or the patients. They must make every effort to incorporate the findings into unit activities so that both staff and patients can benefit from evidence-based care. Nurse managers, as first-line managers, are also in an advantageous position of identifying best nursing practices that can be researched through collaborative efforts of service and educational institutions. Nurse managers can also identify research and practice gaps, support direct care nurses in conducting nursing research, and present their own findings of current evidence-based practice in the literature.

RESEARCH PERSPECTIVE

Perspective 1

Resource: Zori, S., Nosek, L.J., & Musil, C.M. (2010). Critical thinking of nurse managers related to staff RN's perceptions of the practice environment. *Journal of Nursing Scholarship, 42*(3), 305-313.

This descriptive study was conducted at a 490-bed nonprofit tertiary care hospital in the northeastern United States. A convenience sample of 12 nurse managers along with a random sample of 132 of their staff members was used to measure critical thinking skills and staff's perception of the practice environment. Attributes such as critical thinking have been shown to enable nurse manager success in the role as they manage their respective departments. The data were measured for nurse manager critical thinking skills using the California Critical Thinking Disposition Inventory (CCTDI) and the perception of the staff RNs was measured using the Practice Environment Scale (PES). Significant differences in the PES subscale were found for the following five overall dimensions of the practice environment:

1. Staffing and adequacy of resources
2. Participation in hospital activities
3. Nurse manager ability and support
4. Foundations for quality of care
5. Nurse-physician collegiality and communication

Staff RN scores were higher when nurse managers demonstrated a positive nature in four critical-thinking domains (systematicity, open-mindedness, analyticity, and confidence in critical thinking).

Systematicity is defined as organized processes that are related to carefully developed solutions. Open-mindedness is about respect and the ability to engage diverse opinions in discussion while being open to all suggestions. Analyticity is being alert to issues and anticipating consequences so that any necessary interventions are effective. Finally, the critical-thinking confidence scale demonstrates reliance in making strong and sound decisions. The results of the study indicate that the nurse manager plays a critical and pivotal role in creating and sustaining a positive practice environment.

Implications for Practice

Nurse managers face many challenges, and in order to manage teams through these challenges, they must possess a strong skill set with critical thinking at the apex. Without critical-thinking skills, success for the nurse manager is unlikely. A positive work environment developed in tandem with the nursing team can create tremendous quality patient outcomes while optimizing direct care nurse retention.

RESEARCH PERSPECTIVE

Perspective 2

Resource: Warshawsky, N.E., Havens, D.S. & Knafl, G. (2012). The influence of interpersonal relationships on nurse manager's work engagement and proactive work behavior. *The Journal of Nursing Administration, 42*(9), 418-425.

This cross-sectional study was conducted via self-administered electronic survey across 44 states. Participants were a convenience sample of 323 nurse managers working primarily in acute care hospitals for more than 3 months; most were members of the American Organization of Nurse Executives. The definition of frontline nurse manager included 24-hour financial, operational, and performance accountability for a patient care area. The influences of interpersonal relationships on proactive behavior at work and work engagement were examined. Several items were measured for nurse manager engagement using the Utrecht Work Engagement Scale, the Proactive Work Behavior Scale, and the Relational Coordination Scale.

The data revealed that nurse managers were highly engaged in their work, implying that they viewed their work as meaningful

and could manage the daily challenges of their job. Importantly, relationships were highest among the nurse managers and their peer group, followed by their relationships with their nurse administrator. Proactive behavior findings included that nurse managers responded in a proactive manner to medical errors when discovered in their unit. Interestingly, the nurse manager's relationship with their nurse administrator was the greatest predictor of work engagement.

Implications for Practice

Collaborative work environments are essential for nurse managers to proactively work in today's complex healthcare environment in a manner that engages them in their duties. Interpersonal relationships can be fostered with organizational designs that encourage a culture of collaboration, reward and recognition, communication, and mentoring. Reward and recognition should be tied to organizational goals and performance, such as preventing medical errors and ensuring patient care quality.

ORGANIZATIONAL CULTURE

In the ever-changing environment of health care, nurse managers need to know the organizational culture at their workplace and how it is integrated with and supports their unit's mission and goals.

Laschinger, Leiter, Day, Gilin-Oore, and Mackinnon (2012) report the results of a quasi-experimental study of 755 registered nurses in 5 hospitals (41 total units). The study's aim was to analyze a workplace intervention (Civility, Respect, and Engagement in the Workplace [CREW]) and its impact on structural empowerment of the nurse, discourteous co-workers and/or supervisors, and trust in nurse management. Units were surveyed 3 months before implementation of an intervention of CREW sessions and after the 6-month intervention. The CREW intervention involves routine work group sessions for employees, usually once or twice a week for 6 months. Employees work with an experienced facilitator to develop unit goals and improve collaboration and communication on the work unit. An example of CREW goals might be unit teambuilding or promoting interactions that are respectful among the unit staff. After the intervention period, the nursing supervisor's interactions with the nurses became significantly more courteous, and finally, trust in management improved.

MENTORING

Most managers were mentored, formally or informally, at one time in their career by someone of influence. In turn, a manager should be concerned about preparing successors. Cathcart and Greenspan (2012) described the importance of nurse manager growth, especially in the development of moral courage and clinical leadership in order to manage complex situations and personnel challenges. Cherry and Jacob (2014) include the role of mentoring as a significant role that nurses in leadership and management positions must embrace. Mentoring is viewed as an interactive, multifaceted role that assists the staff, especially novice staff, with setting realistic, attainable goals. Through mentoring their staff, nurse managers can help boost staff self-confidence, thereby helping them gain professional satisfaction as they reach their goals. Nurse managers give clinical guidance to their staff, and they can be instrumental in assisting them with their present work and their own career development.

DAY-TO-DAY MANAGEMENT CHALLENGES

The nurse manager who meets the day-to-day management challenges must be able to balance three sources of demand: upper management requests, consumer demands, and staff needs. The manager has a pivotal two-way responsibility to (1) ensure that staff members have opportunities for providing input to upper management regarding changes that may affect them,

and (2) make staff and departmental needs known to upper management. Many consumers of health services today are well educated and accustomed to providing input into care decisions that affect them. The nurse manager needs to respect these requests yet maintain care in the broadest context of safety and efficiency. Staff members also may need coaching to achieve recognition and independence when carrying out their roles and responsibilities. The nurse manager must maintain awareness of when to coach and relinquish control, thus allowing decision making at the point closest to the service. Furthermore, the nurse manager is highly influential in creating a practice environment that enhances direct care nurses' satisfaction with the work environment.

Nurse managers also must be authentic clinicians in the areas they manage, and they must "walk the talk". Critically important for being an excellent nurse manager is understanding the correlation between staff satisfaction and engagement and the achievement of optimal patient outcomes, engaging families in the plan of care, and advocating for the allocation of resources and technology in a fair and ethical manner. The nurse manager as clinician is confronted with complex and ambiguous patient-care situations and must use courage to make decisions to meet one important patient care need at the expense of another. Good communication skills are necessary for engaging staff in understanding and conveying this rationale.

EXERCISE 4-2

Select a department within an organization that has the highest employee satisfaction scores. Observe the nurse manager of that department over a certain time (e.g., 2 to 4 hours) as well as during a staff meeting. What is the style he/she exhibits? Is power shared or centralized? Are interactions positive or negative? What does he/she do to engage the staff? How do your observations relate to managerial, leadership, and followership characteristics?

Workplace Violence

Nurse managers have an added responsibility for the safety of both patients and staff. High-risk areas, such as the emergency departments, require special attention. For the nurse manager, "special attention" translates to his or her staff receiving adequate training to prepare for adverse situations that may erupt. Such training may include effective techniques relating to crisis intervention and de-escalation and handling of highly agitated people who may become violent. From the point of hiring through the potential disciplinary process, nurse managers assess both employees and the workplace to help avert violence and the conditions that may lead to it. Top-level administrators are ultimately responsible for employee violence in their organization; however, managers are the first to identify situations that may become out of control. Managers must ensure that their employees receive training and adhere to policies to prevent any increased risk for nonadherence to state and federal employee selection requirements. Refer to Chapter 25 (Workplace Violence and Incivility) for additional information on this topic.

MANAGING WORK COMPLEXITY AND STRESS

Managing the complexity within healthcare settings is always challenging for the nurse manager, including managing diverse personnel (see the Research Perspective below). The nursing shortage has made this challenge even more difficult. The nurse manager is a key person in creating and maintaining a healthy work setting that keeps stress to a minimum so that the staff can achieve optimal work satisfaction. However, before the manager can help the staff, he or she must be able to work in a relatively stress-free environment. Kath, Stichler, and Ehrhart (2012) state that job satisfaction and intention to leave is affected by workplace stress. Autonomy, predictability, and social support are all important in reducing workplace stress. The better the quality of relationships among nurse managers, their supervisors, and peers, the greater the likelihood of increased job satisfaction of the manager. Improved patient outcomes as well as a positive work environment for everyone is also a probable result.

The historic Institute of Medicine (IOM) report, *Keeping Patients Safe* (2004), spoke to the creation of work environments that are more conducive to nurses providing safer patient care. To enable positive work environments, many changes are required of those in leadership and management roles, beginning with top-level administration and filtering through the hierarchy to department managers. If managers see themselves as change coaches or change agents, they can enable a more positive and receptive work environment for their staff. Managers need to address the five management practices that have been found to be effective when instituting

---

 RESEARCH PERSPECTIVE

Resource: Shirey, M. R., McDaniel, A. M., Ebright, P. R., Fisher, M. L., & Doebbeling, B. N. (2010). Understanding nurse manager stress and work complexity: Factors that make a difference. *The Journal of Nursing Administration, 40*(2), 82–91.

This study provided understanding and insight into coping and stress of the nurse manager in their qualitative descriptive study of 21 nurse managers of 3 acute-care hospitals within the United States. Recommendations from study findings that could reduce stress, aid coping, and control work complexity include:

- Conducting a job analysis and ensuring that the job design is reasonable
- Reviewing span of control and establishing guidelines that are realistic and achieve organizational outcomes
- Determining that the Chief Nursing Officers (CNOs) are receptive to the potential for co-management of a unit
- Establishing formal succession planning models
- Reducing stress related to work load by encouraging work-life balance.
- Implementing structures that support positive organizational environment, such as the ANCC Magnet Recognition Program® or the AACN Healthy Work Environment Initiative

- Encouraging health-related outcomes to reduce work-related stress such as sleeping disorders
- Educating at all levels through on-site programs, certification, and career development
- Partnering between nurse leaders and researchers to develop new findings and disseminating them for staff, leaders, and patients

Implications for Practice

The findings of the study clearly demonstrate that the nurse managers need supportive structures to successfully manage their workplace stress. Enhanced or unrealistic performance expectations in the workplace add to the complexity and coping challenges within the health system. Several factors such as experience, a positive organizational environment, and items within the system such as a realistic span of control and a chief nursing officer that is supportive and empowering, make a tremendous impact on the perception of stress, support, and coping by the manager. Nurse managers are extremely valuable resources, not expendable, and nursing needs to reexamine and develop mechanisms that reduce the stress in these essential management leaders.

change and achieving patient safety in high-risk organizations. These practices are as follows:

1. Managing the change process actively
2. Balancing the tension between efficiency and reliability
3. Creating a learning environment
4. Creating and sustaining trust
5. Involving the workers in the work-redesign and the workflow decision making (IOM, 2004)

Keeping Patients Safe (IOM, 2004) also addressed and supported the use of evidence-based management. Evidence-based practice is supported from systematic research findings, and the same should apply to management practices. Evidence-based management should reflect application of empirical research into everyday managing practices. Another historic and impactful IOM report that remains significant for nurse managers is *Crossing the Quality Chasm: A New Health System for the 21st Century* (2001). This report proposes six "improvement" aims for today's lower-performing healthcare system. Those aims are identified in Chapter 2.

Finally, one of the more recent reports of significance to nursing leaders is the Robert Wood Johnson Foundation Initiative on the Future of Nursing at the Institute of Medicine (IOM, 2011). The report recommends that nurses must be ready to assume leadership roles, and new mentoring and leadership development programs must be developed. Professional and personal growth is encouraged and cultivated so that nurses will rise across their profession and be involved in the redesign of healthcare delivery in the United States. Nurse leaders are encouraged to be full partners in developing areas of improvement and new models of care.

High use and rapid development of technology will continue to modify nurse managers' roles. For example, because of the ability to perform more complex surgery through technology such as robotics, nurse managers will find themselves practicing new skills and learning new applications. With the increased expansion of electronic health records, nurse leaders must continue to encourage the use of clinical data information management to assess practice concerns and to advance and standardize care processes. A key to successful management is interdependence, and a critical component is collaboration, which uses the different strengths of each person. Collaboration requires one to be flexible and broad-minded and to have a strong self-concept. When collaboration is used to solve a conflict or to create new directions, the energies of all parties are focused on solving the problem versus defeating the opposing party, and creating the best possible solution rather than one that is just okay.

Staff members often look to nurse managers to lead them in addressing workplace issues with higher levels of administration. To do this, nurse managers must possess two sets of skills: (1) the ability to address power sources in the work environment and to define power-based strategies, such as in organizing a following of other nurse managers with similar concerns; and (2) the ability to place pressure on the power holders so that needed changes can occur. Employees' "buy in" to a change needs to be thoroughly examined and encouraged.

Staff members look to nurse managers to lead them in ethical, value-based management. No greater stage than the one the manager is on influences staff more, because every employee pays tremendous attention to the actions of the manager. The manager's commitment to the mission, vision, and purpose must be demonstrated in everyday behavior, not merely recited on special occasions. This ongoing commitment lends stability in a time of constant change. In other words, although the approach to an issue may change, the core values remain, and the nurse manager is the one who must manage the group in the changed behavior to reflect the mission, vision, and purpose. Without this evidence that is almost palpable, direct care nurses may be skeptical about the manager's commitment to the organization and to them. The staff will eventually lose faith in the ability of the manager to lead if they do not believe in the authenticity of the manager. This contemporary commitment reflects an understanding of the core values and a relationship with the world as it is today. The nurse manager then must translate this commitment to the staff members so that they know they are valued in accomplishing the work of the unit that furthers the mission of the organization. One way of demonstrating that employees are valued is by recognizing staff through various means. Employees who have gone beyond the scope of their job to meet the needs of the patient, department, or institution deserve recognition. An award may reflect the institution's philosophy, beliefs, and mission, as exemplified in one institution's "Quality Credo"—communication, competent performance, personal leadership, respect, and teamwork.

MANAGING RESOURCES

Each of these concepts inherent in managing resources is addressed in depth elsewhere in this book, but the key point is that the manager must manage all of them and integrate each with the others. The practice settings of tomorrow will no doubt continue to include in-hospital care; however, numerous innovative practice models operating from a community-based framework also may be found. As the Patient Protection and Affordable Care Act (PPACA) is implemented, managing resources is likely to be increasingly challenging. Maintaining and improving quality will remain a high priority at a time when new models will need to be tested, and financial incentives and penalties will alter approaches to care.

Nurse managers must create and foster an environment that supports the continual quest to achieve excellent patient outcomes, thus demonstrating the important economic value that nursing brings to health care. Value-based purchasing was designed to align the financial incentives of providers with demonstration of quality outcomes (Keepnews, 2013). These incentives serve as rewards for achieving positive results and alternatively, penalties are incurred for failing to achieve them. The Patient Protection and Affordable Care Act (PPACA) has propelled Medicare to reimburse hospitals not on data reporting alone, but on how well the hospital performs or betters their performance. An example of Medicare's policy for non-reimbursement of hospitals is the non-payment for hospital-acquired conditions (HACs) (Keepnews, 2013). It is important for nurse managers to stay abreast of healthcare policy and reimbursement changes that are driven by the value of nursing care in improving patient outcomes. Nurse leaders must not only be aware of these financial changes but also lead and encourage the nursing staff to ensure the achievement of positive patient outcome.

The manager is responsible for managing all resources designated to the unit of care including all personnel (professionals and others) under the manager's span of control. The astute manager quickly determines that in order for a unit to function economically, the ways that nursing care is delivered may have to be altered. Consistent with the IOM (2011) report on the future of nursing and the evolving implementation of the PPACA, nurse managers, leaders, and followers will need to serve as change agents in numerous situations.

Budget and personnel have always been considered critical resources. However, as technology improves, informatics must be integrated with budget and personnel as a critical resource element. Basing practice on research findings (evidence-based care), networking through the Internet with other nurse managers, sharing concerns and difficulties, and being willing to step outside of traditional roles can assist future managers in making solid decisions about resource utilization and preservation.

MANAGED CARE

Managed care was introduced in the 1980s. The goal of managed care is to provide needed services efficiently and at an appropriate cost. In essence, this goal requires nurse managers to know and incorporate business principles into patient-care practices. Nurse managers who know business principles become conduits for ensuring safe, effective, affordable care. The same can be said for the Never Events identified by the Centers for Medicare & Medicaid Services (CMS) over the years (2008). The term *Never Events* refers to conditions for which healthcare organizations will not be paid. They are conditions that are acquired while the patient is institutionalized. Examples of some of the Never Events include a stage 3 or 4 pressure ulcer acquired during a hospital stay, a bloodstream infection acquired while hospitalized, a fall occurring during a hospital stay that results in an injury requiring a longer stay, or surgery on the wrong body part or side of the body requiring a return trip to surgery.

CASE MANAGEMENT

Case management is a method used for many years to provide care for patients in outpatient service areas. Increasingly, more traditional acute inpatient care is moving to outpatient service areas (refer to Chapter 7). The key to effective case management is proactive coordination of care from the point of admission, with identified time frames for accomplishing appropriate care outcomes. The nurse manager often provides oversight of or collaboration with the case managers, and in some settings, the nurse manager is the immediate supervisor of the case managers. Case management involves components of case selection, multidisciplinary assessment, collective planning, coordination of events, negotiation, and evaluation and documentation of the outcomes of patient status in measures of cost and quality. Case managers are employed in acute care settings, rehabilitation facilities, subacute care facilities, community-based programs, home care, and insurance companies. These managers must possess a broad range of personal, interpersonal, and management skills.

INFORMATICS

Informatics in health care is in a stage of constant change and growth. With the implementation of the Health Information Technology for Economic and Clinical Health (HITECH) Act (2009), the federal government committed substantial resources to encourage widespread adoption of electronic health records (EHRs) by organizations. The goal of the government was to create a seamless flow of information and to transform health care by enabling smart technology such as tablets, smart phones, and Web-enabled devices to improve communication. EHRs are expected to:

- Increase participation in care by patients
- Increase patient convenience and quality
- Enhance coordination of care
- Improve health outcomes and accuracy of diagnoses
- Improve cost savings and practice productivity (Benefits of EHRs, n.d.)

Today technology changes abound and are available to organizations to assist in improving patient care and work efficiency. The EHR gives quick and ready access to current and retrospective clinical patient data. The use of electronic patient classification systems allows managers to better measure the acuity of nursing areas, as well as assist in budget planning and in matching patient needs with the right resources. Smart beds are actual patient beds being used in hospital settings that replace the manual process of documentation of patients' vital statistics, creating real time for nurses to think critically about what to do regarding the data. Smart beds can actually turn the patient with a prescribed frequency as well as document and collect the information for the nurse. In-home monitoring and consultation along with telehealth changes the role of nurses and provides new opportunities for nurse managers to consider services to a population. The accessibility and use of the Internet facilitates the education of staff, patients, and their families. Nurse managers must stay abreast of the changing technology and informatics available in health care and be ready to defend the need for it to make improvements. In addition, managers must be early adapters of the technology to demonstrate its value in performance to staff and to serve as a change agent in managing generational differences. Older generations of nurses (Veterans and many Baby Boomers) were not exposed to informatics systems for most of their careers and may have a difficult time adapting to new technology, whereas the Generation X-ers and Millennials grew up with technology and would not know how to exist without it.

BUDGETS

Budgetary allocations, whether they are related to the number of dollars available to manage a unit or related to full-time equivalent employee formulas, are the direct responsibility of nurse managers. For highly centralized organizations, only the administrative group at the executive level decides on the budgetary allocations. As healthcare organizations adopt "flat" organizational structures and decentralize responsibilities to the patient care areas, nurse managers must understand, determine, and allocate fiscal resources for their designated unit. In the decentralized organizational model, nurse managers must have the business and financial skills to be able to prepare and justify a detailed budget that reflects the short-term and long-term needs of the unit. The ability to present a logical position, reinforced with data, is critical for the nurse manager to be able to successfully operate their department while gaining the respect of and credibility from financial and operational leaders.

Perhaps the most important aspect of a budget is the provision for a mechanism that allows some self-control, such as decision making at the point-of-service (POS), which does not require previous hierarchical approval and a rationale for budgetary spending. Self-scheduling is one way of allowing staff control; however, the nurse manager must set parameters to guide the scheduling staff so that the department remains within the budget.

> **EXERCISE 4-4**
> Visit an ambulatory surgery center. What type of information system is used? How do patients register? With paper (hard copy) and/or computer? What do you assume about the budget, based on the physical appearance of the setting? Does any equipment appear in disrepair? Do the employees (and perhaps volunteers) seem motivated? Ask two or three employees of the center to tell you, in a sentence or two, the purpose (vision and mission) of the organization. Can you readily identify the nurse manager? What principles does the manager use to manage the three critical resources of personnel, finances, and technologic access?

QUALITY INDICATORS

The nurse manager and the staff are consistently concerned with the quality of care that is being delivered on their unit. The quality indicators developed by the American Nurses Association (ANA), such as the National Database of Nursing Quality Indicators (NDNQI) (n.d.), are excellent resources for the nurse manager. The NDNQI measures are specifically concerned with patient safety and aspects of quality of care that may be affected by changes in the delivery of care or staffing resources. The quality indicators address staff mix and nursing hours for acute-care settings, as well as other care components. The NDNQI project is designed to assist healthcare organizations in identifying links between nursing care and patient outcomes. The Joint Commission (2011) expects organizations, as part of meeting accreditation, to adhere to and strive for improvement in certain core measures. Hospitals are compared across the nation in these measurements. Examples of core measures required by The Joint Commission are practices associated with acute myocardial infarctions, care for the patient with congestive heart failure, care associated with the treatment of pneumonia, and patient satisfaction. As with the NDNQI measures, the core measures are concerned with level of quality of care and outcomes of care. Organizations may also benchmark within their system or within groups of other organizations to compare outcomes and practices.

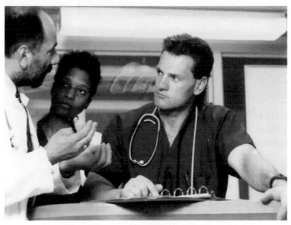

Nurse managers are constantly concerned with the quality of care that is being delivered on their unit.

PROFESSIONALISM

Nurse managers must set examples of professionalism, which include academic preparation, roles and function, and increasing autonomy. The ANA's classic "Nursing's Social Policy Statement" (ANA, 2011) provides significant ideals for all nurses, specifically autonomy, self-regulation, and accountability. Nurses are guided by a humanistic philosophy that includes the highest regard for self-determination, independence, and choice in decision making, whether for staff or for patients. The policy statement can be used by the nurse manager as a framework for a broader understanding of nursing's connection with society and nursing's accountability to those who receive nursing care that facilitates "health and healing" in a caring relationship. For example, a nurse manager's professional philosophy should include the patient's rights. These rights have traditionally identified such basic elements as human dignity, integrity, honesty, confidentiality, privacy, and informed consent.

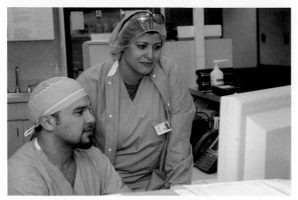

Nurse manager professionalism. (From Miami
Children's Hospital with permission.)

EXERCISE 4-5

Nurse Mary Garrison has been a nurse in the intensive care unit
(ICU) for the last 10 years and she is extremely clinically proficient.
Today she is caring for Mrs. Gonzalez, a young mother of three who
is recovering from injuries sustained in a motor vehicle accident. Mrs.
Gonzalez is worried about being in the hospital so long without seeing
her children and wants to be able to see them, although they are very
young and not typically allowed in the ICU. Mrs. Gonzalez asks the
nurse if they can visit. Nurse Garrison is very busy handling her patient
load and consulting with others who come to her for questions. She
tells Mrs. Gonzalez that it is against the unit's and hospital's rules to
have children in the ICU who are under the age of 12 years and exits
the bedside. Mrs. Gonzalez begins to cry because she knows her family is worried about her and she knows the children have been crying
for her at home. Nurse Gordon gives report to the next 12-hour shift
and reports that Mrs. Gonzalez is trying to go against hospital policy
and that the department needs to be united in adhering to rules. How
would you handle this situation? Was the behavior that Nurse Gordon
exhibited professional or family-centered behavior? What would be
a good solution for Mrs. Gonzalez and her family? How would you
demonstrate professionalism in this example?

Professionalism is all-encompassing and reflects
the manager's professional philosophy as to how he
or she interacts with personnel, other disciplines,
patients, and families. Professional nurses are ethically and legally accountable to the standards of
practice and the accompanying nursing actions
delegated to others. Conveying high standards,
holding others accountable, and shaping the future
of nursing are inherent behaviors in the role of a
manager.

The nurse manager is the closest link with the direct care staff. That individual sets the tone, creates
a positive work environment, and manages within
this context while serving as a professional role model
in the development of future managers and leaders.
Nurse managers must lead by example because they
are highly influential when staff members decide to
stay or leave. Finally, the nurse manager is critical to
the success and quality outcomes of any healthcare
unit or operation.

CONCLUSION

Nurse managers have a responsibility to the patients
they serve by supporting an environment that promotes advocacy for the health and healing of patients within their own emotional and psychosocial
support system. By setting the example of professionalism, the manager leads by influence and models the behaviors that the direct care staff can follow.
The manager must encourage ethical practice and
guide direct care staff in delivering excellent quality care in order to achieve the desired results and
outcomes.

THE SOLUTION

Using the LEAN methodology of process improvement, we started
with a task force focused on improving the preoperative process.
Bringing the frontline staff of coordinators, nurse practitioners, cardiologists, and fellows together in one room, we succeeded in mapping out each step of the preoperative process from patient arrival
to discharge through a value stream map (VSM) showing a time
interval for each step. The map showed a process with 10 different
locations of treatment for our patients across 2 units and potentially
5 areas of infection exposure for our patients. The map highlighted
the inefficiency of our current process. The data collected from

shadowing several patients showed the entire process taking 5 to 6
hours from registration to discharge home. The next steps included
coordinating a working meeting with a representative from each
department influencing the process. The meeting included a nurse
practitioner, a cardiologist, the patient care coordinator, and a supervisor from the registration, laboratory, and radiology departments.
The goal of the process was to become more "patient-centric" and
bring the diagnostics and consultations to the patient, limiting overall travel and process steps. We started by changing the arrival time
of our patients to reduce the delays caused by an influx of patients.

THE SOLUTION—cont'd

This would better meet the needs of our patients and reduce the challenges associated with decreased resources available as the overall volume in the emergency department and hospital increased during the day. Updating our registration process was next, and by using iPads, we were able to move it to the bedside. The phlebotomist, EKG technician, and ECHO technician were then brought to the patient's bedside and scheduled times were allotted for patients to have their chest x-rays done and for the caregivers to consult with the patients so they would prioritize these patients and be available. Since the implementation of the updated process the overall preoperative time has been reduced by almost 50%, six steps and one

unit. Families have commented on the faster process and shorter wait times compared to their previous experience. Patient satisfaction scores have been significantly affected with an achievement of an improved overall score. By using process improvement methods and collaborating with the appropriate caregivers across the organization we have been successful in streamlining care for these fragile patients and their families.

—*Erika Vila*

Would this be a suitable approach for you? Why?

THE EVIDENCE

Scherb, Specht, Loes, and Reed (2011) conducted a descriptive correlational study of 320 RNs from a rural healthcare network located in the Midwest to measure level and the desire of involvement of direct care RNs and nurse managers. The study framework used the ANCC Magnet Recognition Program® and shared governance model. Data collection included demographics, and the Decisional Involvement Scale (DIS) was used to discover the differences between direct care nurse and nurse manager actual and preferred decisional involvement. In studying the differences between the total scores for decisional involvement, the difference was statistically significant between the direct care nurses and nurse managers. The subscales of quality of support staff practices

and unit governance and leadership were also statistically significant. There was a difference between the perceived desired level of direct care nurse involvement between the direct care nurses and the nurse managers. Nurse managers did not perceive that the direct care nurses really needed or wanted more decision making. The dissonance that exists in these findings is a source for potential conflict within a nursing department. The authors suggest that nurse managers must gain comfort in sharing decision making with direct care nurses. As both groups come together and mutual expectations are discussed and fostered, communication and collaboration are enhanced, patient care will likely see positive outcomes from a more structurally empowered workforce.

WHAT NEW GRADUATES SAY

- I want to work in an environment where the manager challenges me to learn, involves me in patient care decisions and seeks to ensure a positive work environment.
- I don't want to work for a manager that I have to worry they are behaving unethically and are not

committed to the organizational mission, vision and purpose.
- I am excited about the value that nurses are able to demonstrate our excellence with new models focused on patient outcomes such as value-based purchasing.

CHAPTER CHECKLIST

The role of the nurse manager is multifaceted, complex, and challenging. Integrating clinical concerns with management functions, synthesizing leadership abilities with management requirements, and addressing human concerns while maintaining efficiency

are the challenges facing a manager. Thus the nurse manager's role is to ensure effective operation of a defined unit of service and to contribute to the overall mission of the organization and quality of care by working through others and being a change agent.

- The definition of management
- Nurse manager role and the intergenerational workforce
- Consuming research
- Organizational culture
- Mentoring
- Day-to-day management challenge
  - Workplace violence
- Managing work complexity and stress
- Managing resources
- Managed care
- Case management
- Informatics
- Budgets
- Quality indicators
- Professionalism

TIPS FOR IMPLEMENTING THE ROLE OF NURSE MANAGER

The role of the nurse manager includes being a leader as well as a follower. The nurse manager must be operationally aware at all times and must collaborate and communicate well within the healthcare team. To implement the role, the nurse manager must profess to the following:

- A management philosophy that values and respects people and incorporates personal and professional integrity
- Commitment to patient-centric safe and quality of care outcomes that are inclusive of customer satisfaction
- The courage to know when to stand and advocate for the patient, staff, or improvements in care
- A desire to grow, innovate, and learn new healthcare trends to serve as a change agent as well as to understand the effects on his or her role and functions

REFERENCES

American Association of Critical-Care Nurses, (2005). *AACN standards for establishing and sustaining healthy work environments: A journey to excellence*. Retrieved April 20, 2013, from, www.aacn.org/WD/HWE/Docs/HWEStandards.pdf.

American Nurses Association NDNQI. (n.d.). *NDNQI Quality improvement solutions from ANA*. Retrieved from, www.nursingquality.org.

American Nurses Association (ANA), (2011). *Nursing's social policy statement (NP-107)*. Washington, DC: American Nurses Publishing.

American Organization of Nurse Executives (AONE), (2004). *Principles & elements of a healthful practice/work environment*. Retrieved September 23, 2009, from, www.aone.org/aone/pdf/PrinciplesandElementsHealthfulWorkPractice.pdf.

American Organization of Nurse Executives, (2006). *Nurse manager learning domain framework*. Retrieved March 30, 2013 from, www.aone.org/resources/leadership%20tools/NMLPframework.shtml.

AORN position statement: Key components of a healthy perioperative work environment. (2009). Retrieved March 31, 2013 from, www.aorn.org/WorkArea/DownloadAsset.aspx?id=21934.

Benefits of electronic health record (EHRs). (n.d.) HealthIT.gov. Retrieved on March 31, 2013 from, www.healthit.gov/providers-professionals/benefits-electronic-health-records-ehrs.

Cathcart, E. B., & Greenspan, M. (2012). A new window into nurse manager development. *Journal of Nursing Administration*, 42(12), 557–561.

Centers for Medicare & Medicaid Services (CMS), (2008). *CMS improves patient safety for Medicare and Medicaid by addressing Never Events*. Retrieved September 23, 2009, from, www.cms.hhs.gov/apps/media/press/factsheet.asp?Counter=3224&intNumPerPage.

Cherry, B., & Jacob, S. R. (2014). *Contemporary nursing, issues, trends and management*. St. Louis: Mosby.

Conway, M. E. (1978). Theoretical approaches to the study of roles. In M. E. Hardy & M. E. Conway (Eds.), *Role theory: Perspectives for health professionals*. New York: Appleton-Century-Crofts.

Drucker, P. F. (1974). *Management tasks, responsibilities and practices*. New York: Harper & Row.

Duffield, C. M., Roche, M. A., Blay, N., & Stasa, H. (2011). Nursing unit managers, staff retention and the work environment. *Journal of Clinical Nursing*, 20, 23–33.

Fennimore, L., & Wolf, G. (2011). Nurse manager leadership development. *Journal of Nursing Administration*, 51(5), 204–210.

Health Information Technology for Economic and Clinical Health (HITECH) Act. (2009). Retrieved from www.hhs.gov/ocr/privacy/hipaa/administrative/enforcementrule/hitechenforcementifr.html.

Institute of Medicine (IOM), *Crossing the quality chasm: A new health system for the 21st century*. (2001). Washington, DC: The National Academy Press.

Institute of Medicine (IOM), *Keeping patients safe: Transforming the work environment of nurses*. (2004). Washington, DC: The National Academy Press.

Institute of Medicine (IOM), *Robert Wood Johnson Foundation's: The future of nursing: Leading change, advancing health*. (2011). Washington, D.C.: The National Academy Press.

Kath, L. M., Stichler, J. F., & Ehrhart, M. G. (2012). Moderators of the negative outcomes of nurse manager stress. *Journal of Nursing Administration*, 42(4), 215–221.

Keepnews, D. M. (2013). *Mapping the economic value of nursing.* Washington State Nurses Association, 1–14.

Laschinger, H., Leiter, M. P., Day, A., Gilin-Oore, D., & Mackinnon, S. (2012). Building empowering work environments that foster civility and organizational trust: Testing an intervention. *Nursing Research*, 61(5), 316–325.

Laschinger, H., & Marie, L. (2013). The influence of authentic leadership and empowerment on new-graduate nurses' perceptions of interprofessional collaboration. *Journal of Nursing Administration*, 43(1), 24–29.

Maslow, A. (1954). *Motivation and personality.* New York: Harper.

McGregor, D. (1960). *The human side of enterprise.* New York: McGraw-Hill.

Newman, B. M., & Newman, P. R. (2012). *Development through life: A psychosocial approach.* Belmont, CA: Cengage Learning, pp. 48-50.

Paris, L. G., & Terhaar, M. (2011). *Using Maslow's pyramid and the national database of nursing quality indicators™ to attain a healthier work environment. The Online Journal of Issues in Nursing*, 16(1). retrieved online from, www.nursingworld.org/MainMenuCategories/ANAMarketplace/ANAPeriodicals/OJIN/TableofContents/Vol-16-2011/No1-Jan-2011/Articles-Previous-Topics/Maslow-and-NDNQI-to-Assess-and-Improve-Work-Environment.html.

Patient Protection and Affordable Care Act, *Public laws 111-148&111-152*. (2010, January 5). Retrieved March 25, 2013 from, www.ncsl.org/documents/health/ppaca-consolidated.pdf.

Porter-O'Grady, T., & Malloch, K. (2011). *Quantum leadership: Advancing innovation, transforming health care* (3rd ed). Sudbury, MA: Jones & Bartlett Learning LLC.

Scherb, C. A., Specht, J. K., Loes, J. L., & Reed, D. (2011). Decisional involvement: Staff nurse and nurse manager perceptions. *Western Journal of Nursing Research*, 33(2), 161–179.

Sherman, R., & Pross, E. (2010). *Growing future nurse leaders to build and sustain healthy work environments at the unit level. Online Journal of Issues in Nursing*, 15(1). Retrieved from, http://gm6.nursingworld.org/MainMenuCategories/ANAMarketplace/ANAPeriodicals/OJIN/TableofContents/Vol152010/No1Jan2010/Growing-Nurse-Leaders.aspx#Sherman.

Shirey, M. R., McDaniel, A. M., Ebright, P. R., Fisher, M. L., & Doebbeling, B. N. (2010). Understanding nurse manager stress and work complexity: Factors that make a difference. *The Journal of Nursing Administration*, 40(2), 82–91.

Stanley, D. (2010). Multigenerational workforce issues and their implication for leadership in nursing. *Journal of Nursing Management*, 18(7), 846–852.

Stefancyk, A., Hancock, B., & Meadows, M. T. (2013). The nurse manager: Change agent, change coach? *Nursing Administration Quarterly*, 37(1), 13–17.

The Joint Commission (TJC), *A comprehensive review of development and testing for national implementation of hospital core measures.* (2011). Retrieved September 23, 2009, from, www.jointcommission.org.

Thornton, P. B. (2013). *Management principles and practice* (5th ed.). Livermore CA: WingSpan Press, pp 4–5.

Warshawsky, N. E., Havens, D. S., & Knafl, G. (2012). The influence of interpersonal relationships on nurse manager's work engagement and proactive work behavior. *The Journal of Nursing Administration*, 42(9), 418–425.

Wieck, L., Dois, J., & Landrum, P. (2010). Retention priorities for the intergenerational nurse workforce. *Nursing Forum*, 45(1), 7–17.

Zori, S., Nosek, L. J., & Musil, C. M. (2010). Critical thinking of nurse managers related to staff RN's perceptions of the practice environment. *Journal of Nursing Scholarship*, 42(3), 305–313.

SUGGESTED READINGS

Codier, E., Kamikawa, C., & Kooker, M. B. (2011). The impact of emotional intelligence development on nurse managers. *Nursing Administration Quarterly*, 35(3), 270–276.

Effken, J. A., Brewer, B. B., Logue, M. D., Gephart, S., & Verran, J. A. (2011). Using cognitive work analysis to fit decision support tools to nurse managers' work flow. *International Journal of Medical Informatics*, 80(10), 698–707.

Robinson, L. D., Paull, D. E., Mazzia, L. M., Falzetta, L., Hay, J., Neily, J., et al. (2010). The role of the operating room nurse manager in the successful implementation of preoperative briefings and postoperative debriefings in the VHA medical team training program. *Journal of Perianesthesia Nursing*, 25(5), 302–306.

Yee, T., Pearson, M., & Parkerton, P. (2011). Nurse manager perceptions of the impact of process improvements by nurses. *Journal of Nursing Care Quality*, 26(3), 226–235.

Legal and Ethical Issues

Ginny Wacker Guido

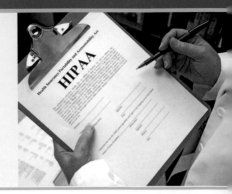

This chapter highlights and explains key legal and ethical issues, especially as they pertain to managing and leading. Nurse practice acts, negligence and malpractice, informed consent, types of liability, selected federal and state employment laws, ethical principles, and related concepts are discussed. This chapter provides specific guidelines for preventing legal liability and guides the reader in applying ethical decision-making models in everyday clinical practice settings.

LEARNING OUTCOMES

- Examine nurse practice acts, including the legal difference between licensed registered nurses and licensed practical (vocational) nurses.
- Apply various legal principles, including negligence and malpractice, privacy, confidentiality, reporting statutes, and doctrines that minimize one's liability, when acting in leading and managing roles in clinical practice settings.
- Evaluate informed-consent issues, including patients' rights in research and health literacy, from a nurse manager's perspective.
- Analyze key aspects of employment law and give examples of how these laws benefit professional nursing practice.
- Analyze ethical principles, including autonomy, beneficence, nonmaleficence, veracity, justice, paternalism, fidelity, and respect for others.
- Apply the *Code of Ethics for Nurses* and the MORAL model from the nurse manager's perspective.
- Discuss moral distress and its implications for nurse managers.
- Analyze the role of institutional ethics committees.
- Analyze decision making when legal and ethical situations overlap, using the Theresa M. Schiavo case as the framework for this analysis.

KEY TERMS

apparent agency	corporate liability	fidelity
autonomy	emancipated minor	foreseeability
beneficence	ethics	Health Care and Education
collective bargaining	ethics committee	Reconciliation Act
confidentiality	failure to warn	health literacy

indemnification	moral distress	respect for others
independent contractor	negligence	respondeat superior
informed consent	nonmaleficence	standard of care
justice	nurse practice act	statute
law	paternalism	veracity
liability	Patient Protection and Affordable	vicarious liability
liable	Care Act	whistle blowing
licensure	personal liability	
malpractice	privacy	

THE CHALLENGE

Acacia Syring, BSN, RN
Staff Nurse Emergency Center, PeaceHealth Southwest
Washington Medical Center, Vancouver, Washington

In my role as a staff nurse in a busy Level 1 trauma emergency center, staff members were often confronted with questions about family presence during lifesaving techniques. Should the family or other loved ones be allowed to be present during cardiopulmonary resuscitation? Did the presence of family members hinder the ability of staff members to provide appropriate and competent care? Did their presence in some way benefit the patient? Was there a legal right for family members to be present at this time?

Currently the issue of family presence is being addressed on a case-by-case basis. The primary healthcare professional has the final say in

whether family can be present, given the option of being present, or the family is tactfully escorted to a another area of the unit. I continued to be ambivalent, especially when an 18-month-old girl was transported to the emergency center after falling from the family boat into a lake. Cardiopulmonary resuscitation was being given as the child was admitted; her mother was with her and her father was coming with other family members. The mother was escorted to the waiting area, crying, "I want to be with my baby!"

What do you think you would do if you were this nurse?

INTRODUCTION

The role of professional nursing continues to expand and incorporate increasingly higher levels of expertise, specialization, autonomy, and accountability from both legal and ethical perspectives. This evolving role has focused new concerns for nurses, nurse managers, and nurse leaders and a heightened awareness of the interaction of legal and ethical principles. Areas of concern include professional nursing practice, legal issues, ethical principles, labor-management interactions, and employment. Each of these areas is individually addressed in this chapter. Although this chapter emphasizes the perspective of the nurse manager, all nurses benefit from understanding the legal and ethical aspects of managing, if only to understand the guidelines their managers are following.

PROFESSIONAL NURSING PRACTICE

Nurse Practice Acts

The scope of nursing practice, those actions and duties that are allowable by the profession, is defined and guided individually by each state in the nurse practice act. The state nurse practice act is the single most important piece of legislation for nursing because it affects all facets of nursing practice. Furthermore, the act is the law within the state or a U.S. territory, and state boards of nursing cannot grant exceptions, waive the act's provisions, or expand practice outside the act's specific provisions.

Nurse practice acts define three categories of nurses: licensed practical or vocational nurses (LPNs and LVNs, respectively), licensed registered nurses (RNs), and advanced practice nurses. The nurse practice acts set educational and examination requirements, provide for licensing by individuals who have met these requirements, and define the functions of each category of nurse, both in general and in more specific terminology. The nurse practice act must be read to ascertain what actions are allowable for the three categories of nurses. In the few states where separate acts for RNs and LPNs/LVNs exist, the acts must be reviewed at the same time to ensure that all allowable actions are included in one of the two acts and that no overlap exists between the acts. In addition, nurse managers should understand that individual state nurse practice acts are not consistent in defining or delineating nursing practice, especially for advanced nursing roles.

Each practice act also establishes a state board of nursing. The main purposes of state boards of nursing are to ensure enforcement of the act and to protect the public. The board enforces the act by regulating those practitioners who come under its provisions and preventing individuals not addressed within the act from practicing nursing. To protect the public, all those who present themselves as nurses must be licensed to practice within the state. The National Council of State Boards of Nursing (NCSBN) serves as a central clearinghouse, further ensuring that individual state actions against a nurse's license are recorded and enforced in all states in which the individual nurse holds licensure.

These various boards of nursing develop and implement rules and regulations regarding the discipline of nursing and must be read in conjunction with the nurse practice act. Often any changes within the state's definition of nursing practice occur through modifications in the rules and regulations rather than in the act itself. This mandates that nurses and their nurse managers periodically review both the state act and the board of nursing rules and regulations.

Because each state has its own nurse practice act and state courts have jurisdiction for the state, nurses are well advised to know and understand the provisions of the state's nurse practice act. This is especially true in the areas of diagnosis and treatment; states vary greatly on whether nurses can diagnose and treat or merely assess and evaluate. Thus an acceptable action in one state may be the practice of medicine in a bordering state.

With the advent of the nurse license compact (NLC), informally known as multistate licensure, the need to know and understand provisions of state nurse practice acts has become even more critical. Multistate licensure permits an RN to be licensed in one state

and to legally practice in states belonging to the NLC without obtaining additional state licenses. For the purposes of the law, the state nurse practice act that regulates the practice of the RN is the state in which the patient or client resides, not the state in which the nurse holds his or her license. Many of the nurses practicing under multistate licensure work with patients in a variety of states through telenursing, using telecommunications technology, such as telephone triage and advice. Others work for agencies or clinics that serve patients across state borders.

All nurses must know applicable state law and use the nurse practice act for guidance and appropriate action. Nurse managers have this same basic responsibility to apply legal principles in their practice. However, they are also responsible for monitoring the practice of employees under their supervision and for ensuring that personnel maintain current and valid licensure. Unless nurses and nurse managers remain current with the nurse practice act in their state or with nurse practice acts in all states in which nurse managers supervise employees, a constant potential for liability exists.

EXERCISE 5-1

Review your state's nurse practice act, including rules and regulations that the state board of nursing has promulgated for the profession. You may need to read two acts if RNs and LPNs/LVNs come under different licensing boards. How does your state address advanced practice? How do the definitions of nursing vary for RNs, LPNs/LVNs, and advanced practice nurses? Describe why it is vital that the nurse manager understands these distinctions.

Negligence and Malpractice

Nurse managers frequently serve as mentors and consultants for the nurses whom they supervise. Nurse managers must have a full appreciation for this area of the law because negligence and malpractice continue to be the major causes of action brought against nursing staff members. Managers cannot guide and counsel their employees unless the managers are fully knowledgeable about this area of the law.

Negligence denotes conduct that is lacking in care and typically concerns nonprofessionals. Many experts equate negligence with carelessness, a deviation from the care that a reasonable person would deliver. Malpractice, sometimes referred to as *professional negligence,* concerns professional actions and is the failure of a person with professional education and skills to act in a reasonable and prudent manner. Issues of malpractice have become increasingly important to the nurse as the authority, accountability, and autonomy of nurses have increased. The same types of actions may be the basis for either negligence or malpractice, though some actions almost always are seen as malpractice because only the professional person would be performing the action. Specific examples include drawing blood for arterial blood gas analysis via a direct arterial puncture or initiating blood transfusions. Common causes of malpractice or negligence among nurses include the failure to follow standards of care, communicate appropriately, access and monitor patients, and act as a patient advocate (Painter et al., 2011).

Negligence and malpractice have two commonalities. Negligence and malpractice both concern actions that are a result of omission (the failure to do something that the reasonable, prudent person or nurse would have done) or commission (acting in a way that causes injury to the patient). They also concern nonintentional actions; though there is some injury to a patient, the individual who caused the harm never intended to hurt the patient.

Six elements must be presented in a successful malpractice suit. All of these factors must be shown before the court will find liability against the nurse and/or institution. These six elements are described in Table 5-1.

Elements of Malpractice
Duty Owed the Patient
The first element is duty owed the patient, which involves both the existence of the duty and the nature

TABLE 5-1 ELEMENTS OF MALPRACTICE

ELEMENTS	EXAMPLES
Duty owed the patient	Failure to monitor a patient's response to treatment
Breach of the duty owed	Failure to communicate change in patient status to the primary healthcare provider
Foreseeability	Failure to ensure minimum standards are met
Causation	Failure to provide adequate patient education
Injury	Fractured hip and head concussion after a patient fall
Damages	Additional hospitalization time; future medical and nursing care needs and costs

of the duty. Existence of the duty of care is generally established by showing the valid employment of the nurse within the institution. The more difficult part is the nature of the duty, which involves the standard of care that represents the minimum requirements for acceptable practice or the minimum requirements for how one conducts oneself. Standards of care are established by reviewing the institution's policy and procedure manual, the individual's job description, and the practitioner's education and skills, as well as pertinent standards established by professional organizations, journal articles, and standing orders and protocols.

Several sources may be used to determine the applicable standard of care. The American Nurses Association (ANA), as well as a cadre of specialty nursing organizations, publishes standards for nursing practice. Accreditation standards, such as those published yearly by The Joint Commission (TJC), also assist in establishing the acceptable standard of care for healthcare facilities. In addition, many states have healthcare standards that affect individual institutions and their employees.

Nurse managers are directly responsible for ensuring that standards of care, as written in the hospital policy and procedure manuals, are current and that all nursing staff follow these standards of care. Should a standard of care be revised or changed, nurse managers must ensure that all staff members who are expected to implement this altered standard are apprised of the revised standard. If the new standard entails new skills, staff members must be educated about this revision and acquire the necessary skills before they implement the new standard. For example, if the institution alters a policy regarding a specific skill to be implemented, the nurse manager must first ensure that all nurses who will be performing this skill understand how to perform the skill safely, know what possible complications that could occur, and know the most appropriate interventions to take should those complications occur. The nurse manager may work with others, such as clinical nurse educators, in attaining the desired outcomes.

Breach of the Duty of Care Owed the Patient
The second element required in a malpractice case is breach of the duty of care owed the patient. Once the standard of care is established, the breach or falling below the standard of care is relatively easy to

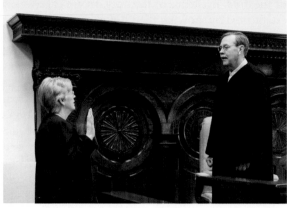

Nurses sometimes serve as expert witnesses whose testimony helps the judge and jury understand the applicable standards of nursing care.

show. To determine the appropriate standard of care to apply, expert witnesses give testimony in court on a case-by-case basis, assisting the judge and jury in understanding nursing standards of care. In nursing malpractice suits, nurses serve as the expert witnesses whose testimony helps the judge and jury understand the applicable standards of nursing care.

Opinions of experts attesting to the standard of care may differ depending on whether the injured party is trying to establish the standard of care or whether the defendant nurse's attorney is establishing an acceptable standard of care for the given circumstances. The injured party will attempt to show that the acceptable standard of care is at a much higher level than that shown by the defendant hospital and staff. An example appears in Case Example Box 5-1.

Foreseeability

The third element needed for a successful malpractice case, foreseeability, involves the concept that certain events may reasonably be expected to cause specific results. The nurse must have prior knowledge or information that failure to meet a standard of care may result in harm. The challenge is to show what was foreseeable given the facts of the case at the time of the occurrence, not when the case finally comes to court. Some of the more common areas concerning foreseeability concern medication errors, patient falls, and failure to enact physician orders. For example, in *Massey v. Mercy Medical Center* (2009), a resident known to be

at high risk for falls was left unattended standing next to his walker. When he attempted to move forward, he lost his balance and sustained a compression fracture at the level of the twelfth thoracic vertebra.

Causation

The fourth element of a malpractice suit is causation: the nurse's actions or lack of actions directly caused the patient's harm. There must be a direct relationship between the failure to meet the standard of care and the patient's injury. It is not sufficient that the standard of care has been breached, but rather that the breach of the standard of care must be the direct cause-and-effect factor for the injury. For example, *O'Shea v. State of New York* (2007) concerned a patient who sustained an accident in which two fingers were severed while using a power saw. The patient permanently lost the two fingers when the nursing staff failed to follow the order for an immediate orthopedist consultation.

Injury

The resultant injury, the fifth malpractice element, must be physical, not merely psychological or transient. In other words, some physical harm must be incurred by the patient before malpractice will be found against the healthcare provider. Although some specific exceptions exist to the requirement that a physical injury must result, they are extremely limited and usually involve specific relationships, such as the parent-child relationship. Pain and suffering are allowed when they accompany actual physical injuries.

Damages

The injured party must be able to prove damages, the sixth element of malpractice. Damages are vital because malpractice is nonintentional. Thus the patient must show financial harm before the courts will allow a finding of liability against the defendant nurse and/or hospital. Acceptable damages may be for immediate as well as future medical costs.

A nurse manager must know the applicable standards of care and ensure that all employees of the institution meet or exceed them. The standards must be reviewed periodically to ensure that the staff members remain current and attuned to advances in technology and newer ways of performing skills. If standards of care appear outdated or absent, the appropriate committee within the institution should be notified so that timely revisions can be made. Finally, the nurse manager must ensure that all employees meet the standards of care. This may be done by (1) performing or reviewing all performance evaluations for evidence that standards of care are met, (2) reviewing randomly selected patient charts for standards of care documentation, and (3) inquiring of employees what constitutes standards of care and appropriate references for standards of care within the institution.

> **EXERCISE 5-2**
> You are the nurse manager for a skilled nursing facility that will now accept patients requiring long-term ventilator support. How should you begin to ensure that all the staff in the facility are educated in the care of ventilator-dependent patients, know what complications to anticipate, and know how to respond should these complications arise? Should all staff members be educated in this skill?

LIABILITY: PERSONAL, VICARIOUS, AND CORPORATE

Personal liability defines each person's responsibility and accountability for individual actions or omissions. Even if others can be shown to be liable for a patient injury, each individual retains personal accountability for his or her actions. The law, though, sometimes allows other parties to be liable for certain causes of negligence. Known as vicarious liability, or *substituted liability,* the doctrine of respondeat superior (let the master answer) makes employers accountable for the negligence of their employees. The rationale underlying the doctrine is that the employee would not have been in a position to have caused the wrongdoing unless hired by the employer, and the injured party would be allowed to suffer a double wrong if the employee was unable to pay damages for the wrongdoings. Nurse managers can best prevent these issues by ensuring that the staff they supervise know and follow hospital policies and procedures and continually deliver safe, competent nursing care or raise issues about policies and procedures through formal channels.

Nurses often believe that the doctrine of vicarious liability shields them from personal liability; the institution may be sued but not the individual nurse or nurses. However, patients injured because of substandard care have the right to sue both the institution and the nurse. This includes potentially suing the direct care nurse's manager if he or she knowingly allowed substandard and unsafe care to be given to a patient. In addition, the institution has the right under indemnification to countersue the nurse for damages paid to an injured patient. The principle of indemnification is applicable when the employer is held liable based solely on the actions of the staff member's negligence and the employer pays monetary damages because of the employee's negligent actions.

Corporate liability is a newer trend in the law and essentially holds that the institution has the responsibility and accountability for maintaining an environment that ensures quality healthcare delivery for consumers. Corporate liability issues include negligent hiring and firing issues, failure to maintain safety in the physical environment, and lack of a qualified, competent, and adequate staff. In *Wellstar Health System, Inc. v. Green* (2002), a hospital was held liable to an injured patient for the negligent credentialing of a nurse practitioner.

Nurse managers play a key role in assisting the institution to avoid corporate liability. For example, nurse managers ensure that staff members remain competent and qualified, that personnel within their supervision have current licensure, and that incompetent, illegal, or unethical practices are reported to the proper persons or agencies. Nurse managers also play a pivotal role in whether a nurse remains employed on the unit or is discharged or reassigned.

Perhaps the key to avoiding corporate liability is ensuring that all members of the healthcare team fully collaborate and work with other disciplines to ensure quality, competent health care, regardless of the care setting. Such collaboration is a competency that must be mastered across disciplines.

CAUSES OF MALPRACTICE FOR NURSE MANAGERS

Nurse managers are charged with maintaining a standard of safe and competent nursing care within the institution. Several potential sources of liability for malpractice among nurse managers may be identified; thus guidelines to prevent or avoid these pitfalls should be developed.

Assignment, Delegation, and Supervision

The field of nursing management involves supervision of various personnel who directly provide nursing care to patients. *Supervision* is defined as the active process of directing, guiding, and influencing the outcome of an individual's performance of an activity. The nurse manager retains personal liability for the reasonable exercise of assignment, delegation, and supervision activities. The failure to assign, delegate, and supervise within acceptable standards of professional nursing practice may constitute malpractice. In addition, in a newer trend in the law, failure to delegate and supervise within acceptable standards may extend to direct corporate liability for the institution.

Delegation, used throughout all of nursing history, has evolved into a complex, work-enhancing strategy that has the potential for varying levels of legal liability. Before the early 1970s, nurses used delegation to direct the multiple tasks performed by the various levels of staff members in a team-nursing model. Subsequently, the concept of primary nursing and assignment became the desirable nursing model in acute care settings, with the focus on an all-professional staff, requiring little delegation but considerable assignment of duties. By the mid-1990s, a nursing shortage had again shifted the nursing model to a multilevel staff, with the return of the need for delegation.

Nurse managers need to know certain definitions regarding this area of the law. *Delegation* involves at least two people, a delegator and a delegatee, with the transfer of authority to perform some type of task or work. A working definition could be that delegation is the transfer of responsibility for the performance of an activity from one individual to another, with the delegator retaining accountability for the outcome. In other words, delegation involves the transfer of responsibility for the performance of tasks and skills without the transfer of accountability for the ultimate outcome. Examples include an RN who delegates patients' personal care tasks to certified nursing aides who work in a long-term care setting. In delegating these tasks, the RN retains the ultimate accountability and responsibility for ensuring that the delegated tasks are completed in a safe and competent manner.

Typically, delegation involves the tasks and procedures that are given to unlicensed assistive personnel, such as certified nursing aides, orderlies, assistants, attendants, and technicians. However, delegation can also occur with licensed to licensed staff members. For example, if one RN has the accountability for an outcome and asks another RN to perform a specific component of the overall function, that is delegation. This is typically the type of delegation that occurs between professional staff members when one member leaves the unit/work area for a meal break.

Delegation is complex because it involves the delegation relationship and communication. It also involves trusting others, because both the delegator and the delegatee have shared accountability for certain tasks and duties. Interventions are needed to improve this relationship and communication effectiveness, which directly affects the quality of competent care delivery. Multiple players, usually with varying degrees of education and experience and different scopes of practice, are involved in the process. Understanding these variances and communicating effectively to the delegatee involve an understanding of competencies and the ability to communicate with all levels of staff personnel.

Assignment is the transfer of both the accountability and the responsibility from one person to another. This is typically what happens between professional staff members. The nurse manager assigns patient care responsibilities to other professional nurses working in the same unit of the institution or community healthcare setting. The level of accountability for the nurse manager who assigns as opposed to delegates is fairly obvious, although some accountability can occur in both instances. The degree of knowledge concerning the skills and competencies of those one supervises is of paramount importance. The doctrine of respondeat superior has been extended to include "knew or should have known" as a legal standard in both assigning and delegating tasks to individuals whom one supervises. If it can be shown that the nurse manager assigned/delegated tasks appropriately and had no reason to believe that the nurse to whom tasks were assigned/delegated was not competent to perform the task, the nurse manager potentially has no or minimal personal liability. The converse is also true; if it can be shown that the nurse manager was aware of incompetence in a given employee or that the assigned/delegated task was outside the employee's capabilities, the nurse manager becomes substantially liable for the subsequent injury to a patient.

Nurse managers have a duty to ensure that the staff members under their supervision are practicing in a safe and competent manner. The nurse manager must be aware of the staff members' knowledge, skills, and competencies and should know whether they are maintaining their competencies. Knowingly allowing a staff member to function below the acceptable standard of care subjects both the nurse manager and the institution to potential liability. This point is illustrated in Case Example Box 5-2.

As this case illustrates, delegation is both process and a condition (Potter, Deshields, & Kuhrik, 2010). It is a process of delegating appropriate tasks and activities to others, and it is a condition because there

---

EXERCISE 5-3

You are the nurse manager on a busy surgical postoperative 38-bed unit. A newly postoperative patient, Mrs. R., requires assistance with feeding, and you note that an unlicensed assistive personnel has been delegated to feed her. Reading Mrs. R.'s care plan, you also note that she is elderly, has had periods of confusion, and has had difficulty swallowing since her surgery. Determine if this is the right circumstances for such delegation. What are your next actions and why?

CASE EXAMPLE BOX 5-2

In *Estate of Travaglini v. Ingalls Health* (2009), an 84-year-old patient was admitted to the hospital with general complaints of "not feeling well." At the time of his admission, the physician told the admitting nurse that the patient had dysphagia and must be observed whenever he was eating or trying to swallow liquids. At 10:00 that evening, an aide came to the patient's room and left a sandwich for him to eat. Shortly afterward, the patient's roommate heard the patient choking and summoned help. At autopsy, it was confirmed that he had aspirated the turkey sandwich, and that this was the cause of the cardiopulmonary arrest that killed the patient. Though liability was found against the aide and her supervisor, the court also upheld a verdict of $500,000 against the hospital.

 RESEARCH PERSPECTIVE

Resource: Saccomano, S.J., & Pinto-Zipp, G. (2011). Registered nurse leadership style and confidence in delegation. *Journal of Nursing Management, 19*(4):522-533.

To be successful nurse managers and leaders, nurses must understand how to delegate appropriately and effectively. This study examined the relationship between nurses' leadership styles, demographic variables, and confidence in delegation. Conducted at a community teaching hospital, the 158 study participants completed two questionnaires, one measuring leadership style and one measuring confidence and intent to delegate. The sample was composed of 82 participants who had either a diploma or an associate degree, and 78 participants who had either a bachelor's or a master's degree in nursing. Participants had an average age of 43.58 years and 15.64 years of nursing experience. Findings indicated that there was no relationship between one's leadership style, categorized in this study as supportive, directive, or participative, and confidence in delegating tasks to unlicensed assistive personnel. The data from

the study did confirm that one's educational preparation and nursing experience play a role in the nurses' confidence level. Confidence in delegating was found to be greater in nurses with at least a bachelor's degree. For those without this degree, years of nursing experience increased their confidence level in delegating tasks to unlicensed assistive personnel. The authors concluded that it is imperative that all nursing curricula address the issues related to delegation.

Implications for Practice

The study demonstrates that nurse managers must acquire confidence in delegating and provide the nurses they oversee with the educational and clinical opportunities necessary to develop these delegation skills. To support optimal patient care, the entire team must work in a coordinated manner. Being able to appropriately and confidently delegate tasks to unlicensed assistive personnel is one means of beginning to meet this goal.

must be mutual understanding by both the delegator and the delegatee of the specific results expected and the means of attaining those results. As the Research Perspective on p. 77 notes, it is also a process that can be affected by one's formal education and clinical experience.

Duty to Orient, Educate, and Evaluate

Most healthcare institutions have continuing education departments to orient nurses who are new to the institution and to supply in-service education addressing new equipment, procedures, and interventions to existing employees. Nurse managers also have a duty to orient, educate, and evaluate. Nurse managers and their representatives are responsible for the daily evaluation of whether nurses are performing safe and competent care. The key to meeting this requirement is reasonableness and is determined by courts on a case-by-case basis. Nurse managers should ensure that they promptly respond to all allegations, whether by patients or staff, of incompetent or questionable nursing care. Nurse managers should thoroughly investigate such allegations, recommend options for correcting the situation, and follow up on recommended options and suggestions.

For example, in *Marinock v. Manor at St Luke's* (2010), the nursing facility had experienced multiple problems with patients falling or being dropped during Hoyer lift transfers because some staff members were unaware of how to properly secure patients in the sling before beginning the transfer. These incidents apparently did not lead to additional training, and subsequently an 82-year-old patient was dropped during a transfer from one bed to another bed, resulting in a femur fracture. The patient's lawsuit resulted in a $310,000 judgment against the facility for failure to properly orient and train its personnel.

EXERCISE 5-4

In a landmark study, the Institute of Medicine (1999) outlined six characteristics for a safe healthcare system, noting that incorporating these six characteristics created a culture of safety. For example, culture focuses on effective systems and teamwork to accomplish the goal of safe, high-quality patient care. Review the Institute of Medicine report and consider how nurse managers might begin to apply the characteristics of a culture of safety to the facts in the *Marinock v. Manor at St. Luke's* (2010) lawsuit.

Failure to Warn

A more recent area of potential liability for nurse managers is failure to warn potential employers of staff incompetence or impairment. Information about suspected addictions, violent behavior, and incompetency is of vital importance to subsequent employers. If the institution has sufficient information and suspicion to warrant the discharge of an employee or force a resignation, subsequent employers should be advised of those issues. In addition, the state board of nursing or agency that oversees disciplinary actions of professional and nonprofessional nursing staff should also be notified whenever there is cause to dismiss an employee for incompetency or impairment unless the employee voluntarily enters a peer-assistance program.

One means of supplying this information is through the use of *qualified privilege* to certain communications. In general, qualified privilege concerns communications made in good faith between persons or entities with a need to know. Most states now recognize this privilege and allow previous employers to give factual, objective information to subsequent employers. Note, however, that the previous employee must have listed the nurse manager or institution as a reference before this privilege arises.

Staffing Issues

Three issues arise under the general term *staffing*. These include (1) maintaining adequate numbers of staff members in a time of advancing patient acuity and limited resources; (2) floating staff from one unit to another; and (3) using temporary or "agency" staff to augment the healthcare facility's current staffing. Though each area is addressed separately, common to all three of these staffing issues is the requisite of collaboration among nurse managers in addressing the needs for the entire institution or healthcare agency.

Accreditation standards, specifically those of TJC and the Community Health Accreditation Program (CHAP), as well as other state and federal standards, mandate that healthcare institutions provide adequate staffing with qualified personnel. This applies not only to the number of staff but also to the legal status of the staff. For instance, some areas of an institution, such as critical care areas, postanesthesia care areas, and emergency care centers, must have greater percentages of RNs than LPNs/LVNs. Other areas, such as the general nursing areas and some long-term care areas, may have equal or lower percentages of RNs to LPNs/LVNs or nursing assistants. Whether understaffing exists in a given situation depends on the number of patients, care acuity scores, and number and classification of staff. Courts determine whether understaffing existed on an individual case basis.

California was the first state to adopt legislation that mandated fixed nurse-to-patient ratios, passing this historic legislation in 1999. These types of ratios require set nurse-to-patient ratios based solely on numbers of patients within given nursing care areas and do not consider issues such as patient acuity, level of staff preparation, or environmental factors. Though a first step toward beginning to ensure adequate numbers of nurses, many states are now moving toward the concept of safe staffing rather than specific nurse-to-patient ratios.

Several states plus the District of Columbia have passed safe staffing measures rather than mandating ratios. Generally, these safe staffing measures call for a committee to develop, oversee, and evaluate a plan for each specific nursing unit and shift based on patient care needs, appropriate skill mix of RNs and other nursing personnel, the physical layout of the unit, and national standards or recommendations regarding nursing staffing. Washington state's plan, for example, also includes a provision that the staffing information is posted in a public area of the nursing unit and updated at least once per shift. The information must also be made available to patients and visitors upon request (Safe Nurse Staffing Legislation, 2008).

Federal legislation regarding safe staffing was first introduced during the 2007-2008 legislative session by Senator Daniel Inouye and Representative Lois Capps. Defeated in that session, the legislation was reintroduced in subsequent legislative sessions. In 2011, it was again introduced as the *Registered Nurse Safe Staffing Act of 2011* and included such provisions as a required public reporting of staffing information, a procedure for receiving and investigating complaints, and allowing the imposition of civil monetary penalties for each known violation. Because staffing has major implications for quality, legislation likely will be introduced and refined over several sessions.

Although the institution is ultimately responsible for staffing issues, nurse managers may also incur liability because they directly oversee numbers of personnel assigned to a given unit. Courts have looked to the constant exercise of professional judgment, rather than reliance on concrete nurse-to-patient ratios, in cases involving staffing issues. Thus nurse managers should exercise sound judgment to ensure patient safety and quality care rather than rely on exact nurse-to-patient ratios. For liability to incur against the nurse manager, it must be shown that a resultant patient injury was directly caused by staffing issues and not by the incompetent or inappropriate actions of an individual staff member. To prevent nurse managers' liability, they must show that sufficient numbers of competent staff were available to meet nursing needs.

Guidelines for nurse managers in inadequate staffing issues include alerting hospital administrators and upper-level managers of concerns. First, however, the nurse manager must do whatever is under his or her control to alleviate the circumstances, such as approving overtime for adequate coverage, reassigning personnel among those areas he or she supervises, and restricting new admissions to the area. Second, nurse managers have a legal duty to notify the chief operating officer, either directly or indirectly, when understaffing endangers patient welfare. One way of notifying the chief operating officer is through formal nursing channels, for example, by notifying the nurse manager's direct supervisor. Upper management must then decide how to alleviate the staffing issue, either on a short-term or a long-term basis. Appropriate measures could be closing a unit or units, restricting elective surgeries, hiring new staff members, or temporarily reassigning personnel from other departments. Once the nurse manager can show that he or she acted appropriately, used sound judgment given the circumstances, and alerted his or her supervisors of the serious nature of the situation, the institution and not the nurse manager becomes potentially liable for staffing issues.

Several states prohibit the use of mandatory overtime by nurses. Generally these laws state that the healthcare facility may not require an employee to work in excess of agreed to, predetermined, and regularly scheduled daily work shifts unless an unforeseeable declared national, state, or municipal emergency or catastrophic event occurs that is unpredicted or unavoidable and that substantially affects or increases the need for healthcare services. In addition, many of these laws define "normal work schedule" as 12 or fewer hours; protect employees from disciplinary action or retribution for refusing to work overtime; and establish monetary penalties for the employer's failure to adhere to the law. Some states also mandate that healthcare facilities are required to have a process for complaints related to patient safety. Note that nothing in these laws negates voluntary overtime.

Floating staff from unit to unit is the second issue that concerns overall staffing. Institutions have a duty to ensure that all areas of the institution are staffed adequately. Units temporarily overstaffed because of low patient census or a lower patient acuity ratio usually float staff to units that are understaffed. Although floating nurses to areas with which they have less familiarity and expertise can increase potential liability for the nurse manager, leaving another area dangerously understaffed can also increase potential liability.

Before floating staff from one area to another, the nurse manager should consider staff expertise, patient-care delivery systems, and patient-care requirements. Nurses should be floated to units as comparable to their own unit as possible. This requires the nurse manager to match the nurse's home unit and float unit as much as possible or to consider negotiating with another nurse manager to cross-float a nurse. For example, a manager might float a critical care nurse to an intermediate care unit and float an intermediate care unit nurse to a general medical-surgical unit. Or the nurse manager might consider floating the general unit nurse to the postpartum unit and floating a postpartum nurse to labor and delivery. Open communications regarding staff limitations and concerns, as well as creative solutions for staffing, can alleviate some of the potential liability involved and create better morale among the floating nurses. A positive option is to cross-train nurses within the institution so that nurses are familiar with two or three areas and can competently float to areas in which they have been cross-trained.

The use of temporary or "agency" personnel has created increased liability concerns among nurses and nurse managers. Until recently, most jurisdictions held that such personnel were considered **independent contractors** and thus the institution was not liable for their actions, although their primary employment agency did retain potential liability. Today, courts have begun to hold the institution liable under the principle of **apparent agency.** *Apparent authority* or *apparent agency* refers to the doctrine whereby a principal becomes accountable for the actions of his or her agent. Apparent agency is created when a person (agent) holds himself or herself out as acting in behalf of the principal; in the instance of the agency nurse, the patient cannot ascertain whether the nurse works directly for the hospital (has a valid employment contract) or is working for a different employer. At law, lack of actual authority is no defense. This principle applies when it can be shown that a reasonable patient believed that the healthcare worker was an employee of the institution. If it appears to the reasonable patient that this worker is an employee of the institution, the law will consider the worker an employee for the purposes of corporate and vicarious liability.

These trends in the law mean that nurse managers must consider the temporary worker's skills, competencies, and knowledge when delegating tasks and supervising the worker's actions. If a manager suspects that the temporary worker is incompetent, he or she must convey this fact to the agency. The nurse manager must also either send the temporary worker home or reassign the worker to other duties and areas. The same screening procedures should be performed with temporary workers as are used with new institutional employees.

Additional areas that nurse managers should stress when using agency or temporary personnel include ensuring that the temporary staff member is given a brief but thorough orientation to institution policies and procedures, is made aware of resource materials within the institution, and is made aware of documentation procedures. Also, nurse managers should assign a resource person to the temporary staff member. This resource person serves in the role of mentor for the agency nurse and serves to prevent potential problems that could arise merely because the agency staff member does not know the institution routine or is unaware of where to turn for assistance. The resource person also serves as a mentor with critical decision making for the agency nurse.

PROTECTIVE AND REPORTING LAWS

Protective and reporting laws ensure the safety or rights of specific classes of individuals. Most states have reporting laws for suspected child and older adult abuse and laws for reporting certain categories of diseases and injuries. Examples of reporting laws include reporting cases of sexually transmitted diseases, abuse of residents in nursing and convalescent homes, and suspected child abuse. Nurse managers are often the individuals who are responsible for ensuring that the correct information is reported to the correct agencies, thus avoiding potential liability against the institution.

Many states now also have mandatory reporting of incompetent practice, especially through nurse practice acts, medical practice acts, and the National Practitioner Data Bank. In addition, the NCSBN has developed an electronic license verification system called *Nursys* that monitors nurses' licensure status in all states and U.S. territories for discipline issues, competency ratings, and renewals. Reporting incompetent practice often is restricted to issues of chemical abuse, and special provisions prevail if the affected nurse voluntarily undergoes drug diversion or chemical-dependency rehabilitation.

Mandatory reporting of incompetent practitioners is a complex process, involving both legal and ethical concerns. Nurse managers must know what the law requires, when reporting is mandated, to whom the report must be sent, and what the individual institution expects of its nurse managers. When in doubt, seek clarification from the state board of nursing, hospital administration, or professional association.

INFORMED CONSENT

Informed consent becomes an important concept for nurse managers in three very different instances. First, direct care nurses may approach the nurse manager with questions about informed consent; thus the nurse manager becomes a consultant for the direct care nurse. Second, and more often, the nurse manager is queried about patients' rights in research studies that are being conducted in the institution. Third, the issue of medical literacy has implications for the provision of valid informed consent by an ever-growing number of patients.

Remember: informed consent is the authorization by the patient or the patient's legal representative to do something to the patient; it is based on legal capacity, voluntary action, and comprehension. Legal capacity is usually the first requirement and is determined by age and competency. All states have a legal age for adult status defined by statute; generally, this age is 18 years. Competency involves the ability to understand the consequences of actions or the ability to handle personal affairs. State statutes mandate who can serve as the representative for a minor or incompetent adult. The following types of minors may be able to give valid informed consent: emancipated minors, minors seeking treatment for substance abuse or communicable diseases, and pregnant minors.

Voluntary action, the second requirement, means that the patient was not coerced by fraud, duress, or deceit into allowing the procedure or treatment. Comprehension is the third requirement and the most difficult to ascertain. The law states that the patient must be given sufficient information, in terms he or she can reasonably be expected to comprehend, to make an informed choice. Inherent in the doctrine of informed consent is the right of the patient to informed refusal. Patients must clearly understand the possible consequences of their refusal. In recent years, most states have enacted statutes to ensure that the competent adult has the right to refuse care and that the healthcare provider is protected should the adult validly refuse care. This refusal of care is most frequently seen in end-of-life decisions. Box 5-1 lists the information needed for obtaining informed consent.

Nurses often ask about issues concerning informed consent that concern the actual signing of the informed consent document, not the teaching and information that make up informed consent. Many nurses serve as witnesses to the signing of the informed consent document; in this capacity, they are attesting only to the voluntary nature of the patient's signature. There is no duty on the part of the nurse to insist that the patient repeat what has been said or what he or she remembers. If the patient asks questions that alert the nurse to the inadequacy of true comprehension on the patient's part or expresses uncertainty while signing the

---

BOX 5-1   INFORMATION REQUIRED FOR INFORMED CONSENT

- An explanation of the treatment/procedure to be performed and the expected results of the treatment/procedure
- Description of the risks involved
- Benefits that are likely to result because of the treatment/procedure
- Options to this course of action, including absence of treatment
- Name of the person(s) performing the treatment/procedure
- Statement that the patient may withdraw his or her consent at any time

document, the nurse has an obligation to inform the primary healthcare provider and appropriate persons that informed consent has not been obtained.

A separate issue with informed consent concerns the patient who is part of a research study. Federal laws regulate this area because patients are generally considered to come under the heading of *vulnerable populations.* Whenever research is involved, such as a drug study or a new procedure, the investigators must disclose the research to the subject or the subject's representative and obtain informed consent. Federal guidelines have been developed that specify the procedures used to review research and the disclosures that must be made to ensure that valid informed consent is obtained.

The federal government mandates the basic elements of information that must be included to meet the standards of informed consent. Elements of informed consent are enumerated in Box 5-2.

BOX 5-2   ELEMENTS OF INFORMED CONSENT IN RESEARCH STUDIES

- A statement that the study involves research, an explanation of the purposes of the research and the expected duration of the subject's participation, a description of the procedures to be followed, and identification of any procedures that are experimental
- A description of any reasonably foreseeable risks or discomforts to the subject
- A description of any benefits to the subjects or others that may reasonably be expected from the research
- A disclosure of appropriate alternative procedures or courses of treatment, if any, that may be advantageous to the subject
- A statement describing the extent, if any, to which confidentiality of records identifying the subject will be maintained
- For research involving more than minimal research, an explanation as to any compensation and an explanation as to whether any medical treatments are available if injury occurs and, if so, what they consist of or where further information may be obtained
- An explanation of whom to contact for answers to pertinent questions about the research and research subjects' rights and whom to contact in the event of a research-related injury to the subject
- A statement that participation is voluntary, refusal to participate will involve no benefits to which the subject is otherwise entitled, and the subject may discontinue participation at any time without penalty or loss of benefits to which the subject is otherwise entitled

Source: *45 Code of Federal Regulations (CFR),* Sec. 46.116 (1991).

BOX 5-3   ELEMENTS OF CONCERN IN RESEARCH STUDIES

- Any additional costs that they might incur because of the research
- Potential for any foreseeable risks
- Rights to withdraw at will, with no questions asked or additional incentives given
- Consequences, if any, of withdrawal before the study is completed
- A statement that any significant new findings will be disclosed
- The number of proposed subjects for the study

Source: *45 Code of Federal Regulations (CFR),* Sec. 46.101(b) (1991).

The information given must be in a language that is understandable by the subject or the subject's legal representative. No exculpatory wording may be included, such as a statement that the researcher incurs no liability for the outcomes of the study or any injury to an individual subject. Subjects should be advised of the elements listed in Box 5-3.

Excluded from these strict requirements were studies that use existing data, documents, records, or pathologic and diagnostic specimens, if these sources are publicly available or the information is recorded so that the subjects cannot be identified. Other studies that involve only minimal risks to subjects, such as moderate exercise by healthy adults, may be expedited through the review process (Protection of Human Subjects, 1991, Section 46.110). Nurse managers must verify that staff members understand any research protocol with which their patients are involved.

The advent of the Health Insurance Portability and Accountability Act (HIPAA) of 1996 (Public Law [P.L.] 104-191) has affected how health record information can now be used in research studies. No separate permission need be secured from the patient to use medical-record information if de-identified information is used. De-identified information is health information that cannot be linked to an individual; most of the 18 demographic items constituting the protected health information (PHI) must be removed before researchers are permitted to use patient records without obtaining the individual patient's permission to use/disclose PHI. The de-identified data set that is permissible for usage may contain the following demographic factors: gender and age of individuals and a three-digit

ZIP code. Note that all individuals 90 years of age or older are listed as 90 years of age.

To prevent the onerous task of requiring patients who have been discharged from healthcare settings to sign such permission forms, researchers are allowed to submit a request for a waiver. The waiver is a request to forego the authorization requirements based on two conditions: (1) the use and/or disclosure of PHI involves minimal risk to the subject's privacy, and (2) the research cannot be done practically without this waiver. Additional information about HIPAA and confidentiality are covered later in this chapter.

Concerns over the past abuses that have occurred in the area of research with children have led to the adoption of federal guidelines specifically designed to protect children when they are enrolled as research subjects. Before proceeding under these specific guidelines, state and local laws must be reviewed for laws regulating research on human subjects. In 1998, Subpart D: Additional Protections for Children Involved as Subjects in Research was added to the code (Protection of Human Subjects, 1998, 46.401 *et seq.*). These sections were added to give further protection to children when they are subjects of research studies and to encourage researchers to involve children, where appropriate, in research.

A final issue with informed consent about which nurses and nurse managers should be cognizant concerns health literacy or the degree to which individuals have the capacity to obtain, process, and understand basic health information, including services needed to make appropriate health decisions. Functional health literacy relates to the person's ability to act upon the basic health information received. Comprehending medical jargon is difficult for well-educated Americans; about 12% or American adults are considered proficient in health literacy (Department of Health and Human Services, 2012). Comprehending medical instructions and terms may be impossible for individuals whose first language is not English, who cannot read at greater than a second-grade level, or who have vision or cognitive problems caused by aging or disabilities. These individuals have difficulty following instructions that are printed on medication labels (both prescription and over-the-counter), interpreting hospital consent forms, and even understanding diagnoses, treatment options, and discharge instructions.

Nurses play a significant role in addressing this growing problem. The first issue to address is awareness of the problem, because many patients and their family members hide the fact that they cannot read or do not understand what healthcare providers are attempting to convey. A second issue involves ensuring that the information and words nurses use to communicate with patients are at a level that the person can comprehend. One means to ensure that patients do understand patient discharge information and medication instructions is to give a patient a bottle of prescription medication and ask him or her to tell you how he or she would take the medication at home.

PRIVACY AND CONFIDENTIALITY

Privacy is the patient's right to protection against unreasonable and unwarranted interference with his or her solitude. This right extends to protection of the person's reputation as well as protection of one's right to be left alone. Within a medical context, the law recognizes the patient's right to protection against (1) appropriation of the patient's name or picture for the institution's sole advantage, (2) intrusion by the institution on the patient's seclusion or affairs, (3) publication of facts that place the patient in a false light, and (4) public disclosure of private facts about the patient by the hospital or staff. Confidentiality is the right to privacy of the health record.

Institutions can reduce potential liability in this area by allowing access to patient data, either written or oral, only to those with a "need to know." Persons with a need to know include physicians and nurses caring for the patient, technicians, unit clerks, therapists, social service workers, and patient advocates. Usually, this need to know extends to the house staff and consultants. Others wishing to access patient data must first ask the patient for permission to review a record. Administrative staff of the institution can access the patient record for statistical analysis, staffing, and quality-of-care review.

The nurse manager is cautioned to ensure that staff members both understand and abide by rules regarding patient privacy and confidentiality. "Interesting" patients should not be discussed with others, and all information concerning patients should be given only in private and secluded areas. All nurses may need to review the current means of giving reports to oncoming shifts and policies about telephone information. Many institutions have now added to the nursing care plan a place to list persons to whom the patient has allowed information to be given. If the caller identifies himself or herself as one of those listed persons, the nurse can give patient information without violating the patient's privacy rights. Patients are becoming more knowledgeable about their rights in these areas, and some have been willing to take offending staff members to court over such issues.

The patient's right of access to his or her health record is another confidentiality issue. Although the patient has a right of access, individual states mandate when this right applies. Most states give the right of access only after the health record is completed; thus the patient has the right to review the record after discharge. Some states do give the right of access while the patient is hospitalized, and therefore individual state law governs individual nurses' actions. When supervising a patient's review of his or her record, the nurse manager or representative should explain only the entries that the patient questions or about which the patient requests further clarification. The nurse makes a note in the record after the session, indicating that the patient has viewed the record and what questions were answered.

Patients also have a right to copies of the record, at their expense. The health record belongs to the institution as a business record, and patients never have the right to retain the original record. This is also true in instances in which a subpoena is obtained to secure an individual's health record for court purposes. A hospital representative will verify that the copy is a "true and valid" copy of the original record.

An issue that is closely related to the health record is that of incident reports or unusual occurrence reports. These reports are mandated by TJC and serve to alert the institution to risk management and quality assurance issues within the setting. As such, incident reports are considered internal documents and thus not discoverable (open for review) by the injured party or attorneys representing the injured party. In most jurisdictions where this question has arisen, however, the courts have held that the incident report was discoverable and thus open to review by both sides of the suit.

Therefore prudent nurse managers complete and have staff members complete incident reports as though they will be open records, omitting any language of liability, such as, "The patient would not have fallen if Jane Jones, RN, had ensured the side rails were in their up and locked position." This document should contain only pertinent observations and care given the patient, such as x-rays that were obtained for a potential broken bone, medication that was given, and consultants who were called to examine the patient. It is also inadvisable to make any notation of the incident report in the official patient record because such a notation incorporates the incident report "by reference," and thus can be seen by the injured party or attorneys for the injured party.

Protected health information (PHI), which includes some 18 individual identifiers, is at the crux of the confidentiality aspect of the law. The privacy standards limit how PHI may be used or shared, mandate safeguards for protecting the health information, and shift the control of health information from providers to the patient by giving patients significant rights. Healthcare facilities must provide patients with a documented Notice of Privacy Rights, explaining how PHI will be used or shared with other entities. This document also alerts patients to the process for complaints if they later determine that their information rights have been violated. Nurse managers have the responsibility to ensure that those they supervise uphold these patient rights as dictated by HIPAA and to take corrective actions should these rights not be upheld.

POLICIES AND PROCEDURES

Risk management is a process that identifies, analyzes, and treats potential hazards within a given setting. The object of risk management is to identify potential

---

EXERCISE 5-5

You are assigned some risk management activities in the nursing facility where you work. In investigating incident reports filed by staff, you discover that this is the third incident this week where a patient has fallen while attempting to get out of bed and sit in a chair. How would you begin to address this issue? Decide how you would start a more complete investigation of this issue. For example, is it a facility-wide issue or one that is confined to one unit? Does it affect all shifts or only one? What safety issues are you going to discuss with your staff, and how are you going to discuss these issues? Do these falls involve the same staff member? Design a unit in-service class for the staff concerning incident reports and patient safety.

hazards and eliminate them before anyone is harmed or disabled. Risk management activities include writing policies and procedures. Written policies and procedures are a requirement of TJC. These documents set standards of care for the institution and direct practice. They must be clearly stated, well delineated, and based on current practice. Nurse managers should review the policies and procedures frequently for compliance and timeliness. If policies are absent or outdated, the nurse manager must request the appropriate person or committee to either initiate or update the policy.

EMPLOYMENT LAWS

The federal and individual state governments have enacted laws regulating employment. To be effective and legally correct, nurse managers must be familiar with these laws and how the individual laws affect the institution and labor relations. Many nurse managers have come to fear the legal system because of personal experience or the experiences of colleagues, but much of this concern may be directly attributable to uncertainty with the law or partial knowledge of the law. By understanding and correctly following federal

employment laws, nurse managers may actually decrease their potential liability by complying with both federal and state laws. Table 5-2 gives an overview of key federal employment laws.

Equal Employment Opportunity Laws

Several federal laws have been enacted to expand equal employment opportunities by prohibiting discrimination based on gender, age, race, religion, handicap, pregnancy, and national origin. The Equal Employment Opportunity Commission (EEOC) enforces these laws. All states have also enacted statutes that address employment opportunities, and the nurse manager should consider both when hiring and assigning nursing employees.

The most significant legislation affecting equal employment opportunities today is the amended Civil Rights Act of 1964. Section 703(a) of Title VII makes it illegal for an employer "to refuse to hire, discharge an individual, or otherwise to discriminate against an individual, with respect to his compensation, terms, conditions, or privileges of employment because of the individual's race, color, religion, sex, or national origin." The Equal Employment Opportunity Act of 1972 also

TABLE 5-2 SELECTED FEDERAL LABOR LEGISLATION

YEAR	LEGISLATION	PRIMARY PURPOSE OF THE LEGISLATION
1935	Wagner Act; National Labor Act	Unions, National Labor Relations Board established; unionization rights established
1947	Taft-Hartley Act	Established a more equal balance of power between unions and management
1962	Executive Order 10988	Allowed public employees to join labor unions
1963	Equal Pay Act	Became illegal to pay lower wages based solely on gender
1964	Civil Rights Act	Protected against discrimination based on race, color, creed, national origin, etc.
1967	Age Discrimination in Employment Act	Protected against discrimination based on age
1970	Occupational Safety and Health Act	Established the development and enforcement of standards for occupational health and safety
1974	Wagner Amendments	Allowed nonprofit organizations to unionize and allowed collective bargaining in nursing
1990	Americans with Disabilities Act	Barred discrimination against workers with disabilities in the workplace
1991	Civil Rights Act	Addressed sexual harassment in the workplace
1993	Family and Medical Leave Act	Allowed work leaves based on family and medical needs
1996	Health Insurance Portability and Accountability Act	Provided for the phased introduction of a comprehensive system of mandated health insurance reforms
2010	Patient Protection and Accountability Act	Provided for the phased introduction of a comprehensive system of mandated health insurance reforms
2010	Health Care and Education Reconciliation Act	Amended the Patient Protection and Affordable Care Act to clarify budget resolutions

amended Title VII so that it applies to private institutions with 15 or more employees, state and local governments, labor unions, and employment agencies.

The amended Civil Rights Act of 1991 further broadened the issue of sexual harassment in the workplace and supersedes many of the sections of Title VII. Sections of the new legislation define sexual harassment, its elements, and the employer's responsibilities regarding harassment in the workplace, especially prevention and corrective action. The Civil Rights Act of 1991 is enforced by the EEOC. The primary activity of the EEOC is processing complaints of employment discrimination. Three phases comprise processing complaints: investigation, conciliation, and litigation. Investigation focuses on determining whether the employer has violated provisions of Title VII. If the EEOC finds "probable cause," an attempt is made to reach an agreement or conciliation between the EEOC, the complainant, and the employer. If conciliation fails, the EEOC may file suit against the employer in federal court or issue to the complainant the right to sue for discrimination under its auspices, including those relating to staffing practices and sexual harassment in the workplace.

The EEOC defines sexual harassment broadly, and this has generally been upheld in the courts. Nurse managers must realize that it is the duty of employers (management) to prevent employees from sexually harassing other employees. The EEOC issues policies and practices for employers to implement, both to sensitize employees to this problem and to prevent its occurrence. Nurse managers should be aware of these policies and practices and seek guidance in implementing them if sexual harassment occurs in their units.

Employers may seek exceptions to Title VII on a number of premises. For example, employment decisions made on the basis of national origin, religion, and gender (never race or color) are lawful if such decisions are necessary for the normal operation of the business, although the courts have viewed this exception very narrowly. Promotions and layoffs based on bona fide seniority or merit systems are permissible, as are exceptions based on business necessity.

Age Discrimination in Employment Act of 1967

The Age Discrimination in Employment Act of 1967 made discrimination against older men and women by employers, unions, and employment agencies illegal.

A 1986 amendment to the law prohibits discrimination against persons older than 40 years. The practical outcome of this act has been that mandatory retirement is no longer allowed in the American workplace.

As with Title VII, some exceptions to this act exist. Reasonable factors other than age may be used when terminations become necessary. Reasonable factors may include a performance evaluation system or certain limited occupational qualifications, such as the tedious physical demands of a specific job.

Americans with Disabilities Act of 1990

The Americans with Disabilities Act (ADA) of 1990 provides protection to persons with disabilities and is the most significant civil rights legislation since the Civil Rights Act of 1964. The purpose of the ADA is to provide a clear and comprehensive national mandate for the elimination of discrimination against individuals with disabilities and to provide clear, strong, consistent, enforceable standards addressing discrimination in the workplace. The ADA is closely related to the Civil Rights Act of 1991 and incorporates the anti-discrimination principles established in Section 504 of the Rehabilitation Act of 1973.

The act has five titles; Table 5-3 depicts the pertinent issues of each title. The ADA has jurisdiction over employers, private and public; employment agencies; labor organizations; and joint labor-management committees. Disability is defined broadly. With respect to an individual, a disability is (1) a physical or mental impairment that substantially limits one or more of the major life activities of such individual, (2) a record of such impairment, or (3) regarded as having such an impairment (ADA Amended Act, 2008). The effects of this amended act were to allow the definition of disability to be as broad as possible, and also to disallow impairments that are transitory (6 month duration or less) and minor. It also allows the definition to include an impairment that is episodic or in remission if the disability substantially limits a major life event when not in remission.

The overall effect of the legislation is that persons with disabilities will not be excluded from job opportunities or adversely affected in any aspect of employment unless they are not qualified or are otherwise unable to perform the job. The ADA thus protects qualified individuals with disabilities in regard to job application procedures, hiring, compensation, advancement, and all other employment matters.

TABLE 5-3 AMERICANS WITH DISABILITIES ACT OF 1990

TITLE	PROVISIONS
I	Employment: defines the purpose of the act and who is qualified under the act as having a disability
II	Public services: concerns services, programs, and activities of public entities as well as public transportation
III	Public accommodations and services operated by private entities: prohibits discrimination against persons with disabilities in areas of public accommodations, commercial facilities, and public transportation services
IV	Telecommunications: intended to make telephone services accessible to individuals with hearing or speech impairments
V	Miscellaneous provisions: certain insurance matters; incorporation of this act with other federal and state laws

Source: Americans with Disabilities Act of 1990, 42 U.S.C. § 12101 et seq. (1990).

CASE EXAMPLE BOX 5-3

This last point was well illustrated by the court in *Zamudio v. Patia* (1997). The court stated that the employer would be required to inform Ms. Zamudio when a position became available for which the reasonable accommodation she required could be met. She would be allowed to apply, but "as a disabled employee seeking reasonable accommodation she did not have to be given preference over other employees without disabilities who might have better qualifications or more seniority" (*Zamudio v. Patia*, 1997, at 808).

The number of lawsuits filed under the ADA since its enactment is extensive. This is due in part to the fact that to prevent the act from being overly narrow, the determination of qualified individuals is done case by case, and the individual must show (1) that he or she has a physical or mental impairment, (2) the impairment must substantially limit one or more major life activities, and (3) the qualified individual must still be able to perform the essential function of the employment position sought or in which the individual is currently employed.

The ADA requires an employer or potential employer to make reasonable accommodations to employ persons with a disability. The law does not mandate that individuals with a disability be hired before fully qualified persons who do not have a disability; it does mandate that those with disabilities not be disqualified merely because of an easily accommodated disability. An example appears in the Case Example Box 5-3 that follows.

Moreover, the court will not impose job restructuring on an employer if the person needing accommodation qualifies for other jobs not requiring such accommodation. In *Mauro v. Borgess Medical Center* (1995), the court refused to impose accommodation on the employer hospital merely because the affected employee desired to stay within a certain unit of the institution. In this case, an operating surgical technician who tested positive for HIV was offered an equivalent position by the hospital in an area where there would be no patient contact. He refused the transfer, desiring accommodation within the operating arena, and was denied such accommodation by the Michigan court.

The act also provides for essential job functions. These are defined by the ADA as those functions that the person must be able to perform to be qualified for employment positions. Courts have assisted in determining these essential job functions. For example, in *Moschke v. Memorial Medical Center of West Michigan* (2003), the court determined that the ability to take "on-call" work is an essential function of a surgical nurse's job. Such on-call work involves the ability of the surgical nurse to be available when emergency cases or scheduling problems require the staff to work beyond their assigned shifts. In *Laurin v. Providence Hospital and Massachusetts Nurses Association* (1998), the ability to work rotating shifts was held to be an essential job function.

The act specifically excludes the following from the definition of disability: homosexuality and bisexuality, sexual behavioral disorders, gambling addiction, kleptomania, pyromania, and current use of illegal drugs (ADA, 1990). Employers may hold alcoholic persons to the same job qualifications and job performance standards as other employees, even if the unsatisfactory behavior or performance is related to the alcoholism (ADA, 1990). As with other federal employment laws, the nurse manager should have a thorough understanding of the law as it applies to the institution and his or her specific job description and should know whom to contact within the institution structure for clarification as needed.

Affirmative Action

The policy of affirmative action (AA) differs from the policy of equal employment opportunity (EEO). AA policy enhances employment opportunities of protected groups of people; EEO policy is concerned with implementing employment practices that do not discriminate against or impair the employment opportunities of protected groups. Thus AA can be seen in conjunction with several federal employment laws. For example, in conjunction with the Vietnam Era Veterans' Readjustment Assistance Act of 1974, AA requires that employers with government contracts take steps to enhance the employment opportunities of veterans with disabilities who served during the Vietnam Era.

Equal Pay Act of 1963

The Equal Pay Act of 1963 makes it illegal to pay lower wages to employees of one gender when the jobs (1) require equal skill in experience, training, education, and ability; (2) require equal effort in mental or physical exertion; (3) are of equal responsibility and accountability; and (4) are performed under similar working conditions. Courts have held that unequal pay may be legal if it is based on seniority, merit, incentive systems, or a factor other than gender. The main cases filed under this law in the area of nursing have been by nonprofessionals.

Occupational Safety and Health Act

The Occupational Safety and Health Administration (OSHA) Act of 1970 was enacted to ensure that healthful and safe working conditions would exist in the workplace. Among other provisions, the law requires isolation procedures, placarding areas containing ionizing radiation, proper grounding of electrical equipment, protective storage of flammable and combustible liquids, and the gloving of all personnel when handling bodily fluids. The statute provides that if no federal standard has been established, state statutes prevail. Nurse managers should know the relevant OSHA laws for the institution and their specific area. Frequent review of new additions to the law also must be undertaken, especially in this era of acquired immunodeficiency syndrome (AIDS) and infectious diseases, and care must be taken to ensure that necessary gloves and equipment as specified are available on each unit.

Violence in the workplace is an issue that OSHA continues to address in its rules. Violence is perhaps the greatest hidden health and safety threat in the workplace today, and nurses, as the largest group of healthcare professionals, are most at risk of assault at work. In 1996, OSHA developed voluntary guidelines to protect healthcare workers and consumers. Relatively few states have laws that mandate employers to report incidents of workplace violence, although more states have enacted laws that strengthen or increase penalties for acts of workplace violence. At least one state has pending legislation that would implement standards of conduct and policies reducing workplace bullying. Additionally, TJC has created standards that address the incidence and prevention of workplace violence, and the American Nurses Association (ANA) has generated a model state bill entitled The Violence Prevention in Health Care Facilities Act (ANA, 2012a).

An issue now being addressed in depth is the issue of safe patient handling, preventing injury to healthcare workers while ensuring that patients are protected as they are transferred or moved in healthcare settings. The ANA (2012b) reported that more than one third of back injuries in nurses are associated with the handling of patients. Given these data and recognizing that there simply is no safe manual patient lifting, the ANA promotes legislation that would require hospitals and other healthcare institutions to develop programs to prevent work-related musculoskeletal disorders and eliminate manual patient lifting. Toward this end, a few states have passed safe patient handling legislation.

Also in 2012, OSHA announced that it had initiated a 3-year National Emphasis Program (NEP) for nursing and residential care facilities in order to focus on the workplace hazards that are the most common in the healthcare industry, including ergonomic stressors related to patient lifting. The desire is that this momentum will lead to federal laws that would require mechanical lifting equipment and friction-reducing devices for all healthcare workers, patients, and residents across all healthcare settings.

Family and Medical Leave Act of 1993

The Family and Medical Leave Act of 1993 was passed because of the large numbers of single-parent and two-parent households in which the single parent or both parents are employed full-time, placing job security and parenting at odds. The law also supports the growing demands that aging parents are placing on their working children. The act was written in an attempt to balance the demands of the workplace with the demands of the family, allowing employed individuals to take leaves for medical reasons, including the birth or adoption of children and the care of a spouse, child, or parent who has serious health problems. Essentially, the act provides job security for unpaid leave while the employee is caring for a new infant or other family healthcare needs. The act is gender-neutral and allows both men and women the same leave provisions. Medical leave may be taken to care for a spouse, son, daughter, or parent of the employee when that person has a serious medical condition. Employees are also permitted to use medical leave for their own serious health condition.

To be eligible under the act, the employee must have worked for at least 12 months and worked at least 1250 hours during the preceding 12-month period. The employee may take up to 12 weeks of unpaid leave. The act allows the employer to require the employee to use all or part of any paid vacation, personal leave, or sick leave as part of the 12-week family leave. Employees must give the employer 30-days notice, or such notice as is practical in emergency cases, before using the medical leave.

On January 28, 2008, President George W. Bush signed the Family and Medical Leave Amended Act of 2008, which became effective January 16, 2009. The amendments permit a spouse, son, daughter, parent, or next of kin to take up to 26 work weeks of leave to care for a member of the U.S. Armed Forces, including a member of the National Guard or Reserves, who is undergoing medical treatment, recuperation, or therapy; is otherwise in outpatient status; or is otherwise on the temporary disability retired list, for a serious injury or illness. In addition, the act permits an employee to take leave for any qualifying exigency arising out of the fact that the spouse or a son, daughter, or parent of the employee is on active duty (or has been notified of an impending call or order to active duty) in the Armed Forces in support of a contingency operation.

Employment-at-Will and Wrongful Discharge

Historically, the employment relationship has been considered a "free will" relationship. Employees were free to take or not take a job at will, and employers were free to hire, retain, or discharge employees for any reason. Many laws, some federal but predominantly state, have been slowly eroding this at-will employment relationship. Evolving case law provides at least three exceptions to the broad doctrine of employment-at-will.

The first exception is a public policy exception. This exception involves cases in which an employee is discharged in direct conflict with established public policy. Under this exception, an employer may not discharge an employee if it would violate the state's public policy doctrine or a state or federal statute. Some examples include discharging an employee for serving on a jury, reporting employers' illegal actions (better known as whistle blowing, or the disclosure of information regarding misconduct within a workplace that either is illegal or endangers the welfare of others), and filing a workers' compensation claim. Most states and the District of Columbia recognize public policy as an exception to the at-will rule.

Several recent court cases attest to the number of terminations in healthcare settings that serve as retaliation for the employer. More commonly known as whistle-blowing cases, the healthcare provider in these cases is terminated for one of three distinct reasons: (1) speaking out against unsafe practices, (2) reporting violations of federal laws, or (3) filing lawsuits against employers. Essentially, whistleblower laws state that no employer can discharge, threaten, or discriminate against an employee regarding compensation, terms, conditions, location, or privileges of employment because the employee in good faith reported or caused to be reported, verbally or in writing, what the employee had a reasonable cause to believe was a violation of a state or federal law, rule, or regulation. Most whistleblowers are internal, that is they report misconduct to a fellow employee or supervisor within the agency. External whistleblowers are those who report misconduct to outside persons or entities. The examples appear in the Case Example Boxes 5-4 and 5-5.

The second exception to wrongful discharge involves situations in which an implied contract exists. The courts have generally treated employee handbooks, company policies, and oral statements made at the time of employment as "framing the employment relationship" (*Watkins v. Unemployment Compensation Board of Review,* 1997). For example, in *Trombley v. Southwestern Vermont Medical Center*

CASE EXAMPLE BOX 5-4

Martell v. Tarpon Springs Hospital (2010) concerned a hospital surgical nursing supervisor with a spotless 14-year record who was fired 10 days after she voiced a complaint that the hospital administrator had falsified records. In these falsified records, the administrator had personally certified a number of hospital nurses' annual cardiopulmonary resuscitation retraining, which neither he nor anyone else had actually done. During the trial, it was further disclosed that this same administrator had been fired from his previous employments for falsifying time records and for poor performance.

The jury in the case awarded the former nursing supervisor $425,000 as damages for compensation for emotional distress and the fact that her new employment paid less, had fewer benefits, and was less personally satisfying than her former position. The jury also noted that complaining about an illegal action by a superior was expressly protected by the state's whistleblower-protection law and that the hospital had no grounds on which to dismiss her.

CASE EXAMPLE BOX 5-5

Perhaps one of the best known whistleblower cases involving nurses is what has become known as the Winkler County Nurses Lawsuit (Yoder-Wise, 2010). The case became nationally known after two registered nurses, Anne Mitchell and Vicki Galle, were terminated by the Winkler County Hospital in Kermit, Texas. The nurses first attempted to report a physician's behavior and negligent healthcare practices through designated hospital channels. When the hospital took no action, they reported the physician to the Texas Medical Board for serious misconduct, substandard care, and an inappropriate business partnership with the sheriff of Winkler County.

Although the usual procedure was for the medical board to investigate and keep the complainants' names confidential, the sheriff used the power of his position to learn that the reporting nurses had worked at the hospital for about 20 years and that each nurse was about 50 years old. That information allowed the sheriff to identify the two nurses; he then used his office to confiscate the nurses' computers, where he found the letter to the Texas Medical Board. The nurses were subsequently terminated and indicted on felony charges of misuse of official information, which could have resulted in their imprisonment for 10 years.

The criminal charges against Vicki Galle were dismissed the day before the trial was to occur, though the trial proceeded against Anne Mitchell. The trial lasted less than 4 days, with the jury returning a not guilty verdict. The nurses later filed successful civil lawsuits against the physician, Winkler County, the hospital and its administrator, the sheriff, and the district and county attorneys of Winkler County (*Mitchell & Galle v. Winkler County et al.*, 2010). Their cause of action included violations of their rights of free speech and due process, whistleblower retaliation, and interference with their business relationship, specifically their employment status.

(1999), the court found that the employee handbook outlined the procedure for progressive discipline, mandating that such procedure be followed before a nurse could be terminated for incompetent nursing care.

The third exception to wrongful discharge is a "good faith and fair dealing" exception. The purpose of this exception is to prevent unfair or malicious terminations, and the courts use the exception sparingly. States also do not favor this exception, and today less than a quarter of the states recognize breach of such implied contracts. Although this exception is rarely seen in nursing, it remains a valid exception to wrongful discharge of an employee.

Nurse managers are urged to know their respective state laws concerning this growing area of the law, particularly in conjunction with whistleblower laws. Managers should review institution documents, especially employee handbooks and recruiting brochures, for unwanted statements implying job security or other unintentional promises. Managers are also cautioned not to say anything during the preemployment negotiations and interviews that might be construed as implying job security or other unintentional promises to the potential employee. To prevent successful suits for retaliation by whistleblowers, nurse managers should carefully monitor the treatment of an employee after a complaint is filed and ensure that performance evaluations are conducted and placed in the appropriate files. The nurse manager should also take steps to correct the whistleblower's complaint or refer the complaint to upper management so that it can effectively be addressed.

Collective Bargaining

Collective bargaining, also called *labor relations*, is the joining together of employees for the purpose of increasing their ability to influence the employer and improve working conditions. Collective bargaining is defined and protected by the National Labor Relations Act of 1935 and its amendments; the National Labor Relations Board (NLRB) oversees the act and those who come under its auspices. The NLRB ensures that employees can choose freely whether they want to be represented by a particular bargaining unit, and it serves to prevent or remedy any violation of the labor laws. Chapter 19 provides further detail regarding collective bargaining and collective action.

PATIENT PROTECTION AND AFFORDABLE CARE ACT AND HEALTH CARE AND EDUCATION RECONCILIATION ACT

The Patient Protection and Affordable Care Act (PPACA) was signed into legislation by President Barack Obama on March 23, 2010 (Public Law 111-148). Citing a need for health insurance reform and a need to insure the millions of uninsured Americans, the PPACA provides for the phased implementation over 4 years of a comprehensive system of mandated health insurance reforms designed to eliminate precondition screenings, premium loading fees and structures, policy cancellation when illnesses appear imminent, and annual and lifetime coverage gaps. The act also sets a minimum ratio of direct healthcare spending to premium income, creates price control measures through the creation of three standard insurance coverage levels to enable side-by-side comparisons by consumers, and creates a Web-based health insurance exchange. The act preserves private insurance and private healthcare providers while instituting more subsidies to enable all individuals to purchase healthcare insurance. Challenged by several states as unconstitutional, the act was fully upheld by the U.S. Supreme Court in June 2012 (*National Federation of Independent Businesses v. Sebelius, Secretary of Health and Human Services, et al.*, 2012).

A week after signing the PPACA into law, President Obama signed the Health Care and Education Reconciliation Act on March 30, 2010 (Public Law 111-152). This subsequent act was passed to amend the earlier act as it related to the federal budgetary resolutions and deficit. Basically, this second act served to increase the tax credits to buy insurance, lower the penalty for not buying health insurance, closed the Medicare Part D "donut hole" provision, and required physicians who treat Medicare patients to be reimbursed at a full rate of payment.

With the passage of this act, nurses and the healthcare delivery systems are projected to be affected in many ways. Though much of the additional coverage will be phased in during subsequent years, new patient care standards should be evident within the next year. Facilities will be required to post notices advising employees of their rights; these rights may not be waived in an employment agreement with the institution. Skilled nursing and nursing facilities will be required to have compliance and ethics training programs to prevent and detect criminal, civil, and administrative violations and to promote quality of care. These programs will encourage employees to report violations by others without fear of retribution. As for all nurses, nurse managers are urged to stay up-to-date with the various provisions of this healthcare reform law to ensure continuing compliance with its provisions.

PROFESSIONAL NURSING PRACTICE: ETHICS

Ethics is an area of professional practice in which nurse managers should have a solid foundation, because it is becoming increasingly more prominent in clinical practice settings. However, it remains an area in which many nurses feel the most inadequate. This is partially because ethics is much more nebulous than are laws and regulations. In ethics, no right and wrong answers are possible, just better or worse answers, and nurses seek mentorship and counseling from nurse managers when they encounter difficult situations. Thus nurse managers must have a deep understanding of ethical principles and their application.

Ethics may be distinguished from the law because ethics is internal to an individual, looks to the ultimate "good" of an individual rather than society as a whole, and concerns the "why" of one's actions. The law, comprising rules and regulations pertinent to society as a whole, is external to oneself and concerns one's actions and conduct. Ethics concerns the individual within society, whereas law concerns society as a whole. Law can be enforced through the courts, statutes, and boards of nursing, whereas ethics is enforced via ethics committees and professional codes.

Today, ethics and legal issues often become entwined, and it may be difficult to separate ethics from legal concerns. Legal principles and doctrines assist the nurse manager in decision making; ethical theories and principles are often involved in those decisions. Thus the nurse manager must be cognizant of both laws and ethics in everyday management concerns, remembering that ethical principles form the essential base of knowledge from which to proceed, rather than giving easy, straightforward answers.

BOX 5-4   ETHICAL PRINCIPLES

- Autonomy
- Beneficence
- Nonmaleficence
- Veracity
- Justice
- Paternalism
- Fidelity
- Respect for others

Ethical Principles

Ethical principles, used daily in patient care situations, are equally paramount to the nurse manager. Ethical principles that nurse managers should consider when making decisions include the eight items listed in Box 5-4. Each of the principles is applied daily in clinical practice, though some principles are used a greater degree than others.

The principle of **autonomy** addresses personal freedom and self-determination; the right to choose what will happen to oneself as well as the accountability for making individual choices. The legal doctrine of informed consent is a direct reflection of this principle. Autonomy involves respect for other's decisions, even if the nurse manager does not agree with the decision chosen. An example could be in the instance of progressive discipline. The employee has the option to meet delineated expectations or accept the consequences of not complying with these delineated expectations.

The principle of **beneficence** states that the actions one takes should promote good; beneficence is the basic obligation to assist others. Nurse managers employ this principle when encouraging employees to seek more challenging clinical experiences or to take on additional responsibilities, such as the position of assistant manager of a specific unit. Progressive discipline incorporates this principle when the employee's positive attributes and qualities are included when developing goals and expected outcomes.

The corollary of beneficence, the principle of **nonmaleficence,** states that one should do no harm. For a nurse manager following this principle, performance evaluation should emphasize an employee's good qualities and give positive direction for growth. Destroying the employee's self-esteem and self-worth would be considered doing harm under this principle.

Veracity concerns telling the truth and demands that the truth be told completely. Nurse managers employ this principle when they give all the facts of a situation truthfully and then assist employees to make appropriate decisions. For example, when encouraging a staff member to accept a promotion to a position of greater responsibility, both the challenges and the benefits of the position must be discussed.

Justice is the principle of treating all persons equally and fairly. This principle most often arises in times of short supplies or when competition for resources or benefits is occurring. This principle is used by nurse managers when they decide which staff members to promote or to recommend for professional development opportunities. The staff member's overall performance and skills should be considered rather than who may have seniority or the popular vote of his/her peer group. Justice is also encountered when deciding who should be floated to another unit/service within the institution or which staff member should be moved to a straight day position rather than remaining on a rotating schedule.

The principle of **paternalism** allows one person to make partial decisions for another and is most frequently deemed to be a negative or undesirable principle. Paternalism, however, may be used to assist persons to make decisions when they do not have sufficient data or expertise. Paternalism becomes undesirable when the entire decision is taken from the employee. Nurse managers employ this principle in a positive manner by assisting employees in deciding major career moves and plans, helping the staff member more fully understand all aspects of a possible career change, or conversely, assisting staff members comprehend why such a potential change could impact their future growth opportunities within the organization.

Fidelity means keeping one's promises or commitments. Nurse managers abide by this principle when they follow through on any promises they have previously made to employees, such as a promised leave, a certain shift to be worked, or a promotion to a preceptor position within the unit.

Many consider the principle of **respect for others** as the highest principle. Respect for others acknowledges the right of individuals to make decisions and to live by these decisions. Respect for others also transcends cultural differences, gender issues, and racial concerns and is the first principle enumerated in the American Nurses Association's *Code of Ethics for Nurses* (2001). Nurse managers positively reinforce this principle daily in their actions with employees, patients, and peers because they serve as leaders and models for staff members and others in the institution.

Codes of Ethics

Professional codes of ethics are formal statements that articulate values and beliefs of a given professional, serving as a standard of professional actions and reflecting the ethical principles shared by its members. Professional codes of ethics generally serve the following purposes:

- Inform the public of the minimum standards acceptable for conduct by members of the discipline and assist the public in understanding a discipline's professional responsibilities
- Outline the major ethical considerations of the profession
- Provide to its members guidelines for professional practice
- Serve as a guide for the discipline's self-regulation

The *Code of Ethics for Nurses* (ANA, 2001) should be the starting point for any nurse faced with an ethical issue. The first American nursing code was adopted in 1950, and it focused on the character of the nurse and the virtues that were essential to the profession. In 1968, the focus shifted to a duty-based ethical focus, and the current *Code of Ethics for Nurses* (ANA, 2001) has blended these duty-based ethics with a historical focus on character and virtue. The *Code of Ethics for Nurses* (ANA, 2001) has nine points that guide nurses in understanding the extent of their commitment to the patient, themselves, other nurses, and the nursing profession. Further provisions in the code assist nurses in understanding that patients, whether as individuals or as members of families, groups, or communities, are their first obligation and that nurses must not only ensure quality care but also protect the safety of these patients. Nurses and their nurse managers should ensure that the provisions of the code are incorporated into nursing care delivery in all clinical settings. Along with establishing the ethical standard for the disciplines, the nursing codes of ethics provide a basis for ethical analysis and decision making in clinical situations.

Ethical Decision-Making Framework

Ethical decision making involves reflection on the following:
- Who should make the choice
- Possible options or courses of action
- Available options
- Consequences, both good and bad, of all possible options
- Rules, obligations, and values that should direct choices
- Desired goals or outcomes (Guido, 2006)

When making decisions, nurses need to combine all of these elements using an orderly, systematic, and objective method; ethical decision-making models assist in accomplishing this goal.

For most nurses, ethical decision-making models are considered only when complex ethical dilemmas present in clinical settings. In truth, however, nurses use ethical decision-making models each time an ethical situation arises, although the decision-making model may not be acknowledged or fully appreciated. Ethical dilemmas involve situations in which a choice must be made between equally unacceptable alternatives that an individual perceives he or she can accept and reasonably justify on a moral plane or in which there is not a more favorable or appropriate choice that dominates the situation.

Ethical decision making is always a process. To facilitate this process, the nurse manager must use all available resources, including the institutional ethics committee, and communicate with and support all those involved in the process. Some decisions are easier to reach and support than others. Allowing sufficient time for the process contributes to a supportable option being reached.

Moral Distress

Nurses experience stress in clinical practice settings as they are confronted with situations involving ethical dilemmas. **Moral distress** most often occurs when faced with situations in which two ethical principles compete, such as when the nurse is balancing the patient's autonomy issues with attempting to do what the nurse knows is in the patient's best interest. Moral distress may occur also when the nurse manager is balancing a direct care nurse's autonomy with what the nurse manager perceives to be a better solution to an ethical dilemma. Though the dilemmas are stressful, nurses must make decisions and implement those decisions.

Seen as a major issue in nursing today, moral distress is experienced when nurses cannot provide what they perceive to be best for a given patient. Examples of moral distress include constraints caused by financial pressures, limited patient care resources, disagreements among family members regarding patient interventions, and/or limitations imposed by primary healthcare providers. Moral distress may also be experienced when actions nurses perform violate their personal beliefs.

The impact of moral distress can be quite serious. McAndrew, Leske, and Garcia (2011) reported that moral distress compromises patient care and that moral distress may be manifested in such behaviors as avoiding or withdrawing from patient care situations. Additional behaviors include failure to act as a patient advocate, which often further contributes to patient discomfort and suffering. The Literature Perspective gives additional information about the seriousness of moral distress and risk factors for ethical issues in clinical practice.

Nurse managers can best assist nurses experiencing moral distress by remembering that such distress may be lessened through adequate levels of

knowledge regarding nursing ethics and its application, acknowledging that such distress does occur, and serving as an advocate for nurses. In this latter role, the nurse manager advocates for improvement in conditions that may directly influence moral distress, such as additional staff during periods of high patient acuity, additional counselors to work with patients' family issues and disputes, and the implementation of ethical in-service education and/or education concerning better communication among all levels of healthcare practitioners. These positive aspects of leadership may significantly reduce the level of moral distress encountered by direct care nurses and greatly increase their job satisfaction.

Ethics Committees

With the increasing numbers of ethical dilemmas in patient situations and administrative decisions, healthcare providers are increasingly turning to hospital ethics committees for guidance. Such committees can provide both long-term and short-term assistance. Ethics committees provide structure and guidelines for potential problems, serve as open forums for discussion, and function as true patient advocates by placing the patient at the core of the committee discussions.

To form such a committee, the involved individuals should begin as a bioethical study group so that all potential members can explore ethical principles and theories. The composition of the committee should include nurses, physicians, clergy, clinical social workers, nutritional experts, pharmacists, administrative personnel, and legal experts. Once the committee has become active, individual patients or patients' families and additional representatives of members of the healthcare delivery team may be invited to committee deliberations.

Ethics committees traditionally follow one of three distinct structures, although some institutional committees blend the three structures. The *autonomy model* facilitates decision making for competent patients. The *patient-benefit model* uses substituted judgment (what the patient would want for himself or herself if capable of making these issues known) and facilitates decision making for the incompetent patient. The *social justice model* considers broad social issues and is accountable to the overall institution.

In most settings, the ethics committee already exists because complex issues divide healthcare

---

 LITERATURE PERSPECTIVE

Resource: Storch, J., Makaroff, K.S., Pauly, B., & Newton, L. (2013). Take me to my leader: The importance of ethical leadership among formal nurse leaders. *Nursing Ethics, 20*(2), 150-157.

Recognizing that formal nurse leaders can and should provide ethical leadership through role modeling, often nurses feel unsupported by their nurse managers. This is true even when direct care nurses undertake informal leadership roles to enhance ethical practices; these informal nurse leader actions cannot be sustained unless they are also supported by nurse managers. Thus nurse managers must begin to work toward ethical leadership by engaging in values that are clear and are shared, where these values direct ethical practice, and where individuals are allowed to express their opinions.

Implications for Practice
To meet these expectations, nurse leaders must understand the vital role they play in ethical leadership. Nurse managers should begin to engage with their fellow nurse managers to understand better ethical responsibilities and develop strategies to ensure that these responsibilities are being met.

workers. In many centers, ethical rounds, conducted weekly or monthly, allow staff members, who may later become involved in ethical decision making, to begin reviewing all the issues and to become more comfortable with ethical issues and their resolution.

Blending Ethical and Legal Issues

Blending legal demands with ethics is a challenge for nursing, and no case better portrays this type of difficult decision making than does the case of Theresa (Terri) M. Schiavo. The Case Example Box 5-6 describes this situation.

Whichever side of the case one supported, the plight of Terri Schiavo created numerous ethical concerns for the nurses caring for her and for the nurse managers in the clinical setting. Issues that created these conflicts ranged from working with feuding family members, to multiple media personnel attempting to cover the story, to constant editorial and news stories invading the privacy of this individual, to masses of people lined at the borders of the hospice center insisting that she be fed, to individual emotions about the correctness of either keeping or removing the feeding tube. One issue remains clear: the nurse managers and nurses caring for this particular patient had a legal obligation to either remove or reinsert the feeding tube based on the prevailing court decision or legislative act. Their individual reflections about the correctness or justice of such court decrees were secondary to the prevailing court orders.

Nurse managers should ensure that nurses whose ethical values differ from court orders are given

---

CASE EXAMPLE BOX 5-6

Ms. Schiavo suffered a cardiac arrest in February 1990, sustaining a period of approximately 11 minutes when she was anoxic. She was resuscitated and, at the insistence of her husband, was intubated, placed on a ventilator, and eventually received a tracheotomy. The cause of her cardiac arrest was determined to be a severe electrolyte imbalance that was directly caused by an eating disorder. In the 6 years preceding the cardiac event, Ms. Schiavo had lost approximately 140 pounds, going from 250 to 110 pounds.

During the first 2 months after her cardiac arrest, Ms. Schiavo was in a coma. She then regained some wakefulness and was eventually diagnosed as being in persistent vegetative state (PVS). She was successfully weaned from the ventilator and was able to swallow her saliva, both reflexive behaviors. However, she was not able to eat food or drink liquids, which is characteristic of PVS. A permanent feeding tube was placed so that she could receive nutrition and hydration.

Throughout the early years of her PVS, there was no challenge to the diagnosis or to the appointment of her husband as her legal guardian. Four years after her cardiac arrest, a successful lawsuit was filed against a fertility physician who failed to detect her electrolyte imbalance. A judgment of $300,000 went to her husband for loss of companionship and $700,000 was placed in a court-managed trust fund to maintain and provide care for Ms. Schiavo.

Sometime after this successful lawsuit, the close family relationship that Ms. Schiavo's husband and her parents had, began to erode and the public first became aware of Ms. Schiavo's plight. As her court-appointed guardian noted (Wolfson, 2005):

> Thereafter, what is for millions of Americans a profoundly private matter catapulted a close, loving family into an internationally watched blood feud. The end product was a most public death

for a very private individual ... Theresa was by all accounts a very shy, fun loving, and sweet woman who loved her husband and her parents very much. The family breach and public circus would have been anathema to her. (p. 17)

The court battles regarding the removal or retention of her feeding tube were numerous. There was adequate medical and legal evidence to show that Ms. Schiavo had been correctly diagnosed and that she would not have wanted to be kept alive by artificial means. Laws in the state of Florida, where Ms. Schiavo was a patient, allowed the removal of tubal nutrition and hydration in patients with PVS. The feeding tube was removed and later reinstated following a court order.

In October 2003, there was a second removal of the feeding tube after a higher court overturned the lower court decision that had caused the feeding tube to be reinserted. With this second removal, the Florida legislature passed what has become to be known as *Terri's Law*. This law gave the Florida governor the right to demand the feeding tube be reinserted and also appoint a special guardian to review the entire case. The special guardian ad litem was appointed in October 2003. Terri's Law was later declared unconstitutional by the Florida Supreme Court, and the U.S. Supreme Court refused to overrule their decision.

In early 2005, during the last weeks of Ms. Schiavo's life, the U.S. Congress attempted to move the issue to the federal rather than Florida state court system. Finally, the Federal District Court in Florida and the 11th Circuit Court of Appeals ruled that there was insufficient evidence to create a new trial, and the U.S. Supreme Court refused to review the findings of these two lower courts (Wolfson, 2005). Ms. Schiavo died on March 31, 2005; she was 41 years old.

opportunities to voice their concerns and feelings, mechanisms for requesting reassignment, and time for quiet reflection. Although no deviance can occur from one's legal obligation, the nurse manager must ensure that the emotional and psychological well-being of those he or she supervises are also recognized. Merely acknowledging that such discord can occur and allowing positive means to express this concern may be the best solution in handling these difficult legal and ethical patient situations.

Future Ethical Concerns for Nurses

Issues of concern in the near future involve autonomy and independent practice among nurses, quality of care in home and community settings, and development of nurses as leaders in the healthcare delivery field. Issues that continue to permeate ethical concerns for nurses include the patient's right to refuse health care; issues surrounding death and dying including the issues of hydration and nutrition for patients in persistent vegetative states; nurses' ability to be patient advocates in today's healthcare structure; and the ability to perform competent, quality nursing care in a system that continuously rewards cost-saving measures rather than quality healthcare delivery. As with ethical dilemmas in patient care, the more expertise and time one has to resolve issues, usually, the better the outcome. The Evidence section reinforces this need for nurse leaders to be proficient in ethical decision making.

CONCLUSION

In addition to knowing legal issues related to clinical concerns, formal leaders and managers need to know employment law, union laws, and numerous other legal findings. Though each state may have distinctive laws governing being a manager and working in a healthcare organization, the key decisions tested in court or laws that govern all healthcare operations within the United States are ones with which we must all be familiar. Legal and ethical aspects present additional opportunities for nurses to exhibit leadership capabilities.

THE SOLUTION

Staff members and nursing leadership began by working together to understand the varied viewpoints of the healthcare team. We attempted to understand why some of the primary healthcare providers allowed family members to be present and other primary healthcare providers insisted that family members not be present during resuscitation efforts. When asked, primary healthcare providers often noted that the behaviors and attitudes of the family members were a factor in their decision, and that one could not know in advance if the family members might be hostile or belligerent and thus distract or prevent the healthcare team from being able to provide necessary care. Additionally, no clear hospital policy existed, many of these primary healthcare providers were more comfortable in not having the family members present, and the current practice was to assign a chaplain and social worker to provide supportive services as well as comfort and information to family members when such situations arose. Thus the family members, though not present within the patient's room, were also not alone during this time and had the opportunity to ask questions.

We then looked at the issue from an ethical perspective. For many patients and family members, being present during this crucial time could have many positive effects, thus beneficence and respect for others were the two ethical principles that most clearly seemed to support family presence. Seeing for themselves and understanding that everything possible was being done to save their loved one's life were the most positive outcomes to support family presence. Family members could later have an opportunity to more fully question why certain aspects were performed, and the nursing staff as well as the primary care provider could then explain in more detail answers to the family members' questions.

Viewing the literature about this topic was enlightening. We discovered that this topic has continually been studied, dating back to the early 1980s. These studies almost uniformly noted that family presence did not alter the effectiveness of the healthcare team's interventions, nor did family presence interfere with the duration of resuscitative efforts or selection of medications. Some of the more recent studies addressed the issue of interference by family members and noted that very few family members were aggressive or in conflict with the team's performance and that family members excluded from being present expressed regret at not having been present during resuscitation. Interestingly, some of the reviewed studies continued to question how to best determine which family members should be given the option of viewing resuscitation measures or if all families should be given this option. At present, we continue to explore possible guidelines concerning family presence during resuscitation, recognizing that such a complex issue cannot be rapidly resolved.

—*Acacia Syring*

Would this be a suitable approach for you? Why?

THE EVIDENCE

Many of the issues challenging nurse managers and leaders in today's environment involve conflict resolution, most often involving ethical conflicts and dilemmas. The evidence, according to Keselman (2012), is that the ethical leader will develop, endorse, and support beneficial outcomes to create a healthy work environment. This demands that nurse managers and leaders have knowledge of the history of ethics so that they can have a better understanding of ethics within society and healthcare organizations and can better assist members of the healthcare team in making ethical decisions. Preventing ethical conflicts in the future will depend on the manager's knowledge and application of ethical principles, the ability to assert leadership and role modeling, periodic ethics assessment within the institution, support for ethical decision making by higher administration and the governing board of the institution, and the development of ethical policies within the institution.

Nurses need to begin now to look at the issues, professional values, and expectations they face and decide the issues they will fight for and those that are acceptable as they are. Once these issues are identified, strategies for promoting quality nursing care can be delineated.

WHAT NEW GRADUATES SAY

- I always thought ethical issues would be rare in clinical practice, but now I know that I encounter them several times each day.
- I am so glad I learned about ethics in school. Who would have thought that we use them so often in clinical settings?
- It is hard to advocate for patients when the physician does not want to listen, but I know that I must continue to advocate for what is best for the patient.
- Legal issues are easier than ethical issues. I know the right answers when it is a legal concern. I often need to ask other nurses when it is an ethical concern

CHAPTER CHECKLIST

This chapter explores multiple legal and ethical issues as they pertain to managing and leading in nursing. Legal areas that nurse managers must understand include the importance of nurse practice acts, elements of negligence and malpractice with particular emphasis on areas of potential liability for nurse managers, informed consent, and selected federal and state employment laws. Ethical areas of concern include ethical theories and principles, codes of ethics, and ethics committees. The chapter concludes with a discussion of a relevant case in which legal and ethical issues overlapped.
- Professional nursing practice
  - Nurse practice acts
  - Negligence and malpractice
  - Elements of malpractice
    - Duty owed the patient
    - Breach of the duty of care owed the patient
    - Foreseeability
  - Causation
  - Injury
  - Damages
- Liability: personal, vicarious, and corporate
- Causes of malpractice for nurse managers
  - Assignment, delegation, and supervision
  - Duty to orient, educate, and evaluate
  - Failure to warn
  - Staffing issues
- Protective and reporting laws
- Informed consent
- Privacy and confidentiality
- Policies and procedures
- Employment laws
  - Equal employment opportunity laws
  - Age discrimination in employment act of 1967
  - Americans with disabilities act of 1990
  - Affirmative action
  - Equal pay act of 1963

- Occupational safety and health act
- Family and medical leave act of 1993
- Employment-at-will and wrongful discharge
- Collective bargaining
- Patient protection and affordable care act and health care and education reconciliation act
- Professional nursing practice: ethics

- Ethical principles
- Code of ethics
- Ethical decision-making framework
- Moral distress
- Ethics committees
- Blending ethical and legal issues
- Future ethical concerns for nurses

TIPS FOR INCORPORATING LEGAL AND ETHICAL ISSUES IN PRACTICE SETTINGS

- Read the state nurse practice act, ensuring compliance with the allowable scope of practice.
- Apply legal principles in all healthcare settings.
- Understand and follow state and federal employment laws.
- Follow the *Code of Ethics for Nurses* (ANA, 2001) in all aspects of healthcare delivery.
- Remember that no right and wrong answers exist in ethical situations, merely better or worse solutions. Consider all aspects and consult with others before proceeding if there are unanswered questions.
- If legal and ethical issues are contradictory, legal aspects are enacted first.

REFERENCES

Age Discrimination in Employment Act of 1967, P.L. 90-202, 29 United States Code 621 (December 15, 1967).

American Nurses Association (ANA). (2001). *Code of ethics for nurses with interpretive statements.* Washington, DC: Author.

American Nurses Association, *Workplace violence.* (2012a). Available at http://nursingworld.org/workplaceviolence.

American Nurses Association, *Safe patient handling.* (2012b). Available at http://www.anasafepatienthandling.org.

Americans with Disabilities Act of 1990, Public Law 101-336, 104 Statutes 327 (July 26, 1990).

Americans with Disabilities Amended Act of 2008, Public Law 110-325 (September 25, 2008).

Civil Rights Act of 1964, P. L. 88-352, 78 Statutes 241, § 703 et seq. (July 2, 1964).

Civil Rights Act of 1991, P. L. 102-166 (November 21, 1991).

Department of Health and Human Services, *Quick guide to health literacy: Fact sheet.* (2012). U.S. Department of Printing and Engraving Washington, D.C.: Author.

Equal Employment Opportunity Act of 1972, 78 Statutes 253; 42 U.S.C. 2000e (March 24, 1972).

Equal Pay Act of 1963, P. L. 88-38, 77 Statutes 56 (June 10, 1963).

Estate of Travaglini v. Ingalls Health, 2009 WL 4432565 (Ill. App., November 24, 2009).

Family and Medical Leave Act of 1993, P. L. 103-3, 107 Statutes 6 (February 5, 1993).

Family and Medical Leave Amended Act of 2008, P. L. 110-181, 122 Statutes 128 (January 28, 2008).

Guido, G. W. (2006). *Legal and ethical issues in nursing* (4th ed.). Upper Saddle River NJ: Prentice Hall.

Health Care and Education Reconciliation Act of 2010, Public Law 111-152, 124 Statutes 1029 (March 30, 2010).

Health Insurance Portability and Accountability Act of 1996, Public Law 104-191, 100 Statutes 2548, (August 21, 1996).

Institute of Medicine. (1999). *To err is human: Building a safer health care system.* Washington, D.C.: The National Academies Press, Institute of Medicine.

Keselman, D. (2012). Ethical leadership. *Holistic Nursing Practice,* 26(5), 259–261.

Laurin v. Providence Hospital and Massachusetts Nurses Association, 150 F.3d 52 (1st Cir., 1998).

Marinock v. Manor at St. Luke's, 2010 WL 3233125 (Ct. Com. Pl. Luzerne Co., Pennsylvania, January 29, 2010).

Mitchell & Galle v. Winkler County et al., CV 00037-RAJ, Document 42, Winkler County Trail Court, filed April 18, 2010.

Martell v. Tarpon Springs Hospital, 2010 WL 5485106 (Cir. Ct. Pinellas Co., Florida, September 29, 2010).

Massey v. Mercy Medical Center, 180 Cal. App. 4th 690, 103 Cal. Rept. 3d 209 (Cal. App., December 22, 2009).

Mauro v. Borgess Medical Center, 4:94 CV 05 (Mich., 1995).

McAndrew, N. S., Leske, J. S., & Garcia, A. (2011). Influence of moral distress on the professional practice environment during prognostic conflict in critical care. *Journal of Trauma Nursing,* 18(4), 221–230.

Moschke v. Memorial Medical Center of West Michigan, 2003 WL 462374 (Mich. App., February 21, 2003).

National Federation of Independent Businesses v. Sebelius, Secretary of Health and Human Services, et al., No. 11-393 (June 28, 2012).

National Labor Relations Act, P. L. 74-198, 49 Statutes 449 (July 5, 1935).

Occupational Safety and Health Administration Act of 1970, P. L. 91-595, 84 Statutes 1590 (December 29, 1970).

O'Shea v. State of New York, WL 1516492 (N.Y. Ct. Cl., January 22, 2007).

Painter, L. M., Dudjak, L. A., Kidwell, K. M., Simmons, R. L., & Kidwell, R. P. (2011). The nurse's role in the causation of compensable injury. *Journal of Nursing Care Quality, 26*(4), 311–319.

Patient Protection and Affordable Care Act of 2010, Public Law 111-148, 124 Statutes 896 (March 23, 2010).

Potter, P., Deshields, T., & Kuhrik, M. (2010). Delegation practices between registered nurses and nursing assistive personnel. *Journal of Nursing Management, 18*, 157–165.

Protection of Human Subjects, 45 Code of Federal Regulations, Sec. 46.111, 46.101(b), 46.110, 46.116 (1991).

Protection of Human Subjects, 45 Code of Federal Regulations, Sec. 46.401 et seq. (1998).

Registered Nurse Safe Staffing Act of 2011. United States House Bill 876/United States Senate Bill 58. Retrieved from http://legiscan.com/US/comments/HB876/2011; http://legiscan.com/US/bill/SB58/2011.

Sabol v. Richmond Heights General Hospital, 676 N. E.2d 958 (Ohio App. 1996).

Safe Nurse Staffing Legislation, Washington State HB 3123 (March, 2008).

Trombley v. Southwestern Vermont Medical Center, 738 A.2d 103 (Vt., 1999).

Vietnam Era Veterans' Readjustment Assistance Act of 1974, 38 United States Code § 4212 (1974).

Watkins v. Unemployment Compensation Board of Review, 689 A.2d 1019 (Pa. Commonwealth, 1997).

Wellstar Health System, Inc. v. Green, WL 31324127 (Ga. App., October 18, 2002).

Wolfson, J. (2005). Erring on the side of Theresa Schiavo: Reflections of the special guardian ad litem. *The Hastings Center Report, 35*(3), 16–19.

Yoder-Wise, P. (2010). More serendipity: The Winkler County trial. *The Journal of Continuing Education in Nursing, 41*(4), 147–148.

Zamudio v. Patia, 956 F. Supp. 803 (N.D. Ill., 1997).

SUGGESTED READINGS

ANA/AONE Principles for collaborative relationships between clinical nurses and nurse managers. (2012). *Nurse Leader, 10*(3), 17–18.

Beauchamp, T. L., & Childress, J. E. (2009). *Principles of biomedical ethics* (6th ed.). New York: Oxford University Press.

Burston, A. S., & Tuckett, A. G. (2013). Moral distress in nursing: Contributing factors, outcomes, and interventions. *Nursing Ethics, 20*(3), 312–324.

Jones, F., Podila, P., & Powers, C. (2013). Creating a culture of safety in the emergency department. *Journal of Nursing Administration, 43*(4), 194–200.

Patient information on Facebook traced to temporary staff. (2012). *Healthcare Risk Management, 34*(3), 25–27.

Pavlish, C., Brown-Saltzman, K., Hersh, M., Shirk, M., & Nudelman, O. (2011). Early indicators and risk factors for ethical issues in clinical practice. *Journal of Nursing Scholarship, 43*(1), 13–21.

Plawecki, L. H., & Amrhein, D. W. (2010). Legal issues: A question of delegation: Unlicensed assistive personnel and the professional nurse. *Journal of Gerontological Nursing, 36*(8), 18–21.

Making Decisions and Problem Solving

Sylvain Trepanier, Jeannette T. Crenshaw

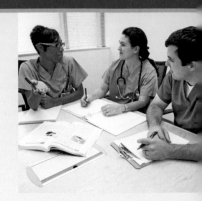

This chapter explores the stages of the decision-making and problem-solving processes and describes the analytical tools used in the application of these processes. Strategies for both individual and group decision making are addressed.

LEARNING OUTCOMES

- Apply a decision-making model to create the best option to solve a problem.
- Evaluate the effect of faulty information gathering on a decision-making experience.
- Analyze the decision-making style of a nurse leader/manager.
- Critique resources on the Internet that focus on critical thinking.

KEY TERMS

autocratic	decision making	problem solving
creativity	optimizing	satisficing
critical thinking	optimizing decision	satisficing decision

Vickie Lemmon, RN, MSN
Director of Clinical Strategies, Operations WellPoint Inc.
Ventura, California

Healthcare managers today are faced with numerous and complex issues that pertain to providing quality services for patients within a resource-scarce environment. Stress levels among staff can escalate when problems are not resolved, leading to a decrease in morale, productivity, and quality service. This was the situation I encountered in my previous job as administrator for California Children Services (CCS). When I began my tenure as the new CCS administrator, staff expressed frustration and dissatisfaction with staffing, workload, and team communications. This was evidenced by high staff turnover, lack of teamwork, customer complaints, unmet deadlines for referral and enrollment cycle times, and poor documentation. The team was in crisis, characterized by infighting, blaming, lack of respectful communication, and lack of commitment to program goals and objectives. I had not worked as a case manager in this program. It was hard for me to determine how to address the problems the staff presented to me. I wanted to be fair but thought that I did not have enough information to make immediate changes. My challenge was to lead this team to greater compliance with state-mandated performance measures.

What do you think you would do if you were this nurse?

INTRODUCTION

Problem solving and decision making are essential skills for effective nursing practice. As one of the contributors to this book often says, "All the easy decisions have already been made." So, the challenges we face often are complex, have critical consequences, require thoughtful consideration, and reflect on us as leaders. These problem-solving and decision-making processes not only are involved in managing and delivering care, but also are essential for engaging in planned change. Technologic, social, political, and economic changes have dramatically affected health care and nursing. Increased patient acuity, shorter hospital stays, shortage of healthcare providers, increased technology, greater emphasis on quality and patient safety, value-based purchasing, "pay for performance," and the continuing shift from inpatient to ambulatory and home health care are some of the changes that require nurses to make rational and valid decisions and identify solutions to problems precipitated by change. Moreover, increased diversity in patient populations, employment settings, and types of healthcare providers requires efficient and effective decision making and problem solving. More emphasis is now placed on recognizing patients as the source of control and as full partners in decision making (shared decision making) and problem solving with interprofessional teams to achieve evidence-based results.

Nurses must possess the basic knowledge and skills required for effective decision making and problem solving. These competencies are especially important for nurses with leadership and management responsibilities.

DIFFERENTIATION OF DECISION MAKING AND PROBLEM SOLVING

Decision making and *problem solving* are not synonymous terms. However, the processes for engaging in decision making and problem solving are similar. Both skills require **critical thinking,** which is a high-level cognitive process, and both can be improved with practice.

Decision making is a purposeful and goal-directed effort that uses a systematic process to choose among options. Some decisions are not prompted by a problem. The hallmark of any type of decision making is the identification and selection of options or alternatives.

Problem solving, which includes a decision-making step, is focused on trying to resolve an issue that can be viewed as the gap between "what currently is" and "the best available option." Often the "what currently is" can be seen as a problem.

Effective decision making and problem solving are based on an individual's ability to think critically. Although critical thinking has been defined in numerous ways, The Critical Thinking Community (2011) defines critical thinking as " a mode of thinking, about any subject, content, or problem, in which the thinker improves the quality of his or her thinking by skillfully analyzing, assessing, and reconstructing it. Critical thinking is self-directed, self-disciplined, self-monitored, and self-corrective thinking." Effective critical thinkers are self-aware individuals who strive to improve their reasoning abilities by asking "why," "what," or "how." A nurse who questions why a patient is restless is thinking critically. Compare the analytical abilities of a nurse who assumes a patient is restless because of anxiety related to an upcoming procedure with those of a nurse who asks if there could be another explanation and proceeds to investigate possible causes. It is important for nurse leaders and managers to assess staff members' ability to think critically and enhance their knowledge and skills through staff-development programs, coaching, and role modeling. Establishing a healthy work environment can promote staff members' ability to think critically.

Creativity is essential for the generation of options or solutions. Creative individuals can conceptualize new and innovative approaches to a problem or issue by employing flexible and independent thinking. It takes just one person to plant a seed for new ideas to generate.

The model depicted in Figure 6-1 demonstrates the relationship among related concepts such as professional judgment, decision making, problem solving, creativity, and critical thinking. Sound clinical judgment requires critical or reflective thinking. Critical thinking is the concept that interweaves and links the other concepts together. An individual, through the application of critical-thinking skills, engages in decision making and problem solving in an environment that may have the effect of either promoting or inhibiting these skills. It is the nurse leader's and manager's task to model these skills and promote the use of these skills by others.

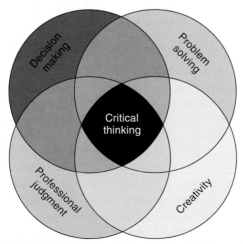

FIGURE 6-1 Problem-solving and decision-making model.

DECISION MAKING

The phases of the decision-making process include defining objectives, generating options, identifying advantages and disadvantages of each option, ranking the options, selecting the option most likely to achieve the predefined objectives, implementing the option, and evaluating the result. Box 6-1 contains a form that can be used to complete these steps. The challenge in this work is weighing the advantages and disadvantages.

Poor-quality decision making is likely if objectives are not clearly identified or if objectives are inconsistent with the values of the individual or organization. Lewis Carroll illustrates the essential step of defining the goal, purpose, or objectives in the following excerpt from *Alice's Adventures in Wonderland:*

> One day Alice came to a fork in the road and saw a Cheshire Cat in a tree. "Which road do I take?" she asked. His response was a question: "Where do you want to go?" "I don't know," Alice answered. "Then," said the cat, "it doesn't matter."

Decision Models

The decision model that a nurse uses depends on specific circumstances. Is the situation routine and predictable, or complex and uncertain? Is the goal to make a decision that is "just good enough" (conservative) or one that is optimal?

If the situation is fairly routine, nurse leaders and managers can use a normative or prescriptive approach. Agency policy, standard procedures, and

BOX 6-1   DECISION-MAKING FORMAT

Objective: _____

OPTIONS	ADVANTAGES	DISADVANTAGES	RANKING

Add more rows as necessary. Rank the priority of options, with "1" being most preferred. Select the best option.

Implementation plan: _____

Evaluation plan: _____

analytical tools can be applied to situations that are structured and in which options and outcomes are known.

If the situation is subjective, non-routine, and unstructured or if outcomes are unknown or unpredictable, the nurse leader and manager may need to take a different approach. In this case, a descriptive or behavioral approach is required. More information will be needed to be gathered to address the situation effectively. Creativity, experience, and group process are useful in dealing with the unknown. In these situations, it is especially important for nurse leaders to seek expert opinion and involve key stakeholders.

Another strategy is satisficing. With this approach, the decision maker selects an acceptable solution, one that may minimally meet the objective or standard for a decision. This approach allows for quick decisions and may be the most appropriate when lack of time is an issue.

Optimizing is a decision style in which the decision maker selects the option that is best, based on an analysis of the pros and cons associated with each option. A better decision is more likely using this approach, although it takes longer to arrive at a decision.

For example, a young nurse contemplates seeking employment in one of three places: an acute care hospital in the city, a community health organization, or a rural, comprehensive clinic/hospital. A satisficing decision might result if the nurse picked the rural hospital that offered a decent salary and benefit packet or the position closest to home. However, an optimizing decision is more likely to occur if the nurse lists the pros and cons of each position being considered, such as salary, benefits, opportunities for advancement, staff development, mentorship programs, and career goals.

Decision-Making Styles

The decision-making style of a nurse manager can be conceptualized using three distinct models: paternalistic, informative, and shared decision making (Moreau et al., 2012). In the paternalistic model the managers decide what is best for their team. The informative model offers the staff the ability to make a decision after the information has been shared and without the active involvement of the manager. In a shared decision model, the decisions are made through an interactive, deliberate process and the staff may express and discuss options and preferences. The shared decision model has been shown to increase work performance and productivity, decrease employee turnover, and enhance employee satisfaction. Managers need to involve nursing personnel in decisions that affect patient care. One mechanism for doing so is by including nursing representation on various committees or task forces.

The autocratic decision-making method results in more rapid decision making and is appropriate in crisis situations. However, followers are generally more satisfied with a shared decision-making approach. Although this approach takes more time, it is more appropriate when conflict is likely to occur or when the problem is unstructured.

Any decision style can be used appropriately or inappropriately. Like the tenets of situational leadership theory, the situation and circumstances should dictate which decision-making style is most appropriate. A Code Blue is not the time for managers to democratically solicit volunteers for chest compressions!

EXERCISE 6-1

Interview colleagues about their most preferred decision-making model and style. What barriers or obstacles to effective decision making have your colleagues encountered? What strategies are used to increase the effectiveness of the decisions made? Based on your interview, is the model effective? Why or why not?

Factors Affecting Decision Making

Numerous factors affect individuals and groups in the decision-making process. In the now classic work, Tanner (2006) conducted an extensive review of the literature to develop a Clinical Judgment Model. Out of the research, she concluded that five principle factors influence decision making. (See the Literature Perspective on p. 104.)

Internal and external factors can influence how a situation is perceived. Internal factors include variables such as the decision maker's physical and emotional state, personal philosophy, biases, values, interests, experience, knowledge, attitudes, and risk-seeking or risk-avoiding behaviors. External factors include environmental conditions, time, and resources. Decision-making options are externally limited when time is short or when the environment is characterized by a "we've always done it this way" attitude.

LITERATURE PERSPECTIVE

Resource: Tanner, C.A. (2006). Thinking like a nurse: A research-based model of clinical judgment in nursing. *Journal of Nursing Education, 45*(6), 204-211.

Tanner engaged in an extensive review of 200 studies focusing on clinical judgment and clinical decision making to derive a model of clinical judgment that can be used as a framework for instruction. The first review summarized 120 articles and was published in 1998. The 2006 article reviewed an additional 71 studies published since 1998. Based on an analysis of the entire set of articles, Tanner proposed five conclusions, which are listed below. Refer to the article for detailed explanation of each of the five conclusions.

The author considers clinical judgment as a "problem-solving activity." She notes that the terms "clinical judgment," "problem solving," "decision making," and "critical thinking" are often used interchangeably. For the purpose of aiding in the development of the model, Tanner defined clinical judgment as actions taken based on the assessment of the patient's needs. Clinical reasoning is the process by which nurses make their judgments (e.g., the decision-making process of selecting the most appropriate option) (Tanner, 2006, p. 204):

- Clinical judgments are more influenced by what nurses bring to the situation than the objective data about a situation.
- Sound clinical judgment rests, to some degree, on knowing the patient and the patient's typical pattern of responses, as well as engaging with the patient and identifying the patient's concerns.
- Clinical judgments are influenced by the context in which a situation occurs and the culture of the nursing care unit.
- Nurses use a variety of reasoning patterns alone or in combination.
- Reflection on practice is often triggered by a breakdown in clinical judgment and is critical for the development of clinical knowledge and improvement in clinical reasoning.

The Clinical Judgment Model involves four steps that are similar to decision-making and problem-solving steps described in this chapter. The model starts with a phase called "noticing." In this phase, the nurse comes to expect certain responses resulting from knowledge gleaned from similar patient situations, experiences, and knowledge. External factors influence nurses in this phase, such as the complexity of the environment and values and typical practices within the unit culture.

The second phase of the model is "interpreting," during which the nurse understands that a situation requires a response. The nurse employs various reasoning patterns to make sense of the issue and to derive an appropriate action plan.

The third phase is "responding," during which the nurse decides on the best option for handling the situation. This is followed by the fourth phase, "reflecting," during which the nurse assesses the patient's responses to the actions taken.

Tanner emphasized that "reflection-in-action" and "reflection-on-action" are major processes required in the model. Reflection-in-action is real-time reflection on the patient's responses to nursing action with modifications to the plan based on the ongoing assessment. On the other hand, reflection-on-action is a review of the experience, which promotes learning for future similar experiences.

Implications for Practice
Nurse educators and managers can use the Clinical Judgment Model with new and experienced nurses to help them understand more about the thought processes involved in decision making. For example, nurses can be encouraged to maintain reflective journals to record observations and impressions from clinical experiences. In clinical post-conferences or staff development meetings, the nurse manager can engage nurses in applying Tanner's five conclusions to their "lived" experiences. The ultimate goal of analyzing their decisions and decision-making processes is to improve clinical judgment, problem-solving, decision-making, and critical thinking skills.

Values affect all aspects of decision making, from the statement of the problem/issue through the evaluation. Values, which are influenced by an individual's cultural, social, and philosophical background, provide the foundation for one's ethical stance. The steps for engaging in ethical decision making are similar to the steps in other decision-making models. However, in ethical decision making, alternatives or options identified in the decision-making process are evaluated with the use of ethical resources. The resources that can facilitate ethical decision making include institutional policy; principles such as autonomy, nonmaleficence, beneficence, veracity, paternalism, respect, justice, and fidelity; personal judgment; trusted co-workers; institutional ethics committees; and legal precedent. The *Guide to the Code of Ethics for Nurses: Interpretation and Application* (American Nurses Association, 2010) provides guidance to this model.

Risk-taking is an essential competency for nurse leaders and influences effective decision making and problem solving. The work environment affects whether one is willing to take risks. According to Crenshaw and Yoder-Wise (2013), effective nurse leaders create a work environment that welcomes considered risk taking and encourages employees to share and discuss new and innovative ideas. This type of environment enables effective decision making and problem solving. Certain personality factors, such as self-esteem and self-confidence, also affect whether one is willing to take risks in solving problems or making decisions. Similarly, the work group, peers, and others can influence how decisions are made. For example, are you inclined to make decisions to satisfy people to whom you are accountable or from whom you feel social pressure?

Characteristics of an effective decision maker include courage, a willingness to take considered risks, self-awareness, energy, creativity, sensitivity, and flexibility. Ask yourself, "Do I prefer to let others make the decisions? Am I more comfortable in the role of 'follower' than leader? If so, what might be the reasons? Am I able to assume the role of leader if no leader emerges?"

EXERCISE 6-2

Identify a current or past situation that involved resource allocation, an end-of-life issues, conflict among healthcare providers or patient/family/significant others, or some other ethical dilemma. Describe how internal and external factors influenced the decision options, the option selected, and the outcome.

Group Decision Making

Two primary criteria make for effective decisions. First, the decision must be of a high quality; that is, it achieves the predefined goals, objectives, and outcomes. Second, those who are responsible for its implementation must accept the decision.

Higher-quality decisions are more likely to result if groups are involved in the decision-making and problem-solving process. In reality, with the increased focus on quality and safety, decisions cannot be made alone. When team members are included in the process, they tend to function more productively and the quality of decisions is generally superior. Taking ownership of the process and outcome provides a smoother transition. Interprofessional teams should be used in the decision-making process, especially if the issue, options, or outcome involves other healthcare professionals.

Research findings suggest that groups are more likely to be effective if members are actively involved, the group is cohesive, communication is encouraged, and members demonstrate some understanding of the group process. In deciding to use the group process

for decision making, consider group size and composition. If the group is too small, a limited number of options will be generated and fewer points of view expressed. Conversely, if the group is too large, it may lack structure, and consensus becomes more difficult. Homogeneous groups may be more compatible; however, heterogeneous groups may be more successful in problem solving. The most productive groups are those that are moderately cohesive. In other words, divergent thinking is useful to create the best decision.

For groups to be able to work effectively, the group facilitator or leader should carefully select members on the basis of their knowledge and skills in decision making and problem solving. Individuals who are aggressive, are authoritarian, or manifest self-serving behaviors tend to decrease the effectiveness of groups.

The nurse leader or manager should provide a nonthreatening and positive environment in which group members are encouraged to participate actively. Using tact and diplomacy, the facilitator can minimize the effect of aggressive individuals who may attempt to monopolize the discussion and can encourage more passive individuals to contribute by asking direct, open-ended questions. Providing positive feedback such as "You raised an interesting point," protecting members and their suggestions from attack, and keeping the group focused on a task are strategies that create an environment conducive to problem solving.

Advantages of Group Decision Making

The advantages of group decision making are numerous. The adage "two heads are better than one" illustrates that when individuals with different knowledge, skills, and resources collaborate to solve a problem or make a decision, the likelihood of a quality outcome is increased. More ideas can be generated by groups and have a synergistic effect. In addition, when followers are directly involved in the process, they are more apt to accept the decision, because they have an increased sense of ownership and commitment to the decision. Implementing solutions becomes easier when individuals have been actively involved in the decision-making process. Involvement can be enhanced by making information readily available to the appropriate personnel, requesting input, establishing committees and task forces with broad representation, and using group decision-making techniques.

The group leader must establish with the participants what decision procedure will be followed. Will the group strive to achieve consensus, or will the majority prevail? In determining which decision rule to use, the group leader should consider the necessity for quality and acceptance of the decision. Achieving both a high-quality and an acceptable decision is possible, but more time and engagement, and approval from individuals affected by the decision, are required.

Groups will be more committed to an idea if it is achieved by consensus rather than as an outcome of individual decision making or as a majority decision. Consensus requires that all participants agree to go along with the final decision. However, achieving consensus does not mean that the final decision will be all participants' "first choice." When striving for consensus, ask group members if they "can live" with the decision. Achieving consensus requires considerable time. However, consensus leads to both high-quality and high-acceptance decisions and reduces the risk of sabotage.

Majority rule can be used to compromise when 100% agreement cannot be achieved. This method saves time, but the solution may only partially achieve the goals of quality and acceptance. In addition, majority rule carries certain risks. First, if the informal group leaders agree with the minority opinion, they may not support the decision of the majority. Disgruntled members may build coalitions to gain support for their position and block the majority choice. After all, the majority may represent only 51% of the group. In addition, group members may support the position of the formal leader because they fear reprisal or they wish to obtain the leader's approval. In general, as the importance of the decision increases, so does the percentage of group members required to approve and implement it.

To secure the support of the group, the leader should maintain open communication with those affected by the decision and be honest about the advantages and disadvantages of the decision. If possible, the leader should also demonstrate how the advantages outweigh the disadvantages. The leader should also suggest ways the unwanted outcomes can be minimized and be available to assist when necessary. Decisions may result in some group members gaining something valued and some group members losing something valued. Loss should be discussed opening and honestly.

Challenges of Group Decision Making

Although group decision making and problem solving have distinct advantages, involving groups also carries certain disadvantages and may not be appropriate in all situations. The time required for making group decisions and for achieving consensus may not be appropriate, especially in a time sensitive situation requiring prompt decisions. In addition, some decision may have been made at the organizational level and discussing the decision as though other options were possible is counter-productive.

Another disadvantage of group decision making relates to unequal power among group members. Dominant personality types may influence passive or less influential group members to conform to their points of view. Furthermore, individuals may expend considerable time and energy defending their positions, resulting in the primary objective of the group effort being lost.

Groups may be more concerned with maintaining group harmony than engaging in active discussion on the issue and generating creative ideas to address it. Group members who manifest a groupthink mentality may be so concerned with avoiding conflict and supporting their leader and other members that important issues or concerns are not raised. Failure to bring up options, explore conflict, or challenge the status quo results in ineffective group functioning and decision outcomes.

Strategies

Strategies to minimize the problems encountered with group decision making and problem solving include techniques such as brainstorming, nominal group techniques, focus groups, and the Delphi technique.

Brainstorming can be an effective method for generating a large volume of creative options. Often, the premature critiquing of ideas stifles creativity, idea generation, and innovation. When members use inflammatory statements, euphemistically referred to as *killer phrases,* the usual response is for members to stop contributing. Some killer phrases are "It will never work," "Administration won't go for it," "What a dumb idea," "It's not in the budget," "If it ain't broke, don't fix it," and "We tried that before."

The hallmark of effective brainstorming is to list all ideas as stated without critique or discussion. The group leader or facilitator should encourage people to build upon or spin off ideas from those already suggested. One idea may be piggybacked on others. Ideas should not be judged, nor should the relative merits or disadvantages of the ideas be discussed while brainstorming. The goal is to generate ideas, no matter how seemingly unrealistic or absurd. It is important for the group leader or facilitator to cut off criticism and be alert for nonverbal behaviors signaling disapproval. Because the emphasis is on the volume of ideas generated, not necessarily the quality, solutions may be superficial and fail to solve the problem. Group brainstorming also takes longer, and the logistics of getting people together may pose a problem. If the facilitator allows the group to establish the rules for discussion, the aspects that impede open discussion often are eliminated by the group's norms or agreements of participation.

The **nominal group technique** allows group members the opportunity to provide input into the decision-making process. Participants are asked to not talk to each other as they write down their ideas to solve a predefined problem or issue. After a period of silent generation of ideas, generally no more than 10 minutes, each member is asked to share an idea, which is displayed on a flip chart. Comments and elaboration are not allowed during this phase. Each member takes a turn sharing one idea each until all ideas are presented, after which, discussion is allowed. Members may "pass" if they have exhausted their list of ideas. During the next step, ideas are clarified and the merits of each idea are discussed. In the third and final step, each member privately assigns a priority rank to each option. Group members can then place colored stickers on the flip chart next to their first, second, and third choices or they may use pieces of paper to record their choices. The solution chosen is the option that receives the highest ranking by the majority of participants. The advantage of this technique is that it allows equal participation among members and minimizes the influence of dominant personalities. The disadvantages of this method are that it is time-consuming and requires advance preparation. A similar process can be facilitated via the use of web conferencing technologies.

The purpose of **focus groups** is to explore issues and generate information. Focus groups can be used to identify problems or to evaluate the effects of an intervention. The groups meet face-to-face to discuss issues. Under the direction of a moderator or facilitator, participants are able to validate or disagree with ideas expressed. Depending on the purpose of a focus group, it may be helpful for an objective individual to facilitate the discussion (e.g., someone other than the manager). Because the interaction is face-to-face, potential disadvantages include the logistics of getting people together, time, and issues related to group dynamics. Nevertheless, if managed effectively, the experience can yield valuable information.

Another group decision-making strategy is the **Delphi technique**. It involves systematically collecting and summarizing opinions and judgments on a particular issue from respondents, such as members of expert panels, through interviews, surveys, or questionnaires. Opinions of the respondents are repeatedly reported back to them with a request to provide more refined opinions and rationales on the issue or matter under consideration. Between each round, the results are tabulated and analyzed so that the findings can be reported to the participants. This allows the participants to reconsider their responses. The goal is to achieve a consensus.

Different variations on the Delphi technique exist. The procedure includes anonymous feedback, multiple rounds, and statistical analyses. One advantage of this technique is the ability to involve a large number of respondents, because the participants do not need to physically convene. Indeed, participants may be located throughout the country or world. Also, the questionnaire or survey requires little time commitment on the part of the participants. This technique may actually save time because it eliminates the off-the-subject digressions typically encountered in face-to-face meetings. In addition, the Delphi technique prevents the negative or unproductive verbal and nonverbal interactions that can occur when groups work together. Although the Delphi technique has its advantages, using it may result in a lower sense of accomplishment and involvement because the participants are detached from the overall process and do not communicate with each other.

Nursing lore places value on actions based on intangible and invisible "gut feeling" responses, referred to as *nursing intuition*. What is nursing intuition? Like critical thinking, many definitions exist. Nursing intuition is a valid form of knowledge (see the Literature

Perspective that follows). Green (2012) describes four component of nursing intuition:

- Embodied knowledge (e.g., like riding a bicycle)
- Highly attuned sensory perception of complex (and sometimes rapidly changing) situations
- Conceptual knowledge
- Consistent efforts to achieve the best patient outcomes

LITERATURE PERSPECTIVE

Resource: Pretz, J.E., & Folse, V.N. (2011). Nursing experience and preference for intuition in decision making. *Journal of Clinical Nursing, 20,* 2878-2889.

Pretz and Folse (2011) conducted a study aimed at answering two primary questions: Is preference for intuition a construct that transcends all domains and areas of life or is it a more domain-specific construct? Is preference for intuition strengthened with increased experience in the domain? The authors invited nurses (n = 145, 78% females) to complete a secured online survey. Of the participants, 78 had completed a bachelor's degree; 49, master's; 6, doctorate; 1 associate's; and 1, diploma program. The authors used the following instruments: Rational-Experiential Inventory (REI); Myers-Briggs Type Indicator® (MBTI); Types of Intuition Scale (TIntS); Miller Intuitiveness Instrument; Acknowledges Use of Intuition in Nursing Scale; and Smith Intuition Instrument. Using multiple step regressions, relationships were examined.

Experience was associated to preference for nursing intuition ($p<.001$). Students were less "innovative" and "willing to act" on intuition than nurses with 4 or more years of experience ($p=.053$). In addition, nurses with experience had a stronger preference for intuition in nursing and this preference also extended to other areas of life. The analysis offered two types of nursing intuition: skilled innovator and physical/spiritual. Further research is required to identify whether a specific type of nursing intuition may be associated with improved clinical outcomes.

Implications for Practice

Helping experienced nurses share how they developed their intuition with less experienced nurses may move that group to greater levels of intuition. Providing opportunities to test intuitive thinking with an experienced nurse may also help develop the experiences that contribute to intuition.

Decision-Making Tools

Nurse leaders and managers can use a variety of decision-making tools such as decision grids and Strength, Weakness, Opportunity, Threat (SWOT) analyses in the decision-making process. These tools are most appropriately used when information is available and options are known. To be part of the solution, followers must be a part of making the decisions.

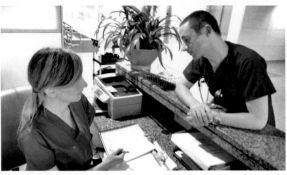

To be part of the solution, followers must be a part of making the decisions.

Decision grids facilitate the visualization of the options under consideration and allow comparison of options using common criteria. Criteria, which are determined by the decision makers, may include time required, ethical or legal considerations, equipment needs, and cost (Figure 6-2). The relative advantages and disadvantages should be listed for each option. For example, the manager of a hospital education department is assessing whether it is better to retain the services of an outside consultant to coordinate an advanced cardiac life support (ACLS) course in the hospital, pay the per-person fees to send the staff to another hospital for the training, or train staff in the agency as ACLS instructors to be able to provide the training in-house. The type of information this manager might compile includes a breakdown of the costs for the three options, equipment needs, benefits of each option, the number of nurses needing the course, future training needs, and feasibility of training hospital staff to conduct the course.

A SWOT analysis is commonly used in strategic planning or marketing efforts but can also be used by individuals and groups in decision making. Using the SWOT analysis, the individual or team lists the Strengths, Weaknesses, Opportunities, and Threats related to the situation under consideration. Strengths and weaknesses are internal to the individual, group, or organization, whereas the opportunities and threats are external factors (Manktelow & Carlson, 2013). For example, Estella has worked in a medical-surgical unit for 5 years and is considering whether to request a transfer to the intensive care unit (ICU). Box 6-2 is a

Options Under Consideration	Time	Cost	Legal/Ethical Considerations	Equipment Needed

FIGURE 6-2 Decision grid.

BOX 6-2 SWOT ANALYSIS

Strengths
- Familiar with the healthcare system
- Clinically competent and has received favorable performance appraisals
- Good communication skills; well liked by her peers
- Recently completed 12-lead electrocardiogram (ECG) interpretation class

Weaknesses
- Has not attended the critical care class
- Has had a prior unresolved conflict with one of the surgeons who frequently admits to the intensive care unit (ICU)
- Is uncertain whether she wants to work full-time, 12-hour shifts

Opportunities
- Anticipated staff openings in the ICU in the next several months
- Critical care course will be offered in 1 month
- Advanced cardiac life support (ACLS) course is offered four time a year
- A friend who already works in ICU has offered to mentor her

Threats
- Possible bed closures in another critical care unit may result in staff transfers, thus eliminating open positions
- Another medical-surgical nurse is also interested in transferring

SWOT analysis outlining potential or actual strengths, weaknesses, opportunities, and threats.

Examples of decision-making tools can be viewed in the Internet Resources section on p. 116. One of the Internet resources, *http://www.mindtools.com*—a commercial Website—provides links to software and other resources. Many of the tools are free to download. Click on the links to "Decision Making" and/or "Problem Solving."

EXERCISE 6-3

Design a decision grid for a current situation you are experiencing. Identify the components you need to explore in the decision-making process, such as cost, time, resources, advantages, and disadvantages, for the various options you are considering.

PROBLEM SOLVING

As Albert Einstein allegedly said, "If I were given one hour to save the planet, I would spend 59 minutes defining the problem and one minute resolving it." Thus the effective leader anticipates problems and develops methods for dealing with them. The leader of

group who defines the problem well has the potential to create a solid solution.

Problem solving includes the decision-making process; the trigger for action is the existence of a "problem" or issue. Before attempting to solve a problem, a nurse must ask certain key questions:

1. Is it important?
2. Do I want to do something about it? (e.g., Do I "own" the problem?)
3. Am I qualified to handle it?
4. Do I have the authority to do anything?
5. Do I have the knowledge, interest, time, and resources to deal with it?
6. Can I delegate it to someone else?
7. What benefits will be derived from solving it?

If the answers to questions 1 through 5 are "no," why waste time, resources, and personal energy? At this juncture, a conscious decision is made to ignore the problem, refer or delegate it to others, or consult or collaborate with others to solve it. On the other hand, if the answers are "yes," the nurse leader or manager chooses to accept the problem and assume responsibility for it.

After identifying the problem, nurse leaders and managers must decide whether the problem is within their control and whether it is significant enough to require intervention. Sometimes individuals believe they need to "solve" every problem brought to their attention. Some situations, such as some interpersonal conflicts, are best resolved by the individuals who own the problem. Known as *purposeful inaction,* a "do nothing" approach might be indicated when other persons should resolve problems or when the problem is beyond one's control. Consider the following scenario:

Mary complains to the nurse manager that Sam, a fellow nurse, was rude and abrupt with her when passing in the hall. How should the nurse manager handle Mary's complaint? Should the manager discuss the problem with Sam? Should Mary be present during the discussion? What are the possible risks or benefits of such an approach? Alternatively, should the manager assist Mary in developing her communication skills so that Mary can address the problem herself?

EXERCISE 6-4

Using the decision-making format presented in Box 6-1 on p. 102, list other options for this scenario and the advantages and disadvantages of each approach. Rank the options in order of most desirable to least desirable and select the best option. Determine how you would implement and evaluate the chosen option.

Some decisions are "givens" because they are based on firmly established criteria in the institution, which may be based on the traditions, values, doctrines, culture, or policy of the organization. Every manager has to live with mandates from persons higher in the organizational structure. Although managers may not have the authority to control certain situations, they may be able to influence the outcome. For example, because of losses in revenue, administration has decided to eliminate the clinical educator positions in a home health agency and place the responsibility for clinical education with the senior home health nurses. It is beyond the manager's control to reverse this decision. Nevertheless, the manager can explore the nurses' fear and concerns regarding this change and facilitate the transition by preparing them for the new role.

In these examples, it is a misnomer to refer to the approach as *do nothing,* because there is deliberate action on the part of the manager. This approach should not be confused with the laissez-faire (hands off) approach taken by a manager who chooses to do nothing when intervention is indicated. Rather, a conscious decision was made.

Problem-Solving Process

Several models or approaches to problem solving exist. A problem-definition model is illustrated in Figure 6-3. In this figure, a series of questions is provided to help the nurse leader or manager increase the likelihood of successfully defining a problem by finding the best solution. (See the following Research Perspective.)

RESEARCH PERSPECTIVE

Resource: Spradlin, D. (2012). Are you solving the right problem? *Harvard Business Review, 90*(9), 85-93.

Spradlin (2012) reported that energy should be focused on defining a problem to ensure a suitable solution. In fact, failure to correctly define a problem may result in a team trying to solve the wrong problem. He further explains the importance of asking questions until you get to the root cause of a problem. In order to ensure a successful process, Spradlin offers a four-step model: establish the need for a solution, justify the need, contextualize the problem, and write a problem statement. In order to use all of the four steps, he offers sample questions to ensure success:
- What is the basic need?
- What is the desired outcome?
- Who stands to benefit and why?
- Is the effort aligned with our strategy?
- What are the desired benefits for the company, and how will we measure them?
- How will we ensure that a solution is implemented?
- What approaches have we tried?
- What have others tried?
- What are the internal and external constraints on implementing a solution?
- Is the problem actually many problems?
- What requirements must a solution meet?
- Which problem solvers should we engage?
- What do solvers need to submit?

Implications for Practice
Expert clinicians such as clinical nurse specialists, clinical nurse leaders, unit-based nurse managers, and clinical educators can adapt this approach in mentoring new staff on a unit. Reviewing the novice nurses' responses to the questions can yield valuable information about their critical-thinking, problem-solving, and decision-making skills and serve as a foundation for ongoing staff development, mentoring, and support. Asking each question when trying to resolve a problem has the potential to yield highly innovative solutions to everyday problems.

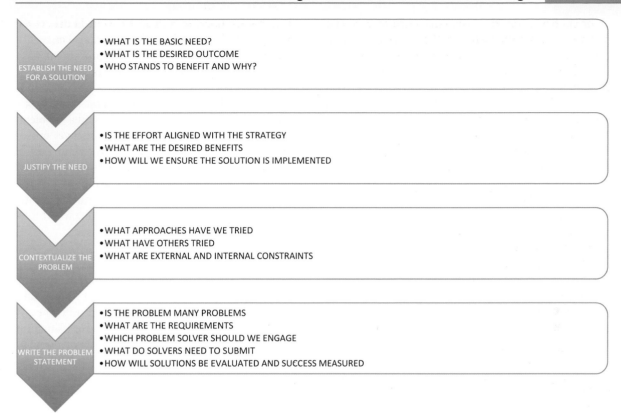

ESTABLISH THE NEED FOR A SOLUTION
- WHAT IS THE BASIC NEED?
- WHAT IS THE DESIRED OUTCOME
- WHO STANDS TO BENEFIT AND WHY?

JUSTIFY THE NEED
- IS THE EFFORT ALIGNED WITH THE STRATEGY
- WHAT ARE THE DESIRED BENEFITS
- HOW WILL WE ENSURE THE SOLUTION IS IMPLEMENTED

CONTEXTUALIZE THE PROBLEM
- WHAT APPROACHES HAVE WE TRIED
- WHAT HAVE OTHERS TRIED
- WHAT ARE EXTERNAL AND INTERNAL CONSTRAINTS

WRITE THE PROBLEM STATEMENT
- IS THE PROBLEM MANY PROBLEMS
- WHAT ARE THE REQUIREMENTS
- WHICH PROBLEM SOLVER SHOULD WE ENGAGE
- WHAT DO SOLVERS NEED TO SUBMIT
- HOW WILL SOLUTIONS BE EVALUATED AND SUCCESS MEASURED

FIGURE 6-3 The problem-definition process.

Define the Problem, Issue, or Situation

The main principles for diagnosing a problem are (1) know the facts, (2) separate the facts from interpretation, (3) be objective and descriptive, and (4) determine the scope of the problem. Nurses also need to determine how to establish priorities for solving problems. For example, do you tend to work on the problems that are encountered first, the problems that appear to be the easiest to resolve, the problems that take the shortest amount of time to resolve, or the problems that have the greatest urgency?

The most common cause for failure to resolve problems is the improper identification of the problem/issue; therefore problem recognition and identification are considered the most vital steps. The quality of the outcome depends on accurate identification of the problem, which is likely to recur if the true underlying causes are not targeted. Problem identification is influenced by the information available; by the values, attitudes, and experiences of those involved; and by time. Sufficient time should be allowed for the collection and organization of data. Too often, an inadequate amount of time is allocated for this essential step, resulting in unsatisfactory outcomes. Nurse leaders and managers should remember the power of asking questions. One method is to use the "5 Why" (Institute for Healthcare Improvement). After answering the first question as to why a problem occurred, ask why again, and so on until "why" has been asked at least five times. This is particularly helpful for problems that keep resurfacing over time because it gets to the actual root causes of problems.

It is important to differentiate between the actual problem and the symptoms of a problem. Consider the problem of an inadequately stocked emergency cart from which emergency medications often are missing and equipment often fails to function properly. Individuals charged with resolving this problem may discover that this is symptomatic of the underlying problem, perhaps inadequate staffing or staffing mix. Based on the proper identification of the problem in this scenario, a possible solution might be to assign the task of checking and stocking the emergency cart to the unlicensed personnel in the unit.

In work settings, problems often fall under certain categories that have been described as the *four M's: m*anpower, *m*ethods, *m*achines, and *m*aterials. Manpower issues might include inadequate staffing or staffing mix and knowledge or skills deficits. Methods issues could include communication problems or lack of protocols. Machine issues could include lack of equipment or malfunctioning equipment. Last, problems with materials could include inadequate supplies or defective materials. A fishbone diagram, also known as a *cause-and-effect diagram,* is a useful model for categorizing the possible causes of a problem. The diagram graphically displays, in increasing detail, all of the possible causes related to a problem to try to discover its root causes. This tool encourages problem solvers to focus on the content of the problem and not be sidetracked by personal interests, issues, or agendas of team members. It also collects a snapshot of the collective knowledge of the team and helps build consensus around the problem. The "effect" is generally the problem statement, such as decreased morale, and is placed at the right end of the figure (the "head" of the fish). The major categories of causes are the main bones, and these are supported by smaller bones, which represent issues that contribute to the main causes. An example of a fishbone diagram appears in Figure 6-4.

EXERCISE 6-5

Using a fishbone diagram (see p. 113 as a point of reference), identify all the factors (causes) that are at the root of a problem you are currently facing in the workplace. After you have listed as many issues as possible, share the diagram with a work colleague. Are there other issues you did not consider? Where do most of the factors influencing the problem fit: manpower, methods, machines, or materials?

Gather Data

After the general nature of the problem is identified, individuals can focus on gathering and analyzing data to resolve the issue. Assessment, through the collection of data and information, is done continuously throughout this dynamic process. The data gathered consist of objective (facts) and subjective (feelings) information. Information gathered should be valid, accurate, relevant to the issue, and timely. Moreover, individuals involved in the process must have access to information and adequate resources to make cogent decisions.

Analyze Data

Data are analyzed to further refine the problem statement and identify possible solutions or options. It is important to differentiate a problem from the symptoms of a problem. For example, a nurse manager is dismayed by the latest quality improvement (QI) report indicating nurses are not documenting patient teaching. Is this evidence that patient teaching is not being done? Is lack of documentation the actual problem? Perhaps it is a symptom of the actual problem. On further analysis, the manager may discover nurses do not know how to document patient teaching using the new computerized documentation system. By distinguishing the problem from the symptoms of the problem, a more appropriate solution can be identified and implemented. This example is one where asking the five whys could be effective.

Develop Solutions

The goal of generating options is to identify as many choices as possible. Occasionally, rigid "black and white" thinking hampers the quality of outcomes. A nurse who is unhappy with his or her work situation and can think of only two options—stay or resign—is displaying this type of thinking. That "either/or" thinking limits the possibilities for solutions.

Being flexible, open-minded, and creative—attributes of a critical thinker—is critical to being able to consider a range of possible options. Everyone has preconceived notions and ideas when confronted with certain situations. Although putting these notions on hold and considering other ideas is beneficial, it is difficult to do. However, asking questions such as the following can allow a person to consider other viewpoints:

- Am I jumping to conclusions?
- If I were (insert name of role model), how would I approach it?
- How are my beliefs and values affecting my decision?

Select a Solution

The decision maker should then objectively weigh each option according to its possible risks and consequences as well as positive outcomes that may be derived. Criteria for evaluation might include variables such as cost-effectiveness, time, and legal or ethical considerations. The options should be ranked in the order in which they are likely to result in the desired goals or objectives. The solution selected should be the one that is most feasible and satisfactory and has the fewest undesirable consequences. Nurses must consider whether they are choosing the solution because it is the best solution or because it is the most

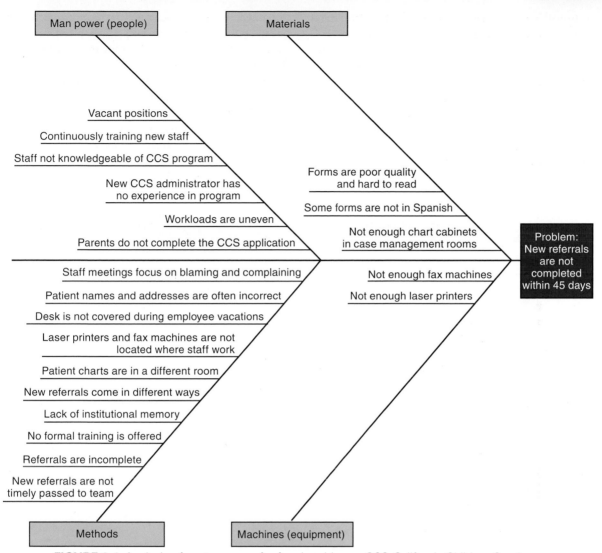

FIGURE 6-4 Analysis of root causes of referral problems. *CCS,* California Children Services.

expedient. Being able to make cogent decisions based on a thorough assessment of a situation is an important indicator of a nurse's effectiveness.

Implement the Solution

The planned solution is implemented using a defined and often phased strategy. Implementation may include revising policies and procedures, education, and documentation. The nurse leader or manager should remember that the implementation phase requires a contingency plan to deal with negative

consequences if they arise and be prepared to implement a "plan B."

Evaluate the Result

Considerable time and energy are usually spent on identifying the problem or issue, generating possible solutions, selecting the best solution, and implementing the solution. However, not enough time is typically allocated for evaluation and follow-up. It is important to establish early in the process how evaluation and monitoring will take place, who will be responsible for it, when it will take place, and what the desired outcome is. Be prepared to make mistakes and take responsibility for them. The key is to learn from mistakes and use the experiences to help guide future actions. Henry Ford said, "Failure is only the opportunity to begin again more intelligently."

CONCLUSION

Sometimes, individuals and groups do not adopt a structured problem-solving approach because it takes too much time, the process may be boring, stakeholders are too busy to get involved, or participants may perceive there is little or no recognition for their participation. Leaders should be cognizant of these potential barriers and should be prepared to prevent or minimize them.

All nurses, whether they are managers, leaders, or followers, need adequate decision-making and problem-solving skills to be effective in their roles. Regardless of the problem-solving approach, the use of a systematic approach will help address issues in an organized and focused manner.

THE SOLUTION

In a previous job, I had used interprofessional process improvement teams which consisted of key stakeholders, to initiate process improvement. I chose to try this concept in this setting. Our team consisted of the public health nurse (PHN) case managers, the CCS case workers, the billing and claims staff, the CCS medical director, clerical and support staff, and me. I believed that a group approach to these problems would yield the most information and gain the greatest support for any changes that would be made. The team met weekly for an hour. We began by identifying our customers and key stakeholders and their expectations. This was extensive and took a few months to complete. Key stakeholders included the patients (children) and their parents; the providers (physicians and hospitals); pharmacists; vendors; representatives from schools, insurance plans, and other agencies; taxpayers (state and county); and our own team members. The expectations for each stakeholder were listed, discussed for clarity, and recorded. During this exercise, the team learned a great deal about each person's job duties (there were a few surprises) and how each stakeholder's role affected other team members' ability to do their job. As the team began understanding each person's job and issues, they focused less on blaming and more on how to change our processes.

Next, the team brainstormed (divergent thinking) a list of issues. The numerous issues were then grouped according to similarity, and duplicates were eliminated. Multi-voting was then used to determine the three highest-priority issues. Our number one problem related to cycle time. When a client is referred to CCS, determination of eligibility, opening (or denying) the case, and authorizing care are key cycles. Patient care is often coordinated based on the client's eligibility, and delays in service can result when the process is not completed in a timely manner. The reasons for our failure to meet these deadlines seemed overwhelming and beyond our ability to resolve. We needed a method to find the root causes to improve our performance. We chose to use a fishbone diagram, also known as a cause-and-effect diagram (see Figure 6-4). Our problem was "New referrals are not completed within 45 days." We categorized our known barriers on the four bones of the fish, manpower, methods,

machines, and materials. Once we had identified the factors contributing to our problem, we prioritized them and generated action plans for each major factor. These action plans were extensive and involved implementing training and education programs, redesigning work space for greater efficiency, purchasing more equipment, revising job descriptions, increasing provider outreach activities, and more. Performance data did not improve during the initial year of our process improvement initiative, and I chose not to share it with staff to avoid demoralizing them. My management team and I were taking a leap of faith that our process would eventually result in the desired outcome of meeting the performance metrics.

It took 18 months for CCS to "turn the curve," but once improvement started, it was exponential. The cycle time measure for "referral to case open" was initially 57 days. Two years later, it was 30 days. The cycle time "referral to deny" began at 97 days, and 2 years later was down to 39 days. Most important, the cycle time "referral to first authorization" decreased from an initial 189 days to just 49 days! It was at this time that I shared the outcome data with the team. They were ecstatic! I asked the team to list the problems they believed we had solved through our process improvement team's efforts. They listed (1) improved staffing, (2) increased staff morale and decreased turnover (all the positions were now filled), (3) better understanding of the job expectations and the rationale behind those expectations, (4) improved teamwork, and (5) more efficient and effective work space. They have maintained enthusiastic support of the PIT, and participation remains high. The team is still highly focused on problem solving. I have learned that when assuming leadership of a department in which one has no experience, a structured team approach to information gathering, assessment of data, identification of problems, and implementation of action plans can be highly effective in the resolution of priority problems.

—*Vickie Lemmon*

Would this be a suitable approach for you? Why?

THE EVIDENCE

According to Porter-O'Grady and Malloch, authors of *Quantum Leadership* (2010), the three essential components to effective problem solving within organizations are tactical methods, strategic approaches, and cultural changes. Too often, nurse leaders and managers use a "firefighting" approach to problems, which is ineffective and generally causes more problems than it resolves.

Tactical methods for dealing with problems include getting assistance from someone with a fresh perspective, trying something new, and triaging problems (Porter-O'Grady & Malloch, 2010). Getting assistance may require sharing some "dirty laundry" outside of the unit or organization, but a new point of view is helpful to bring clarity to a situation. Sometimes nurse leaders and managers rely on specific problem-solving methods out of habit, so a new approach may help resolve a difficult issue. After triaging problems, the urgent and most important can be addressed first.

Strategic approaches include strategies such as prioritizing problems to deal with critical issues first and developing learning scenarios to develop staff to take ownership of problems, and to develop the skills to deal with them independently. This will address the tendency of staff to expect their manager to fix everything for them.

Cultural changes within the organization are necessary to create an environment that supports effective decision making and problem solving. The organization needs to avoid "patching" as a problem-solving approach. Porter-O'Grady and Malloch (2010) describe patching as focusing on the symptoms of a problem instead of the actual issue. They emphasize that deadlines are irrelevant if the methodology used to solve problems is effective. The authors emphasized that firefighting should not be rewarded within the organization.

WHAT NEW GRADUATES SAY

- I feel much better when things are explained to me. This way I can better support my manager.
- Sometimes I am not sure what to do. I wish I knew exactly what to do in all situations.
- I like it when my managers ask me my opinion about work. I feel important and engaged in the decision-making process.
- I am amazed of the power of asking questions. Asking why fives times really allows us to get to the root of any problem.
- I did not realize how many decisions a nurse can make in one work shift.

CHAPTER CHECKLIST

The ability to make good decisions and encourage effective decision making in others is a hallmark of nursing leadership and management. A nurse manager or leader is in a position to facilitate effective decision making by individuals and groups. This requires good communication skills, conflict resolution and mediation skills, knowledge of the vagaries of group dynamics, and the ability to foster an environment conducive to effective problem solving, decision making, and creative thinking.

- Differentiation of decision making and problem solving
- Decision making
  - Decision models
  - Decision-making styles
- Factors affecting decision making
- Group decision making
- Advantages of group decision making
- Challenges of group decision making
- Strategies
- Decision-making tools
- Problem solving
  - Problem-solving process
    - Define the problem, issue, or situation
    - Gather data
    - Analyze data
    - Develop solutions
    - Select a solution
    - Implement the solution
    - Evaluate the result

TIPS FOR DECISION MAKING AND PROBLEM SOLVING

- Seek additional information from other sources, even if they do not support the preferred action.
- Learn how other people approach problem situations.
- Talk to colleagues and superiors who you believe are effective problem solvers and decision makers. Observe positive role models in action such as

clinical nurse specialists, clinical nurse leaders, educators, and managers.
- Research journal articles and relevant sections of textbooks to increase your knowledge base.
- Risk using new approaches to problem resolution through experimentation, and calculate the risk to self and others.

REFERENCES

American Nurses Association (ANA), *Guide to the code of ethics for nurses: Interpretation and application.* (2010). Silver Springs, MD: American Nurses Association.

Crenshaw, J. T., & Yoder-Wise, P. (2013). Creating an environment for innovation: The risk-taking leadership competency. *Nurse Leader, 11*(1), 24–27.

Green, C. (2012). Nursing intuition: A valid form of knowledge. *Nursing Philosophy, 13*(2), 98–111.

Manktelow, J., & Carlson, A. (2013). *SWOT analysis.* Retrieved on February 3, 2013 from, www.mindtools.com/pages/article/newTMC_05.htm.

Moreau, A., Carol, L., Dedianne, M. C., Dupraz, C., Perdrix, C., Laine, X., et al. (2012). What perceptions do patients have of decision making (DM)? Toward an integrative patient-centered care model. A qualitative study using focus-group interviews. *Patient Education and Counseling, 87*(2), 206–211.

Porter-O'Grady, T., & Malloch, K. (2010). *Quantum leadership* (3rd ed.). Boston: Jones & Bartlett.

Pretz, J. E., & Folse, V. N. (2011). Nursing experience and preference for intuition in decision making. *Journal of Clinical Nursing, 20,* 2878–2889.

Spradlin, D. (2012). Are you solving the right problem? *Harvard Business Review, 90*(9), 85–93.

Tanner, C. A. (2006). Thinking like a nurse: A research-based model of clinical judgment in nursing. *Journal of Nursing Education, 45*(6), 204–211.

The Critical Thinking Community. (2011). *Our concept and definition of critical thinking.* Retrieved February 3, 2013 from, http://www.criticalthinking.org/pages/defining-critical-thinking/410.

SUGGESTED READINGS

Green, C. (2012). Nursing intuition: A valid form of knowledge. *Nursing Philosophy, 13*(2), 98–111.

Holtz, B., Morrish, W., & Krein, S. (2013). A nurse-patient shared decision support tool. *American Journal of Nursing, 113*(1), 47–52.

May, N., Becker, D., Frankel, R., Haizlip, J., Harmon, R., Plews-Ogan, M., et al. (2011). *Appreciative inquiry in healthcare: Positive questions to bring the best.* Brunswick, OH: Crown Custom Publishing.

Sherwood, G. D., & Horton-Deutsch, S. (2012). *Reflective practice: Transforming education and improving outcomes.* Indianapolis, IN: Sigma Theta Tau International.

INTERNET RESOURCES

Institute for Healthcare Improvement. www.ihi.org/IHI/Topics/Improvement/ImprovementMethods/Tools/.

Mind Tools. www.mindtools.com/.

Robert Wood Johnson Foundation. www.rwjf.org (search on transforming care at the bedside).

The Joint Commission. *Framework for conducting a root cause analysis and action plan.* www.jointcommission.org/SentinelEvents/Forms/.

7

Healthcare Organizations

Mary E. Mancini

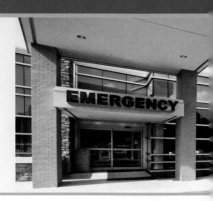

This chapter presents an overview of existing and emerging healthcare organizations, their characteristics, and their designs. Economic, social, and demographic factors that influence organizational development are discussed. A major emphasis is placed on management and leadership responses that professional nurses must consider in planning the delivery of nursing care in the changing environment. Leaders, managers, followers, and nursing students engaged in active practice must be aware of the changing dynamics if they are to be effective healthcare professionals and advocate for patients, families, and community.

LEARNING OUTCOMES

- Identify and compare characteristics that are used to differentiate healthcare organizations.
- Classify healthcare organizations by major types.
- Analyze economic, social, and demographic forces that drive the development of healthcare organizations.
- Describe the impact of the evolution of healthcare organizations on nursing leadership and management roles.

KEY TERMS

accountable care organization	managed care	secondary care
accreditation	networks	teaching institution
consolidated systems	preferred provider organization	tertiary care
deeming authority	primary care	third-party payers
fee-for-service	private non-profit (or not-for-	vertical integration
for-profit organization	profit) organization	
horizontal integration	public institution	

INTRODUCTION

Organizations are collections of individuals brought together in a defined environment to achieve a set of predetermined objectives. Economic, social, and demographic factors affect the purpose and structuring of the system, which in turn interact with the mission, philosophy, and structure of healthcare organizations.

Healthcare organizations provide two general types of services: illness care (restorative) and wellness care (preventive). Illness care services help the sick and injured. Wellness care services promote better health as well as illness and accident prevention. In the past, most organizations (e.g., hospitals, clinics, public health departments, community-based organizations, and physicians' offices) focused their attention on illness services. Recent economic, social, and demographic changes have placed emphasis on the development of organizations that focus on the full spectrum of health, especially wellness and prevention, to meet consumers' needs in more effective ways. Emphasis is being placed on the role of the nurse as both a designer of these restructured organizations and a healthcare leader and manager within the organizations. For example, the manner in which chronic and acute illnesses are managed is dramatically different from such a decade ago. Nurses take a much more active and independent role in providing these services. Similarly, as population numbers increase and the demand for nurses exceed the supply, we can anticipate more changes in how nurses function within the healthcare system. An increased focus on continuous performance improvement and benchmarking demands that organizations constantly consider their own practices and make appropriate changes, including those related to the organization's culture and the role of nurses within the organization.

Nurses practice in many different types of healthcare organizations. Nursing roles develop in response to the same social, cultural, economic, legislative, and demographic factors that shape the organizations in which they work. As the largest group of healthcare professionals providing direct and indirect care services to consumers, nurses have an obligation to be involved in the development of healthcare, social, and economic policies that shape healthcare organizations.

CHARACTERISTICS AND TYPES OF ORGANIZATIONS

Responding to the rapidly changing nature of the economic, social, and demographic environment at the national, state, and local level, the United States healthcare system is in a continual state of flux as are the organizations within this system. Organizations either anticipate or respond to these environmental changes.

Institutional Providers

Acute care hospitals, long-term care facilities, and rehabilitation facilities have traditionally been classified as institutional providers. Major characteristics that differentiate institutional providers as well as other healthcare organizations are (1) types of services provided, (2) length of direct care services provided, (3) ownership, (4) teaching status, and (5) accreditation status.

Types of Services Provided

The type of services offered is a characteristic used to differentiate institutional providers. Services can be classified as either general or special care. Facilities that provide specialty care offer a limited scope of services, such as those targeted to specific disease entities or patient populations. Examples of special care facilities are those providing psychiatric care, burn care, children's care, women's and infants' care, and oncology care. Alternatively, facilities such as general hospitals provide a wide range of services to multiple segments of the population.

Length of Direct Care Services Provided

Another characteristic that is used to differentiate healthcare organizations is the duration of the care provided. According to the American Hospital Association (AHA) (2012), most hospitals are acute care facilities giving short-term, episodic care. The AHA defined an acute care hospital as a facility in which the average length of stay is less than 30 days. Chronic care or long-term facilities provide services for patients who require care for extended periods in excess of 30 days. In acute care institutions, patients are discharged as soon as their conditions are stabilized. An example of a long-term care facility is a geriatric organization that provides care services from onset of impairment until death. Many institutions have components of both

short-term and long-term services. They may provide acute care, home care, hospice care, ambulatory clinic care, day surgery, and an increasing number of other services, such as day care for dependent children and adults or focused services such as Meals-on-Wheels. The term *healthcare network* refers to interconnected units that either are owned by the institution or have cooperative agreements with other institutions to provide a full spectrum of wellness and illness services. The spectrum of care services provided is typically described as primary care (first-access care), secondary care (disease-restorative care), and tertiary care (rehabilitative or long-term care). Table 7-1 describes the continuum of care and the units of healthcare organizations that provide services in the three phases of the continuum.

EXERCISE 7-1

Using the local telephone directory, determine the types and numbers of primary care, secondary care, and tertiary care services available. Table 7-2 provides an example of a format for collecting data.

TABLE 7-1   CONTINUUM OF HEALTHCARE ORGANIZATIONS

TYPE OF CARE	PURPOSE	ORGANIZATION OR UNIT PROVIDING SERVICES
Primary	• Entry into system • Health maintenance • Long-term care • Chronic care • Treatment of temporary nonincapacitating malfunction	• Ambulatory care centers • Physicians' offices • Preferred provider organizations • Nursing centers • Independent provider organizations • Health maintenance organizations • School health clinics
Secondary	• Prevention of disease complications	• Home health care • Ambulatory care centers • Nursing centers
Tertiary	• Rehabilitation • Long-term care	• Home health care • Long-term care facilities • Rehabilitation centers • Skilled nursing facilities • Assisted living programs/retirement centers

TABLE 7-2   CHARACTERISTICS AND TYPES OF HEALTHCARE ORGANIZATIONS

HEALTHCARE ORGANIZATION	TYPE	SERVICES	OWN	FIN	TCG	MULTI
Veterans Administration	Institution	General	Federal	NP	Y	Y
Academic Medical Center	Institution	General	Private	NP	Y	Y
Community General	Institution	General	Private	NP	N	Y
Public Hospital	Institution	General	County	NP	Y	N
Shriners Burn Hospitals	Institution	Specialty	Private	NP	N	N
Prepaid Health Plan	HMO	General	Private	NP-P	N	N
Public Health Department	Community	General	State	NP	N	N
Women's and Infants' Project	Community	Specialty	State	NP	N	N
Geriatric Corporation	Institution	Long term	Private	NP	N	Y
Visiting Nurses Association	Community	Specialty	Private	NP	N	N

Fin, Financing; *HMO*, health maintenance organization; *Multi*, multiunit; *N*, no; *NP*, non-profit; *Own*, ownership; *P*, profit; *TCG* teaching status; *Y*, yes.

Ownership

Ownership is another characteristic used to classify healthcare organizations. Ownership establishes the organization's legal, business, and mission-related imperative. Healthcare organizations have three basic ownership forms: public, private non-profit, and for-profit. Public institutions provide health services to individuals under the support and/or direction of local, state, or federal government. These organizations must answer directly to the sponsoring government agency or boards and are indirectly responsible to elected officials and taxpayers who support them. Examples of these service recipients at the federal level are veterans, members of the military, Native Americans, and inmates of correctional facilities. State-supported organizations may be health service teaching facilities, chronic care facilities, and prisoner facilities. Locally supported facilities include county-supported and city-supported facilities. Table 7-2 shows how several common healthcare organizations are classified.

Private non-profit (or not-for-profit) organizations—often referred to as *voluntary agencies*—are controlled by voluntary boards or trustees and provide care to a mix of paying and charity patients. In these organizations, excess revenue over expenses is redirected into the organization for maintenance and growth rather than returned as dividends to stockholders. These organizations are required to serve people regardless of their ability to pay. Non-profit organizations located in impoverished urban and rural areas are often economically disadvantaged

by the amount of uncompensated care that they provide. Historically, non-profit organizations have been exempt from paying taxes because they commit to providing an important community service. The owners of such organizations include churches, communities, industries, and special interest groups such as the Shriners. The ownership influences how organizations are structured, what services they provide, and which patients they serve.

For-profit organizations are also referred to as *proprietary* or *investor-owned organizations*. These organizations operate with the specific intent of earning a profit by providing healthcare services to individuals who can afford to pay for these services. Organizations such as private or public insurers who provide healthcare insurance coverage are known as third-party payers. Many for-profit organizations, like the not-for-profit ones, receive supplementary funds through private and public sources to provide special services and research. This funding allows them to provide financial assistance to patients who can afford ordinary care but are not in a position to finance catastrophic occurrences such as vital organ failure, birth of premature or sick infants, or transplant operations.

The Patient Protection and Affordable Care Act of 2010 established accountable care organizations (ACOs) to coordinate care and chronic disease management and improve the overall quality of care provided to Medicare patients. ACOs are designed as seamless healthcare delivery systems that bring together physicians, hospitals, and other caregivers focused on improving the health of individuals and communities while decreasing costs. ACOs continue to emerge to provide cost-effective care (*www.cms.gov/ Medicare/Medicare-Fee-for-Service-Payment/ACO/ index.html?redirect=/aco/*). These patient-centered organizations are designed for the healthcare team and patients to be true partners in caring. Participation in the program is voluntary and payments to ACOs are tied to achieving explicit healthcare quality goals and outcomes. Five quality measures are targeted: patient-caregiver experience of care, care coordination, patient safety, preventive health, and frail elderly health (*https://www.healthcare.gov/glossary/accountable-care-organization/*). To maximize the desired outcomes from forming ACOs, nurses at all levels of the organization, especially the nurse executive, must be well versed in their structure and goals (Cady, 2011; Ritter-Teitel, 2012).

Ownership can impact efficiency and quality. Although hospital ownership is defined legally, significant differences are found within the three sectors related to teaching status, location, bed size, and corporate affiliation. For-profit hospitals, which represent approximately 15% of the beds in short-term acute care hospitals, are typically nonteaching, suburban facilities with small to medium bed capacity and have the ability to access group purchasing cooperatives that lower non-salary expenses. For-profit hospitals tend to have higher hospital charges and lower wage and salary costs that most likely represent an aggressive approach to maximizing return on investment (ROI).

Ownership results in differential treatment relative to regulatory requirements. Public and non-profit hospitals are tax exempt and have a concomitant responsibility to provide mandated community service such as delivering care to the poor and indigent. Thus one can expect operational differences between and among the three ownership sectors. Ownership impacts the organization's level of effort in regard to the provision of uncompensated care. Those organizations with taxing authority or direct support from local or state government have a clear mandate to care for indigent patients and receive at least some level of dedicated funds to do so. For-profit hospitals offer fewer unprofitable services and actively seek to avoid providing uncompensated care and are required to pay taxes that can have an impact on their

bottom line. To keep a non-profit status, facilities must make a good-faith effort to provide community service and charity care. Unfortunately, the literature provides conflicting and inconclusive evidence in regard to the impact of ownership on hospital financial performance.

Teaching Status

Teaching status is a characteristic that can differentiate healthcare organizations. The term **teaching institution** is applied to academic health centers (those directly affiliated with a school of medicine and at least one other health profession school) and affiliated teaching hospitals (those that provide only the clinical portion of a medical school teaching program). Although care is usually more costly at teaching hospitals than at nonteaching hospitals (estimates range from 12% higher in Canada to 27% higher in the United States), teaching hospitals generally offer better care because of their access to state-of-the-art technology and researchers. The higher costs of teaching hospitals have been attributed to the unique missions these institutions tend to pursue, including graduate medical education, biomedical research, and the maintenance of stand-by capacity for highly specialized patient care (Doyle, Graves, Gruber, & Kleiner, 2012).

Traditionally, teaching hospitals have received government reimbursement to cover these additional costs. However, intrinsic costs of providing a medical training program are not fully reimbursed by the government. Maintaining a teaching program places a financial burden on hospitals relative to the direct cost of the program and the indirect cost of the inefficiencies surrounding the training process. These inefficiencies include (1) salaries of physicians who supervise students' care delivery and participate in educational programs such as teaching rounds and seminars, (2) duplicated tests or procedures, and (3) delays in processing patients related to the teaching process. Currently, these expenses are reimbursed based on a formula that considers the cost of caring for the low-income and uninsured patients who populate most academic teaching programs. This reimbursement is being revised as states reduce subsidies for the education of physicians. Hospitals make strategic decisions about their level of participation in physician training. Because of the additional costs, few for-profit hospitals sponsor teaching programs. Teaching hospitals are usually located close to their affiliated medical school. They tend to be larger and located in more urban and economically depressed inner-city areas than their nonteaching counterparts. Teaching hospitals, therefore, tend to exhibit weaker economic performance compared with nonteaching hospitals.

> **EXERCISE 7-2**
> Return to the data you started in the first exercise and add financial and teaching status information.

Accreditation Status

Another characteristic that can be used to distinguish one organization from another is whether a healthcare organization has been accredited by an external body as having the structure and process necessary to provide high-quality care. Private organizations play significant roles in establishing standards and ensuring care delivery compliance with standards by accrediting healthcare organizations. Examples of these organizations are The Joint Commission and The National Committee for Quality Assurance (NCQA). The Joint Commission provides accreditation programs for ambulatory care, behavioral health care, acute care and critical access hospitals, laboratory services, long-term care, and hospital-based surgery. The NCQA is a non-profit organization that accredits, certifies, and recognizes a wide variety of healthcare organizations, services, and providers. More information on accrediting organizations is provided in the "Accrediting Bodies" section on pp. 127-128.

Consolidated Systems and Networks

Healthcare organizations are being organized into consolidated systems through both the formation of for-profit or not-for-profit multihospital systems and the development of networks of independently owned and operated healthcare organizations.

Consolidated Systems

Consolidated systems tend to be organized along five levels. The first level includes the large national hospital companies, most of which are investor owned.

The second level involves large voluntary affiliated systems, which provide members with access to capital, political power, management expertise, joint venture opportunities, and links to health insurance services or, as in Canada, to a national healthcare coverage program. The third level involves regional hospital systems that cover a defined geographic area, such as an area of a state. The fourth level involves metropolitan-based systems. The fifth level is composed of the special interest groups that own and operate units organized along religious lines, teaching interests, or related special interests that drive their activities. This level often crosses over the regional, metropolitan, and national levels already described. Through the creation of multiunit systems, an organization has greater marketing, policy, and contracting potentials.

Networks

Healthcare markets with 100,000 or more residents are generally served by one to three health networks. The networks usually follow one of three organizational models: public utilities, for-profit businesses, or loose alliances. Public utility models are organized and governed just like today's public utilities (e.g., the county water department). Their aim is serving large regional populations. In most markets, two or three competing markets have emerged that require significant capital, causing many traditional not-for-profit providers to shift to for-profit status. Loose alliances take the shape of loosely connected "virtual" networks that emulate integrated health systems through contracts and linked computer systems.

Ambulatory-Based Organizations

Many health services are provided on an ambulatory basis. The organizational setting for much of this care has been the group practice or private physician's office. Prepaid group practice plans, referred to as *managed care systems,* combine care delivery with financing and provide comprehensive services for a fixed prepaid fee. A goal of these services is to reduce the cost of expensive acute hospital care by focusing on out-of-hospital preventive care and illness follow-up care. Group practice plans take various forms. One form has a centralized administration that directs and pays salaries for physician practice (e.g., health maintenance organizations [HMOs]).

The HMO is a configuration of healthcare agencies that provide basic and supplemental health maintenance and treatment services to voluntary enrollees who prepay a fixed periodic fee without regard to the amount of services used. To be federally qualified, an HMO company must offer inpatient and outpatient services, treatment and referral for drug and alcohol problems, laboratory and radiology services, preventive dental services for children younger than 12 years, and preventive healthcare services in addition to physician services.

Independent practice associations (IPAs) (or professional associations [PAs]) are a form of group practice in which physicians in private offices are paid on a **fee-for-service** basis by a prepaid plan to deliver care to enrolled members. **Preferred provider organizations (PPOs)** operate similarly to IPAs; contracts are developed with private practice physicians, but fees are discounted from their usual and customary charges. In return, physicians are guaranteed prompt payment.

Nurse practitioners' leadership in managing patients in group practices has contributed greatly to their success. Examples of this can be found by reviewing literature related to nurses' activities at Kaiser Permanente HMO, the Harvard Pilgrim Health Plan, and Minute Clinics.

Increasing evidence shows that nurse-run clinics as well as ambulatory care centers can succeed whether they are integrated within a larger medical complex or physically and administratively separate organizations. Examples of freestanding organizations include surgicenters, urgent care centers, primary care centers, and imaging centers. Benefits and risks are associated with geographic and administrative separation between organizations. For example, when an ambulatory surgery center is located separately from an acute care facility, addressing emergency response teams and seamless transfer of patients in need of a higher level of care is critical. On the other hand, having the ambulatory surgery center apart from the acute care hospital typically provides the opportunity for more patient-focused amenities such as parking and family waiting. Often, the nurse manager in these facilities is charged with identifying the strategies to maximize the benefits and minimize the risks or challenges inherent in the characteristics of the facility and organization.

> **EXERCISE 7-3**
> Again return to the data started in the first exercise and add information about the status of the multiunit systems that are in place.

Other Organizations

Although hospitals, nursing homes, health departments, visiting nurse services, and private physicians' offices have made up the traditional primary service delivery organizations, the critical role being played by other organizations that may be freestanding or units of hospitals or other community organizations is also important. These include community service organizations, subacute facilities, and a proliferating number of home health agencies, long-term care facilities, and hospices. In addition, nurse-owned/nurse-organized services and self-help voluntary organizations contribute to the overall service provision. Growth in these organizations was spurred by the implementation of the prospective payment

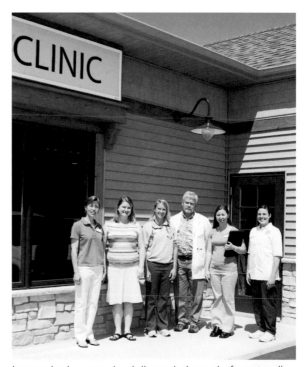

Increasingly, care is delivered through freestanding clinics or community or hospital-affiliated services.

system, which resulted in early discharge of many patients from acute care facilities. These patients require highly technical continuing nursing care to maintain a stable status. The focus of these organizations is on the care of individuals and their family and significant others rather than on the community as a whole. Many of these organizations are functioning as PPOs, and this is expected to be a continuing pattern in the future.

Community Services

Community services, including public health departments, are focused on the treatment of the community rather than that of the individual. The historical focus of these organizations has been on control of infectious agents and provision of preventive services under the auspices of public health departments. Local, state, and federal governments allocate funds to health departments to provide a variety of necessary services. These funds provide personal health services that include maternal and child care, care for communicable diseases such as acquired immunodeficiency syndrome (AIDS) and tuberculosis, services for children with birth defects, mental health care, and investigation of epidemiology and treatment of bioterrorism threats and attacks such as anthrax. Monies are allocated also for environmental services (e.g., ensuring that food services meet established standards) and for health resources (e.g., control of reproduction, promotion of safer sex, and breast cancer screening programs). Local health departments have been provided some autonomy in determining how to use funds that are not assigned to categorical programs.

School health programs whose funds are also allocated to them by local, state, and federal governments traditionally have been organized to control infectious disease outbreaks; to detect and refer problems that interfere with learning; to treat on-site injuries and illnesses; and to provide basic health education programs. Increasingly, schools are being seen as primary care sites for children.

Visiting nurse associations, which are voluntary organizations, have provided a large amount of the follow-up care for patients after hospitalization and for newborns and their mothers. Some are organized by cities, and others serve entire regions. Some operate for profit; others do not.

Subacute Facilities

As hospitals began to discharge patients earlier in their recuperation, the subacute facility emerged as a healthcare organization. Initially, many of these facilities were old-style nursing homes refurbished with the high-tech equipment necessary to deal with patients who have just come out of surgery or who are still acutely ill and have complex medical needs. Today, many are newly built centers or new businesses that have taken over existing clinical facilities.

Home Health Organizations

Home health organizations have numerous configurations; they may be freestanding or owned by a hospital and may be for-profit or not-for-profit organizations. Professional nurses with expert skills in assessing patients' self-care competencies and in building structures to overcome patients' and families' social and emotional deficits in providing sick and palliative care are needed to meet home care needs. Home care agencies staffed appropriately with adequate numbers of professional nurses have the potential to keep older adults, those with disabilities, and persons with chronic illnesses comfortable and safe at home. An increasing number of restrictions on home care by managed care companies, as well as changing financial reimbursement strategies, are threatening the adequate performance of this function.

Home care is the fastest growing segment in health care. The organizational design will likely change to the integration of a functional and divisional structure because the home health service industry is becoming more complex and is changing rapidly. For example, reimbursement for home care is primarily an arrangement of contract pricing and capitation. The integration of clinical, financial, human resources, and patient outcome information will influence the organizational design of the home care agency in the future.

Long-Term Care and Residential Facilities

Long-term care (LTC) facilities may also be known as *skilled nursing facilities*. These organizations provide long-term rehabilitation and professional nursing services. In residential facilities, no skilled care is provided but residents who have special needs are offered safe, sheltered environments in which to live.

Hospice

The concept of hospice or palliative care was launched at St. Christopher Hospice in London. Hospices can be located on inpatient nursing units, such as the kind commonly found in Canada, the United Kingdom, and Australia, or in the home or residential centers in the community. Hospices focus on confirming rather than denying the reality of death and thus provide care that ensures dignity and comfort.

Nurse-Owned and Nurse-Organized Services

Nursing centers, which are nurse-owned and nurse-operated places where care is provided by nurses, are another form of community-based organizations. Many nursing centers are administered by schools of nursing and serve as a base for faculty practice and research and clinical experience for students. Others are owned and operated by groups of nurses. These centers have a variety of missions. Some focus on care for specific populations, such as the homeless, or on care for people with AIDS. Others have taken responsibility for university health services. Some have assumed responsibility for school health programs in the community, and others operate employee wellness programs, hospices, and home care services. Some are freestanding, and others are units within hospitals. Church-affiliated organizations, sometimes operating as parish or shul (a service of synagogues) nursing facilities, are also examples of nurse-based organizations.

Self-Help Voluntary Organizations

Other organizations are the self-help/self-care organizations. These organizations also come in various forms. They are often composed of and directed by peers who are consumers of healthcare services. Their purpose is most often to enable patients to provide support to each other and raise community consciousness about the nature of a specific physical or emotional disease. AIDS support groups and Alcoholics Anonymous are two examples. Community geriatric organizations, frequently sponsored by healthcare organizations and offering multiple services for promoting wellness and rehabilitation, are increasing rapidly.

Supportive and Ancillary Organizations

Organizations involved in the direct provision of health care are supported by a number of other organizations whose operations have a significant effect on provider organizations, as well as on the overall performance of the health system. These organizations include regulatory organizations, accrediting bodies, third-party financing organizations, pharmaceutical and medical equipment supply corporations, and various professional, educational, and training organizations.

EXERCISE 7-4

Identify supportive and ancillary organizations operating in your community. Can you determine whether nurses are playing leadership or staff roles in those organizations and what functions are incorporated into existing nursing roles?

Regulatory Organizations

Regulatory organizations set standards for the operation of healthcare organizations, ensure compliance with federal and state regulations developed by governmental administrative agencies, and investigate and make judgments regarding complaints brought by consumers of the services and the public. They approve organizations for licensure as providers of health care. Healthcare organizations are regulated by a number of different federal, state, and local agencies to protect the health and safety of the patients and communities they serve. A number of different regulatory agencies monitor functions in healthcare organizations. These include the Centers for Medicare & Medicaid Services (CMS), the U.S. Food and Drug Administration, the Occupational Health and Safety Administration, the U.S. Equal Employment Opportunity Commission, and state licensing boards for various health professions. Regardless of the type of organization in which they work, nurses are often involved in these processes. Therefore all nurses need to be familiar with the regulations that impact their organization.

Established in 1965, Medicare is the country's largest and most influential health insurance program, providing healthcare funding for more than 40 million individuals. This makes the federal government the primary payer of healthcare costs in the United States. The Medicare program is not limited to individuals age 65 years or older. Persons with certain permanent illnesses, such as end-stage renal disease, also receive Medicare health benefits. Because of the size of the Medicare market, the federal government serves as the leading regulator of healthcare services in this country.

The CMS administers the Medicare and Medicaid programs. Participation in these programs is regulated by a complex set of rules outlined in a lengthy set of guidelines—the Conditions of Participation (CoP). These guidelines are established to improve quality and protect the health and safety of Medicare and Medicaid beneficiaries by specifying the requirements that organizations must meet to be eligible to receive Medicare and Medicaid reimbursement.

To be in compliance with the CoP, healthcare organizations must meet certain quality assessment and performance improvement requirements. Through its Quality Improvement Organization program (formerly called *Peer Review*), CMS contracts with one organization in each state (typically the state's Department of Health & Human Services) to work with healthcare organizations to improve the quality, efficiency, and effectiveness of care provided in that state to Medicare beneficiaries. CMS provides a financial incentive for hospitals to report quality data. These data are used to establish minimum quality standards for healthcare facilities and by patients to help them make decisions about where to seek healthcare. The program is designed to ensure that healthcare organizations systematically examine the quality of care provided and that they use the data obtained to develop and implement projects that improve quality, enhance patient safety, and reduce medical errors. To help reach these quality goals, CMS sponsors the Medicare Quality Improvement Community (MedQIC). The MedQIC website contains information and tools to support healthcare providers and organizations in creating community-based approaches to quality improvement.

Nurses are actively involved in CMS patient safety and quality improvement processes. The level of their participation may be as participants in facility-based quality or utilization management activities, or they may be involved as case managers. Nurse case managers can serve in a number of different roles, but they frequently serve as the organization's interface with the physician. In this role, these case managers routinely monitor for appropriate physician documentation of medical necessity and other required CoP elements. In the ambulatory or acute care setting, nurses in the role of case managers typically work with physician advisors to ensure that patient care follows recognized standards and facilitates patient flow to the appropriate setting for care.

Nurses also play key roles in developing, implementing, and evaluating the review processes of these regulatory agencies. As members of healthcare organizations providing both direct and indirect services to patients and as members of or advisors to regulatory agencies, baccalaureate-prepared nurses in roles of direct care nurse and nurse managers have active roles in monitoring and improving quality as well as establishing standards and ensuring that organizations comply with standards

Accrediting Bodies

Accreditation refers to the approval, recognition, or certification by an official review board that an organization has met certain standards. CMS is responsible for the enforcement of its standards through its certification activities. For a healthcare organization to participate in and receive payment from either Medicare or Medicaid, the organization must be certified as complying with the CoP. One manner that an organization can be recognized as complying with the CoP is through a survey process conducted by a state agency on behalf of CMS. Alternatively, an organization can be surveyed and accredited by a national accrediting body holding "deeming authority" for CMS. To obtain deeming authority, an accreditation organization must undergo a comprehensive evaluation by CMS to ensure that the standards of the accrediting organization are at least as rigorous as CMS standards. (See Table 7-3 for a list of organizations with deeming authority.) Healthcare organizations accredited by an organization with CMS deeming authority are therefore deemed as meeting Medicare and Medicaid certification requirements. A number of states accept national accreditation by an approved accrediting agency in lieu of other types of regulatory activity. For these reasons, healthcare organizations often seek accreditation by an accrediting body with deeming authority rather than through a multiple survey process conducted by state agencies and CMS.

Acute care healthcare organizations commonly seek accreditation by The American Osteopathic Association (AOA) or The Joint Commission. Both of these organizations have been granted deeming authority by CMS. The AOA is a professional association specifically for osteopathic healthcare organizations. It accredits osteopathic acute care hospitals, mental health facilities, substance abuse centers, and physical rehabilitation centers. The Joint Commission is an independent,

TABLE 7-3   ACCREDITING ORGANIZATIONS WITH DEEMING AUTHORITY FOR CMS

ACCREDITING ORGANIZATION	SERVICES ACCREDITED
Accreditation Association for Ambulatory Health Care (AAAHC)	ASCs
Accreditation Commission for Health Care (ACHC)	HHAs, hospice
American Association for Accreditation of Ambulatory Surgery Facilities (AAAASF)	ASCs, OPTs, RHCs
American Osteopathic Association's Healthcare Facilities Accreditation Program (AOA/HFAP)	ASCs, CAHs, hospitals
Community Health Accreditation Program (CHAP)	HHAs, hospice
Det Norske Veritas Healthcare, Inc. (DNV Healthcare) Mechanical Circulatory Support Certification Program	Hospitals and CAHs
The Joint Commission (TJC)	ASCs, CAHs, HHAs, hospice, hospitals, psychiatric hospitals

Retrieved from *www.cms.gov/Medicare/Provider-Enrollment-and-Certification/SurveyCertificationGenInfo/downloads/AOContactInformation.pdf.*
ASC, Ambulatory surgery center; *CAH,* critical access hospital; *HHA,* home health agency; *OPT,* outpatient physical therapy; *RHC,* rural health clinics.

not-for-profit organization that accredits more than 15,000 healthcare organizations in the United States and internationally. The explicit mission of The Joint Commission is to continuously improve the safety and quality of care provided to the public through the provision of healthcare accreditation and related services that support improvement of performance in healthcare organizations. The Joint Commission accredits approximately 80% of acute care hospitals in the United States, as well as numerous ambulatory surgicenters, clinical laboratories, critical access hospitals, HMOs, PPOs, home healthcare agencies, and hospices.

Third-Party Financing Organizations

Organizations that provide financing for health care comprise another subset of supportive and organizations.

As noted earlier, the government, through CMS, finances a large portion of the population and represents the largest third-party organization involved in healthcare provision. Private health insurance carriers, who account for most of the remaining financing, are composed of not-for-profit and for-profit components. Commercial insurance companies represent the private sector.

Third-party financing organizations have a major effect on the actual delivery of health care. They do so by identifying those procedures, tests, services, or drugs that will be covered under their healthcare insurance programs. In addition, they indirectly affect the configuration of the healthcare delivery system through the use of their significant political influence. As the cost of health care increases and the number of medically uninsured and underinsured grows, pressure increases for significant changes in healthcare reimbursement. Under the Affordable Care Act of 2010, reconfiguration of the current system is certain to bring with it restructuring of the organizations responsible for delivery of healthcare services.

Pharmaceutical and Medical Equipment Supply Organizations

About one tenth of all healthcare expenditures is allocated to drugs and medical equipment, and this is increasing. When other healthcare supply organizations, such as healthcare information system corporations, are considered, the estimated percentage may rapidly escalate toward the one-quarter mark. Nurses in direct care, manager, and leadership role are primary users of these products. They play a significant role in healthcare organizations in setting standards for safe and efficient products that meet both consumers' and organizations' needs in a cost-effective manner. Supply organizations often seek nurses as customers and as participants in market surveys for the design of new products, services, and marketing techniques. Nurses are employed by these organizations as designers of new products, marketing representatives, and members of the sales and research staffs. Examples of the roles nurses play can be seen by studying organizations that employ nurses to design new products and market them through production and distribution of a newsletter and ongoing continuing education presentations.

Integration

As the healthcare industry faces continuing and increasing pressure to improve patient safety as well as to be efficient and effective, healthcare organizations are entering into a number of different organizational relationships such as accountable care organizations. Organizations can come together to form affiliations, consortiums, and consolidations that result in multihospital systems and/or multi-organizational arrangements. When organizations that provide similar services come together, the arrangement is referred to as **horizontal integration.** An example of horizontal integration is a group of acute care facilities that come together to provide coverage for an expanded region. When organizations align to provide a full array or continuum of services, the arrangement is referred to as **vertical integration.** Organizations brought together in a vertical integration might include an acute care facility, a rehabilitation facility, a home care agency, an ambulatory clinic, and a hospice. Benefits attributed to vertical integration include enhanced coordination of services, efficiency, and customer services.

Acquisitions and Mergers

The economic forces of capitated payments and **managed care** have caused healthcare organizations to reorganize, restructure, and reengineer to decrease waste and economic inefficiency. Many organizations are forming multi-institutional alliances that integrate healthcare systems under a common organizational infrastructure. These alliances are accomplished through acquisitions or mergers. Acquisitions involve one organization directly buying another. Mergers involve combining two or more organizations and their assets to form a new entity. Mergers can also happen within organizations as departments or patient care units come together. People, structure, culture, and political issues or organizational change can be very traumatic and lead to dysfunctional outcomes if it is not managed well.

FORCES THAT INFLUENCE HEALTHCARE ORGANIZATIONS

Economic, social, and demographic factors provide the input for future development and act as major forces driving the evolution of healthcare organizations.

Economic Factors

Overall economic conditions as well as decisions surrounding the financing of health care have shaped the supply, configuration, and distribution of healthcare organizations and substantially changed the provision of health care in the United States. The radical restructuring of the healthcare system that is required to reduce the continuing escalation of economic resources into the system and to make health care accessible to all citizens will necessitate ongoing changes in healthcare organizations. As the impact of healthcare reform legislation unfolds, more people will be covered by insurance, and more services will be needed. As the Literature Perspective points out, nurses have great potential to be engaged with more services and to revamp the approach to care.

In addition to struggling to respond to the increasing numbers of uninsured patients and the concomitant increase in the amounts of uncompensated care, healthcare organizations are being confronted daily with the financial pressures associated with rapidly escalating drug costs, expensive new technology, and spiraling personnel costs. In 2013, the Henry J. Kaiser Family Foundation reported that U.S. healthcare

 LITERATURE PERSPECTIVE

Resource: Hassmiller, S. (2010). Nursing's role in healthcare reform. *American Nurse Today, 5*(9). Retrieved December 9, 2013, from www.americannursetoday.com/article.aspx?id=7086.

Nurses have great potential to influence how health care is delivered and to alter the way nurses are prepared and function. Dr. Hassmiller identified nine challenges, some of which relate directly to healthcare organizations. Using nurse-led innovations allows lower-cost and equally effective care to be delivered. With the addition of multiple patients to an already challenged system, this approach will be vital to meet the increased demand for care. Creating evidence, something nurses already do well, provides the opportunity to determine additional effective care strategies. Expanding the scope of nursing (at all levels) will increase the capacity of the profession to meet the needs of the care recipients. This includes registered nurses without advanced practice standing. Enhancing nurses' potential for leadership also increase the ability of nurses to create more effective systems of care.

Implications for Practice
The opportunities afforded to nursing as a result of healthcare reform are enormous. The challenge lies in our readiness and ability to respond to the opportunities.

spending reached 17.6% of the gross domestic product (GDP). According to the World Health Organization, the United States' healthcare expenditures as a percent of its GDP ranks it third highest among the 308 countries reporting (range, 1.6% to 19.5%). (See *http://apps.who.int/nha/database* for the most recent updates.)

The complexity of controlling costs remains a major issue driving changes in the healthcare system. Beyond coverage and cost issues, revised Medicare rules related to implementation of electronic medical records (EMRs) and other health information technology (HIT) requirements are driving substantial change in the organization of healthcare services. Adoption of EMRs and HIT are long-term journeys toward improvement as opposed to quick fixes to endemic problems. Despite the challenges associated with acquiring and implementing these complex information systems, reflecting upon the importance of informatics to patient safety, the IOM identified that using information technology is one of the five core competencies for all health professions.

Another concept associated with maximizing quality and minimizing costs is regionalization of services in which local coalitions consisting of community health providers, consumers, and corporations act to unify business initiatives in healthcare cost containment and to provide consumers with input into health planning and policy development. Wellness programs designed to modify consumers' use of and demand for services (e.g., health-promotion campaigns, ergonomic programs to reduce work-related injuries such as carpal tunnel syndrome, and fitness and exercise programs) are other industrial corporate initiatives being introduced to reduce costs. Again, nurses are assuming key roles in managed care and in organizing and directing wellness programs.

Nurses have a major role to play in demonstrating that access to care and quality management are essential components of cost control. With the increasing involvement of industry, business management techniques will assume greater emphasis in healthcare organizations. Nurses will need to lead efforts to redesign roles and restructure healthcare organizations. Nurse leaders and managers will need to go beyond obtaining education in business techniques to gaining skill in adapting that knowledge to meet the specific needs of delivery of cost-effective, quality care. The increasing focus on preparing registered nurses at the levels of

clinical nurse leader (CNL) and doctor of nursing practice (DNP) reflects the clear need for practicing nurses, nurse managers, and nurse administrators to be able to work efficiently and effectively in a constantly changing healthcare environment (Stanley et al., 2008). The evidence section, which reflects some specific research, on p. 133 describes the role and impact of the CNL.

Social Factors

Increasing consumer attention to disease prevention and promotion of healthful lifestyles is redefining relationships of healthcare organizations and their patients. Patients are becoming increasingly active in care planning, implementation, and evaluations and are seeking increased participation with their providers. Demands will be made of healthcare organizations for more personal, responsive, and coordinated care. As such, development of strategies that allow patients to become empowered controllers of their own health status is essential. Responsive structural changes in service delivery will be needed to maintain congruence with new missions and philosophies developed in response to cultural demands and social changes. Continuous evaluation will be needed to assess cost and quality outcomes related to these changes. Maintaining focus on the quality of care provided as well as access to care will be required so that bottom-line costs do not overshadow quality care provisions. Nursing's history of work with the development of patient-centered interactive strategies places nurses in a position to assume leadership roles in this area of organizational development.

Demographic Factors

Geographic dispersion, regional access to care, incomes of the population, aging of the population, and immigration trends are among the demographic factors influencing the design of healthcare organizations. Changing economic and demographic characteristics of many communities are resulting in a larger number of uninsured and underinsured individuals. Geographic isolation often limits access to necessary health services and impedes recruitment of healthcare personnel. Community-based rural health networks that provide primary care links to urban health centers for teaching, consultation, personnel sharing, and the provision of high-tech services are one solution for meeting needs in rural areas. Federal and state funding, which includes incentives for healthcare personnel to work in rural areas, is another approach. Strategic planning by nursing is critical to address community needs.

A major influence exerted on healthcare organizations comes from the aging of the population. By the year 2025, more than 18% of the population is expected to be older than 65 years. The number of "the old-old," those older than 80 years, is increasing dramatically. In response to this demographic shift, the CMS provides the Program of All-inclusive Care for the Elderly (PACE) to ensure that quality care is provided to impaired and frail elderly who are nursing home eligible. PACE aims to keep this population out of nursing homes by providing access to a full continuum of comprehensive community-based care. Although this segment of the population does not necessarily have dependency needs, a need exists for more long-term beds, supportive housing, and community programs. To meet these emerging needs of older adults, new healthcare organizations will continue to evolve, be evaluated, and be restructured based on findings. New roles for nurses as leaders and managers of the care of older adults are evolving. An example is the role of advanced nurse practitioners to direct the care of patients who have become members of geriatric care organizations such as retirement centers.

Another significant effect on the system will come from the increasing number of individuals and families who cannot afford care to meet even their most basic needs. These individuals may be truly indigent or may be the working poor who are but one paycheck or illness from being hungry or homeless. Without a broad array of basic healthcare services that are affordable and available to these individuals, failure to treat a minor problem such as high blood pressure can result in a high-cost illness such as a cerebrovascular accident. This lack of healthcare provision is compounded by the number of people excluded from coverage because of preexisting health conditions, job loss, or immigration status.

A THEORETICAL PERSPECTIVE

Systems Theory

Systems theory attempts to explain productivity in terms of a unifying whole as opposed to a series of unrelated parts (Thompson, 1967). Systems can be either closed (self-contained) or open (interacting with both internal and external forces). In systems theory, a system is described as comprising four elements: structure, technology, people, and their environment. Systems theorists focus on the interplay among these elements in a framework of (1) inputs—resources such as people, money, or materials; (2) throughputs—the processes that produce a product from the inputs; and (3) outputs—the product of inputs and throughputs.

The theoretical concepts of systems theory have been applied to nursing and to organizations. Systems theory presents an explanation of organizational evolution that is similar to biological evolution. Systems theory produces a model that explains the process of healthcare organization evolution (Figure 7-1). The survival of the organization, as portrayed throughout this chapter, depends on its evolutionary

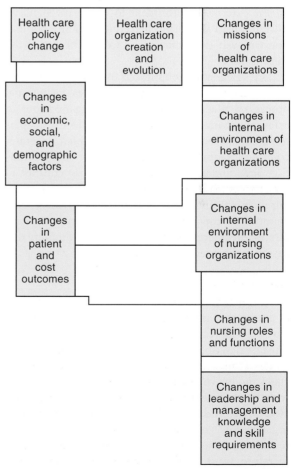

FIGURE 7-1 Healthcare organizations as open systems.

response to changing environmental forces; it is seen as an open system. The response to environmental changes brings about internal changes, which produce changes that alter environmental conditions. The changes in the environment, in turn, act to bring about changes in the internal operating conditions of the organization.

A very simplified example of this can be seen in the implementation of the prospective payment system that was caused by the economic driving force of escalating healthcare costs in the 1990s. Ambulatory surgery, same-day admissions, and hospital- and community-based home care organizations are some of the internal healthcare organization changes that resulted from an environmentally driven policy change—the cap that was placed on reimbursing expenses incurred by hospitalized patients. These internal organizational developments placed pressure on the external environment to create mechanisms to respond to increasing percentages of the population with self-care deficits who were returning to the community.

This open systems approach to organizational development and effectiveness emphasizes a continual process of adaptation of healthcare organizations to external driving forces and a response to the adaptations by the external environment, which generates continuing inputs for further healthcare organization development. This open system is in contrast to a closed system approach that views a system as being sufficient unto itself and thus untouched by what happens around it. (The effects of external forces on internal structures of healthcare organizations are discussed in Chapter 8.)

Chaos Theory

Unfortunately, health care as an industry is not always as predictable and orderly as systems theorists would have us believe. In contrast to the somewhat orderly universe described in systems theory, in which an organization can be viewed in terms of a linear, cause-and-effect model, chaos theory sees the universe as filled with unpredictable and random events (Hawking, 1998). According to the proponents of chaos theory, organizations must be self-organizing and adapt readily to change in order to survive. Organizations, therefore, must accept that change is inevitable and unrelenting. When one embraces the tenets of chaos

THEORY BOX
Systems and Chaos Theories

Systems theory	• Definition: A system comprises four elements (structure, technology, people, and environment) forming a unified whole • Viewed as inputs, throughputs, and outputs • Closed systems—self-contained • Open systems—interacting with internal and external forces
Chaos theory	• Definition: The universe is chaotic and requires organizations to be self-organizing and adaptive to survive • Viewed as unpredictable and random events • Constant change resulting in little long-term stability

theory, one gives up on any attempt to create a permanent organizational structure. Using creativity and flexibility, successful managers will be those who can tolerate ambiguity, take risks, and experiment with new ideas in response to each day's unique situation or environment. They will not rest upon a successful transition or organizational model because they know the environment that it flourished in is fleeting. The successful nurse leaders will be those individuals who are committed to lifelong learning and problem solving. The Theory Box notes key elements of systems and chaos theories.

NURSING ROLE AND FUNCTION CHANGES

Leadership and management roles for nurses are proliferating in healthcare organizations that are developing or evolving in response to environmental driving forces. With the expansion of accountable care organizations, the proportion of nursing positions in the community is increasing, as are various care management positions, clinical nurse leaders, and advanced practice nurses. Filling these roles require knowledge and skills to coordinate the care of patients or communities with the many other disciplines and organizational units that are providing the continuum of care. Our society needs nurses who can engage in the political process of policy development, coordinate care across disciplines and settings, use conflict management techniques to create win-win situations for patients and providers in resolving the healthcare system's delivery problems, and use business savvy to market and prepare financial and organizational plans for the delivery of cost-effective care.

Economic, social, and demographic changes are not limited to patients and communities. These shifts are affecting the workplace as well. To be effective, nurse managers and leaders need to consider how these phenomena affect the workplace in the same way they consider it when seeking to address the needs of their patients and the communities they serve. To be efficient and effective, nurse leaders must be not only patient-centered but also employee-centered. Establishing healthy work environments where employee engagement is maximized results in increased job satisfaction and positive patient outcomes. (Shared governance as an organizing structure is discussed in Chapter 8.)

CONCLUSION

Whether influenced by systems or chaos theory, today's healthcare organizations are in a dynamic state. Nurses must be continuously alert to assessing both the internal and external environment for forces that act as inputs to changes needed in their healthcare organization and for the effects of changes that are made. Awareness of the changing status of healthcare organizations and the ability to play a leading role in creating and evaluating adaptation in response to changing forces will be central functions of nurse leaders and managers in healthcare organizations. Nurses need to develop a foundation of leadership and management knowledge that they can build on through a planned program of continuing education. Even in tumultuous times within the healthcare industry, nursing leaders have demonstrated their ability to strengthen the quality of both their organizations and the practice of nursing. As healthcare organizations continue to undergo transformation, tomorrow's nurses—whether leaders, managers, or followers—need to carry these lessons forward.

THE SOLUTION

I contacted the hospital case manager, who arranged for this patient to have access to special programs in the hospital to fund the medications and support the case management expenses. We arranged for the patient to be seen by a state agency that provides emergency funds for utilities and phone service and assisted him with a Medicaid application with a request for a retroactive initiation date. Finally, we contacted hospice and the American Cancer Society to support the tube-feeding expenses and worked with other agencies to delay billings until Medicaid was available. Clearly, today's nurse manager has to be connected with the extended resources in the community to ensure care for patients who require assistance.

—Beth A. Smith

Would this be a suitable approach for you? Why?

THE EVIDENCE

The American Association of Colleges of Nursing introduced the role of the master's-prepared clinical nurse leader (CNL) in 2004 as a response to the need for more evidence-based, collaborative, cost effective, patient-centered care. Bender, Connelly, Glaser, and Brown (2012) assessed the impact of CNLs on a progressive care unit as measured by patient satisfaction with their care.

Introduction of the CNL role resulted in significantly improved patient satisfaction with admission processes ($r=+.63$, $p=.02$), nursing care ($r=+.75$, $p=.004$), skill level of nurses ($r=.83$, $p=.003$), and keeping patients informed ($r=.70, p=.003$).

The evidence supports the positive impact of organizational designs that include expanded roles for nurses, such as the CNL.

WHAT NEW GRADUATES SAY

- I didn't know that the ownership and governance of a hospital could determine the level of care patients receive.
- I like working in a teaching hospital. Interacting with students and residents helps keep a focus on evidence-based practice.
- We are caring for an increasing number of uninsured patients on my unit. It is often a challenge to coordinate the transitions of care to home when there are limited services available. I wish I had learned more about the financing of health care while I was in nursing school.
- There are increasing numbers of options for nurses working in primary care. I expect to focus my career in this area.

CHAPTER CHECKLIST

Knowledge of types of healthcare organizations and characteristics used to differentiate healthcare organizations provides a foundation for examining the operation of the healthcare system. Understanding the economic, social, and demographic forces driving changes in healthcare organizations identifies needs that organizations must be designed to fit. Recognizing that alterations in the environment and in healthcare organizations are mutually interactive is necessary to determine the effects of change and the steps that need to be taken in response to the constant changes. Changes in nursing roles as well as in the settings in which services are provided require that nurses expand their knowledge and skills. These changes are part of a continual evolution that demands a foundation in leadership and management knowledge that serves as a basis for future development.

- Characteristics and types of organizations
  - Institutional providers
    - Types of services provided
    - Length of direct care services provided
    - Ownership
    - Teaching status
    - Accreditation status
  - Consolidated systems and networks
    - Consolidated systems
    - Networks
  - Ambulatory-based organizations
  - Other organizations
    - Community services
    - Subacute facilities
    - Home health organizations
    - Long-term care and residential facilities
    - Hospice
    - Nurse-owned and nurse-organized services
    - Self-help voluntary organizations
  - Supportive and ancillary organizations
    - Regulatory organizations
    - Accrediting bodies
    - Third-party financing organizations
    - Pharmaceutical and medical equipment supply organizations
    - Integration
    - Acquisitions and mergers
- Forces that influence healthcare organizations
  - Economic factors
  - Social factors
  - Demographic factors
- A theoretical perspective
  - Systems theory
  - Chaos theory
- Nursing role and function changes

TIPS FOR HEALTHCARE ORGANIZATIONS

- Knowledge of economic, social, and demographic changes is essential to redesigning healthcare organizations to meet society's needs.
- Increasing consolidation of healthcare services that provide all levels of care necessitates the development of communication systems that provide

information on patients receiving services at the various points of care in the network.

• Diversified positions will be available for professional nurses in the various organizations that are developing to enhance the provision of care.

• New configurations of healthcare delivery will demand that professional nurses continually acquire new knowledge and skills in leadership and management.

REFERENCES

American Hospital Association. *AHA Hospital Statistics*. (2012 ed.). Chicago: American Hospital Association.

Bender, M., Connelly, C. D., Glaser, D., & Brown, C. (2012). Clinical nurse leader impact on microsystem care quality. *Nursing Research*, *61*(5), 326–332.

Cady, R. F. (2011). Accountable care organizations: What the nurse executive needs to know. *JONA's Healthcare Law, Ethics and Regulation*, *13*(2), 55–60.

Doyle, J. J., Graves, J. A., Gruber, J., & Kleiner, S. (2012). *Do high-cost hospitals deliver better care? Evidence from ambulance referral patterns*. National Bureau of Economic Research (NBER). Working Paper 17936. March 2012, www.nber.org/papers/w17936.pdf.

Hawking, S. (1998). *A brief history of time*. London: Bantam Press.

Henry J. Kaiser Family Foundation. (2013). *The uninsured*. Washington, DC: Author.

Ritter-Teitel, J. (2012). Evolving forms of accountable care organizations: Implications for nurse leaders. *Nurse Leader*, *10*(6), 36–38.

Stanley, J. M., Gannon, J., Gabaut, S., Adams, N., Mayes, C., Shouse, G. M., et al. (2008). The clinical nurse leader: A catalyst for improving quality and patient safety. *Journal of Nursing Management*, *16*(5), 612–622.

Thompson, J. D. (1967). *Organization in action*. New York: McGraw-Hill.

SUGGESTED READINGS

Aiken, L. H., Sloane, D. M., Clarke, S., Poghosyan, L., Cho, E., You, L., et al. (2011). Importance of work environments on hospital outcomes in nine countries. *International Journal for Quality in Health Care*, *23*(4), 357–364.

Etheridge, P. (1997). The Carondelet experience. *Nursing Management*, *28*(3), 26–28.

Kaiser Commission on Medicaid and the Uninsured, *Health care coverage in America*. (2012). Washington, DC: Henry J. Kaiser Family Foundation.

Kast, F. E., & Rosenweiz, J. E. (1991). General systems theory: Applications for organizations and management. In M. J. Ward & S. A. Price (Eds.), *Issues in nursing administration: Selected readings* (pp. 60–73). St. Louis: Mosby.

Smith, M., Saunders, R., Stuckhardt, L., & McGinnis, J. M. (Eds.). (2012). Committee on the Learning Health Care System in America. *Best care at lower cost: The path to continuously learning health care in America*. Washington, DC: National Academies Press.

Porter-O'Grady, T. (1996). The seven basic rules for successful redesign. *Journal of Nursing Administration*, *26*(1), 46–55.

INTERNET RESOURCES

Centers for Medicare & Medicaid Services (CMS). www.cms.gov.

Community Health Assessment Program (CHAP). www.chapinc.org.

Institute for Healthcare Improvement (IHI). www.ihs.gov.

Kaiser Family Foundation—Kaiser Commission on Medicaid and the Uninsured. www.kff.org/.

Medicare Quality Improvement Community (MedQIC). www.qualitynet.org.

National Committee on Quality Assurance (NCQA). www.ncqa.org.

National PACE Association (NPA). www.npaonline.org.

QualityNet. www.qualitynet.org.

The Joint Commission. www.jointcommission.org.

8

Understanding and Designing Organizational Structures

Mary E. Mancini

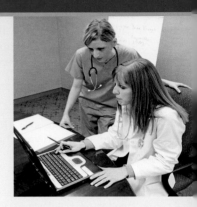

This chapter explains key concepts related to organizational structures and provides information on designing effective structures. This information can be used to help nurse managers and baccalaureate-prepared nurses function in an organization and to design structures that support work processes. An underlying theme is designing organizational structures that will respond to the continuous changes taking place in the healthcare environment.

LEARNING OUTCOMES

- Analyze the relationships among mission, vision, and philosophy statements and organizational structure.
- Analyze factors that influence the design of an organizational structure.
- Compare and contrast the major types of organizational structures.
- Describe the differences between redesigning, restructuring, and reengineering of organizational systems.

KEY TERMS

accountable care organization	mission	restructuring
bureaucracy	organization	service-line structures
chain of command	organizational chart	shared governance
flat organizational structure	organizational culture	span of control
functional structure	organizational structure	staff function
hierarchy	organizational theory	system
hybrid	philosophy	systems theory
line function	redesign	vision
matrix structure	reengineering	

THE CHALLENGE

Anonymous

I am the director of a thriving nursing service. We specialize in three to four product lines and are highly effective at serving our market. We are a subsidiary of a more generalized healthcare service and are probably envied by them because our return on investment far exceeds theirs. Our business is growing and theirs is stagnating or even decreasing. I have been asked to have the more generalized healthcare service provide support services so that the income and expenses associated with my service can enhance the other service.

In addition, the equivalent of a merger is being proposed. Because of the relationship with the more generalized healthcare service, I am really obligated to function within the guidelines this group sets. I envision my budget growing to support the other group and am concerned that my services will be diluted and thus not provide the same quality we have in the past. I can easily move onto another position but I am very committed to the staff and the people we serve.

What do you think you would do if you were this nurse?

INTRODUCTION

Since time began, people have organized themselves into groups. The term **organization** has multiple meanings. It can refer to a business structure designed to support specific business goals and processes, or it can refer to a group of individuals working together to achieve a common purpose. Regardless of how the term is used, learning to determine how an organization accomplishes its work, how to operate productively within an organization, and how to influence organizational processes is essential to a successful professional nursing practice.

Organizational theory (sometimes called *organizational studies*) is the systematic analysis of how organizations and their component parts act and interact. Organizational theory is based largely on the systematic investigation of the effectiveness of specific organizational designs in achieving their purpose. Organizational theory development is a process of creating knowledge to understand the effect of identified factors, such as (1) organizational culture; (2) organizational technology, which is defined as all the work being carried out; and (3) organizational structure or organizational development. A purpose of such work is to determine how organizational effectiveness might be predicted or controlled through the design of the organizational structure.

Specific organizational theories provide insight into areas such as effective organizational structures, motivation of employees, decision-making, and leadership. A common framework in health care for analysis and application of organizational theory is **systems theory.** A **system** is an interacting collection of components or parts that together make up an integrated whole. The basic tenet of systems theory is that the individual components of any system interact with each other and with their environment. To be effective, baccalaureate-prepared nurses need to understand the specific part—role and function—they play within a system and how they interact, influence, and are influenced by other parts of the system.

An organization's mission, vision, and philosophy form the foundation for its structure and performance as well as the development of the professional practice models it uses. An organization's **mission,** or reason for the organization's existence, influences the design of the structure (e.g., to meet the healthcare needs of a designated population, to provide supportive and stabilizing care to an acute care population, or to prepare patients for a peaceful death). The **vision** is the articulated goal to which the organization aspires. A vision statement conveys an inspirational view of how the organization wishes to be described at some future time. It suggests how far to strive in all endeavors. Another key factor influencing structure is the organization's **philosophy.** A philosophy expresses the values and beliefs that members of the organization hold about the nature of their work, about the people to whom they provide service, and about themselves and others providing the services.

EXERCISE 8-1

Consider how you might use the information in the Introduction:
1. To analyze an organization that you are considering joining to determine whether it fits your professional goals,
2. To assess the functioning of an organization of which you are already a member
3. To make a plan to reengineer the structure or philosophy to better accomplish the mission of the organization.

MISSION

The mission statement defines the organization's reason or purpose for being. The mission statement identifies the organization's customers (individuals, families, populations, or communities) and the types of services offered, such as outreach, comprehensive care management, acute care, rehabilitation, or home care. It enacts the vision statement.

The mission statement sets the stage by defining the services to be offered, which, in turn, identify the kinds of technologies and human resources to be employed. The mission statement of accountable care organizations (a group of providers and healthcare organizations who are organized to give comprehensive, coordinated care focused on improving patient outcomes) are focused on providing comprehensive coordinated care in order to improve the health and well-being of a group of individuals. An example of a mission statement appears in Box 8-1. Hospitals' missions are primarily treatment-oriented; the missions of ambulatory care group practices combine treatment, prevention, and diagnosis-oriented services; long-term care facilities' missions are primarily maintenance and social support–oriented; and the missions of nursing centers are oriented toward promoting optimal health status for a defined group of people. The definition of services to be provided

---

BOX 8-1 MISSION, VISION, AND PHILOSOPHY FOR A NEUROSURGICAL UNIT

Mission Statement

This unit's purpose is to provide high-quality nursing care for neurosurgical patients during the acute phase of their illness that facilitates their progression to the rehabilitation phase. We strive to cultivate a multidisciplinary approach to the care of the neurosurgical patient and provide multiple educational opportunities for the professional development of neurosurgical nurses.

Vision Statement

To be the premier neurosurgical nursing unit in the state.

Philosophy

The philosophy is based on Roy's Adaptation Model and on the American Association of Neurosurgical Nursing conceptual framework.

Patients

We believe

- It is the right of the patients to make informed choices concerning their treatment.
- Patients have a right to high-quality nursing care and opportunities for improving their quality of life, regardless of the potential outcomes of their illness.
- The patient/family/significant other has a right to exercise personal options to participate in care to the extent of individual abilities and needs.

Nursing

We believe

- Neuroscience nursing is a unique area of nursing practice because neurosurgical interventions and/or neurological dysfunction affect all levels of human existence.
- The goal of the neuroscience nurse is to engage in a therapeutic relationship with his or her patients to facilitate adaptation to changes in physiological, self-concept, role performance, and interdependent modes.

- The ultimate goal for the neuroscience nurse is to foster internal and external unity of patients to achieve optimal health potentials.

Nurse

We believe

- The nurse is the integral element who coordinates nursing care for the neurosurgical patient using valuable input from all members of the patient care team.
- The nurse has an obligation to assume accountability for maintaining excellence in practice.
- The nurse has three basic rights: human rights, legal rights, and professional rights.
- The nurse has a right to autonomy in providing nursing care based on sound nursing judgment.

Nursing Practice

We believe

- Nursing practice must support and be supported by activities in practice, education, research, and management.
- Insofar as possible, patients must be assigned one nurse who is responsible and accountable for their care throughout their stay on the neurosurgical unit.
- The primary nurse is responsible for consulting and collaborating with other healthcare professionals in planning and delivering patient care.
- The contributions of all members of the nursing team are valuable, and an environment must be created that allows each member to participate fully in the delivery of care in accord with his or her abilities and qualifications.
- The nursing process is the vehicle used by nurses to operationalize nursing practice.
- Data generated in nursing practices must be continually and consistently collected and analyzed for the purpose of managing the quality of nursing practice.

Courtesy Upstate Medical University, University Hospital, Syracuse, NY (W. Painter, J. Van Nest-Kinne).

and the implications for technologies and human resources greatly influence the design of the organizational structure, that is, the arrangement of the work group.

Nursing, as a profession providing a service within a healthcare agency, formulates its own mission statement that describes its contributions to achieve the agency's mission. One of the purposes of the nursing profession is to provide nursing care to patients. The statement should define nursing based on theories that form the basis for the model of nursing to be used in guiding the process of nursing care delivery. Nursing's mission statement tells why nursing exists within the context of the organization. This statement is written so that others within the organization can know and understand nursing's role in achieving the agency's mission. The mission should be the guiding framework for decision making. It should be known and understood by other healthcare professionals, by patients and their families, and by the community. It indicates the relationships among nurses and patients, other personnel in the organization, the community, as well as health and illness. The mission provides direction for the evolving statement of philosophy and the organizational structure. It should be reviewed for accuracy and updated routinely. Various work units that provide specific services such as intensive care, women's health services, or hospice care may also formulate mission statements that detail their specific contributions to the overall organization.

VISION

Vision statements are future-oriented, purposeful statements designed to identify the desired future of an organization. They serve to unify all subsequent statements toward the view of the future and to convey the core message of the mission statement. Typically, vision statements are brief, consisting of only one or two phrases or sentences. An example of a vision statement is provided in Box 8-1.

PHILOSOPHY

A philosophy is a written statement that articulates the values and beliefs held about the nature of the work required to accomplish the mission and the nature and rights of both the people being served and those providing the service. A nursing philosophy states the vision of what nursing practice should be within the organization and how it contributes to the health of individuals and communities. For example, the organization's mission statement may incorporate the provision of individualized care as an organizational purpose. The philosophy statement would then support this purpose through an expression of a belief in the responsibility of nursing staff to act as patient advocates and to provide quality care according to the wishes of the patient, family, and significant others.

Philosophies are evolutionary in that they are shaped both by the social environment and by the stage of development of professionals delivering the service. Nursing staff reflect the values of their time. The values acquired through education are reflected in the nursing philosophy. Philosophies require updating to reflect the extension of rights brought about by such changes. Box 8-1 shows an example of a philosophy developed for a neurosurgical unit.

> **EXERCISE 8-2**
> Obtain a copy of the philosophy of a nursing department. Identify behaviors that you observe on a unit of the department that relate or do not relate to the beliefs and values expressed in the document.

ORGANIZATIONAL CULTURE

An organization's mission, vision, and philosophy both shape and reflect organizational culture. Organizational culture is the reflection of the norms or traditions of the organization and is exemplified by behaviors that illustrate values and beliefs. Examples include rituals and customary forms of practice, such as celebrations of promotions, degree attainment, professional performance, weddings, and retirements. Other examples of norms that reflect organizational culture are the characteristics of the people who are recognized as heroes by the organization and the behaviors—either positive or negative—that are accepted or tolerated within the organization.

In organizations, culture is demonstrated in two ways that can be either mutually reinforcing or conflict-producing. Organizational culture is typically expressed in a formal manner via written mission, vision, and philosophy statements; job descriptions; and policies and procedures. Beyond formal documents and verbal descriptions given by administrators and managers, organizational culture is also represented in the day-to-day experience of staff and patients. To many, it is the lived experience that reflects the true organizational culture. Do the decisions that are made within the organization consistently demonstrate that the organization values its patients and keeps their needs at the forefront? Are the employees treated with trust and respect, or are the words used in recruitment ads simply empty promises with little evidence to back them up? When a lack of congruity exists between the expressed organizational culture and the experienced organizational culture, confusion, frustration, and poor morale often result (Casida and Parker, 2011; Tsai, 2011).

Organizational culture can be effective and promote success and positive outcomes, or it can be ineffective and result in disharmony, dissatisfaction, and poor outcomes for patients, staff, and the organization. A number of workplace variables are influenced by organizational culture. When seeking employment or advancement, nurses need to assess the organization's culture and develop a clear understanding of existing expectations as well as the formal and informal communication patterns. Various techniques and tools are available to assist the nurse in performing a cultural assessment of an organization (Cummings, Midodzi, Wong, & Estabrooks, 2010). With a solid understanding of organizational culture, nurses will be better able to be effective change agents and help transform the organizations in which they work. The Research Perspective presents a study on the effect of authentic leadership and structural empowerment on the emotional exhaustion and cynicism of new graduates and experienced nurses.

FACTORS INFLUENCING ORGANIZATIONAL DEVELOPMENT

To be most effective, organizational structures must reflect the organization's mission, vision, philosophy, goals, and objectives. Organizational structure defines how work is organized, where decisions are made, and the authority and responsibility of workers. It provides a map for communication and outlines decision-making paths. As organizations change through acquisitions and mergers, it is essential that structure changes to accomplish revised missions.

Probably the best theory to explain today's nursing organizational development is chaos (complexity, nonlinear, quantum) theory. (See Chaos Theory in the Index.) In essence, chaos theory suggests that lives—and organizations—are web-like. Pulling on one small segment rearranges the web, a new pattern emerges, and yet the whole remains. This theory, applied to nursing organizations, suggests that differences logically exist between and among various organizations and that the constant environmental forces continue to affect the structure, its functioning, and the services. See the Theory Box for Chapter 7, p. 132.

Ongoing changes in the U.S. healthcare delivery system, such as the *Patient Protection and Affordable Care Act (http://housedocs.house.gov/energycommerce/ppacacon.pdf)*, revise reimbursement regulation and develop networks for delivery of health care. These modifications have profound effects on organizational structure designs. Consumerism, the consumer demand that care be customized to meet individual needs, necessitates that decision making be done where the care is delivered. Increased consumer knowledge and greater responsibility for selecting healthcare providers and options have resulted in consumers who demand immediate access to customized care. Information from Internet sources and direct-to-consumer advertising are significantly altering the

---

 RESEARCH PERSPECTIVE

Resource: Laschinger, H.K.S, Wong, C.A., & Grau, A.L, (2012). Authentic leadership, empowerment, and burnout: a comparison in new graduates and experienced nurses. *Journal of Nursing Management, 21*(3) Article first published online: 15 APR 2012. DOI: http://dx.doi.org/10.1111/j.1365-2834.2012.01375.x.

This study involved examining the concept of authentic leadership and the effects on new graduates and experienced nurses in acute care settings in Canada. The major finding was that authentic leadership significantly affected both emotional exhaustion and cynicism in a negative manner for both groups. This means that authentic leadership has a positive impact on both new and experienced nurses in acute care settings.

Implications for Practice

Development for new and existing managers should focus on authentic leadership because it positively affects the work environment.

expectation and behaviors of healthcare consumers. For example, Hospital Compare *(www.hospitalcompare. hhs.gov)* is a tool that consumers can use to access a searchable database of information describing how well hospitals care for patients with certain medical and surgical conditions. Access to this information allows consumers to make informed decisions about where they seek their health care. In response to consumer expectations, facilities concentrate on consumer satisfaction and delivery of patient-focused care. Changes in both facility design and care delivery systems are likely to continue as efforts are made to reduce cost while still striving to meet or exceed consumer expectations and improve patient outcomes.

Competition for patients is another factor influencing structure design. These three factors—change including federal mandates, consumerism, and competition—necessitate reengineering healthcare structures. Whereas **redesign** is a technique to analyze tasks to improve efficiency (e.g., identifying the most efficient flow of supplies to a nursing unit) and **restructuring** is a technique to enhance organizational productivity (e.g., identifying the most appropriate type and number of staff members for a particular nursing unit), **reengineering** involves a total overhaul of an organizational structure. It is a radical reorganization of the totality of an organization's structure and work processes. In reengineering, fundamentally new organizational expectations and relationships are created. An example of where reengineering is required is technologic change, particularly in information services, that provides a means of customizing care. Its potential for making all information concerning a patient immediately accessible to direct care givers has the potential for a profound positive impact on healthcare decision-making.

The Transforming Care at the Bedside (TCAB) initiative is an example of redesigning the work environment from the bottom up. The initiative, funded by the Robert Wood Johnson Foundation and the Institute for Healthcare Improvement, was started in 2003 to develop and validate an evidence-based process for transforming care in acute care facilities. Reports from TCAB facilities demonstrate the value of nurse involvement in the process as well as the value to nurses in terms of their participation (Chaboyer, Johnson, Hardy, Gehrke, & Panuwatwanich, 2010; Unruh, Agrawal, & Hassmiller, 2011).

Regardless of the level of changes made within an organization—redesign, restructuring, or reengineering—staff and patients alike feel the impact. Some of the changes result in improvements, whereas others may not; some of the impacts are expected, whereas others are not. It is critical, therefore, that nurse managers as well as direct care nurses are vigilant for both anticipated and unanticipated results of these changes. Nurses need to position themselves to participate in change discussions and evaluations. Ultimately, it is their day-to-day work with their patients that is affected by the decisions made in response to a rapidly changing environment.

EXERCISE 8-3

Arrange to interview a nurse employed in a healthcare agency or use your own experience to identify examples of changes taking place that necessitate reengineering. These may include changes associated with implementation of new reimbursement strategies, development of policies to carry out legislative regulations related to patient confidentiality, or development of chest pain centers. Identify examples of how previous systems of communication and decision making were either adequate or inadequate to cope with these changes.

CHARACTERISTICS OF ORGANIZATIONAL STRUCTURES

The characteristics of different types of organizational structures provide a catalog of options to consider in designing structures that fit specific situations. Knowledge of these characteristics help leaders, managers, and nursing staff understand the expectations and structures in which they currently function.

Organizational designs are often classified by their characteristics of complexity, formalization, and centralization. *Complexity* concerns the division of labor in an organization, the specialization of that labor, the number of hierarchical levels, and the geographic dispersion of organizational units. *Division of labor* and *specialization* refer to the separation of processes into tasks that are performed by designated people. The horizontal dimension of an **organizational chart,** the graphic representation of work units and reporting relationships, relates to the division and specialization of labor functions attended by specialists. Hierarchy connotes lines of authority and responsibility. Chain of command is a term used to refer to the hierarchy and is depicted in vertical dimensions of organizational charts. Hierarchy vests authority in positions on an ascending line away from where work is performed and allows control of work. Staff members are often placed on a bottom level of the organization, and those in authority, who provide control, are placed in higher levels. Span of control refers to the number of subordinates a supervisor manages. For budgetary reasons, span of control is often a major focus for organizational restructuring. Although cost implications are present when a span of control is too narrow, when a span of control becomes too large, supervision can become less effective. The Research Perspective describes the effect of span of control.

 RESEARCH PERSPECTIVE

Resource: Wong, C.A., Elliott-Miller, P., Laschinger, H., Cuddihy, M., Meyer, R.M., Keatings, M., Burnett, C., Szudy, N. (2013). Examining the relationships between span of control and manager job and unit performance outcomes. *Journal of Nursing Management*. Jul 5. DOI: http://dx.doi.org/10.1111/jonm.12107. [Epub ahead of print]

This non-experimental predictive survey was designed to assess frontline nurse managers and span of control from the standpoint of effects on the managers and on unit outcomes. Fourteen Canadian hospitals participated in this study and 121 managers responded. The important finding was that only span of control predicted adverse outcomes. Neither span of control nor self evaluation predicted unit turnover.

Implications for Practice
To be effective, nurse managers need to have reasonable spans of control. The span of control often increases when organizations downsize; so nurse leaders need to be alert to the effects on patient care outcomes.

Geographic dispersion refers to the physical location of units. Units of work may be in one building; in several buildings in one location; spread throughout a city; or in different counties, states, or countries. The more dispersed an organization is, the greater are the demands for creative designs that place decision-making related to patient care close to the patient and, consequently, far from corporate headquarters. A similar type of complexity exists in organizations that deliver care at multiple sites in the community; for example, the care delivery sites of an accountable care organization may be at great distances from the corporate office that has overall responsibility for the programs.

Formalization is the degree to which an organization has rules, stated in terms of policies that define a member's function. The amount of formalization varies among institutions. Formalization is often inversely related to the degree of specialization and the number of professionals within the organization.

EXERCISE 8-4
Review a copy of a nursing department's organizational chart and identify the divisions of labor, the hierarchy of authority, and the degree of formalization.

Centralization refers to the location where a decision is made. Decisions are made at the top of a centralized organization. In a decentralized organization, decisions are made at or close to the patient-care level. Highly centralized organizations often delegate *responsibility* (the obligation to perform the task) without the *authority* (the right to act, which is necessary to carry out the responsibility). For example, some hospitals have delegated both the responsibility and the authority for admission decisions to the charge nurse (decentralized), whereas others require the nurse supervisor or chief nurse executive to make such decisions (centralization). As the Center for Medicare & Medicaid Services (CMS) evolved guidelines to facilitate the delivery of health care, CMS identified that non-physicians, including registered nurses can write orders to admit patients so long as the practice fits with state laws and organizational policies.

BUREAUCRACY

Many organizational theories in use today find their basis in the works of early twenty-first century theorists Max Weber, a German sociologist who developed the basic tenets of bureaucracy (Weber, 1947), and Henri Fayol, a French industrialist who crafted 14 principles of management (Fayol, 1949). Initially, bureaucracy referred to the centralization of authority in administrative bureaus or government departments. The term has come to refer to an inflexible approach to decision making or an agency encumbered by red tape that adds little value to organizational processes. The Literature Perspective presents information about high-value organizations.

LITERATURE PERSPECTIVE

Resource: Bohmer, R.M. (2011). The four habits of high-value health care organizations. *New England Journal of Medicine,* *365*(22):2045-2047.

The author acknowledges that organizations vary in structure, resources, and culture. However most have a similar approach to managing care. He identifies four habits that could be translated across organizations and that would promote better care. The habits are:

1. Specification and planning: This includes both operational decisions and clinical decisions. These decisions are based on specific criteria.
2. Infrastructure design: This element includes microsystems such as technology, physical design, and policies and procedures.
3. Measurement and oversight: High-performing organizations seem to collect more data—and use it—than other organizations.
4. Self study: This habit involves introspection about any deviations from expected results, both positive and negative. The goal is to increase the positive deviations and intervene when the deviations are negative. Outcomes are viewed as critical to the organization, not just to an individual or unit.

The difference of high-value organizations seems to revolve around two things. First is the systematic use of the habits, and the second is that they are integrated into the processes and outcomes in the organizations.

Implications for Practice

Nursing has demonstrated these approaches in organizations that provide excellent care. Integrating these into the culture of the nursing organization can improve the outcomes nursing produces for health care.

Bureaucracy is an administrative concept imbedded in how organizations are structured. The concept arose at a time of societal development when services were in short supply, workers' and clients' knowledge bases were limited, and technologies for sharing information were undeveloped. Characteristics of bureaucracy arose out of a need to control workers and were centered on the division of processes into discrete tasks. Weber (1947) proposed that organizations could achieve high levels of productivity and efficiency only by adherence to what he called "bureaucracy." Weber believed that bureaucracy, based on the sociological concept of rationalization of collective activities, provided the idealized organizational structure. Bureaucratic structures are formal and have a centralized and hierarchical command structure (chain of command). Bureaucratic structures have a clear division of labor and well-articulated and commonly accepted expectations for performance. Rules, standards, and protocols ensure uniform actions and limit individualization of services and variance in workers' performance. In bureaucratic organizations, as shown in Figure 8-1, communication and decisions flow from top to bottom. Although bureaucracy enhances consistency, by nature, it limits employee autonomy and thus the potential for innovations and client-centric service.

In developing his 14 principles of management, Fayol (1949) outlined structures and processes that guide how work is accomplished within an organization. Consistent with theories of bureaucracy, his principles of management include division of labor or specialization, clear lines of authority, appropriate levels of discipline, unity of direction, equitable treatment of staff, fostering of individual initiative, and promotion of a sense of teamwork and group pride. More than 60 years after they were described, these principles remain the basis of most organizations. Therefore, to be effective organizational leaders and followers, nurses need to be familiar with the theory and concepts of bureaucracy.

At the time that bureaucracies were developed, these characteristics promoted efficiency and production. As the knowledge base of the general population and employees grew and technologies developed, the bureaucratic structure no longer fit the evolving situation. Increasingly, employees and consumers functioning in bureaucratic situations complain of red tape, procedural delays, and general frustration.

Regardless of the form an organization takes (acute care hospital, ambulatory setting, accountable care organization, free-standing clinic, etc.), the characteristics of bureaucracy can be present in varying degrees. An organization can demonstrate bureaucratic characteristics in some areas and not in others. For example, nursing staff in intensive care units may be granted autonomy in making and carrying out direct patient care decisions, but they may not be granted a voice in determining work schedules or financial reimbursement systems for hours worked. One method to determine the extent to which bureaucratic tendencies

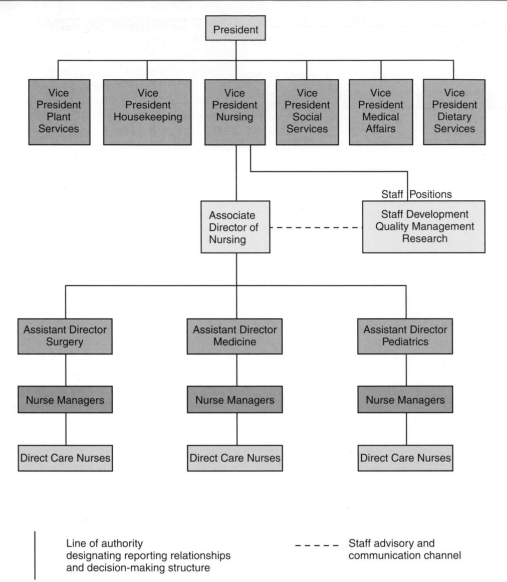

FIGURE 8-1 A bureaucratic organizational chart depicting specialization of labor, centralization, hierarchical authority, and line and staff responsibilities.

exist in organizations is to assess the organizational characteristics of the following:

- Labor specialization (the degree to which patient care is divided into highly specialized tasks)
- Centralization (the level of the organization on which decisions regarding carrying out work and remuneration for work are made)
- Formalization (the percentage of actions required to deliver patient care that is governed by written policy and procedures)

Decision making and authority can be described in terms of line and staff functions. **Line functions** are those that involve direct responsibility for accomplishing the objectives of a nursing department, service, or unit. Line positions may include registered nurses, licensed practical/vocational nurses, and unlicensed assistive (or nursing) personnel who have the responsibility for carrying out all aspects of direct care. **Staff functions** are those that assist individuals in line positions in accomplishing the primary objectives.

In this context, the term *staff positions* should not be confused with specific jobs that include "staff" in their names, such as staff nurse or staff physician. Staff positions include individuals, such as professional or staff development personnel, researchers, and special clinical consultants, who are responsible for supporting line positions through activities of consultation, education, role modeling, and knowledge development, with limited or no direct authority for decision-making. Line personnel have authority for decision making, whereas personnel in staff positions provide support, advice, and counsel. Organizational charts usually indicate line positions through the use of solid lines and staff positions through broken lines (reminder: in this context, the term *staff (or direct care) position* does not reference titles such as staff nurses). Line structures have a vertical line, designating reporting and decision-making responsibility. The vertical line connects all positions to a centralized authority (see Figure 8-1).

To make line and staff functions effective, decision-making authority is clearly spelled out in position descriptions. Effectiveness is further ensured by delineating competencies required for the responsibilities, providing methods for determining whether personnel possess these competencies, and providing means of maintaining and developing the competencies.

EXERCISE 8-5

Organizational structures vary in the extent to which they have bureaucratic characteristics. Using observations in a clinical setting, place a check mark in the "Present" column beside the bureaucratic characteristics that you believe apply to this agency. What does this analysis indicate about the bureaucratic tendency of the agency? Do the environment and technologies fit the identified bureaucratic tendency? (Consider the state of development of information systems, method of care delivery, patient characteristics, worker characteristics, regulatory status, and competition.)

CHARACTERISTIC	PRESENT
• Hierarchy of authority	____
• Division of labor	____
• Written procedures for work	____
• Limited authority for workers	____
• Emphasis on written communication related to work performance and workers' behaviors	____
• Impersonality of personal contact	____

TYPES OF ORGANIZATIONAL STRUCTURES

In healthcare organizations, several common types of organizational structures exist: functional, service line, matrix, or flat. Nursing organizations often combine characteristics of these structures to form a hybrid structure. Shared governance is an organizing structure designed to meet the changing needs of professional nursing organizations.

Functional Structures

Functional structures arrange departments and services according to specialty. This approach to organizational structure is common in healthcare organizations. Departments providing similar functions report to a common manager or executive (Figure 8-2). For example, a healthcare organization with a functional structure would have vice presidents for each major function: nursing, finance, human resources, and information technology.

This organizational structure tends to support professional expertise and encourage advancement. It may, however, result in discontinuity of patient care services. Delays in decision making can occur if a silo mentality develops within groups. That is, issues that require communication across functional groups typically must be raised to a senior management level before a decision can be made.

Service-Line Structures

In service-line structures (sometimes called *product lines*), the functions necessary to produce a specific service or product are brought together into an integrated organizational unit under the control of a single manager or executive (Figure 8-3). For example, a cardiology service line at an acute care hospital might include all professional, technical, and support personnel providing services to the cardiac patient population. The manager or executive in this service line would be responsible for the chest pain evaluation center situated within the emergency department, the coronary care unit, the cardiovascular surgery intensive care unit, the telemetry unit, the cardiac catheterization lab, and the outpatient cardiac rehabilitation center. In addition to managing the budget and the facilities for these areas, the manager typically would be responsible for coordinating services for physicians and other providers who care for these patients.

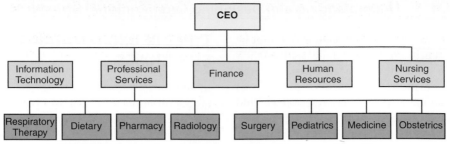

FIGURE 8-2 Functional structure. *CEO,* Chief executive officer.

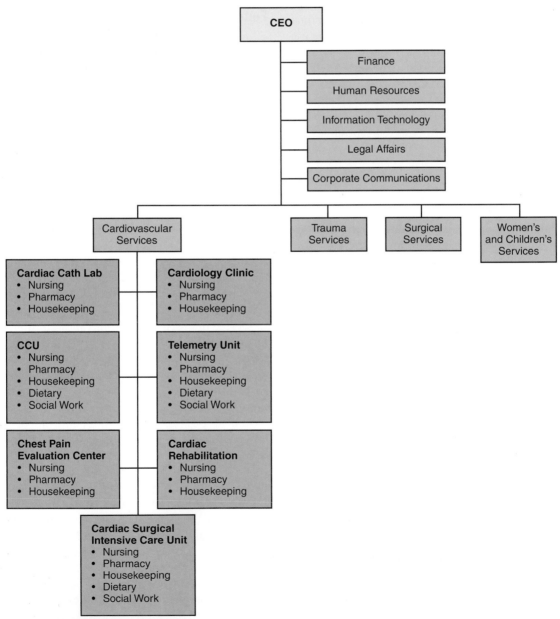

FIGURE 8-3 Service-line structure. *CCU,* Coronary care unit; *CEO,* chief executive officer.

The benefits of a service-line approach to organizational structure include coordination of services, an expedited decision-making process, and clarity of purpose. The limitations of this model can include increased expense associated with duplication of services, loss of professional or technical affiliation, and lack of standardization.

Matrix Structures

Matrix structures are complex and designed to reflect both function and service in an integrated organizational structure. In a matrix organization, the manager of a unit responsible for a service reports to both a functional manager and a service or product line manager. For example, a director of pediatric nursing could report to both a vice president for pediatric services (the service-line manager) and a vice president of nursing (the functional manager) (Figure 8-4).

Matrix structures can be effective in the current healthcare environment. The matrix design enables timely response to the forces in the external environment that demand continual programming, and it facilitates internal efficiency and effectiveness through the promotion of cooperation among disciplines.

A matrix structure combines both a bureaucratic structure and a flat structure; teams are used to carry out specific programs or projects. A matrix structure superimposes a horizontal program management over the traditional vertical hierarchy. Personnel from various functional departments are assigned to a specific program or project and become responsible to two supervisors—their functional department head and a program manager. This approach creates an interdisciplinary team.

A line manager and a project manager must function collaboratively in a matrix organization. For example, in nursing, an organization may have

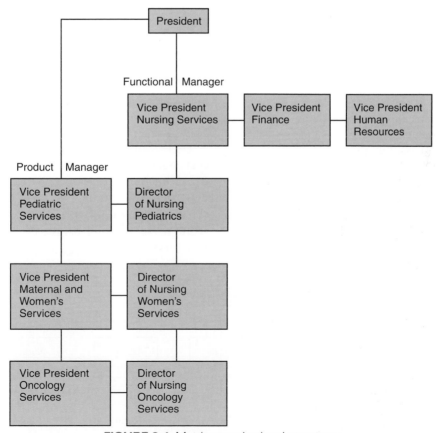

FIGURE 8-4 Matrix organizational structure.

a chief nursing executive, a nurse manager, and direct care nurses in the line of authority to accomplish nursing care. In the matrix structure, some of the nurse's time is allocated to project or committee work. Nursing care is delivered in a teamwork setting or within a collaborative model. The nurse is responsible to a nurse manager for nursing care and to a program or project manager when working within the matrix overlay. Well-developed collaboration and coordination skills are essential to effective functioning in a matrix structure. With the expansion of accountable care organizations, the nature of these organizations with their complex interrelationships requires nurses with high levels of knowledge and skill in interprofessional collaborative practice. (Interprofessional Education Collaborative Expert Panel, 2011).

One example of the matrix structure is the patient-focused care delivery model. Another example is the program focused on specialty services such as geriatric services, women's services, and cardiovascular services. A matrix model can be designed to cover both comprehensive patient-focused care and a specialty service. Other examples within a healthcare facility include discharge planning, quality management, and cardiopulmonary resuscitation teams.

Flat Structures

The primary organizational characteristic of a flat structure is the delegation of decision making to the professionals doing the work. The term *flat* signifies the removal of hierarchical layers, thereby granting authority to act and placing authority at the action level (Figure 8-5). Decisions regarding work methods, nursing care of individual patients, and conditions under which employees work are made where the work is carried out. In a **flat organizational structure,** decentralized decision making replaces the centralized decision making typical of functional structures. Providing staff with authority to make decisions at the place of interaction with patients is the hallmark of a flat organizational structure. Magnet™ hospitals have recognized the benefits of decentralized decision making and its impact on both nursing satisfaction and patient outcomes (Goode, Blegen, Park, Vaughn, & Spetz, 2011). An example of a flat organizational structure is that at Buurtzorg Netherlands, a home care organization where nurses manage themselves, control their schedules, and operate with few policies or procedures (Monsen & de Blok, 2013).

Flat organizational structures are less formalized than hierarchical organizations. A decrease in strict adherence to rules and policies allows individualized decisions that fit specific situations and meet the needs created by the increasing demands associated with consumerism, change, and competition. Work supported by the Institute for Healthcare Improvement *(www.ihi.org/IHI/)*, as an example, capitalizes on decisions being made at the unit level. The focus of this work is to improve patient safety and outcomes. Therefore nurses on a clinical unit can make changes in real time rather than use the traditional organizational hierarchy that includes committees and administrative channels.

Decentralized structures are not without their challenges, however. These include the potential for inconsistent decision making, loss of growth opportunities, and the need to educate managers to communicate effectively and demonstrate creativity in working within these nontraditional structures.

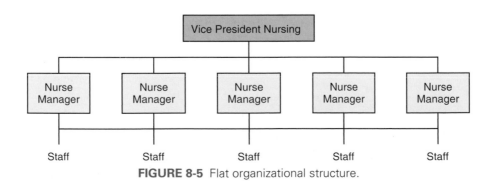

FIGURE 8-5 Flat organizational structure.

The degree of flattening varies from organization to organization. Those that are decentralizing often retain some bureaucratic characteristics. They may at the same time have units that are operating as matrix structures. A **hybrid** structure is one that has characteristics of several different types of structures.

As organizational structures change, some managers are hesitant to relinquish their traditional role in a centralized decision-making process. This reluctance, when combined with recognition of the need to move to a more facilitative role, is partially responsible for the development of hybrid structures. Managers are unsure of what needs to be controlled, how much control is needed, and which mechanisms can replace control. They fear that chaos will ensue without tight managerial control. These fears stem from loss of centralized control because authority, with its concomitant responsibilities, moves to the place of interaction. Registered nurses prepared at the higher educational level develop and use leadership techniques that empower themselves and others to take responsibility for their work and develop skills associated with effective leadership and followership. The evolutionary development of shared-governance structures in nursing departments demonstrates a type of flat structure being used to replace hierarchical control.

Shared Governance

Shared governance goes beyond participatory management through the creation of organizational structures that facilitate nursing staff having more autonomy to govern their practice. Accountability forms the foundation for designing professional governance models. To be accountable, authority to make decisions concerning all aspects of responsibilities is essential. This need for authority and accountability is particularly important for nurses who treat the wide range of human responses to wellness states and illnesses. Organizations in which professional autonomy is encouraged have demonstrated higher levels of staff satisfaction, enhanced productivity, and improved retention (Goode et al., 2011).

The historic early Magnet™ hospital study (McClure, Poulin, Sovie, & Wandelt, 1983), which identified characteristics of hospitals successful in recruiting and retaining nurses, found that the major contributing characteristic to success was a nursing department structured to provide nurses the opportunity to be accountable for their own practice. Studies of Magnet™ hospitals demonstrate that governance structures that promote nurse's accountability will be effective in recruiting and retaining nursing staff while also meeting consumer demands and remaining competitive. Magnet™ characteristics are now accepted as affecting the quality of not only the work environment but also the patient care (Kekky, McHugh, & Aiken, 2011; McHugh, Kelly, Smith, Wu, Vanak & Aiken 2013).

Shared or self-governance structures, sometimes referred to as *professional practice models,* go beyond decentralizing and diminishing hierarchies. In an organization that embraces shared governance, the structure's foundation is the professional workplace rather than the organizational hierarchy. Shared governance vests the necessary levels of authority and accountability for all aspects of the nursing practice in the nurses responsible for the delivery of care. The management and administrative level serves to coordinate and facilitate the work of the practicing nurses. Mechanisms are designed outside of the traditional hierarchy to provide for the functional areas needed to support professional practice. These functions include areas such as quality management, competency definition and evaluation, and continuing education. Changing nurses' positions from dependent employees to accountable professionals is a prerequisite for the radical redesign of healthcare organizations that is required to create value for patients. This change requires administrators, managers, and staff to abandon traditional notions regarding the division of labor in healthcare organizations. Shared governance structures require new behaviors of all staff, not just new assignments of accountability. The areas of interpersonal relationship development, conflict resolution, and personal acceptance of responsibility for action are of particular importance. Education, experience in group work, and conflict management are essential for successful transitions. Understanding the criteria for Magnet™ facilities (American Nurses Credentialing Center, 2012), irrespective of structure, could form the basis for evaluating nursing services.

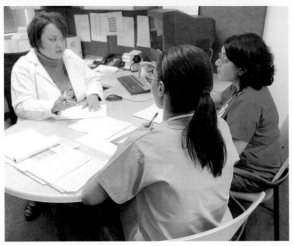

Nurses must have the ability to work with other members of the organization to design organizational models for care delivery that meet patient/customer needs and priorities.

EMERGING FLUID RELATIONSHIPS

As the continuum of care moves health services outside of institutional parameters, different skill sets, relationships, and behavioral patterns will be required. Healthcare organizations are losing their traditional boundaries. Old boundaries of hierarchy, function, and geography are disappearing. Vertical integration aligns dissimilar but related entities such as hospital, home care agency, rehabilitation center, long-term care facility, insurance provider, and medical office/clinic. New technologies, fast-changing markets, and global competition are revolutionizing relationships in health

care, and the roles that people play and the tasks that they perform have become blurred and ambiguous.

In the future, more nurses will practice in settings that extend beyond the walls of a single unit or building. Reframing or changing current static organizations into vibrant learning organizations will require significant effort. To be successful in the future, nurses must participate as active members in these living-learning organizations. Nurses, whether leaders, managers, or followers, must have the ability to work with other members of the organization and with society at large to design organizational models for care delivery that meet patient/customer needs and priorities. It is essential to take a new look at the nature of the work of nursing and propose innovative models for nursing practice that consider emerging laborsaving assistive technologies and rapidly changing healthcare needs. Employee participation and learning environments go hand in hand, and work redesign needs to be regarded as a continuous process. Nurses must value their and others' autonomy to deal successfully in these new structures.

CONCLUSION

Highly successful nursing organizations have grasped the importance of a mission, vision, and philosophy that are meaningful to the practice of nursing and reflect those of the organization. Organizations may be structured in various ways to provide service, and no one approach is "best" for all in all circumstances. The culture of the organization derives from these critical documents, and when embedded, they are reflected in the care delivered.

THE SOLUTION

I met with the director of the other service and differentiated my services from theirs. I clarified the legal and ethical ramifications of how our businesses could work together and when we needed to be separate. I gathered my key team together to seek their input about additional strategies to consider. We conducted a survey to define how we were seen by the broader community, and we sought legal advice about how we could serve our people and simultaneously support a related organization. The intricacies of the relationships were clarified in documents so that both sets of staff would be clear about our projected future relationship.

—Anonymous

Would this be a suitable approach for you? Why?

THE EVIDENCE

A theory being used to explain healthcare systems today is chaos theory. This theory suggests that differences logically exist between and among various organizations as well as between and among the units within an organization. The constantly changing forces of people and the environment affect organizational structure, its functioning, and the services provided in ways that are not often well understood or predicted. Healthcare organizations are examples of complex, unpredictable systems where individuals (healthcare professionals, patients, families, etc.) interact in ways that are nonlinear yet interconnected in substantive and important ways. Chaos theory (complexity science) is increasingly being cited in the nursing literature and is beginning to be used as a theoretical framework for nursing practice in complex adaptive systems (CASs).

An article by Hast, Digioia, Thompson, and Wolf (2013) provides an example of how understanding complexity can provide a framework for clinical intervention. In this study, the authors applied complexity science to improve the preoperative preparation experience of patients undergoing total joint arthroplasty. Using a six-step process, the authors report on the redesign of the preoperative preparation experience. They note that understanding the interrelationships within a complex adaptive system is necessary to improve outcomes.

WHAT NEW GRADUATES SAY

- Next time I apply for a job I will ask for a copy of the organization's mission statement and philosophy of nursing. These will help me know how well I'm likely to fit in.
- Working in a Magnet™-designated facility means I have more control over the decisions that impact my patients.
- I prefer working in a hospital with a flat organizational structure. I have the chance to work with the decision makers in nursing.

CHAPTER CHECKLIST

The mission, vision, and philosophy of the organization determine how nursing care is delivered in a healthcare organization. Changes occurring in the organization's mission affect both the culture of the workplace and the philosophies regarding the work required to accomplish the mission. Actualizing new missions and philosophies requires reengineered organizational structures that place decision-making authority and responsibility where care is delivered. Decision-making responsibility requires staff to understand the organization's mission and to participate in the development of mission and philosophy statements.

- Mission
- Vision
- Philosophy
- Organizational culture
- Factors influencing organizational development
- Characteristics of organizational structures
- Bureaucracy
- Types of organizational structures
- Emerging fluid relationships

TIPS FOR UNDERSTANDING ORGANIZATIONAL STRUCTURES

- Professional nurses in staff or followership positions need to understand the mission, vision, philosophy, and structure at the organization and unit level to maximize their contributions to patient care.
- The overall mission of the organization and the mission of the specific unit in which a professional nurse is employed or is seeking employment provide information concerning the major focus of

the work to be accomplished and the manner in which it will be accomplished.

- Understanding the philosophy of the organization and/or unit where work occurs provides knowledge of the behaviors that are valued in the delivery of patient care and in interactions with persons employed by the organization.
- Formal organizational structures describe the expected channels of communication and decision making.

- Matrix organizations typically have more than one person responsible for the work, and therefore it requires understanding both the service and the function.
- For a shared-governance structure to function effectively, the professionals providing the care must put mechanisms in place to promote decision-making about patient care.

REFERENCES

American Nurses Credentialing Center. (2012). *Health care organization instructions and application process manual*. Washington, DC: Author.

Casida, J., & Parker, J. (2011). Staff nurse perception of nurse manager leadership styles and outcomes. *Journal of Nursing Management*, 19(4), 478–488.

Chaboyer, W., Johnson, J., Hardy, L., Gehrke, T., & Panuwatwanich, K. (2010). Transforming care strategies and nursing-sensitive patient outcomes. *Journal of Advanced Nursing*, 66(5), 1111–1119.

Cummings, G. G., Midodzi, W. K., Wong, C. A., & Estabrooks, C. A. (2010). The contribution of hospital nursing leadership styles to 30-day patient mortality. *Nursing Research*, 59(5), 331–339.

Fayol, H. (1949). *General and industrial management*. London: Pitman.

Goode, C. J., Blegen, M. A., Park, S. H., Vaughn, T., & Spetz, J. (2011). Comparison of patient outcomes in Magnet and non-Magnet hospitals. *The Journal of Nursing Administration*, 41(12), 517–523.

Hast, A. S., Digioia, A. M., Thompson, D., & Wolf, G. (2013). Utilizing complexity science to drive practice change through patient- and family-centered care. *The Journal of Nursing Administration*, 43(1), 44–49.

Interprofessional Education Collaborative Expert Panel. (2011). *Report of an expert panel*. Washington, DC: The Collaborative.

Kekky, L. A., McHugh, M. D., & Aiken, L. H. (2011). Nurse outcomes in Magnet® and non-Magnet hospitals. *The Journal of Nursing Administration*, 41(10), 428–433.

Laschinger, H. K. S., Wong, C. A., & Grau, A. L. (2012). Authentic leadership, empowerment, and burnout: A comparison in new graduates and experienced nurses. *Journal of Nursing Management*, 21(3), 541–552.

McClure, M. L., Poulin, M. A., Sovie, M. D., & Wandelt, M. A. (1983). *Magnet hospitals, attrition and retention of professional nurses*. Kansas City, MO: American Nurses Association.

McHugh, M. D., Kelly, L. A., Smith, H. L., Wu, E. S., Vanak, J. M., & Aiken, L. H. (2013). Lower mortality in Magnet hospitals. *Medical care*, 51(5), 382–388. doi:10.1097/MLR.0b013e3182726cc5.

Monsen, K., & deBlok, J. (2013). A nurse-led model of care has revolutionized home care in the Netherlands. *American Journal of Nursing*, 113(8), 55–59.

Tsai, Y. (2011). Relationship between organizational culture, leadership behavior, and job satisfaction. *BMC Health Services Research*, 11, 98.

Unruh, L., Agrawal, M., & Hassmiller, S. (2011). The business case for transforming care at the bedside among the "TCAB 10" and lessons learned. *Nursing Administration Quarterly*, 35(2), 97–109.

Weber, M. (1947). *The theory of social and economic organization*. Parsons, NY: Free Press.

SUGGESTED READINGS

Capezuti, E., Boltz, M., Cline, D., Dickson, V. V., Rosenberg, M. C., Wagner, L., et al. (2012). Nurses Improving Care for Healthsystem Elders – a model for optimizing the geriatric nursing practice environment. *Journal of Clinical Nursing*, 21(21–22), 3117–3125.

Cummings, G. G., MacGregor, T., Davey, M., Lee, H., Wong, C. A., Lo, E., et al. (2010). Leadership styles and outcome patterns for the nursing workforce and work environment: A systematic review. *International Journal of Nursing Studies*, 47(3), 363–385.

Kirwan, M., Matthews, A., & Scott, P. A. (2013). The impact of the work environment of nurses on patient outcomes: A multi-level modelling approach. *International Journal of Nursing Studies*, 50(2), 253–263.

Kramer, M., Schmalenberg, C., & Maguire, P. (2010). Nine structures and leadership practices essential for a magnetic (healthy) work environment. *Nursing Administration Quarterly*, 34(1), 4–17.

Rittenhouse, D. R., Shortell, S. M., & Fisher, E. S. (2009). Primary care and accountable care – Two essential elements of delivery-system reform. *New England Journal of Medicine*, 361(24), 2301–2303.

Weberg, D. (2012). Complexity leadership: A healthcare imperative. *Nursing Forum*, 47(4), 268–277.

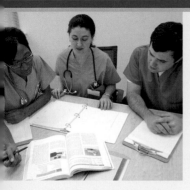

Cultural Diversity in Health Care

Karen A. Esquibel, Dorothy A. Otto

This chapter focuses on the importance of cultural considerations for patients and staff. Although it does not address comprehensive details about any specific culture, it does provide guidelines for actively incorporating cultural aspects into the roles of leading and managing. Diverse workforces are discussed, as well as how to capitalize on their diverse traits and how to support differences to work more efficiently. The chapter presents concepts and principles of transculturalism, describes techniques for managing a culturally diverse workforce, emphasizes the importance of respecting different lifestyles, and discusses the effects of diversity on staff performance. Scenarios and exercises to promote an appreciation of cultural richness are also included.

LEARNING OUTCOMES

- Describe common characteristics of any culture.
- Evaluate the use of concepts and principles of acculturation, culture, cultural diversity, and cultural sensitivity in leading and managing situations.
- Analyze differences between cross-cultural, transcultural, multicultural, and intracultural concepts and cultural marginality.
- Evaluate individual and societal factors involved with cultural diversity.
- Value the contributions a diverse workforce can make to the care of people.

KEY TERMS

acculturation	cultural imposition	ethnicity
cross-culturalism	cultural marginality	ethnocentrism
cultural competence	cultural sensitivity	multiculturalism
cultural diversity	culture	transculturalism

THE CHALLENGE

Sally C. Fernandez, RN, MSN, ANP
Nurse Manager, Emergency Center, The University of Texas
M.D. Anderson Cancer Center, Houston, Texas

I work with a large staff of men and women from several cultures, and they have different perspectives about their assignments. Hispanics, Asians, Asian Indians, and Nigerians provide a challenge for me. If I try to address a work issue, such as assignments, some become defensive. Some men feel that they are superior to me. It might be because I am a woman. In contrast, I have noticed that some Asians are more submissive and do better with female-to-female

interactions. We frequently have a high patient census in the emergency department. There are times when either the charge nurse or I tell staff members to complete a task more quickly within their assignment because of the number of patients waiting to be seen in the emergency department. This does not set well with some staff, who tend to become defensive. For example, a male staff member of one culture felt he was being "overpowered" by the charge nurse from another culture.

What do you think you would do if you were this nurse?

INTRODUCTION

Culture influences leadership from two perspectives. One is the way in which we meet patient needs; the other is the way in which we work together in a diverse workforce. Effective leaders can shape the culture of their organization to be accepting of persons from all races, ethnicities, religions, ages, lifestyles, and genders. These interactions of acceptance should involve a minimum of misunderstandings. Multicultural phenomena are cogent for each person, place, and time. Connerley and Pedersen (2005) provided 10 examples for leading from a complicated culture-centered perspective. For example, "3. Explain the action of employees from their own cultural perspective; 6. Reflect culturally appropriate feelings in specific and accurate feedback" (p. 29). Therefore culture-centered leadership provides organizational leaders, such as nurse managers and effective team members, the opportunity to influence cultural differences and similarities among their unit staff.

CONCEPTS AND PRINCIPLES

What is culture? Does it exhibit certain characteristics? What is cultural diversity, and what do we think of when we refer to cultural sensitivity? Are culture and ethnicity the same? Various authors have different views.

Cultural background stems from one's ethnic background, socio-economic status, and family rituals, to name three key factors. Ethnicity, according to The

Merriam-Webster Dictionary (Merriam-Webster Inc., 2013), is defined as related to groups of people who are "classified" according to common racial, tribal, national, religious, linguistic, or cultural backgrounds. This description differs from what is commonly used to identify racial groups. This broader definition encourages people to think about how diverse the populations in the United States are.

Inherent characteristics of culture are often identified with the following four factors:
1. Culture develops over time and is responsive to its members and their familial and social environments.
2. A culture's members learn it and share it.
3. Culture is essential for survival and acceptance.
4. Culture changes with difficulty.

For the nurse leader or manager, the characteristics of ethnicity and culture are important to keep in mind because the underlying thread in all of them is that staff's and patients' culture and ethnicity have been with them their entire lives. All people view their cultural background as normal; the diversity challenge is for others to view it as normal also and to assimilate it into the existing workforce. Cultural diversity is the term currently used to describe a vast range of cultural differences among individuals or groups, whereas cultural sensitivity describes the affective behaviors in individuals—the capacity to feel, convey, or react to ideas, habits, customs, or traditions unique to a group of people.

Spector (2009) addressed three themes involved with acculturation. (1) *Socialization* refers to growing up within a culture and taking on the characteristics of that group. All of us are socialized to some culture. (2) **Acculturation** refers to adapting to a particular culture. An example of this might be what a particular society calls a particular food or how healthcare organizations are changing to blame-free environments to encourage safety disclosures. The overall process of acculturation into a new society is extremely difficult. "America" has a core culture and numerous subcultures. For example, think how differently people in rural American regions dress from those in urban centers, or how a city looks on Saturday night versus Sunday morning. In other words, subcultures expand on how the core culture might be described. (3) *Assimilation* refers to the change that occurs when nurses move from another country to the United States, or from one part of the country to another. They face different social and nursing practices, and individuals now define themselves as members of the dominant culture. An example of this might be when nurses no longer say they are from their country of origin. They say they are from where they live and practice.

Providing care for a person or people from a culture other than one's own is a dynamic and complex experience. The experience according to Spence (2004) might involve "prejudice, paradox and possibility" (p. 140). Spence used *prejudice* as conditions that enabled or constrained interpretation based on one's values, attitudes, and actions. By talking with people outside their "circle of familiarity," nurses can enhance their understanding of personally held prejudices.

Prejudices "enable us to make sense of the situations in which we find ourselves, yet they also constrain understanding and limit the capacity to come to new or different ways of understanding. It is this contradiction that makes prejudice paradoxical" (Spence, 2004, p. 163). *Paradox,* although it may seem incongruent with prejudice, describes the dynamic interplay of tensions between individuals or groups. We have the responsibility to acknowledge the "possibility of tension" as a potential for new and different understandings derived from our communication and interpretation. *Possibility* therefore presumes a condition for openness with a person from another culture (Spence, 2004).

> **EXERCISE 9-1**
> In a group, discuss the values and beliefs of justice and equality. As a nurse, you may have strong values and beliefs, but you may never have observed their application in health care. Consider language, skin color, dress, and gestures of patients and staff from other cultures. How will you learn and value what differences exist?

Cultural marginality is defined as "situations and feelings of passive betweenness when people exist between two different cultures and do not yet perceive themselves as centrally belonging to either one" (Choi, 2001, p. 193). This "betweenness" is a time when managers might perceive disinterest in cultural considerations. This situation might actually reflect cognitive processing of information that isn't yet reflected in effective behaviors.

Ethnocentrism "refers to the belief that one's own ways are the best, most superior, or preferred ways to act, believe, or behave" (Leininger, 2002b, p. 50), whereas **cultural imposition** is defined as "the tendency of an individual or group to impose their values, beliefs, and practices on another culture for varied reasons" (Leininger, 2002b, p. 51). Such practices constitute a major concern in nursing and "a largely unrecognized problem as a result of cultural ignorance, blindness, ethnocentric tendencies, biases, racism or other factors" (Leininger, 2002b, p. 51).

Providing quality of life and human care is difficult to accomplish if the nurse does not have knowledge of the recipient's culture as it relates to care. Leininger believed that "culture reflects shared values, beliefs, ideas, and meanings that are learned and that guide human thoughts, decisions, and actions. Cultures have manifest (readily recognized) and implicit (covert and ideal) rules of behavior and expectations. Human cultures have material items or symbols such as artifacts, objects, dress, and actions that have special meaning in a culture" (Leininger, 2002b, p. 48). Leininger (2002b) stated that her views of cultural care are "a synthesized construct that is the foundational basis to understanding and helping people of different cultures in transcultural nursing practices" (p. 48). (See the Theory Box on p. 157.) Accordingly, "quality of life" must be addressed from an emic (insider) cultural viewpoint and compared with an etic (outsider) professional's perspective. By comparing these two viewpoints, more meaningful nursing practice interventions will evolve. This comparative analysis will require nurses to include global views in their cultural studies that consider the social and environmental context of different cultures.

EXERCISE 9-2

As a small group activity, assess several clinical settings. Do these settings have programs related to cultural diversity? Why? What are the programs like? If there are no programs, why do you think they have not been implemented?

THEORY

How do leaders, managers, or followers take all of the expanding information on the diversity of healthcare beliefs and practices and give it some organizing structure to provide culturally competent and culturally sensitive care to patients or clients? Purnell and Paulanka (2008), Campinha-Bacote (1999, 2002), Giger and Davidhizar (2002), and Leininger (2002a) provided an overview of each of their theoretical models to guide healthcare providers for delivering culturally competent and culturally sensitive care in the workplace.

Purnell and Paulanka's (2008) Model for Cultural Competence provides an organizing framework. The model uses a circle with the outer zone representing global society, the second zone representing community, the third zone representing family, and the inner zone representing the person. The interior of the circle is divided into 12 pie-shaped wedges delineating cultural domains and their concepts (e.g., workplace issues, family roles and organization, spirituality, and healthcare practices). The innermost center circle is black, representing unknown phenomena. Cultural consciousness is expressed in behaviors from "unconsciously incompetent—consciously incompetent—consciously competent to unconsciously competent" (p. 10). The usefulness of this model is derived from its concise structure, applicability to any setting, and wide range of experiences that can foster inductive and deductive thinking when assessing cultural domains. Purnell (2009) described the dominant cultural characteristics of selected ethnocultural groups and a guide for assessing their beliefs and practices. The Purnell Model for Cultural Competence serves as an organizing framework for providing cultural care, which is based on 20 major assumptions.

Campinha-Bacote's (1999, 2002) culturally competent model of care identifies five constructs: (1) awareness, (2) knowledge, (3) skill, (4) encounters,

and (5) desire. She defined **cultural competence** as "the process in which the healthcare provider continuously strives to achieve the ability to effectively work within the cultural context of a client (individual, family, or community)" (Campinha-Bacote, 1999, p. 203). Cultural awareness is the self-examination and in-depth exploration of one's own cultural and professional background. It involves the recognition of one's bias, prejudices, and assumptions about the individuals who are different (Campinha-Bacote, 2002). "One's world view can be considered a paradigm or way of viewing the world and phenomena in it" (Campinha-Bacote, 1999, p. 204). Cultural knowledge is the process of seeking and obtaining a sound educational foundation about diverse cultural and ethnic groups. Obtaining cultural information about the patient's health-related beliefs and values will help explain how he or she interprets his or her illness and how it guides his or her thinking, doing, and being (Campinha-Bacote, 2002). The skill of conducting a cultural assessment is learned while assessing one's values, beliefs, and practices to provide culturally competent services. The process of cultural encounters encourages direct engagement in cross-cultural interactions with individuals from other cultures. This process allows the person to validate, negate, or modify his or her existing cultural knowledge. It provides culturally specific knowledge bases from which the individual can develop culturally relevant interventions. Cultural desire requires the intrinsic qualities of motivation and genuine caring of the healthcare provider to "want to" engage in becoming culturally competent (Campinha-Bacote, 1999).

The Giger and Davidhizar Transcultural Assessment Model identified phenomena to assess provision of care for patients who are of different cultures (2002). Their model includes six cultural phenomena: communication, time, space, social organization, environmental control, and biological variations. Each one is described based on several premises (e.g., culture is a patterned behavioral response that develops over time; is shaped by values, beliefs, norms, and practices; guides our thinking, doing, and being; and implies a dynamic, ever-changing, active or passive process).

Leininger's (2002a) central purpose in her theory of transcultural nursing care is "to discover and explain diverse and universal culturally based care factors influencing the health, well-being, illness, or death of individuals or groups" (p. 190). She uses her classic "Sunrise Model" to identify the multifaceted theory and provides five enablers beneficial to "teasing out vague ideas," two of which are The Observation, Participation, and Reflection Enabler and the Researcher's Domain of Inquiry. Nurses can use Leininger's model to provide culturally congruent, safe, and meaningful care to patients or clients of diverse or similar cultures. See the following Theory Box.

NATIONAL AND GLOBAL DIRECTIVES

The American Nurses Association (ANA) has a long and vital history related to ethics, human rights, and numerous efforts to eliminate discriminatory practices against nurses as well as patients. The ANA *Code of Ethics for Nurses with Interpretive Statements,* Provision 8, states, "The nurse collaborates with other health professionals and the public in promoting community, national, and international efforts to meet health needs" (2008, p. 23). This provision helps the nurse recognize that health care must be provided to culturally diverse populations in the United States and on all continents of the world. Although a nurse may be inclined to impose his or her own cultural values on others, whether patients or staff, avoiding this imposition affirms the respect and sensitivity for the values and healthcare practices associated with different cultures. This provision is reinforced by the ANA position statement (2010), *The Nurse's Role in Ethics and Human Rights: Protecting and Promoting Individual Worth, Dignity, and Human Rights in Practice Settings.* The value of human rights is placed in the forefront for nurses whose specific actions are to promote and protect the human rights of every individual in all practice care environments.

Similar statements are made with an international emphasis and a specialty emphasis. *The ICN Code of Ethics for Nurses* (2012) states:

The nurse ensures that the individual receives accurate, sufficient and timely information in a culturally appropriate manner on which to base consent to care and related treatment.

The nurse shares with society the responsibility for initiating and supporting action to meet the health and social needs of the public, in particular those of vulnerable populations.

The nurse demonstrates professional values such as respectfulness, responsiveness, compassion, trustworthiness and integrity. (p. 3)

Nurse educators, as a specialty example, are expected to recognize "multicultural, gender, and experiential influences on teaching and learning"; "identify individual learning styles and unique learning needs of international, adult, multicultural, educationally disadvantaged, physically challenged, at-risk, and second degree learners"; and ensure "that the curriculum reflects institutional philosophy and mission, current nursing and health care trends, and community and societal needs so as to prepare graduates for practice in a complex, dynamic, multicultural health care environment." (National League for Nursing, 2005, pp. 1, 2, 4)

These examples illustrate a global concern for cultural sensitivity. Although the emphasis has been on recipients of care, the same attentiveness is needed in the workforce. Patients are aware of how they are treated; and they also see how staff interact with each other.

SPECIAL ISSUES

Health disparities between majority and ethnic minority populations are not new issues and continue to be problematic because they exist for multiple and complex reasons. Causes of disparities in health care include poor education, health behaviors of the minority group, inadequate financial resources, and environmental factors. Disparities in health care that relate to quality of care include provider/patient

THEORY BOX		
THEORY/CONTRIBUTOR	**KEY IDEAS**	**APPLICATION TO PRACTICE**
Leininger (2002a) is credited with developing and advancing a theory of transcultural nursing care since the mid-1950s.	The theory is explicitly focused on the close relationships of culture and care on well-being, health, illness, and death; it is holistic and multidimensional, generic (emic, folk) and professional (etic) care and has a specifically designed research method (ethnonursing).	Care is the essence of nursing, and culturally based care is essential for well-being, health, growth, and survival and for facing handicaps or death.

relationships, actual access to care, treatment regimens that necessarily reflect current evidence, provider bias and discrimination, mistrust of the healthcare system, and refusal of treatment (Baldwin, 2003). Health disparities in ethnic and racial groups are observed in cardiovascular disease, which has a 40% higher incidence in U.S. blacks than in U.S. whites; cancer, which has a 30% higher death rate for all cancers in U.S. blacks than in U.S. whites; and diabetes in Hispanics, who are twice as likely to die from this disease than non-Hispanic whites. Native Americans have a life expectancy that is less than the national average, whereas Asians and Pacific Islanders are considered among the healthiest population groups. However, within the Asian and Pacific Islander population, health outcomes are more diverse. Solutions to health and healthcare disparities among ethnic and racial populations must be accomplished through research to improve care. Consider how these disparities in disease and in healthcare services might affect the healthcare providers in the workplace in relationship to their ethnic or racial group. It is necessary to increase healthcare providers' knowledge of such disparities so that they can more effectively manage and treat diseases related to ethnic and racial minorities, which increasingly might include themselves.

The healthcare system in the United States has consistently focused on individuals and their health problems, but it has failed to recognize the cultural differences, beliefs, symbolisms, and interpretations of illness of some people as a group. As health care moves toward provision of care for populations, culture can have an even greater influence on approaches to care. Commonly, patients for whom healthcare practitioners provide care are newcomers to health care in the United States. Similarly, new staff are commonly neither acculturated nor assimilated into the cultural values of the dominant culture.

Currently, accessibility to health care in the United States is linked to specific social strata. This challenges nurse leaders, managers, and followers who strive for worth, recognition, and individuality for patients and staff regardless of their ascribed economic and social standing. Beginning nurse leaders, managers, and followers may sense that the knowledge they bring to their job lacks "real-life" experiences that provide the springboard to address staff and patient needs.

In reality, although lack of experience may be slightly hampering, it is by no means an obstacle to addressing individualized attention to staff and patients. The key is that if the nurse manager and staff respect people and their needs, economic and social standings become moot points. This challenge will intensify as the implications of the Patient Protection and Affordable Care Act of 2010 unfold. If nothing else happens, the diversity of insured patients will increase.

LANGUAGE

Translating a message in one language to another language to ensure equivalence includes maintaining the same meaning of the word or concept. Equivalency is accomplished through interpretation, which extends beyond "word-for-word" translation to explain the meaning of concepts. When providing care to a language diverse patient, the nurse must realize that the process of translation of illness/disease conditions and treatment is complex and requires certain tasks. Two important tasks are "(a) transferring data from the source language to the target language and (b) maintaining or establishing cross-cultural semantic equivalence" (International Council of Nurses, 2008, p. 5).

The current practice seems to be one of using interpreters rather than translators when speaking with non–English-speaking patients and clients. Why? Purnell and Paulanka (2008) advocate that trained healthcare providers as interpreters can decode words and provide the right meaning of the message. However, the authors also suggest being aware that interpreters might affect the reporting of symptoms, using their own ideas or omitting information. It is important to allow time for translation and interpretation and to clarify information as needed.

Promotion of culturally competent care with a translator has legal implications in the United States. The legal foundation for language access lies in Title VI of the 1964 Civil Rights Act, which states:

> No person in the United States, on the ground of race, color, or national origin, be excluded from participation in, be denied the benefit of, or be subjected to discrimination under any program or activity receiving federal financial assistance (Chen, Youdelman, Brooks, 2007, p. 362).

The federal government has interpreted and treated language as a proxy for national origin, and language assistance should be pursued. These activities supported by the Civil Rights Act include access to health care. Additionally, once a healthcare provider accepts any federal funds (e.g., Medicaid payments), the provider is responsible for providing language access to all the provider's patients.

MEANING OF DIVERSITY IN THE ORGANIZATION

Leading and managing cultural diversity in an organization means managing personal thinking and helping others to think in new ways. According to Noone (2008), nursing leaders need a workforce that can provide culturally competent care. In addition, nursing's goal is to create a workforce that reflects the population it serves. This diversity can occur across roles, including advanced practice registered nurses, managers, and chief nurse executives.

Managing issues that involve culture—whether institutional, ethnic, gender, religious, or any other kind—requires patience, persistence, and much understanding. One way to promote this understanding is through shared stories that have symbolic power.

EXERCISE 9-3

Think of a recent event in your workplace, such as a project, task force, celebration, or something similar. What meaning did people give the event? Was it viewed as being a symbol of some quality of the workplace, such as its effectiveness, its values and beliefs, or its innovations? Or was it seen as a meaningless gesture? What makes an event relevant and value-centric?

Staff who know what is valuable to patients and to themselves can act accordingly and derive satisfaction from work. Having a clear mission, goals, rewards, and acknowledgment of efforts leads to greater productivity from a culturally diverse staff who aspire to unity and uniqueness. (The following Research Perspective illustrates this point in providing end-of-life care.) When assessing staff diversity, the nurse leader or manager can ask these two questions:

- What is the cultural representation of the workforce?
- What kind of team-building activities are needed to create a cohesive workforce for effective healthcare delivery?

 RESEARCH PERSPECTIVE

Resource: Periyakoil, V.S., Stevens, M., & Kramer, H. (2013). Multicultural long-term care nurses' perceptions of factors influencing patient dignity at the end of life. *Journal of American Geriatrics Society, 61*(3), 440-446.

The goal of this mixed methods study was to view the perceptions of multicultural long-term care nurses about patient dignity at the end of life (EOL). This study was conducted in a large, urban, long-term care (LTC) facility. Participants were 45 LTC nurses and 26 terminally ill nursing home residents. Nurses completed an open-ended interview about their perceptions of the concept "dying with dignity." The data were analyzed using grounded theory methods. The main themes included promoting resident dignity at the EOL, which meant treating them with respect, helping them prepare for the EOL, promoting shared decision-making, and providing high quality care. Cultural and religious backgrounds of the nurses influenced their perceptions of dignity-conserving care. Foreign-born nurses stressed the need for EOL rituals; however, this was significantly absent in the statements of U.S.-born nurses. Foreign-born Catholic nurses stated the dying experience should not be altered by analgesics to relieve suffering or by attempts to hasten death by forgoing curative therapy or by other means.

Nurses and terminally ill individuals completed the Dignity Care-sort Tool (DCT). A comparison of the DCT responses of the LTC nurses with those of the terminally ill participants showed that the nurses felt that patient dignity was lessened when patient wishes were not followed and when they were treated with a lack of respect. By contrast, EOL long-term care patients felt that poor medical care and loss of ability to choose care options were the most significant factors directing the lessening of dignity.

Implications for Practice

Nurses should advocate for their culturally diverse patients when providing EOL care by promoting the themes identified in the research study.

Nurses, foreign-born or U.S.-born, need to assess and use their abilities to determine the challenges that will help them provide care that is most important to the patients in a long-term care facility.

The challenge for the manager is to capitalize on such information as presented in the Research Perspective so that patients benefit. Box 9-1 lists some of the techniques that may be effective when managing a culturally diverse nursing staff with multicultural patients in a long-term care facility.

CULTURAL RELEVANCE IN THE WORKPLACE

Although the literature has addressed multicultural needs of patients, it is sparse in identifying effective methods for nurse managers to use when dealing with multicultural staff. Differences in education and culture can impede patient care, and uncomfortable situations may emerge from such differences. For example, staff members may be reluctant to admit language problems that hamper their written communication. They may also be reluctant to admit their lack of understanding when interpreting directions. Psychosocial skills may be problematic as well, because non-Westernized countries encourage emotional restraint. Staff may have difficulty addressing issues that relate to private family matters. Non-Asian nurses may have difficulty accepting the intensified family involvement of Asian cultures. The lack of assertiveness and the subservient physician-nurse relationships of some cultures are other issues that provide challenges for nurse managers. Unit-oriented workshops arranged by the nurse manager to address effective assertive techniques and family involvement as it relates to cultural differences are two ways of assisting staff with cultural work situations. Respecting cultural diversity in the team fosters cooperation and supports sound decision making.

Nurse leaders and managers who ascribe to a positive view of culture and its characteristics effectively acknowledge cultural diversity among patients and staff. This includes providing culturally sensitive care to patients while simultaneously balancing a culturally diverse staff. For example, cultural diversity might mean being sensitive to or being able to embrace the emotions of a large multicultural group comprising staff and patients. Unless we understand the differences, we cannot come together and make decisions that are in the best interest of the patient.

Transculturalism sometimes has been considered in a narrow sense as a comparison of health beliefs and practices of people from different countries or geographic regions. However, culture can be construed more broadly to include differences in health beliefs and practices by gender, race, ethnicity, economic status, sexual preference, age, and disability or physical challenge. Thus, when concepts of transcultural care are discussed, we should consider differences in health beliefs and practices not only between and among countries but also between genders and among, for example, races, ethnic groups, and different economic strata. This requires us to consider multiple factors about all individuals.

The range of attitudes toward culturally diverse groups can be viewed along a continuum of intensity (Lenburg et al., 1995, p. 4) from hate to contempt to tolerance to respect and ending with celebration/affirmation. Managers need to be aware of this continuum so that they can apply strategies appropriately to the workforce—for example, contempt versus affirmation. These responses are equally reflected in employee groups.

Variables that may influence the nurse's response may include how the illness is perceived by the culture and the cultural competency of the healthcare provider. If the nurse's culture is different from the patient's, whose cultural perspective dominates? It might not be possible to adapt care totally to the patient's perspective. However, knowing that a difference exists allows for a mutual conversation related to the rationale for care. Similarly if a workplace dispute occurs, trying to see "the other view" can create new insights into a situation.

To make cultural competence relevant to clinical practice, Engebretson, Mahoney, and Carlson (2008) linked a cultural competency continuum, in which they identified the levels of competence, to values in health care. They cited the levels as cultural destructiveness, cultural incapacity, cultural blindness, cultural pre-competence and proficiency that would be complementary to patient care. The "clinically relevant continuum" included behaviors of maleficence, incompetence, standardization, and outcomes focused (positive health outcomes). A model was developed that integrated the cultural competence continuum with the clinically relevant continuum and the components of evidence-based care; namely, best research practice, clinical expertise, and patient's values and circumstances. Their goal was to suggest how to make cultural concerns relevant to clinical practitioners at the level of the patient-provider encounter.

To understand, value, and use diversity, nurse managers need to approach every staff person as an individual. This same strategy works for all of us. Although staff of different cultural groups may be diverse in appearance, values, beliefs, communication patterns, and mannerisms, they have many things in common. Staff members want to be accepted by others and to succeed in their jobs. With fairness and respect, nurse managers should openly support the competencies and contributions of staff members from all cultural groups with a goal of achieving quality patient care. Nurse managers hold the key to allowing the full potential of each person on the staff.

Body movements, eye contacts, gestures, verbal tone, and physical closeness when communicating are all part of a person's culture. For the nurse manager, understanding these cultural behaviors is critical in accomplishing effective communication within the diverse workforce population. As if language differences aren't challenging enough, add on the slang, idioms, and fads inherent to U.S. culture. It is no surprise that culturally sensitive communications is difficult to achieve. Nurses need to ensure that ineffective communication among staff, with patients, and with others does not lead to misunderstandings and eventual alienation.

Failure to address cultural diversity leads to negative effects on performance and staff interactions. Nurse managers can find many ways to address this issue. For example, in relation to performance, a nurse manager can make sure messages about patient care are received. This might be accomplished by sitting down with a nurse and analyzing a situation to ensure that understanding has occurred. In addition, the nurse manager might use a communication notebook that allows the nurse to slowly "digest" information by writing down communication areas that may be unclear. For effective staff interaction, the nurse manager also can make a special effort to pair mentors and mentees who have different ethnic backgrounds and encourage staff to learn another language, one prominent among the population served. Even a "word a day" approach could alter a team's ability to interact with patients.

EXERCISE 9-4

During one of your group meetings, have everyone share one or two slang words that may have a different meaning for different groups of people. After this meeting, have one in your group post a list of the words and meanings discussed in the meeting. Allow everyone to continue to add slang words that staff members use that may create confusion or misunderstanding. Reviewing the list regularly allows staff to understand phrases and, in some instances, to gain a cultural perspective connected to the phrase.

INDIVIDUAL AND SOCIETAL FACTORS

Nurse managers must work with staff to foster respect of different lifestyles. To do this, nurse managers need to accept three key principles: **multiculturalism,** which refers to maintaining several different cultures; **cross-culturalism,** which means mediating between/among cultures; and **transculturalism,** which denotes bridging significant differences in cultural practices. Each of those principles operates in the workplace. Sometimes we want to keep distinct cultures. For instance, we may advocate for equality unless a particular unit has excellent safety scores. Anyone who wanted to make all cultures alike, and thus increase safety incidents, would be seen as foolish. Healthcare organizations have, as an example, provided various ways to celebrate holy days based on the cultural mix of staff and patients. These practices are designed to acknowledge the individuals who comprise the organization.

EXERCISE 9-5

Create a group of 4 to 6 people. Ask each group member to write down four to six cultural beliefs that he or she values. When everyone has finished writing, have the group members exchange their lists and discuss why these beliefs are valued. When everyone has had a chance to share lists, have a volunteer compile an all-encompassing list that reflects the values of your workforce. (The key to this exercise is that many of the values are similar or perhaps even identical.)

Cultural differences among groups should not be taken in the context that all members of a certain group or subgroup are indistinguishable. For example, regarding gender differences, women are perceived to have a more participative management style; however, this does not mean that all male managers use an authoritative management model. Likewise, female managers may use multiple sources of information to make decisions, and this does not mean that all male managers make decisions on limited data. Thus the norm for gender recognition should be that women and men be hired, promoted, rewarded, and respected for how successfully they do the job, not for who they are, where they come from, whom they know, or the gender they represent.

In today's workplace, female-male collaboration should provide efficacious models for the future. Gender does not determine response in any given situation. However, men reportedly seem to be better at deciphering what needs to be done, whereas women are better at collaborating and getting others to collaborate in accomplishing a task. Men tend to take neutral, logical, and objective stands on problems, whereas women become involved in how the problems affect people. Women and men bring separate perspectives to resolving problems, which can help them function more effectively as a team on the nursing unit. Men and women must learn to work together and value the contributions of the other and the differences they bring to any situation. Similar kinds of comparisons can be made related to other elements of diversity. Nurses have embraced information related to generational differences and have used religious and ethnic contexts as ways to begin dialogs about values and beliefs.

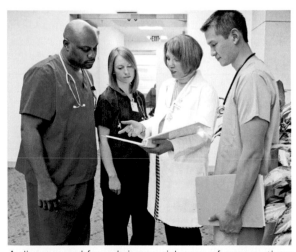

A diverse workforce brings a richness of perspectives to care.

DEALING EFFECTIVELY WITH CULTURAL DIVERSITY

The first individuals in most organizational structure who have to address cultural diversity are the leaders and managers. They have to give unwavering support to embracing diversity in the workplace rather than using a standard cookie-cutter approach. Creating a culturally sensitive work environment involves a long-term vision and financial and healthcare-provider commitment. Leaders and managers need to make the strategic decision to design services and programs especially to meet the needs of diverse cultural, ethnic, and racial differences of staff and patients. Policies in healthcare organizations prohibit discrimination based on several aspects. Such policies, however, don't necessarily succeed at promoting a culturally aware environment.

Nurse managers hold the key to making the best use of cultural diversity. Managers have positions of power to begin programs that enrich the diversity among staff. For example, capitalizing on the knowledge that all staff bring to the patient is possible for better quality care outcomes. One method that can be used is to allow staff to verbalize their feelings about particular cultures in relationship to personal beliefs. Another is to have two or three staff members of different ethnic origins present a patient-care conference, giving their views on how they would care for a specific patient's needs based on their own ethnic values.

Mentorship programs should be established so that all staff can expand their knowledge about cultural diversity. Mentors have specific relationships with their mentees. The more closely aligned a mentor is with the mentee (e.g., same gender, age-group, ethnicity, and primary language), the more effective the relationship. Programs that address the staff's cultural diversity should not try to make people of different cultures pattern their behavior after the prevailing culture. Nurse managers must carefully select those mentors who ascribe to transcultural, rather than ethnocentric, values and beliefs. A much richer staff exists when nurse managers build on the valuable culture of all staff members and when diversity is rewarded. The pacesetter for the cultural norm of the unit is the nurse manager. For example, to demonstrate commitment to cultural diversity, a nurse manager might make a special effort to ensure that U.S. black, Asian-American, and Hispanic holidays or other cultural representations on the unit are recognized by the staff. Staff members who are active participants in these programs can then be given positive reinforcement by the nurse manager. These activities promote a better understanding and appreciation of individuals' cultural heritage.

Nurse managers are aware of the increasing shortage of nurses, demanding work environment with its surrounding influences, and statistics indicating that almost 50% of all new nurses leave their first professional nursing position by the first year because of job dissatisfaction and level of stress. This period may be even more challenging for individuals whose culture differs from the predominant unit culture.

Continuing-education programs should help nurses learn about the care of different ethnic groups. For example, professional organizations related to cultural groups (National Black Nurses Association, National Hispanic Nurses Association, Philippine Nurses Association of America) and institutions might develop or sponsor a workshop or conference on cross-cultural nursing for nursing service staff and faculty in schools of nursing who have had limited preparation in cultural care or cultural beliefs in healing.

> **EXERCISE 9-6**
>
> Identify a situation in which working with culturally diverse staff had positive or negative outcomes. If a negative outcome resulted, what could you have done to make it a positive one? If a positive outcome resulted, what strategies could you use in another situation?

Muslims are one of the fastest growing populations in the United States and worldwide. For example, Muslim nurses may feel uncomfortable without long sleeves because of their Islamic dress code. Jewish nurses likely would find a pulled pork barbeque an inappropriate celebration. Males may feel awkward participating in a unit baby shower. The point of all of these examples is to think proactively, ask for input, and consider how best to exhibit cultural sensitivity.

Choices, decisions, and behaviors reflect learned beliefs, values, ideals, and preferences. The goal of communication is maintenance or restoration of personal integrity and recognition of worth and respect of individuals or groups.

The two scenarios described in Box 9-2 illustrate how problem-solving communication can promote

---

BOX 9-2   PROBLEM-SOLVING COMMUNICATION: HONORING CULTURAL ATTITUDES TOWARD DEATH AND DYING

Scenario 1: Staff and a Patient's Family

What nurses often call interference with the care of a patient commonly reflects family attitudes toward death and dying. Often, Hispanic families rush to the hospital as soon as they hear of a relative's illness. Because most Hispanics believe that death is the passing of an individual to a life that offers tranquility and everlasting happiness, being at the bedside offering prayers and encouragement is the norm rather than the unusual exception. The nurse manager in this situation, herself a non–American-educated nurse manager, had worked extensively at helping her staff understand different cultures. A consensus compromise was worked out between the staff and one such Hispanic family. The family, consisting of three generations, was given the authority to decide what family members could stay at the loved one's side and for how long. By doing this, the family felt they had control of the environment and quickly developed a priority list of family members who could stay no more than 5 minutes at the patient's side. As the family member left the bedside, his or her task was to report the condition of the patient to other family members "camping" in the visitors' lounge. Although their loved one did not survive a massive intracranial hemorrhage, all of the family felt that they were a part of their loved one's "passage of life."

Scenario 2: A Nurse Manager and Another Staff Member

Eastern World cultures that profess Catholicism as their faith celebrate the death of a loved one 40 days after the death. The nurse manager needs to recognize that time off for the nurse involved in this celebration is imperative. Such an occurrence had to be addressed by a nurse manager of Asian descent. The nurse manager quickly realized that the nurse, whose mother died in India, did not ask for any time off to make the necessary burial arrangements but, rather, waited 40 days to celebrate his mother's death. The celebration included formal invitations to a church service, as well as a dinner after the service. One day during early morning rounds, the nurse explained how death is celebrated by Eastern World Catholics. The Bible's description of the Ascension of the Lord into heaven 40 days after his death served as the conceptual framework for the loved one's death. The grieving family believed their loved one's spirit would stay on earth for 40 days. During these 40 days, the family held prayer sessions meant to assist the "spirit" to prepare for its ascension into heaven. When the 40 days have passed, the celebration previously described marks the ascension of the loved one's spirit into heaven.

Because this particular unit truly espoused a multicultural concept, the nurses had no difficulty in allowing the Indian nurse 2 weeks of unplanned vacation so that his mother's "passage of life" celebration could be accomplished in a respectful, dignified manner.

mutual understanding and respect. The first scenario involves a compromise between staff members and a patient's family, and the second involves a nurse manager and a staff member from a different culture.

EXERCISE 9-7

Identify a situation involving a staff member requesting additional days of leave that required a culturally sensitive decision. What religious or ethnic practices did you learn about in regard to this request and decision?

Passages of life that culminate in happy events also can challenge the nurse manager, for example, the quinceañera observed by Hispanic families. This event is the celebration for 15-year-old girls to be introduced into society. A nurse whose daughter is celebrating this event must have time to make plans for this festive celebration. Because of the significance of the celebration and the pride that the parents take in their daughter, inviting "key" staff to the quinceañera is common. Nurse managers who understand and value cultural rituals can help individuals meet their needs and help staff, in general, learn and accept various cultural practices and perspectives.

EXERCISE 9-8

Holiday celebrations have cultural significance. Select a specific holiday such as Chinese Lunar New Year (China and Chinatowns) or Araw ng mga Patay (Philippines) or Diwali (India). What is the cultural meaning of the specific holiday? How do staff members of the respective culture celebrate the festive day? Does the nursing unit engage in recognition of special holidays?

IMPLICATIONS IN THE WORKPLACE

Considering culture from a healthcare staff person and the nursing workforce perspective is a daunting task, one that can lead to a more solidly aligned service-community relationship. Even if the workforce is not as diverse as one might desire, learning about the cultures of the groups within the workforce is important. Making clear that diversity is valued, in fact celebrated, attracts others to engage in the complexity of care. One way is to make clear how staff are valued as people, not as representatives of some group. Showing respect to all patients irrespective of their cultural differences tells the staff that their differences also can be valued. The key is for managers and leaders to attend to the workforce issues with the same zest as they do the patient issues. Cultural differences enrich all of us when we make deliberate efforts to include them in our daily values.

Embracing these differences will also enhance the American Association of Colleges of Nursing (AACN) Quality and Safety Education for Nurses (QSEN) Initiative. The overall goal of the QSEN Initiative is to prepare nurses with the knowledge, skills, and attitudes (KSAs) needed to continuously deliver quality and safe patient care (American Association of Colleges of Nursing, 2013). With this initiative we see the need to respect all patients and staff irrespective of their cultural differences to empower Patient/Family Centered Care, which is one of the QSEN initiative competencies. This component recognizes the patient or designee as the source of control and full partner in providing compassionate and coordinated care based on respect for patient's preferences, values, and needs (American Association of Colleges of Nursing, 2013).

CONCLUSION

Understanding and valuing cultural differences benefits both patients and colleagues. Culture is a broad term encompassing many diversities. This broadness both enriches our perspective of diversity and provides a complex challenge. All nurses, regardless of their titles or positions, have a role in improving the workplace and patient care by attending to the implications of culture in healthcare.

THE SOLUTION

As a nurse manager, I prefer to talk on a one-to-one basis. I had a meeting with the male staff member to learn from him. "What made you upset with the charge nurse when she made your assignment?" In our discussion, he told me, "The charge nurse used words [slang] for which I did not know the meaning ... I did not understand why she said it ... she was trying to overpower me ... I didn't like it ... so I was defensive about it." We talked about being sensitive to cultural communication and the need to understand meanings of words and to ask for immediate clarification when such situations arise with members of two different cultures.

—*Sally C. Fernandez*

Would this be a suitable approach for you? Why?

THE EVIDENCE

Acknowledging cultural diversity in patients and staff requires leaders to be proactive.

Working with minority nursing organizations enhances opportunities for successful recruitment and retention.

Taking deliberate actions to acknowledge and celebrate culturally related events helps employees from various groups feel valued.

WHAT NEW GRADUATES SAY

- I went to work in an inner-city hospital and quickly learned that a diabetic diet is very different there from what I learned in school. I'm constantly learning about another new dish and how to help my patients adapt.

- In my new position, I am working with several nurses from outside the United States. Their approach to care is very different. We are constantly learning from each other.

CHAPTER CHECKLIST

All potential or current nurse leaders or managers must acknowledge and address cultural diversity among staff and patients. Culture lives in each of us. It determines how we think, what we value, how we behave, and how we communicate with each other. Leaders, managers, and followers have the potential to capitalize on the diversity in any situation.
- Concepts and principles
- Theory
- National and global directives
- Special issues
- Language
- Meaning of diversity in the organization
- Cultural relevance in the workplace
- Individual and societal factors
- Dealing effectively with cultural diversity
- Implications in the workplace

REFERENCES

American Association of Colleges of Nursing. (2013). *Quality and Safety Education for Nurses (QSEN) initiative.* Robert Wood Johnson Foundation.

American Nurses Association (ANA). (2008). *Code of ethics for nurses with interpretative statements.* Washington, DC: American Nurses Publishing.

American Nurses Association (ANA). (2010). *Position statement: The nurse's role in ethics and human rights: Protecting and promoting individual worth, dignity, and human rights in practice settings.* American Nurses Association, Inc.

Baldwin, D. (2003). Disparities in health and health care: Focusing efforts to eliminate unequal burdens. *Online Journal of Issues in Nursing, 8*(1), 2.

Campinha-Bacote, J. (1999). A model and instrument for addressing cultural competence in health care. *Journal of Nursing Education, 38*(5), 203–207.

Campinha-Bacote, J. (2002). The process of cultural competence in a delivery of healthcare services: A model of care. *Journal of Transcultural Nursing, 13*(3), 181–184.

Chen, A. H., Youdelman, M. K., & Brooks, J. (2007). The legal framework for language access in healthcare settings: Title VI and beyond. *Journal of General Internal Medicine, 22*(Suppl. 2), 362–367.

Choi, H. (2001). Cultural marginality: A concept analysis with implications for immigrant adolescents. *Issues in Comprehensive Pediatric Nursing, 24,* 193–206.

Connerley, M. L., & Pedersen, R. B. (2005). *Leadership in a diverse and multicultural environment: Developing awareness, knowledge and skills.* Los Angeles: Sage Publications.

Engebretson, J., Mahoney, J., & Carlson, E. D. (2008). Cultural competence in the era of evidence-based practice. *Journal of Professional Nursing, 24*(3), 172–178.

Giger, J. N., & Davidhizar, R. (2002). The Giger and Davidhizar transcultural assessment model. *Journal of Transcultural Nursing, 13*(3), 185–188.

International Council of Nurses. (2008). *Translation guidelines for International Classification for Nursing Practice (ICNP).* Geneva, Switzerland. Retrieved April 1, 2009, from www.icn.ch.

International Council of Nurses. (2012). *The ICN code of ethics for nurses.* Geneva, Switzerland: ICN-International Council of Nurses (pp. 1–11).

Leininger, M. 2002a. Cultural care theory: A major contribution to advance transcultural nursing knowledge and practice. *Journal of Transcultural Nursing, 13*(3), 189–192.

Leininger, M. (2002b). Essential transcultural nursing care concepts, principles, examples, and policy statements. Cited in In Leininger, M. & McFarland, M. R. (Eds.), *Transcultural nursing: Concepts, theories, research & practice*. (3rd ed.). New York: McGraw-Hill Medical Publishing Division.

Lenburg, C. B., Lipson, J. G., Demi, A. S., Blaney, D. R., Stern, P. N., Schultz, P. R., et al. (1995). *Promoting cultural competence in and through nursing education: A critical review and comprehensive plan for action*. Washington, DC: American Academy of Nursing.

Merriam-Webster Inc. (2013). *The Merriam-Webster dictionary*. Springfield, Mass: Merriam-Webster.

National League for Nursing. (2005). *Core competencies of nurse educators with task statements*. New York, NY: National League for Nursing. Retrieved 1/5/2013.

Noone, J. (2008). The diversity imperative: Strategies to address a diverse nursing workforce. *Nursing Forum*, *43*(3), 133–143.

Periyakoil, V. S., Stevens, M., & Kramer, H. (2013 March). Multicultural long-term care nurses' perceptions of factors influencing patient dignity at the end of life. *Journal of the American Geriatric Society*, *61*(3), 440–446. Retrieved 5/18/2013 http:/ncbi.nln.nih.gov/pubmed/23496266.

Purnell, L. D. (2009). *Guide to culturally competent health care* (2nd ed.). Philadelphia: FA Davis.

Purnell, L. D., & Paulanka, B. J. (2008). *Transcultural health care: A culturally competent approach* (3rd ed.). Philadelphia: FA Davis.

Spector, R. E. (2009). *Cultural diversity in health and illness* (7th ed.). Upper Saddle River, NJ: Pearson Prentice Hall.

Spence, D. (2004). Prejudice, paradox and possibility: The experience of nursing people from cultures other than one's own. In K. H. Kavanaugh & V. Knowlden (Eds.), *Many voices: Toward caring culture in healthcare and healing*. Madison, WI: The University of Wisconsin Press.

SUGGESTED READINGS

American Association of Colleges of Nursing. (2008). *Cultural competency in baccalaureate nursing education*. Website www.aacn.nche.edu/Education/cultural.htm.

Bonder, B., Martin, L., & Miracle, A. (2002). *Culture in clinical care*. Thorofare, NJ: Slack.

Corlese, I. B., Nicholas, P. K., & Nokes, K. M. (2001). Issues in cross-cultural quality-life research. *Journal of Nursing Scholarship*, *33*(1), 15–20.

Engebretson, J., Mahoney, J., & Carlson, E. D. (2008). Cultural competence in the era of evidence-based practice. *Journal of Professional Nursing*, *24*(3), 172–178.

Hagman, L. W. (2006). Cultural self-efficacy of licensed registered nurses in New Mexico. *Journal of Cultural Diversity*, *13*(2), 105–112.

National Quality Forum. (2009). *A comprehensive framework and preferred practices for measuring and reporting cultural competence: A consensus report*. Washington, DC. Website: www.qualityforum.org/Search.aspx?keyword=A+comprehensive+framework+and+preferred+practices+for+measuring+and+reporting+cultural+competence%3a+A+concensus+report.

Numer, M., Macleod, A., Sinclair, D., & Frank, B. (2008). Interprofessional educations for faculty and staff—A review of the changing worlds: Diversity and health care project. *Journal of Interprofessional Care*, *22*(Suppl. 1), 83–90.

Singleton, K., & Krause, E. M. S. (September 30, 2009). Understanding cultural and linguistic barriers to health literacy. *The Online Journal of Issues in Nursing*, pp. 1–13. Retrieved October 28, 2009, from www.nursingworld.org/MainMenuCategories?ANAMarketplace/ANAPeriodicals/OJIN/TableofCo….

University of Washington Medical Center Patient and Family Education services. (n.d.). *Culture clues. Tip sheets regarding diverse cultures*. Website: http://depts.washington.edu/pfes/CultureClues.htm.

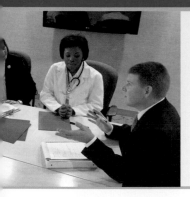

10

Power, Politics, and Influence

Karen Kelly

This chapter describes how power and politics influence the roles of leaders, managers, and followers, and how leaders and managers use power and politics to be influential. Contemporary concepts of power, empowerment, types of power exercised by nurses, key factors in developing a powerful image, personal and organizational strategies for exercising power, and the power of nurses to shape health policy by taking action in the arena of legislative politics are explored. Engaging in the politics of the workplace is critical for effective nursing leadership and management.

LEARNING OUTCOMES

- Explore the concepts of professional and legislative politics related to nursing.
- Value the concept of power as it relates to leadership and management in nursing.
- Use different types of power in the exercise of nursing leadership.
- Develop a power image for effective nursing leadership.
- Choose appropriate strategies for exercising power to influence the politics of the work setting, professional organizations, legislators, and the development of health policy.

KEY TERMS

coalitions	negotiating	politics
empowerment	policy	power
influence		

THE CHALLENGE

Anonymous, a retired emergency department staff nurse

Our hospital was trying hard to improve customer service. The emergency department (ED) had been receiving frequent calls that were not relevant to the work of the ED, such as asking how long to cook a turkey and where the closest 24-hour veterinary clinic is. In some cases, in efforts to provide good customer service, the ED staff provided phone numbers (e.g., the Butterball turkey talk-line®; the phone number for a 24-hour animal hospital). Often we had to tell callers we could not provide them with the information requested; these responses were met with hostile and even obscene reactions from some callers. Other calls (e.g., calls to determine how much a 20-minute late-night visit to the ED or an X-ray would cost) were also met with hostility at times. Staff requested an in-service class on how to handle such calls while providing good customer service. Our director provided us with such a program. We learned to deal with verbal hostility with assertive communication.

Shortly after the in-service class, late on a Friday morning, I took a call from a woman who wanted to know how to treat an infected wound on her cat's back. I gave her the name and phone number of the 24-hour animal clinic. The woman responded by screaming obscenities at me, indicating she had taken the cat to a veterinarian and wasn't going to go back. She screamed so loudly that the ED's medical director and other staff heard the woman's tirade. Feeling

empowered, I used my new skills to assertively end the conversation. A secretary paged our nursing director to come to the ED while the call was in progress. She arrived just as the call ended. I was debriefed by the director. The others who overheard the call gave her the same account of the call. I began to write an incident report on the event before my director was paged to go to the office of the vice president (VP) of nursing.

The VP had just gotten off the phone with the chief executive officer (CEO) of the hospital. The woman with the cat called him to accuse me of calling her obscene names and refusing to help her. The director told my VP what I had told her. She emphasized that the caller was the one using obscenities, not me. The VP directed her to suspend me immediately to placate the CEO; my director insisted that I had done nothing wrong and refused to suspend me, based on the information the others had given her. The VP came to the ED after the director left her office. She then confronted me, threatening to fire me unless I called the woman and apologized. The VP left only when the medical director of the ED insisted that I had used no obscenities and had not responded to the call inappropriately. Badly shaken, I paged the director to come back to the ED as soon as the VP left.

What do you think you would do if you were this nurse?

INTRODUCTION

The profession of nursing developed in the United States at a time when women had limited legal rights (e.g., most were prohibited from voting, and many could not own property). Women were viewed as neither powerful nor political; in the late nineteenth century, *feminine* and *powerful* were practically contradictory terms. During the twentieth century, as the status and role of women changed, so did the status and role of nurses. Moving into the twenty-first century, the economic and social power of women has evolved, as has the power of nurses. This is significant because nursing historically has been and continues to be a discipline comprised primarily of women.

In the twenty-first century, nurses must exercise their power to create a strong voice for nursing in shaping an evolving healthcare environment. In an era of rapid change with a dramatic nursing shortage like none before, healthcare reform offers new opportunities for nurses at the bedside and in the community, for those just entering the profession and those in advance nursing roles. Nurses must use their collective

power and flex their political muscles to create a preferred future for an evolving healthcare system, healthcare consumers, and the profession of nursing.

HISTORY

The word *power* comes from the Latin word *potere*, meaning "to be able." Simply defined, **power** is the ability to influence others in an effort to achieve goals. Power was once considered almost a taboo in nursing. In nursing's formative years, the exercise of power was considered inappropriate, unladylike, and unprofessional. In nursing's earliest decades in the United States, many decisions about nursing education and practice were made by persons outside of nursing (Ashley, 1976). Nurses began to exercise their collective power with the rise of early nursing leaders such as Lillian Wald, Isabel Stewart, Annie Goodrich, Lavinia Dock, M. Adelaide Nutting, Mary Eliza Mahoney, and Isabel Hampton Robb and the development of organizations that evolved into the American Nurses Association (ANA) and the National League for Nursing (NLN) (Lewenson, 2012).

Many social, technologic, scientific, and economic trends have shaped nursing and nurses and nursing's ability to exercise power during the twentieth and early twenty-first centuries. The American Medical Association (AMA), in 1988, proposed a new category of healthcare worker (the registered care technologist or RCT) to replace nurses during a nursing shortage. Nurses and nursing organizations responded powerfully. Nursing leaders came together in "summit meetings" to formulate powerful responses to the AMA and implemented a range of actions, including public education and the education of legislators. A new healthcare worker did not materialize from this proposal. Today, in an era of expanding nursing roles (e.g., advanced practice nurses and new roles for graduates of doctor of nursing practice [DNP] programs), nurses must continue to exercise their power to shape the continuing development of the profession of nursing and the future of the healthcare system and manage the efforts of medicine and others to control nursing practice.

The media, politicians, organized medicine, some healthcare executives, and some nurses have traditionally viewed nurses and nursing as powerless. That view began to change dramatically in the 1990s as nurses began to appear more often on local and national news and on talk shows as experts on health care, the changes occurring in the healthcare system, and the effect of these changes on the public. Nurses have become increasingly visible in political campaigns on the local, state, and national levels, both as candidates and as political influentials. For example, Congresswoman Lois Capps, MA, BSN, RN, represents a California congressional district, assuming the office held by her husband upon his death. A former school nurse, Congresswoman Capps has since been reelected by her constituents to the House seat. The 113th Congress (2013-2015) included six nurses, including one licensed practical nurse (LPN) (American Nurses Association [ANA], 2013a). Nurses and nursing have gained new respect in the political arena in recent years. Sheila Burke, MPA, RN, FAAN, served as Chief of Staff for Senator Robert Dole while he was Senate Majority Leader in the United States Congress, making her one of the most powerful congressional staff people in Washington. Mary Wakefield, PhD, RN, FAAN, was appointed the administrator of the Health Resources and Services Administration (HRSA) under President Barack Obama. She served in the 1990s as chief of staff to North Dakota senators Kent

Conrad and Quentin Burdick. And Marilyn Taveneer, RN, was named the chief administrator of the Centers for Medicare and Medicaid Services in 2013.

INTO THE TWENTY-FIRST CENTURY

Thirty years ago Roberts (1983) addressed the historical evidence of oppressed group behavior among nurses, based on models developed from the study of politically and economically oppressed populations. Oppressed group behavior is apparent when a population is dominated by another group; this population begins to take on the characteristics of the dominant group; and the oppressed population rejects the characteristics of their own group (Roberts 1983), often bullying and abusing their peers. In the twenty-first century, bullying and incivility have become epidemic in both nursing education and clinical settings (Clark, Landrum, & Nguyen, 2010; Croft & Cash, 2012; McNamara, 2012; Vessey, DeMarco, & DiFazio, 2011). Bullying reflects the abuse of power and a fear of the power of others (see Theory Box, p. 171). Bullying and incivility disrupt the healthcare workplace. The problems of bullying and incivility have been tied to patient safety (McNamara, 2012), requiring that The Joint Commission finally address this workplace issue through a Leadership Standard issued in 2009 and clarified in 2012 (The Joint Commission, 2012). The Joint Commission standard demands that leaders ensure that a code of conduct is implemented to ensure patient safety and a culture of quality. This requires leaders to be proactive in addressing the potential for incivility and bullying in the healthcare workplace.

POLICY, POWER, AND ACTIVISM

Schools of nursing too often fail to socialize students to be activists and to prepare them for leadership demands. Students need to be exposed to the concepts of political action and public and health policy to ready as nurse leaders to deal with issues within nursing and health care. A **policy** is just a plan for action related to an issue that affects a group's well-being or ability to function. All nurses need to continue to expand their understanding of the concept of power and to develop their skills in exercising power. Avoiding involvement in the politics of nursing in the workplace, in the profession at large, or in the area of public and health policy limits the power of the individual nurse and the profession as a whole.

Some nurses are still uncomfortable with politics and the use of power, treating "politics" as if it was a dirty word. Historically, politics has been viewed with some disdain. Writer Robert Louis Stevenson noted, "Politics is perhaps the only profession for which no preparation is thought necessary." But contemporary nursing's need to thrive within a healthcare system demands that nursing education prepare nurses to engage in professional, workplace, and legislative politics.

Politics can be defined in many ways. One simple definition of politics that this author uses when teaching health policy and politics in nursing is "a process of human interaction within organizations." Politics permeates all organizations, including workplaces, legislatures, professions, and even families. Young children often learn that one parent is more likely to readily give permission for special activities or more likely to buy toys and other desired items. They quickly learn to ask permission or ask for a desired item from that parent before asking the other. This is an unwritten political rule in many families. Political activism should be an unwritten rule in nursing (see the Literature Perspective). The American Association of Colleges of Nursing (AACN) identifies health policy as one of the essentials for baccalaureate, graduate, and doctoral education (AACN, 2006, 2008, 2011).

📖 LITERATURE PERSPECTIVE

Resource: Leavitt, J.K., Chaffee, M.W., & Vance, C. (2013). Learning the ropes of policy, politics, and advocacy. In D.J. Mason, J.K. Leavitt, & M.W. Chaffee (Eds.), *Policy & politics in nursing and health care* (pp. 19-28, 6th ed.). St. Louis: Elsevier/Saunders.

Political activism is a learned skill that is critical to nurses and the future of nursing. For some, there is an "aha" moment that gets them involved in the politics of nursing and health care. It might be a clinical situation when a patient is denied care because of an institutional or regulatory policy. For others it was the work of a mentor or graduate studies that excited them about working in the area of policy and politics. Florence Nightingale, the mother of modern nursing, was a political activist who viewed all of nursing as forms of advocacy, a political process. A nurse can develop and expand policy, advocacy, and political skills in several ways: continuing education, academic programs (e.g., graduate and DNP programs), learning by doing through active membership in professional associations (e.g., American Nurses Association and one's state nurses association), volunteer work on political campaigns and in a legislator's office, and self-study.

FOCUS ON POWER

Some nurses, including both new graduates and seasoned veterans, have too often viewed power as if it were something immoral, corrupting, and totally contradictory to the caring nature of nursing. However, the definition in this chapter (the ability to influence others in an effort to achieve goals) demonstrates the essential nature of power to nursing. Nurses routinely influence patients to improve their health status. When nurses provide health teaching to patients and their families, the goal is to change patient/family behavior to promote optimal health. That is an exercise of power in nursing practice. Coaching other nurses to improve their performances is an exercise of power. Serving as the chief nursing officer of a hospital or health-related corporation, managing a multimillion dollar budget, demonstrates another exercise of power.

EXERCISE 10-1

Recall a recent opportunity in which you observed the work of an expert nurse. Think about that nurse's interactions with patients, family members, nursing students, nursing colleagues, and other professionals. What kinds of power did you observe this nurse using? What did the nurse do that told you, "This is a powerful person"?

Social scientists have studied the use and abuse of power in human organizations. They have analyzed and categorized the sources and applications of power in human experience. Hersey, Blanchard, and Natemeyer (1979) offered a classic formulation on the bases of social power. Leavitt, Mason, and Whelan (2012) offered a revised view of types of power that readily applies to the efforts of nurses in the workplace, in professional organizations, and in politics (see the Theory Box on p. 171). These types of power are not mutually exclusive. They are often used in concert to exert influence on individuals or groups.

Having a high-status position in an organization immediately provides stature, but power depends on the ability to accomplish goals from that position. Although some may think that "knowledge is power," acting on that knowledge is where the real power lies. Sharing knowledge expands one's power and, in turn,

THEORY BOX

Sources of Power

KEY IDEAS	APPLICATION TO PRACTICE
Expert power: Based on one's reputation for expertise and ones' credibility. The knowledge and skills the nurse possesses that are needed by others.	The leader of a state nurses' association (SNA) may have access to the leaders of the state legislature based on the leader's expert power, which has enabled years of work with members of the legislature. The SNA president has always delivered on promises of support and provided useful information to legislators on matters of health policy.
Position power: Possessed by virtue of one's position within an organization or status within a group.	The dean of a college of nursing is viewed on campus as powerful because this dean leads the fastest growing academic unit on campus.
Information power: Stems from one's possession of selected information that is needed by others.	A direct care nurse demonstrates great skill in teaching patients difficult self-care activities and is sought out by colleagues to help them teach their patients.
Connection power: Gained by association with people who are powerful or who have links to powerful people.	At a National Nurses' Week celebration, nurses take advantage of the opportunity to have extended, informal conversations with those who report to the chief nursing officer.
Referent power: Granted by association with a powerful person.	A graduating senior nursing student asks a well-respected nurse manager to be her preceptor for the senior leadership course. The student wants to work in this agency upon graduation.
Coercive power: Stems from fear of someone's real or perceived fear of another person.	A nurse who lacks confidence in her performance in a new position is worried about an upcoming review with the nursing director.
Reward power: One is perceived as being able to provide rewards or favors.	An instructor is perceived positively by a nursing student who received an *A* for a clinical course.
Empowerment: The nurse is a source of shared power to build the exercise of power by others.	The chief nurse executive develops a model of shared governance to enable nurses to have a stronger voice in patient care decisions.

Source: Leavitt, J. K., Mason, D. J., Whelan, E. (2012). Political analysis and strategies. In D. J. Mason, J. K. Leavitt, & M. W. Chaffee (Eds.), Policy & politics in nursing and health care (6th ed., pp. 65-78). St. Louis: Elsevier/Saunders.

Nurses can use all of these types of power while implementing a wide range of nursing activities. Nurses who teach patients use expert and information power when teaching patients; they also exercise position power as registered nurses, accorded a certain status by society, by virtue of their education and license. Members of a state nurses' association who lobby members of the state legislature use expert, information, and position power when gaining legislators' support for healthcare legislation. New graduates, employed on probationary status until they demonstrate the initial clinical competencies, may view the nurse manager as exercising position, expert, and either coercive or reward power related to their initial evaluations. Nursing faculty and skilled clinicians exercise expert, position, and information power as students emulate their behavior. Connection power is evident at any social gathering in the workplace. People of high status (e.g., vice presidents, directors, deans) within an organization may be sought out for conversation by those who want to move up the organizational hierarchy.

empowers others, including colleagues and patients, by giving them information or skills that they need to take action in a situation.

Influence is the process of using power. Influence can range from the punitive power of coercion to the interactive power of collaboration. Coaching a new graduate to complete a complicated nursing procedure successfully demonstrates the ability of the experienced nurse to influence that orientee. The coach uses expert, positional, and informational power to influence the orientee not only at that moment but also perhaps over the span of a career. Nurses

can use personal, expert, and perceived power while working on the campaigns of legislators who support nursing and healthcare issues.

EMPOWERMENT

Empowerment is a term that has come into common usage in nursing. That term has been used extensively in the nursing literature related to administration and management; it is also highly relevant to the domain of clinical practice. Empowerment is the process of exercising one's own power to facilitate the participation of others in decision making and taking action so they are free to exercise power (Leavitt, Mason, & Whelan, 2012). Empowerment is consistent with the contemporary view of leadership, a paradigm that is exemplified by behaviors characteristic of all nurse leaders: facilitator, coach, teacher, and collaborator. Nursing leaders, in employment settings or in professional organizations, exercise power in making professional judgments in their daily work.

These leadership skills are also essential to effective followers. Powerful nurse managers enable nurses to exercise power, influencing them to grow professionally. Powerful nurses support their patients and families so they can participate actively in their own care. Hence these leadership skills can be viewed as an essential component of professional nursing practice whether one is a clinician, an educator, a researcher, or an executive/manager.

Sharing Power

Nurses, including some leaders, sometimes view power as a finite quantity: "If I give you some of my power, I will have less." Empowerment emphasizes the notion that power grows when shared. Envision the exercise of shared power along a spectrum from low to high levels of sharing. The opposing ends of the spectrum can be characterized by two very different groups of nurses:

- Nurses who view power as finite will avoid cooperation with their colleagues and refuse to share their expertise.
- Nurses who view power as infinite are strong collaborators who gain satisfaction by helping their colleagues expand their expertise and their power base.

Empowered nurses make professional practice possible, creating a culture that satisfies all nurses. Empowered clinicians are essential for effective nursing management, just as empowered managers set the stage for excellence in clinical practice. Encouraging a reticent colleague to be an active participant in committee meetings serves to empower that nurse and to shape practice policy with the institution. Guiding a novice nurse in exercising professional judgment empowers both the senior nurse and the novice clinician. Coaching a patient on how to be more assertive with a physician who is reluctant to answer the patient's questions is another form of empowerment.

> **EXERCISE 10-2**
> Think about a recent clinical experience in which you empowered a patient. What did you do for and/or with the patient (and family) that was empowering? How did you feel about your own actions in this situation? How did the patient (or family) respond to your efforts?

PERSONAL POWER STRATEGIES

Developing a collection of power strategies or tools is a critical aspect of personal empowerment. These strategies are used in situations that demand the exercise of leadership. Such strategies support one's professional power base and developing political skills within an organization (Boxes 10-1 and 10-2). These strategies also indicate to others that one is a powerful nurse and a leader. These boxes identify personal

---

BOX 10-1   POWER STRATEGIES FOR NURSING LEADERS AND ASPIRING LEADERS

Developing a Powerful Image
- Self-confidence
- Body language
- Self-image, including grooming, dress, and speech
- Career commitment and continuing professional education
- Attitudes, beliefs, and values

Additional Personal Power Strategies
- Be honest.
- Be courteous; it makes other people feel good!
- Smile when appropriate; it puts people at ease.
- Accept responsibility for your own mistakes, and then learn from them.
- Be a risk taker.
- Win and lose gracefully.
- Learn to be comfortable with conflict and ambiguity; they are both normal states of the human condition.
- Give credit to others where credit is due.
- Develop the ability to take constructive criticism gracefully; learn to let destructive criticism "roll off your back."
- Use business cards when introducing yourself to new contacts, and collect the business cards of those you meet when networking.
- Follow through on promises.

BOX 10-2   DEVELOPING POLITICAL SKILLS

- Build a working relationship with a legislator, such as one's state senator or representative or member of the U.S. Congress and the legislative staff members.
- Join and be an active member of your state nurses' association affiliate of the ANA.
- Join a specialty nursing organization related to your clinical specialty (e.g., critical care, pediatrics) or specialty role in nursing (nurse practitioner, manager).
- Invite a legislator to a professional organization meeting.
- Invite a legislator or staff person from the legislator's office to spend a day with you at work.
- Register to vote, and vote in every election.
- Join your state nurses' association's government relations or legislative committee and political action committee (PAC); join ANA's PAC.
- Be in touch with your federal and state legislators on nursing and healthcare issues, especially related to specific bills, by writing letters, making telephone calls, or sending e-mails.
- Participate in Nurse Lobby Day and meet with your state legislators.
- Work on a federal or state legislative campaign.
- Visit your U.S. senators and member of Congress if visiting in the Washington, D.C., area to discuss federal legislation related to nursing and health care, or visit their local offices.
- Get involved in the local group of your political party.
- Run for office at the local, county, state, or congressional level.
- Enhance the image of nursing in all your policy efforts.
- Communicate your message effectively and clearly.
- Develop your expertise in shaping policy.
- Seek appointive positions or elective office to shape policy more effectively.

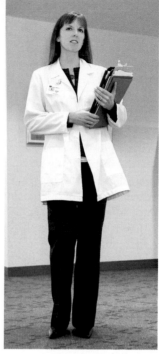

Dressing in an appropriate manner helps to convey an image of power.

power strategies beyond those discussed in this section. These "power tools" have been developed and collected by this author during more than 40 years of nursing experience and observation of successful, effective, powerful nurses.

Strategies for Developing a Powerful Image

Consider the words of Lady Margaret Thatcher, former prime minister of Great Britain: "Being powerful is like being a lady. If you have to tell people you are, you aren't." You don't have to wear a sign around your neck to show that you are powerful!

The most basic power strategy is the development of a powerful image. If nurses think they are powerful, others will view them as powerful; if they view themselves as powerless, so will others. A sense of self-confidence is a strong foundation in developing one's "power image," and is essential for successful political efforts in the workplace, within the profession, and within the public policy arena. Several key factors contribute to one's power image:

- Self-image: thinking of oneself as powerful and effective
- Grooming and dress: ensuring that clothing, hair, and general appearance are neat, clean, and appropriate to the situation
- Good manners: treating people with courtesy and respect
- Body language: maintaining good posture, using gestures that avoid too much drama, maintaining good eye contact, and being confident in movement
- Speech: using a firm, confident voice; good grammar and diction; an appropriate vocabulary; and strong communication skills

EXERCISE 10-3

Think about a powerful public figure you admire. What key factors contribute to this person's powerful image? Think about a powerful nurse you have met. Identify this person's key image factors. Think about nurses who work in wrinkled scrubs, whose hair is pulled back haphazardly into ponytails, and who fail to make eye contact with patients or their family members. What kind of power image message do they send?

Concern about a powerful image may seem superficial. However, the impressions we make on people influence the way they view us now and in the future, as well as how they value what we do and say. We get only one chance to make a first impression. Given similar educational and experiential backgrounds, who is more likely to be hired for a nursing position: the candidate who comes dressed in a suit or the candidate who arrives in jeans and sandals (Chaffee, 2012a)? Who will be seen as the more competent professional by a patient: the nurse in wrinkled scrubs or the nurse in neat street clothes and a freshly laundered lab coat? Who will have a greater positive impact on a member of the state legislature: the nurse who visits in a sweatshirt and shorts or the nurse in business attire? A powerful image signals to others that one is professionally competent, influential, powerful, and capable of exercising appropriate judgments.

Attitudes and beliefs are other important aspects of a powerful image; they reflect one's values. Believing that power is a positive force in nursing is essential to one's powerful image. A firm belief in nursing's value to society and the centrality of nursing's contribution to the healthcare delivery system is also important. Powerful nurses do not allow the phrase "I'm just a nurse" in their vocabulary Instead, powerful nurses can enhance the profession by responding to statements of appreciation with the phrase, "I'm a nurse; it's what we do," as one of this book's contributors says. Behavior reflects one's pride in the profession of nursing. This not only increases a nurse's own power but also helps empower nursing colleagues.

Make a Commitment to Nursing as a Career

Nursing is a profession; professions offer careers, not just a series of jobs. Decades ago, nursing marketed itself to recruits as the perfect preparation for marriage and family. Some people still view nurses only as members of an occupation who drop in and out

of employment, not as members of a profession with a long-term career commitment. Having a career commitment does not preclude leaving employment temporarily for family, education, or other demands. Having a career commitment means that nurses view themselves first and foremost as members of the discipline of nursing with an obligation to make a contribution to the profession. Status as an employee of a particular hospital, home health agency, long-term care facility, or other venue is secondary to one's status as a member of the profession of nursing.

Value Continuing Nursing Education

Valuing education is one of the hallmarks of a profession. The continuing development of one's nursing skills and knowledge is an empowering experience, preparing nurses to make decisions with the support of an expanding body of evidence. Seminars, workshops, and conferences offer opportunities for continued professional growth and empowerment. Seeking advanced nursing degrees or postbaccalaureate/postgraduate certificates is also a powerful growth experience and reflects commitment to the profession. At one time, some nurses sought to get ahead in nursing by seeking education outside of nursing at the baccalaureate and graduate level. To develop expertise in nursing, one must be educated in the discipline of nursing. This evolution is now seen in employment policies that specify degrees in nursing as opposed to a generic statement about bachelor's or master's degree.

Communication Skills

The most basic tool is effective communication skills (Chaffee, 2012a). These same communication skills ensure nurses' effective interaction with patients and families. Listening skills are essential leadership skills. Just as the clinician listens to the patient to collect assessment data, the leader uses listening skills to assess and evaluate. Managers and other leaders who are good listeners develop reputations for being fair and consistent. Listening for recurring themes related to minor issues of staff dissatisfaction in informal conversations can enable a manager to take action before a staff crisis occurs.

Verbal and nonverbal skills are important personal power strategies; the ability to assess these messages is a critical power strategy. Experts in communication estimate that 90% of the messages we communicate to others are nonverbal. When nonverbal and verbal messages are in conflict, the nonverbal message is always more powerful. The basic lessons on the power of nonverbal communication that most nurses learn in an introductory psychiatric nursing course are relevant in all areas of nursing!

Networking

Networking is an important power strategy and political skill (Chaffee, 2012; Leavitt, Mason, & Whelan, 2012). A network is the result of identifying, valuing, and maintaining relationships with a system of individuals who are sources of information, advice, and support. Networking supports the empowerment of participants through interaction and the refinement of their interpersonal skills. Many nurses have relatively limited networks within the organizations where they are employed. They tend to have lunch or coffee with the people with whom they work most closely. One strategy to expand a workplace network is to have lunch or coffee with someone from another department, including managers from non-nursing departments, at least two or three times a month.

Active participation in nursing organizations is the most effective method of establishing a professional network outside one's place of employment. Although only a minority of nurses actively participate in professional organizations, such participation can propel a nurse into the politics of nursing, including involvement in shaping health policy. State nurses' associations offer excellent opportunities to develop a network that includes nurses from various clinical and functional areas (Shinn, 2012). Membership in specialty organizations, including organizations for nurse managers and executives, provides the opportunity to network with nurses with similar expertise and interests. In addition, membership in civic, volunteer, and special interest groups and participation in educational programs (e.g., formal academic programs and conferences) also provide networking opportunities. Use of social media, like LinkedIn and Twitter, also can expand one's professional network around the globe. The nurse must be cautious to avoid mixing one's personal life and professional life in social media.

The successful networker identifies a core of networking partners who are particularly skilled, insightful, and eager to support the development of colleagues. These colleagues need to be nurtured through such strategies as sharing information with them that relates to their interests; introducing them to persons who have comparable interests or who are connected with others of influence; staying connected through notes, e-mail, phone calls, social media, or text messages; and meeting them at important events. Successful networkers are not a burden to others in making requests for support, and they do not refuse the support that is provided.

Mentoring

Mentoring has become an important force in nursing (Leavitt, Chaffee, & Vance, 2013). Mentors are competent, experienced professionals who develop a relationship with less experienced nurses for the purpose of providing advice, support, information, and feedback to encourage the development of that person. Mentoring has been an important element in the career development of men in business, academia, and selected professions. Mentoring has become a significant power strategy for women in general and for nurses in particular during the past 30 years. Mentoring provides expanded access to information, power, and career opportunities. Mentors have been a critical asset to novice nurses trying to negotiate workplace and professional politics.

Effective mentoring in nursing benefits both the mentor and the mentee. Mentors benefit by expanding their own professional development and that of their colleagues, improving their own self-awareness, experiencing the intrinsic benefits of teaching another, nurturing their own interpersonal skills, and expanding their political savvy. Mentees receive one-on-one nurturing and coaching from the mentor, gain insight or savvy about the political rules of the organization and learn about organizational culture from an insider, can expand their self-confidence in a supportive relationship, receive career development advice, profit from the mentor's professional network, and have a unique opportunity for individualized professional development.

Mentoring is an empowering experience for both mentors and protégés. The process of seeking out mentors is an exercise in growth for protégés. Mentors often come from one's professional networks. Mentors sometimes select their protégés; at other times, the reverse is true. Protégés learn new skills from influential mentors and gain self-confidence. Mentors share their influence through the influence of those they mentor and gain satisfaction by experiencing the evolution of those nurses into experienced nurses.

Goal-Setting

Goal-setting is another power strategy. Every nurse knows about setting goals. Students learn to devise patient care goals or patient outcomes as part of the care-planning process. Nurses may be expected to write annual goals for performance reviews at work. Even a project at home (e.g., painting the bedrooms) may necessitate setting goals (e.g., painting a room each day of one's vacation). Goals help one know if what was planned was actually accomplished. Likewise, a successful nursing career needs goals to define what one wants to achieve as a nurse. Without such goals, one can wander endlessly through a series of jobs without a real sense of satisfaction. To paraphrase what the Cheshire Cat told Alice during her trip through Wonderland: Any road will take you there if you don't know where you are going.

Well-defined, long-term goals may be hard to formulate early in a career. For example, few new graduates know specifically that they want to be chief nurse executives, deans, managers, or researchers; yet, eventually, some will choose those career paths. However, developing such a vision early in a career is an important personal power strategy. Once this career vision is developed, one must create opportunities to move toward that vision. Such planning is empowering—putting the nurse in charge rather than letting a career unfold by chance. Having this sense of vision is consistent with a commitment to a career in nursing, part of developing a power image. This vision is always subject to revision as new opportunities are encountered and new interests, knowledge, and skills are gained. Education and work experiences are tools for achieving the vision of one's career.

Developing Expertise

As noted earlier in this chapter, expertise is one of the bases of power. Developing expertise in nursing is an important power strategy. Nursing expertise must not be limited to clinical knowledge. Leadership and communication skills, for example, are essential to the effective exercise of power. Education and practice provide the means for developing such expertise in any domain of nursing—clinical practice, education, research, and management. Developing expertise expands one's power among nursing colleagues, other professional colleagues, and patients. A high level of expertise can make one nearly indispensable within an organization. This is a powerful position to have within any organization, whether it is the workplace or a professional association. A high level of expertise can also lead to a high level of visibility within an organization.

High Visibility

The strategy of high visibility within an organization can begin with volunteering to serve as a member or the chairperson of committees and task forces. High visibility can be nurtured by attending open meetings in the workplace, professional associations, or the community. Even if you are not a member, if meetings deal with local health issues, you must be visible. Review the agendas of these meetings if they are circulated or posted online ahead of time. Use opportunities both before and after meetings to share your expertise and provide valuable information and ideas to members and leaders of such groups. Share your expertise at open meetings when appropriate. Speak up confidently, but have something relevant to say. Be concise and precise; members of the committee will ask for more information if they need it. Create your own business cards using a computer and sheets of business card stock (purchased in any office supply store). Give members of these committees your personal card so that they can contact you later for information.

EXERCISING POWER AND INFLUENCE IN THE WORKPLACE AND OTHER ORGANIZATIONS

To use influence effectively in any organization, one must understand how the system works and develop organizational strategies. Developing organizational savvy includes identifying the real decision makers and those persons who have a high level of influence with the decision makers. Recognize the informal leaders within any organization. An influential senior clinical nurse may have more decision-making power related to direct patient care than the nurse manager.

The senior clinical nurse may have more clinical expertise and a greater knowledge about the history of the unit and its personnel than a nurse manager with excellent management and leadership skills who is new to the unit.

For example, the executive assistants of chief nursing officers (CNOs) are usually very powerful people, although they are not always recognized as such. The CNO's assistant has control over information, making decisions about who gets to meet with the nurse executive and when screening incoming and outgoing mail, letting the CNO know when a document needs immediate attention, or placing a memo under a stack of mail for review at a later time.

Collegiality and Collaboration

Nursing does not exist in a vacuum, nor do nurses work in isolation from one another, other professionals, or support personnel. Nurses function within a wide range of organizations, such as schools, hospitals, community health organizations, governments, insurance companies, professional associations, and universities. Nurses have been divided too long over the appropriate educational level for entry into practice. Nurses are also noted for their failure to join nursing organizations.

Developing a sense of unity requires each nurse to act collaboratively and collegially in the workplace and in other organizations (e.g., professional associations). Collegiality demands that nurses value the accomplishments of nursing colleagues and express a sincere interest in their efforts. Turning to one's colleagues for advice and support empowers them and expands one's own power base at the same time. Unity of purpose does not contradict diversity of thought. One does not have to be a friend to everyone who is a colleague. Collegiality demands mutual respect, not friendship.

Collaboration and collegiality require that nurses work collectively to ensure that the voice of nursing is heard in the workplace and the legislature. Volunteer to serve on committees and task forces in the workplace, not only within the nursing department but also on organization-wide committees. Become an active member of nursing organizations, especially state nursing organizations and specialty organizations consistent with one's clinical specialty (e.g., AACN) or functional role (e.g., American Organization of Nurse Executives [AONE]). If eligible, become a member of a chapter of Sigma Theta Tau International, nursing's honor society. Get involved in the politics of organizations, in the workplace, and in professional associations.

If the workplace uses shared governance or other participatory models, get involved in these councils, committees, task forces, and work groups to share your energy, ideas, and expertise. Many organizations have interdisciplinary committees that bring together nurses, physicians, and other healthcare professionals to improve the quality of professional collaboration and the quality of patient care. Become an active, productive member of such groups within the workplace and in the professional associations and community groups dealing with healthcare issues and problems.

An Empowering Attitude

Demonstrate a positive and professional attitude about being a nurse to nursing colleagues, patients and their families, other colleagues in the workplace, and the public, including legislators. This attitude facilitates the exercise of power among colleagues while educating others about nurses and nursing. A powerful image is an important aspect of demonstrating this positive professional attitude. The current practice of nurses to identify themselves by first name may only decrease their power image in the eyes of physicians, patients, and others. Physicians are always addressed as "Doctor." When they address others only by their first names, inequality of power and status is evident. The use of first names among colleagues is not inappropriate so long as everyone is playing by the same rules. Managers may want to enhance the empowerment of their staff members by encouraging them to introduce themselves as "Dr.," "Ms.," or "Mr." Arriving at work, appointments, or meetings on time; looking neat and appropriately attired for the work setting or other professional situation; and speaking positively about one's work are examples of how easy it is to demonstrate a positive, powerful, and professional attitude.

Magnet™ institutions, as recognized by the American Nurses Credentialing Center (ANCC), are characterized by work environments that empower nurses (ANCC, 2013). Leadership activities have been identified as a critical element of the work culture in Magnet™ hospitals; and quality of leadership is one of the "forces of magnetism."

Developing Coalitions

The exercise of power is often directed at creating change. Although an individual can often be effective at exercising power and creating change, creating certain changes within most organizations requires collective action. Coalition building is an effective political strategy for collective action (Askoy, 2010; Bowers-Lanier, 2012). Coalitions are groups of individuals or organizations that join together temporarily around a common goal. This goal often focuses on an effort to effect change. The networking among organizations that results in coalition building requires members of one group to reach out to members of other groups. This often occurs at the leadership level and may come through formal mechanisms such as letters that identify an issue or problem—a shared interest—around which a coalition could be built. For example, a state nurses association may invite the leaders of organizations interested in child health (e.g., organizations of pediatric nurses, public health nurses and physicians, elementary school teachers, daycare providers) and consumers (e.g., parents) to discuss collaborative support for a legislative initiative to improve access to immunization programs in urban and rural areas. Such coalitions of professionals and consumers are powerful in influencing public policy related to health care.

Collaboration among groups and individuals with common interests and goals often results in greater success in effecting change and exercising power in the workplace and within other organizations, including legislative bodies. A group of diverse nursing organizations may come together as a coalition to support a modification of the state nursing practice act. Expanding networks in the workplace, as suggested earlier in this chapter, facilitates creating a coalition by developing a pool of candidates for coalition building before they are needed. Invite people with common goals to lunch or coffee to begin building a coalition around an issue. Discuss this shared interest, and gain the commitment of the individuals. Meet informally with members of the committee or task force that is working on this issue. Attend the open meetings of professional groups that share the same interests as the organization to which you belong. Share ideas on how to create the desired change most effectively while building coalitions.

Coalition building is an important skill for involvement in legislative politics. Nursing organizations often use coalition building when dealing with state legislatures and Congress. Changes in nurse practice acts to expand opportunities for advanced nursing practice have been accomplished in many states through coalition building. State medical societies or the state agencies that license physicians often oppose such changes. Efforts by a single nursing organization (e.g., a state nurses' association or a nurse practitioners' organization), representing a limited nursing constituency, often lack the clout to overcome opposition by the unified voice of the state's physicians. However, the unified effort of a coalition of nursing organizations, other healthcare organizations, and consumer groups can be powerful in effecting change through legislation.

Negotiating

Negotiating, or bargaining, is a critically important skill for organizational and political power (Kritek, 2002). It is a process of making trade-offs. Children are natural negotiators. Often, they will initially ask their parents for more than what they are willing to accept in the way of privileges, toys, or activities. The logic is simple to children: Ask for more than is reasonable and negotiate down to what you really want!

Negotiating often works the same way within organizations. People will sometimes ask for more than they want and be willing to accept less. In other situations, both sides will enter negotiations asking for radically different things but each may be willing to settle for a position that differs markedly from the respective original position. In the simplest forms of bargaining, each participant has something that the other party values: goods, services, or information. At the "bargaining table," each party presents an opening position. The process moves on until they reach a mutually agreeable result or until one or both parties walk away from a failed negotiation.

Bargaining may take many forms. Individuals may negotiate with a supervisor for a more desirable work schedule or with a peer to effect a schedule change so that one can attend an out-of-town conference. A nurse manager may sit at the bargaining table with the department director during budget planning to expand education hours for the nursing unit in the next year's budget. Representatives of a coalition of nursing organizations meeting with a legislator may negotiate with the legislator over sections of a proposed healthcare-related bill in an effort to eliminate or modify those sections not viewed by the nursing coalition as in the best interests of nurses, patients, or the healthcare system. Nurses may bargain with nursing and hospital administration over wages, staffing levels, other working conditions, and the conditions and policies that govern clinical practice. This is called *collective bargaining,* a specific type of negotiating that is regulated by both state and federal labor laws and that usually involves representation by a state nurses association or a nursing or non-nursing labor union (see Collective Action in Chapter 19).

Successful negotiators are well informed about not only their own positions but also those of the opposing side. Negotiators must be able to discuss the pros and cons of both positions. They can assist the other party in recognizing the costs versus the benefits of each position. These skills are also essential to exercising power effectively with the arenas of professional and legislative politics. When lobbying a member of the legislature to support a bill that is desired by nurses, one must understand the position of those opposed to the bill to respond effectively to questions that the legislator may ask.

Taking Political Action to Influence Policy

In the 1990s, Carolyn McCarthy was an LPN from New York when a tragedy turned her life around. Her husband was killed and her son injured by a gunman on the Long Island Railroad. She sought the support of her congressman on gun control legislation as a result of her personal tragedy. He refused to support such legislation. She took extraordinary action, changing her party affiliation from Republican to Democrat and then running against the incumbent for his seat in Congress. She is still an LPN, and served as Congresswoman Carolyn McCarthy (D-NY) until 2014. Taking action may include such simple acts as working in a legislative campaign or volunteering to work on a church committee to establish a parish health ministry. Extraordinary actions like those taken by Carolyn McCarthy are also essential for nursing's voice to be heard loudly and clearly in the uncertain future (Chaffee, 2012b).

Gaining political skills, like any other skill set, is a developmental process. Some suggested strategies for developing political skills are presented in Box 10-2 on p. 173. Learning one's strengths and areas for improvement requires self-study. The Political Astuteness Inventory (Goldwater & Zusy, 1990) is a helpful tool in determining how well prepared you are to influence legislative politics and public policy, especially public policy related to health care (Box 10-3).

The personal power strategies mentioned earlier in this chapter are also important for building one's political power. Nurses can no longer be passive observers of the political world. Political involvement is a professional responsibility, not just a privilege; political advocacy is a mandate (Priest, 2012). Nurses' perspectives of the critical issues for improving the healthcare system can shape the policy agenda of the nation's political leadership. Healthcare reform offers much opportunity for nurses and the profession if nurses are ready to move forward with reform (see the Research Perspective on p. 180).

BOX 10-3   POLITICAL ASTUTENESS INVENTORY

Place a check mark next to those items for which your answer is "yes." Then give yourself one point for each "yes." After completing the inventory, compare your total score with the scoring criteria at the end of the inventory.
1. I am registered to vote.
2. I know where my voting precinct is located.
3. I voted in the last general election.
4. I voted in the last two elections.
5. I recognized the names of the majority of the candidates on the ballot and was acquainted with the majority of issues in the last election.
6. I stay abreast of current health issues.
7. I belong to the state professional or student nurse organization.
8. I participate (e.g., as a committee member, officer) in this organization.
9. I attended the most recent meeting of my district nurses' association.
10. I attended the last state or national convention held by my organization.
11. I am aware of at least two issues discussed and the stands taken at this convention.

Continued

BOX 10-3   POLITICAL ASTUTENESS INVENTORY—cont'd

12. I read literature published by my state nurses' association, a professional journal/magazine/newsletter, or other literature on a regular basis to stay abreast of current health issues.
13. I know the names of my senators in Washington, D.C.
14. I know the name of my representative in Washington, D.C.
15. I know the name of the state senator from my district.
16. I know the name of the state representative from my district.
17. I am acquainted with the voting record of at least one of the previously mentioned state or federal representatives in relation to a specific health issue.
18. I am aware of the stand taken by at least one of the previously mentioned state or federal representatives in relation to a specific health issue.
19. I know whom to contact for information about health-related issues at the state or federal level.
20. I know whether my professional organization employs lobbyists at the state or federal level.
21. I know how to contact these lobbyists.
22. I contribute financially to my state and national professional organization's political action committee (PAC).
23. I give information about effectiveness of elected officials to assist the PAC's endorsement process.
24. I actively supported a senator or representative during the last election.
25. I have written to one of my state or national representatives in the last year regarding a health issue.
26. I am personally acquainted with a senator or representative or member of his or her staff.
27. I serve as a resource person for one of my representatives or his or her staff.

28. I know the process by which a bill is introduced in my state legislature.
29. I know which senators or representatives are supportive of nursing.
30. I know which house and senate committees usually deal with health-related issues.
31. I know the committees of which my representatives are members.
32. I know of at least two health issues related to my profession that are currently under discussion.
33. I know of at least two health-related issues that are currently under discussion at the state or national level.
34. I am aware of the composition of the state board that regulates my profession.
35. I know the process whereby one becomes a member of the state board that regulates my profession.
36. I know what DHHS stands for.
37. I have at least a vague notion of the purpose of the DHHS.
38. I am a member of a health board or advisory group to a health organization or agency.
39. I attend public hearings related to health issues.
40. I find myself more interested in political issues now than in the past.

Scoring:

0-9: Totally unaware politically/apathetic

10-19: Slightly more aware of the implications of the politics of nursing/buy-in

20-29: Beginning political astuteness/self-interest to political sophistication

30-40: Politically astute, an asset to nursing/leading the way

From Goldwater, M., & Zusy, M.J.L. (1990). *Prescription for nurses: Effective political action.* St. Louis: Mosby; with permission by M. Goldwater.

 ## RESEARCH PERSPECTIVE

Resource: Buerhaus, P.I., DesRoches, C., Applebaum, S., Hess, R., Norman, L.D., & Donelan, K. (2012). Are nurses ready for health care reform? A decade of survey research. *Nursing Economic$, 30,* 318-329.

The implementation of the Patient Protection and Affordable Care Act (ACA) has changed and will continue to change the American healthcare system, particularly related to finance and systems for healthcare delivery. New models, such as accountable care organizations and medical homes, will pave the way for expanding health care access to about 32 million people by 2014. Before the passage of the ACA, there was a sharp national focus on a growing nursing shortage. Shortly after the ACA became law, the Institute of Medicine (IOM) released its report: *The Future of Nursing: Leading Change and Advancing Health* (IOM, 2011). Other initiatives have

emerged to study the shortage and to expand the nursing workforce, especially in view of the dramatic increase in the number of people who will be able to access care as the ACA rolls out more benefits in 2014.

This study reviewed the differences over nearly a decade in the responses of nurses to a biennial survey (The National Survey of Registered Nurses [NSRN] conducted in 2002, 2004, 2006, 2008, and 2010). The surveys were sent to random samples of 1500 registered nurses throughout the United States. Response rates ranged from 37% in 2008 to 56% in 2010. The mean age of responders ranged from 39 years in 2004 to 47 years in 2010. For each survey, 6% to 7% of the respondents were men. None of the 2004 respondents held a doctoral degree; 1% of the 2010 sample held a doctoral degree. The mean hours worked per week ranged from 35.8 in 2006 to 36.7 in 2008. In all surveys, most responders were married (68% to 71%). Average hourly wage ranged from $27.10 in 2004 to $35.30 in 2010.

Nurses in the 2002 survey did not rate their opportunities for influencing workplace decisions highly; only 15% gave excellent or good ratings. In 2010, nurses rated their opportunities for influence at 25%. The 2002 respondents rated their opportunities to influence quality of care in their institutions as excellent or good 23% of the time; in 2010 the sample rated their opportunities as excellent or good 33% of the time. In 2002, only 35% of the nurses reported being very satisfied with being a nurse, whereas 52% were satisfied; in 2010, 57% reported being very satisfied, with 31% satisfied. In 2002, only 59% of the respondents indicated that they definitely or probably would recommend nursing as a career. In 2010, 86% indicated that they definitely or probably would recommend nursing as a career.

These and other survey findings indicated a nursing work environment in need of improvement, including nurse-physician relationships, workplace violence, and risk of injury to nurses in the course of providing care. Concerns that the influx of new healthcare consumers will overwhelm acute care nurse staffing that is already stretched to its limits were evident, a lack of understanding of the ACA, and a perception by only a minority of nurses that they have influence over decision making about care can undermine the positive changes that the ACA offers.

Implications for Practice

The authors of the study (Buerhaus et al., 2012) noted that several foundations (e.g., Josiah Macy) have invested significant funding in initiatives to strengthen nursing in a time of nursing shortage and growth in healthcare access for Americans, including greater need for nursing care. These initiatives seek to improve nursing leadership, support expanded access to higher education in nursing, and innovate to improve the quality of care. Making such changes demands that nurses exercise their power to change the healthcare system and empower nurses to practice to the fullest extent of their education.

CONCLUSION

Power is played out every day in every setting. Politics are played and often for the good of health care and patients. The abuse of either is what is disheartening. Recognizing the sources of power and using them effectively is a critical aspect to every nurse's role.

THE SOLUTION

The director gave me the rest of the shift off with pay. I decided to use the weekend off to consider whether I should resign. My director went back to the VP's office with my incident report about the phone call and presented it to the VP. She indicated that this was a true and accurate report of the event, now known as the "cat lady call." All the witnesses had signed the report, including the medical director. She calmly told the VP that she understood how the VP was being pressured by the CEO to take some immediate action. But she restated her belief that I handled the situation appropriately and that the caller was not honest with the CEO. She asserted that there would be no apology issued by her or by me. The VP said she would talk to us on Monday, after consulting with the hospital's legal counsel. From experience, we all knew that this meant the VP was considering firing both of us.

On Monday morning, the director received a new incident report. The report noted that the local police had brought an elderly woman into the ED on Saturday night. She was covered with scratches, many of which were infected. She was an animal hoarder and had created a disturbance in her neighborhood that resulted in the police bringing her into the hospital and removing dozens of cats from her home. She kept telling the ED staff that she didn't want to be cared for by the nurse she talked to on Friday. She was our "cat lady caller." She was verbally and physically abusive to the ED staff and the police. She was treated and released to family.

The director gave the VP this incident report, which vindicated me. She asked the VP how she would like to proceed with this issue. The VP's face reddened with embarrassment, and she told the director to apologize to me for her. I had already heard from the night staff about the woman's visit to the ED over the weekend by the time my director came to the ED. She was disappointed that the VP would not apologize to me in person. Because of my director's powerful response to the VP, I remained a hospital employee until my retirement a few years later. The VP's misuse of positional power was blocked by my director's use of personal and informational power. Her support empowered me.

—Anonymous

Would this be a suitable approach for you? Why?

THE EVIDENCE

The 2011 Institute of Medicine study, *The Future of Nursing: Leading Change, Advancing Health,* provides the best evidence of the need for nurses to use their power to influence change.

An interdisciplinary panel reviewed the literature to determine how nursing should move forward to meet the needs of a changing healthcare system. The 2-year initiative was conducted with the Robert Wood Johnson Foundation (RWJF).

The IOM study offers four key messages:

- Nurses should practice to the full extent of their education and training.
- Nurses should achieve higher levels of education and training through an improved education system that promotes seamless academic progression.
- Nurses should be full partners, with physicians and other healthcare professionals, in redesigning health care in the United States.
- Effective workforce planning and policy making require better data collection and an improved information infrastructure.

These messages and the eight recommendations of the IOM study demand political action from nurses in order to reshape nursing education and practice to enable nurses to practice to the full extent of their educations. Nurses should have access to a seamless system of educational programs so that they can perform more complex nursing roles and act as full partners in reshaping and leading the healthcare system. Nurses around the country are now participating in state-based work groups to fulfill the recommendations of the IOM study through state action coalitions, working with an initiative of the RWJF and the American Association of Retired Persons called Future of Nursing: Campaign for Action. These action coalitions are working with colleges and universities, state government agencies to include state boards of nursing, nursing organizations, other healthcare professions and their organizations, and funding sources. The state coalitions are developing plans to break down the silos in nursing and health care to ensure that nurses can advance their education to fill advanced nursing roles and be a strong voice in shaping a reformed healthcare delivery system.

WHAT NEW GRADUATES SAY

- I didn't know that politics has anything to do with nursing. Now I see why it's important.
- I just thought "someone" else was responsible for "running" nursing. I guess I am that someone.
- Even nursing has "office politics" like other kinds of business.

CHAPTER CHECKLIST

Power was once a taboo issue in nursing. The exercise of power in nursing conflicted sharply with the historical feminine stereotypes that surrounded nursing. The evolving social and political status of women has also opened nursing to the exercise of power. Power is essential to the effective implementation of both the clinical and the managerial roles of nurses.

- History
- Into the twenty-first century
- Policy, power, and activisim
- Focus on power
- Empowerment
  - Sharing power
- Personal power strategies
  - Strategies for developing a powerful image

  - Make a commitment to nursing as a career
  - Value continuing nursing education
- Communication skills
- Networking
- Mentoring
- Goal-setting
- Developing expertise
- High visibility
- Exercising power and influence in the workplace and other organizations
  - Collegiality and collaboration
  - An empowering attitude
  - Developing coalitions
  - Negotiating
  - Taking political action to influence policy

TIPS FOR USING INFLUENCE

- Become an active member of selected nursing organizations, especially one's state nurses' association and a specialty organization (e.g., special role organization or clinical specialty organization).
- Remember that "power" is not a dirty word.
- Develop a powerful personal/professional self-image.

- Invest in your nursing career by continuing your education.
- Make nursing your career, not just a job.
- Develop networking skills.
- Be visible and competent in the organizations in which you work and network.

REFERENCES

American Association of Colleges of Nursing. (2006, October). *The essentials of doctoral education for advanced nursing practice.* Retrieved from, www.aacn.nche.edu/dnp/Essentials.pdf.

American Association of Colleges of Nursing. (2008, October). *The essentials of baccalaureate education for professional nursing practice.* Retrieved from, www.aacn.nche.edu/education-resources/BaccEssentials08.pdf.

American Association of Colleges of Nursing. (2011, March). *The essentials of master's education in nursing.* Retrieved from, www.aacn.nche.edu/education-resources/MastersEssentials11.pdf.

American Nurses Association. (2013a). *Nurses currently serving in Congress.* Retrieved from, http://nursingworld.org/mainmenucategories/policy-advocacy/federal/nurses-in-congress.

American Nurses Credentialing Center. (2013). *Program overview.* Retrieved from, www.nursecredentialing.org/Magnet/ProgramOverview.

Ashley, J. A. (1976). *Hospitals, paternalism, and the role of the nurse.* New York: Teachers College Press.

Askoy, D. (2010). "It takes a coalition": Coalition potential and legislative decision making. *Legislative Studies Quarterly, 35*(4), 519–541.

Bowers-Lanier, R. R. (2012). Coalitions: A powerful political strategy. In D. J. Mason, J. K. Leavitt, & M. W. Chaffee (Eds.), *Policy & politics in nursing and health care* (pp. 626–632) (6th ed.). St. Louis: Elsevier/Saunders.

Buerhaus, P. I., DesRoches, C., Applebaum, S., Hess, R., Norman, L. D., & Donelan, K. (2012). Are nurses ready for health care reform? A decade of survey research. *Nursing Economic$, 30,* 318–329.

Chaffee, M. W. (2012a). Communication skills for success in policy and politics. In D. J. Mason, J. K. Leavitt, & M. W. Chaffee (Eds.), *Policy & politics in nursing and health care* (pp. 105–113) (6th ed.). St. Louis: Elsevier/Saunders.

Chaffee, M. W. (2012b). Is there a nurse in the House? The nurses in the United States Congress. In D. J. Mason, J. K. Leavitt, & M. W. Chaffee (Eds.), *Policy & politics in nursing and health care* (pp. 572–578) (6th ed.). St. Louis: Elsevier/Saunders.

Clark, C. M., Landrum, E., & Nguyen, D. T. (2010). Development and description of the Organizational Civility Scale (OCS). *The Journal of Theory Construction & Testing, 17*(1), 11–17.

Croft, R. K., & Cash, P. A. (2012). Deconstructing contributing factors to bullying and lateral violence in nursing using a postcolonial feminist lens. *Contemporary Nurse, 42*(2), 226–242.

Goldwater, M., & Zusy, M. J. L. (1990). *Prescription for nurses: Effective political action.* St. Louis: Mosby.

Hersey, P., Blanchard, K., & Natemeyer, W. (1979). Situational leadership, perception and impact of power. *Group and Organization Studies, 4,* 418–428.

Institute of Medicine. (2011). *The future of nursing: Leading change and advancing health.* Washington, DC: National Academies Press.

Joint Commission. (2012, January). *Leadership standard clarified to address behaviors that undermine a safety culture.* Retrieved from, www.jointcommission.org/assets/1/6/Leadership_standard_behaviors.pdf.

Leavitt, J. K., Chaffee, M. W., & Vance, C. (2013). Learning the ropes of policy, politics, and advocacy. In D. J. Mason, J. K. Leavitt, & M. W. Chaffee (Eds.), *Policy & politics in nursing and health care* (pp. 19–28) (6th ed.). St. Louis: Elsevier/Saunders.

Leavitt, J. K., Mason, D. J., & Whelan, E. (2012). Political analysis and strategies. In D. J. Mason, J. K. Leavitt, & M. W. Chaffee (Eds.), *Policy & politics in nursing and health care* (pp. 65–78) (6th ed.). St. Louis: Elsevier/Saunders.

Lewenson, S. B. (2012). A historical perspective on policy, politics, and nursing. In D. J. Mason, J. K. Leavitt, & M. W. Chaffee (Eds.), *Policy & politics in nursing and health care* (pp. 12–18) (6th ed.). St. Louis: Elsevier/Saunders.

McNamara, S. A. (2012). Incivility in nursing: Unsafe nurse, unsafe patients. *AORN Journal, 95*(4), 535–540.

Priest, C. (2012). Advocacy in nursing and health care. In D. J. Mason, J. K. Leavitt, & M. W. Chaffee (Eds.), *Policy & politics in nursing and health care* (pp. 31–38) (6th ed.). St. Louis: Elsevier/Saunders.

Roberts, S. J. (1983). Oppressed group behavior: Implications for nursing. *Advances in Nursing Sciences, 5,* 21–30.

Shinn, L. (2012). Current issue in nursing associations. In D. J. Mason, J. K. Leavitt, & M. W. Chaffee (Eds.), *Policy & politics in nursing and health care* (pp. 602–608) (6th ed.). St. Louis: Elsevier/Saunders.

Vessey, J. A., DeMarco, R., & DiFazio, R. (2010). Bullying, harassment, and horizontal violence in the nursing workforce. *Annual Review of Nursing Research, 28*(1), 133–157.

SUGGESTED READINGS

Abood, S. (2007). Influencing health care in the legislative arena. *The Online Journal of Issues in Nursing, 12*(1). Retrieved October 1, 2009, from, www.nursingworld.org/MainMenuCategories/ANAMarketplace/ANAPeriodicals/OJIN/TableofContents/Volume122007/No1Jan07/tpc32_216091.aspx.

American Nurses Association. (2013b). *Policy & advocacy*. Retrieved from, http://nursingworld.org/MainMenuCategories/Policy-Advocacy.

Ashley, J. A. (1980). Power in structured misogyny: Implications for the politics of care. *Advances in Nursing Science, 2*, 3–22.

Buerhaus, P. I., Ulrich, B., Donelan, K., & DesRoches, C. (2008). Registered nurses' perspectives on health care and the 2008 presidential election. *Nursing Economic$, 26*, 227–235, 257.

Cohen, S. S., Mason, D. J., Kovner, C., Leavitt, J. K., Pulcini, J., & Sochalski, J. (1996). Stages of nursing political development: Where we've been and where we ought to go. *Nursing Outlook, 44*, 259–266.

Cronenwett, L., Sherwood, G., Barnsteiner, J., Disch, J., Johnson, J., Mitchell, P., et al. (2007). Quality and safety education for nurses. *Nursing Outlook, 55*(3), 122–131.

Cunningham, M. P. (2000). Breaking the mold: The many legacies of nurses in progressive movements. *American Journal of Nursing, 100*(10), 121–136 (passim).

Gebbie, K. M., Wakefield, M., & Kerfoot, K. (2000). Nursing and health policy. *Journal of Nursing Scholarship, 32*, 307–315.

Heim, P., & Goliant, S. K. (2005). *Hardball for women: Winning at the game of business*. Los Angeles: Plume Books.

Kelly, K. (2007). From apathy to savvy to activism: Becoming a politically active nurse. *American Nurse Today, 2*(8), 55–56.

Kritek, P. B. (2002). *Negotiating at an uneven table: A practical approach to working with differences and diversity* (2nd ed.). San Francisco: Jossey-Bass.

Mason, D. J., Leavitt, J. K., & Chaffee, M. W. (2012). *Policy & politics in nursing and health care* (6th ed.). St. Louis: Elsevier/Saunders.

Newhouse, R. P., Weiner, J. P., Stanik-Hull, J., White, K. M., Johantgen, M., Steinwachs, D., et al. (2012). Policy implications for optimizing advanced practice registered nurse use nationally. *Policy, Politics & Nursing Practice, 13*(2), 81–89.

QSEN Institute. (n.d.). *Competencies*. Retrieved from: http://qsen.org/competencies/.

PART 2

Managing Resources

11

Caring, Communicating, and Managing with Technology

Janis B. Smith, Ashley Sediqzad, Jana Wheeler

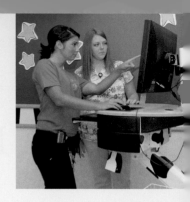

This chapter describes current technology that allows nurses to effectively and efficiently use data gathered at the point of care. It discusses nurses as knowledge workers who use biomedical and information technology to care for patients. It includes sections on biomedical, information, and knowledge technology with subsections that discuss informatics competencies, information systems hardware, the science of informatics, and patient care safety and quality. Nurses build knowledge for practice by comparing and contrasting not only current patient data with previous data for the same patient but also data across patients with the same diagnosis. Information tools and skills are essential for these decision-making processes now and in the future.

LEARNING OUTCOMES

- Articulate the role of technologies in patient safety.
- Describe the core components of informatics: data, information, and knowledge.
- Analyze three types of technology for capturing data at the point of care.
- Discuss decision support systems and their impact on patient care.
- Explore the issues of patient safety, ethics, and information security and privacy within information technology.

KEY TERMS

bar-code technology
biomedical technology
clinical decision support
clinical decision support systems
communication technology
computerized provider order
   entry (CPOE)
data

database
electronic health record (EHR)
electronic medical record (EMR)
informatics
information
information technology
knowledge technology
knowledge worker

meaningful use (MU)
QSEN: Quality and Safety
   Education for Nurses
smart card
speech recognition (SR)
telehealth

THE CHALLENGE

Janis B. Smith, RN, DNP
Senior Director, Clinical Informatics & Professional Practice
Children's Mercy Hospitals and Clinics, Kansas City, Missouri

The nursing, pharmacy, and information systems teams in our hospital are collaborating bar-code medication administration (BCMA) documentation. Our organization has had computerized patient order entry (CPOE) and electronic medication administration documentation for more than 2 years. In addition, we have sophisticated pharmacy technology in place to safeguard medication preparation and dispensing. BCMA should "close the loop" on medication safety by providing a double check of the five rights of medication administration at the point nurses actually give patients their ordered

medications. An important consideration, as we prepare, is to determine the best hardware option for our organization. Our team has several questions to consider:

1. What evidence exists in the literature that might inform our hardware selection decisions?
2. Are BCMA work-arounds associated with a particular type of hardware more than another?
3. Are available technologies equally reliable and easy to use?
4. How important is mobility for nurses? Does mobility trump reliability?

What do you think you would do if you were this nurse?

INTRODUCTION

Technology surrounds us! Intravenous pumps are "smart," biomedical monitoring is no longer exclusively an intensive care practice, and computers are used at the bank, at the grocery checkout, in our cars, and in almost every other aspect of daily living, including the provision of health care. Health care is both a technology and an information intensive business; therefore the success of nurses using biomedical technology, information technology (IT), and knowledge technology will contribute to their personal and professional development and career achievement.

Although information technology abounds in the nursing workplace, students and nurses may not perceive that they are receiving sufficient education about its application in health care, though they report an overall positive attitude toward technology. The Quality and Safety Education for Nurses (QSEN) project identified informatics competency as a necessary component of the knowledge, skills, and attitudes necessary to continuously improve the quality and safety of health care (Cronenwett et al., 2009). Nurses will likely be able to use information and technology to communicate, manage knowledge, mitigate error, and support decision making (AACN, 2012).

The TIGER Initiative, an acronym for **T**echnology **I**nformatics **G**uiding **E**ducation **R**eform, was formed in 2004 to bring together nursing stakeholders to develop a shared vision, strategies, and specific actions for improving nursing practice, education, and the delivery of patient care through the use of health information technology.

The TIGER Informatics Competencies Collaborative (TICC) Team was formed to develop informatics recommendations for all practicing nurses and graduating nursing students. The Team created the TIGER Nursing Informatics Competencies Model, which has three parts:

1. Basic computer competencies
2. Information literacy
3. Information management

Details of each can be found at The Tiger Initiative (2010): *www.tigersummit.com/uploads/3.Tiger.Report_ Competencies_final.pdf*.

In the hospital of the future, technology will be the foundation of patient care planning, organization, and delivery (Parker, 2005). Many leaders in health care see technology as a means to facilitate decision making, improve efficacy and efficiency, enhance patient safety and quality, and decrease healthcare costs (Ball, Weaver, & Abbot, 2003; Institute of Medicine [IOM], 2000, 2001, 2004, 2011). If appropriately implemented and fully integrated, technology has the potential to improve the practice environment for nurses, as well as for patients and their families. However, we are also cautioned by patient safety and quality experts that technology is not a panacea (IOM, 2004, 2011).

Good decision making for patient care requires good information. Nurses are **knowledge workers,** who need **data** and **information** to provide effective and efficient patient care. Knowledge work is not routine or repetitive but, instead, requires considerable cognitive activity and critical thinking (Drucker, 1993). Data and information must be accurate, reliable, and presented in an actionable form. Technology can facilitate and extend nurses' decision-making abilities and support nurses in the following areas: (1) storing clinical data, (2) translating clinical data into information, (3) linking clinical data and domain knowledge, and (4) aggregating clinical data (Snyder-Halpern, Corcoran-Perry, & Narayan, 2001).

TYPES OF TECHNOLOGIES

As nurses, we commonly use and manage three types of technologies: biomedical technology, information technology, and knowledge technology. **Biomedical technology** involves the use of equipment in the clinical setting for diagnosis, physiologic monitoring, testing, or administering therapies to patients. **Information technology** entails recording, processing, and using data and information for the purpose of delivering and documenting patient care. **Knowledge technology** is the use of expert systems to assist clinicians to make decisions about patient care. In nursing, these systems are designed to mimic the reasoning of nurse experts in making patient care decisions.

Biomedical Technology

Biomedical technology is used for (1) physiologic monitoring, (2) diagnostic testing, (3) intravenous fluid and medication dispensing and administration, and (4) therapeutic treatments.

Physiologic Monitoring

Physiologic monitoring systems measure heart rate, blood pressure, and other vital signs. They also monitor cardiac rhythm; measure and record central venous, pulmonary wedge, intracranial, and intra-abdominal pressures; and analyze oxygen and carbon dioxide levels in the blood.

Data about adverse events in hospitalized patients indicate that a majority of physiologic abnormalities are not detected early enough to prevent the event, even when some of the abnormalities are present for hours before the event occurs (Considine & Botti, 2004; Akre et al., 2010). Patient surveillance systems are designed to provide early warning of a possible impending adverse event. One example is a system that provides wireless monitoring of heart rate, respiratory rate, and attempts by a patient at risk for falling to get out of bed unassisted; this monitoring is via a mattress coverlet and bedside monitor.

Innovative technology permits physiologic monitoring and patient surveillance by expert clinicians who may be distant from the patient. The remote or virtual intensive care unit (vICU) is staffed by a dedicated team of experienced critical care nurses, physicians, and pharmacists who use state-of-the-art technology to leverage their expertise and knowledge over a large group of patients in multiple intensive care units (Breslow, 2007; Myers & Reed, 2008).

Intracranial pressure (ICP) monitoring systems monitor the cranial pressure in critically ill patients with closed head injuries or postoperative craniotomy patients. The ICP, along with the mean arterial blood pressure, can be used to calculate perfusion pressure. This allows assessment and early therapy as changes occur. When the ICP exceeds a set pressure, some systems allow ventricular drainage. Similarly, monitoring pressure within the bladder has recently been demonstrated to accurately detect intra-abdominal hypertension while measures of maximal and mean intra-abdominal pressures and abdominal perfusion pressure are made. Intra-abdominal hypertension occurs with abdominal compartment syndrome and other acute abdominal illnesses and has been demonstrated to be independently associated with mortality in these patients (Malbrain et al., 2005; Vidal et al., 2008).

Continuous dysrhythmia monitors and electrocardiograms (EKGs) provide visual representation of electrical activity in the heart and can be used for surveillance and detection of dysrhythmias and for interpretation and diagnosis of the abnormal rhythm. Although not a new technology, these systems have grown increasingly sophisticated. More important, integration with wireless communication technology permits new approaches to triaging alerts to nurses about cardiac rhythm abnormalities. Voice technology and integrated telemetry and nurse paging systems have both been demonstrated to close the communication loop and dramatically decrease response time to dysrhythmia alarms (Bonzheim, 2006).

Biomedical devices for physiologic monitoring can be interfaced with clinical information systems. Monitored vital signs and invasive pressure readings are downloaded directly into the patient's electronic medical record, where the nurse confirms their accuracy and affirms the data entry.

Diagnostic Testing

Dysrhythmia systems can also be diagnostic. The computer, after processing and analyzing the EKG, generates a report that is confirmed by a trained professional. EKG tracings can be transmitted over telephone lines from remote sites, such as the patient's home, to the physician's office or clinic. Patients with implantable pacemakers can have their cardiac activity monitored without leaving home.

Other systems for diagnostic testing include blood gas analyzers, pulmonary function systems, and ICP monitors. Contemporary laboratory medicine is virtually all automated. In addition, point-of-care testing devices extend the laboratory's testing capabilities to the patient's bedside or care area. In critical care areas, for example, blood gas, ionized calcium, hemoglobin, and hematocrit values often are measured from unit-based "stat labs." Point-of-care blood glucose monitors can download results of bedside testing into an automated laboratory results system and the patient's electronic record. Results can be communicated quickly and trends analyzed throughout patients' hospital stays and at ongoing ambulatory care visits. Results can calculate the necessary insulin doses based on evidence for tight blood glucose control and evoke electronic orders for administration. This is an example of integrating a diagnostic test result with the appropriate orders-based intervention.

Intravenous Fluid and Medication Administration

Intravenous (IV) fluid and medication distribution and dispensing via automated dispensing cabinets (ADCs) were introduced in the 1980s and are used in a majority of hospitals today. ADCs can decrease the amount of time before a medication is available on patient care units for administration, ensure greater protection of medications (especially controlled substances), and efficiently and accurately capture drug charges. Most importantly, ADCs can reduce the risk of medication errors but only when safeguards are available and used. The Institute for Safe Medication Practices (ISMP) has developed guidelines for safest use of ADCs (ISMP, 2008). The guidelines contain 12

core practices associated with safe ADC use and are available on the ISMP Website *(www.ismp.org/Tools/guidelines/ADC/default.asp)*. Some ADC machines have the ability to communicate in real time within the electronic health record (EHR), allowing the nurse to see all patient information at the point of care. This closes the loop in the medication process by having all members of the care team using one single patient file and source of truth.

IV smart pumps are used to deliver fluids, blood and blood products, and medications either continuously or intermittently at rates between 0.01 and 999 mL per hour. Twenty-first century pumps offer safety features, accuracy, advanced pressure monitoring, ease of use, and versatility. These pumps have rate-dependent pressure detection systems, designed to provide an early alert to IV cannula occlusion with real-time display of the patient-side pressure reading in the system. Smart pumps can be programmed to calculate drug doses and medication infusion rates from an internal database or "drug library," as well as determine the volume and duration of an infusion. Nurses, when programming the smart pump, can receive soft and hard stop alerts to significant programming errors or contradiction based on entered details.

Therapeutic Treatments

Treatments may be administered via implantable infusion pumps that administer medications at a prescribed rate and can be programmed to provide boluses or change doses at set points in time. These pumps are commonly used for hormone regulation, treatment of hypertension, chronic intractable pain, diabetes, venous thrombosis, and cancer chemotherapy.

Therapeutic treatment systems may be used to regulate intake and output, regulate breathing, and assist with the care of the newborn. Intake and output systems are linked to infusion pumps that control arterial pressure, drug therapy, fluid resuscitation, and serum glucose levels. These systems calculate and regulate the IV drip rate.

Increasingly sophisticated mechanical ventilators are used to deliver a prescribed percentage of oxygen and volume of air to the patient's lungs and to provide a set flow rate, inspiratory-to-expiratory time ratio, and various other complex functions with less trauma to lung tissue than was previously possible. Computer-assisted ventilators are electromechanically controlled by a closed-loop feedback system to analyze and control lung volumes and alveolar gases. Ventilators also provide sophisticated, sensitive alarm systems for patient safety.

In the newborn and intensive care nursery, computers monitor the heart and respiratory rates of the babies there. In addition, newborn nursery systems can regulate the temperature of the infant's environment by sensing his or her temperature and the air of the surrounding environment. Alarms can be set to notify the nurse when preset physiologic parameters are exceeded. Computerized systems monitor fetal activity before delivery, linking the EKGs of the mother and baby and the pulse oximetry, blood pressure, and respirations of the mother.

Biomedical technology affects nursing as nurses provide direct care to patients treated with new technologies: monitoring data from new devices, administering therapy with new techniques, and evaluating patients' responses to care and treatment. Nurses must be aware of the latest technologies for monitoring patients' physiologic status, diagnostic testing, drug administration, and therapeutic treatments. Nurses need to identify the data to be collected, the information that might be gained, and the many ways that these data might be used to provide new knowledge. More importantly, nurses must remember that biomedical technology supplements, but does not replace, the skilled observation, assessment, and evaluation of the patient.

Biomedical technology is designed to help keep patients safe and to alert staff of changes in the patient's condition. A Sentinel Event Alert from The Joint Commission (2013a) brought attention to alarm fatigue or alarm desensitization from biomedical technology. The overuse of alarms from infusion pumps, feeding devices, monitors, and ventilators can cause sensory strain. Staff who are overwhelmed by the sheer number of alarms can miss or delay responding, leading to sentinel events or even patient death. Desensitization to the alarms is quickly becoming a national problem (Wood, 2013; Pevtzow, 2013; Harrison, 2013).

Nursing leaders must be aware of how these technologies fit into the delivery of patient care and the strategic plan of the organization in which they work.

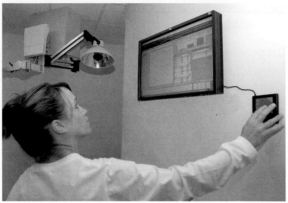

Patient data displayed with computerized systems to provide meaningful information and trends.

They must have a vision for the future and be ready to suggest solutions that will assist nurses across specialties and settings to improve patient care safety and quality.

EXERCISE 11-1

List the types of biomedical technology available for patient care in your organization. List ways that you currently use the data and information gathered by these systems. How do these help you care for patients? Can you think of other ways to use the technology? Can you think of other ways to use the data or information? For example, data from biomedical devices might be sent directly to the electronic health record, negating the need for transcription of a result into the patient's chart. Nurses spend many hours learning to use biomedical devices and to interpret the data gained from them. Have we come to rely too heavily on technology rather than on our own judgment? You might consider using your computer skills to draw a concept map to illustrate the relationships between the types of biomedical, diagnostic, therapeutic, and information technologies available in healthcare organizations you have worked in.

Information Technology

Health care is an information-intensive and knowledge-intensive enterprise. Information technology can help healthcare providers acquire, manage, analyze, and disseminate both information and knowledge. Health care in the twenty-first century should be safe, effective, patient-centered, timely, efficient, and equitable (IOM, 2001). Comprehensive data on patients' conditions, treatments, and outcomes are at the foundation of such care (Stead & Lin, 2009).

Computers offer the advantage of storing, organizing, retrieving, and communicating digital data with accuracy and speed. Patient care data can be entered once, stored in a database, and then quickly and accurately retrieved many times and in many combinations by healthcare providers and others. A database is a collection of data elements organized and stored together. Data processing is the structuring, organizing, and presenting of data for interpretation as information. For example, vital signs for one patient can be entered into the computer and communicated on a graph; many patients' blood pressure measurements can be compared with the number of doses of anti-hypertension medication. Vital signs for male patients between the ages of 40 and 50 years can be correlated and used to show relationships with age, ethnicity, weight, presence of co-morbid conditions, and so on.

Humans process data continuously, but in an analog form. Computers process data in a digital form, process data faster and more accurately than humans,

and provide a method of storage so that data can be retrieved as needed. The Theory Box provides key concepts of information processing, and Box 11-1 describes the development of information management skills from novice to expert.

BOX 11-1   DEVELOPMENT OF INFORMATION MANAGEMENT SKILLS: NOVICE TO EXPERT PRACTICE

Novice nurses focus on learning what data to collect, the process of collecting and documenting the data, and how to use this information. They learn what clinical applications are available for use and how to use them. Computer and informatics skills focus on applying concrete concepts.

As nurses grow in expertise, they look for patterns in the data and information. They aggregate data across patient populations to look for similarities and differences in response to interventions. Expert nurses integrate theoretical knowledge with practical knowledge gained from experience.

Expert nurses know the value of personal professional reflection on knowledge and synthesize and evaluate information for discovery and decision making.

THEORY BOX

Information Theory

KEY CONTRIBUTOR	KEY IDEAS	APPLICATION TO PRACTICE
Locsin (2005): *Technological Competency as Caring in Nursing: A Model for Practice*	The realities of continuously advancing technologies in health care necessitate that contemporary nursing practice incorporates both the concepts of technology and caring. Nurses practice in environments requiring technological expertise. Technology has transformed the practice of nursing with the coexistence of caring and technology. Competency with technology is demonstrated by registered nurses in skillful, intentional, deliberate, and authentic activities which engage technology in caring for patients and families. Nurses can build a strong connection with patients and families through the competent use of technology.	Nurses at all stages of professional development need to acquire the skills to use technology competently. When nurses are adept in the use of technology they engage it to care for patients. For example, the best online resources for patient/family education can be linked to clinical information systems and accessed when the ideal teaching moment is identified. Nurses can influence patients and families to engage in their own care. Providing patients an electronic copy of their record or making patients aware of a patient portal, enrolling them with a portal account, and teaching them how to use it, are steps toward strengthening patient access to their health information and engagement in their own health care.

Locsin, R.C. (2005). *Technological competency as caring in nursing: A model for practice.* Indianapolis, IN: Sigma Theta Tau International.

Knowledge Technology

Knowledge technology consists of systems that generate or process knowledge and provide clinical decision support (CDS). Defined broadly, CDS is a clinical computer system, computer application, or process that helps health professionals make clinical decisions to enhance patient care. The clinical knowledge embedded in computer applications or work processes can range from simple facts and relationships to best practices for managing patients with specific disease states, new medical knowledge from clinical research, and other types of information. Among the most common forms of CDS are drug-dosing calculators—computer-based programs that calculate appropriate doses of medications after a clinician inputs key data (e.g., patient weight or the level of serum creatinine). These calculators are especially useful in managing the administration of medications with a narrow therapeutic index. Allergy alerts, dose range checking, drug-drug interaction, and duplicate order checking are other common applications of CDS.

Clinical (or diagnostic) decision support systems (CDSSs) are interactive computer programs designed to assist health professionals with decision-making tasks by mimicking the inductive or deductive reasoning of a human expert. The basic components of a CDSS include a knowledge base and an *inferencing mechanism* (usually a set of rules derived from the experts and evidence-based practice). The knowledge base contains the knowledge that an expert nurse would apply to data entered about a patient and information to solve a problem. The inference engine controls the application of the knowledge by providing the logic and rules for its use with data from a specific patient.

Box 11-2 illustrates the use of an expert system for determining the maximum dose of pain medication that can safely be given to a patient after an invasive procedure. The knowledge base contains eight items that are to be considered when giving the maximum dose. The inference engine controls the use of the knowledge base by applying logic that an expert nurse would use in making the decision to give the maximum dose. This decision frame states that if pain is severe (A) or a painful procedure is planned (B), and there is an order for pain medication (C) and the time since surgery is less than 48 hours (H) and the time since the last dose is greater than 3 hours (G), and there are no contraindications to the medication (D) or history of allergy (E) or contraindication to the maximum dose (F), then the "decision" would be to

---

BOX 11-2 **EXPERT DECISION FRAME FOR "GIVE MAXIMUM DOSE OF PAIN MEDICATION"**

The Knowledge Base
A. Pain score
B. Invasive procedure scheduled
C. Opiate analgesic ordered
D. Contraindications to the medication
E. History of allergic reaction to opiate analgesics
F. Contraindication to maximum dose of opiate analgesic
G. Time since last dose of opiate analgesic administered
H. Time since surgical procedure

The Inference Engine
Give the maximum dose of pain medication if (A or B) and (C and H <48 hours and G >3 hours) and not (D or E or F)
or:
(C and H <48 hours and G >4 hours) and not (D or E or F)

---

give the dose of pain medication. The rules are those that expert nurses would apply in making the decision to give pain medication.

EXERCISE 11-2
Mr. Jones's heart rate is 54 beats per minute. Tony is about to give Mr. Jones his scheduled atenolol dose. When Tony scans Mr. Jones's armband and the medication bar codes, the computer warns him that atenolol should not be given to a patient with a heart rate less than 60 beats per minute. What should Tony do?

One of the benefits of CDSSs is that they permit the novice nurse to advantage the decision-making expertise and judgment of an expert. Nursing leaders must be aware of the usefulness of decision support systems for nursing, as the development of CDS applicable to nursing practices is just beginning (IOM, 2011). Clinical experts are needed to develop both the knowledge in the database and the logic used to develop the rules for its application to a particular patient in a particular circumstance. Advanced critical thinking skills are needed to develop logic and rules. When these are in place, patient care quality can be standardized and improved.

A critical use of information has been in the area of the medication management process. These processes are high-risk and high-volume activities (Malashock, Smith-Shull, & Gould, 2004). New applications provide support for all aspects of the process, thereby improving safety and efficiency (Box 11-3).

BOX 11-3   INFORMATION TECHNOLOGY: TRENDS IN THE MEDICATION MANAGEMENT PROCESS

Various information technology (IT) devices and software applications are designed to support the medication management process. Each has unique functionality and targets a specific phase of the medication process.

Computerized Provider Order Entry (CPOE)

- Decision support and clinical warnings (e.g., alerts the provider of allergies, pertinent laboratory data, drug-drug and drug-food interactions)
- Automatic dose calculation
- Link to up-to-date drug reference material
- Automatic order notification
- Standardized formulary-compliant order sets
- Legible, accurate, and complete medication orders
- Decreased variations in practice
- Less time clarifying orders
- Fewer verbal orders
- No manual transcription errors

Electronic Medication Administration Record (e-MAR)

- Integration with clinical documentation (in the electronic record)
- Link to up-to-date drug reference material
- Automatic reminders and alarms for approaching or missed medication administration times
- Prompts for associated tasks or additional documentation requirements
- Alert when cumulative dosing exceeds maximum
- Legible record
- Accessible to multiple users
- Improved accuracy of pharmacokinetic monitoring (administration times are reliable)
- Record matches the pharmacy profile
- Generated reports to track medication errors with visibility of near misses
- Perpetual interface with pharmacy inventory system
- Increase the accuracy of charge capture (at the time of administration vs. when drug is dispensed)

Bar Coding and Radio Frequency Identification (RFID) Scanning

- Medication documentation captured electronically at the time of administration (populates the e-MAR)

- Five rights verified
- Positive patient identification
- Clinician alerted to discrepancies (e.g., wrong drug, wrong dose, wrong time, wrong patient, expired drug)
- Automatic tracking of medication errors and provides visibility to near misses

"Smart" Infusion Pumps (Medication Infusion Delivery System)

- Reduced need for manual dose/rate calculation
- Institution defined standardized drug library (drugs, concentrations, dosing parameters)
- Software filter prevention of programming errors/programming within pre-established minimum and maximum limits before infusion can begin
- Device infusion parameter limits based on patient type or care area
- Interface with the patient's pharmacy profile with capabilities to program the pump electronically
- User alerts to pump setting errors, wrong channel selection, and mechanical failures
- Electronic notification to pharmacy when fluids/medications need to be dispensed
- Interface with the patient's e-MAR (accurate documentation of administration times and volumes infused)
- Memory functions for settings and alarms with a retrievable log
- Electronic recording of reprogramming and limit override activity

Automated Dispensing Unit/Cabinets

- Secured drug storage
- Controlled user access—biometric identification
- Interface with the pharmacy profile—access restricted until order reviewed
- Quick access once medication order reviewed by pharmacist
- Ability to monitor controlled substance waste and utilization patterns
- Perpetual interface with pharmacy inventory

Pharmacy Automation and Robotics

- Increased accuracy and speed of dispensing

From Bell, M.J. (2005). Nursing information of tomorrow. *Healthcare Informatics, 22*(2), 74-78; Larrabee, S., & Brown, M.M. (2003). Recognizing the institutional benefits of bar-code point-of-care technology. *Joint Commission Journal on Quality and Safety, 29*(7), 345-353.

INFORMATION SYSTEMS

A patient information system can be manual or computerized—in fact, we have collected and recorded information about patients and patient care since the dawn of health care. Computer information systems manage large volumes of data, examine data patterns and trends, solve problems, and answer questions. In other words, computers can help translate data into information. Ideally, data are recorded at the point in the care process where they are gathered and are available to healthcare providers when and where they are needed. This is accomplished, in part, by networking computers both within and among organizations to form larger systems. These networked systems might link inpatient care units and other departments, hospitals, clinics, hospice centers, home health agencies, and/or physician practices. Data from all patient encounters with the healthcare system are stored in a central data repository, where they are accessible to authorized users located anywhere in the world. These provide the potential for automated patient records, which contain health data from birth to death.

Adopting the technology necessary to computerize patient care information systems is complex and must be accomplished in stages. The Healthcare Information and Management Systems Society (HIMSS) has described seven stages of adoption—the seventh of which marks achievement of a fully electronic healthcare record. The seven stages of adoption are listed and described in Table 11-1. About 5.2% of U.S. hospitals have achieved stage 6, 1.2% have achieved stage 7, and less than 10% are at stage 0 (HIMSS Analytics, 2012).

Nurses care for patients in acute care, ambulatory, and community settings, as well as in patients' homes. In all settings, nurses focus not only on managing acute illnesses but also on health promotion, maintenance, and education; care coordination and continuity; and monitoring chronic conditions. Ideally, information systems support the work of nurses in all settings.

Communication networks are used to transmit data entered at one computer and received by others in the network. These networks can reduce the clerical functions of nursing. They can provide patient demographic and census data, results from tests, and lists of medications. Nursing policies and procedures can be linked to the network and accessed, when needed, at the point of care. Links can be provided between the patient's home, hospital, and/or physician office with computers, handheld technologies, and point-of-care devices. Day-to-day events can be recorded and downloaded into the patient record remotely in community nursing settings or at the point of care in the hospital or clinic.

EXERCISE 11-3

Select a healthcare setting with which you are familiar. What information systems are used? Make a list of the names of these systems and the information they provide. How do they help you in caring for patients or in making management decisions? Think about the communication of data and information among departments. Do the systems communicate with each other? If you do not have computerized systems, think about how data and information are communicated. How might a computer system help you be more efficient?

As an example, assume that an abdominal magnetic resonance imaging (MRI) with contrast has been ordered. In a paper-based system, handwritten

---

TABLE 11-1 ELECTRONIC MEDICAL RECORD ADOPTION MODEL*

US EMR ADOPTION MODEL℠

STAGE	CUMULATIVE CAPABILITIES	2010 Q4	2011 Q4
Stage 7	Complete EMR; CCD transactions to share data; Data warehousing; Data continuity with ED, ambulatory, OP	1.0%	1.2%
Stage 6	Physician documentation (structured templates), fill CDSS (variance & compliance), full R-PACS	3.2%	5.2%
Stage 5	Closed loop medication administration	4.5%	8.4%
Stage 4	CPOE, Clinical Decision Support (clinical protocols)	10.5%	13.2%
Stage 3	Nursing/clinical documentation (flow sheets), CDSS (error checking), PACS available outside Radiology	49.0%	44.9%
Stage 2	CDR, Controlled Medical Vocabulary, CDS, may have Document Imaging; HIE capable	14.6%	12.4%
Stage 1	Ancillaries – Lab, Rad, Pharmacy – All Installed	7.1%	5.7%
Stage 0	All Three Ancillaries Not Installed	10.1%	9.0%
Data from HIMSS Analytics® Database ©2011		N=5.299	N=5.337

*From HIMSS Analytics, Healthcare Information and Management Systems Society. 2012 HIMSS Analytics Report. (2012). *Quality and safety linked to advanced information technology enabled processes.* Retrieved February 12, 2012 from http://www.himssanalytics.org/emram/emram.aspx.

requisitions are sent to nutrition services, pharmacy, and the radiology department. With a computerized system, the MRI is ordered and the requests for dietary changes, bowel preparation medications, and the diagnostic study itself are automatically sent to the appropriate departments. Radiology would compare its schedule openings with the patient's schedule and automatically place the date and time for the MRI on the patient's automated plan of care. The images and results of the diagnostic procedure are available online.

Nurses caring for patients in home health care and hospice must complete documentation necessary to meet government and insurance requirements. Computers assist with direct entry of all required data in the correct format. Portable computers are used to download files of the patients to be seen during the day from a main database. During each visit, the computer prompts the nurse for vital signs, assessments, diagnosis, interventions, long-term and short-term goals, and medications based on previous entries in the medical record. Nurses enter any new data, modifications, or nursing information directly. Entries can be transmitted by telephone line to the main computer at the office or downloaded from the device at the end of the day. This action automatically updates the patient record and any verbal order entry records, home visit reports, federally mandated treatment plans, productivity and quality improvement reports, and other documents for review and signature. Portable and wireless computers have made recording patient care information more efficient and have improved personnel productivity and compliance with necessary documentation.

Placing computers or handheld devices "patient-side" permits nurses to enter data once, at the point of care. Documentation of patient assessments and care provided patient-side saves time, gives others more timely access to the data, and decreases the likelihood of forgetting to document vital information. Point-of-care devices and systems that fit with nurses' workflow, personalize patient assessments, and simplify care planning are available. Patient care areas with point-of-care computers have improved the quality of patient care by decreasing errors of omission, providing greater accuracy and completeness of documentation, reducing medication errors, providing more timely responses to patient needs, and improving

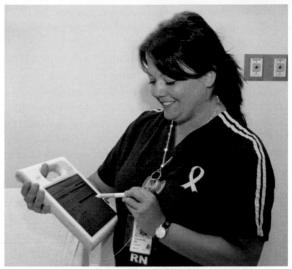

A handheld computer permits point-of-care documentation.

discharge planning and teaching. These systems can eliminate redundant charting and facilitate patient hand-offs from shift to shift or between care areas (Laws & Amato, 2010).

EXERCISE 11-4

Think about the data you gather as you care for a patient through the day. How do you communicate information and knowledge about your patient to others? Does the information system support the way you need this information organized, stored, retrieved, and presented to other healthcare providers? For example, if a patient's pain medication order is about to expire and you want to assess the patient's use and response to the pain medication during the past 24 hours, can the information system generate a graph that compares the time, dose, and pain score for this period? If your assessment is that the medication order needs to be renewed, how do you communicate that message to the prescriber?

Meaningful Use

The potential of electronic health records (EHRs) to benefit caregivers, patients, and their families depends on how they are used. Meaningful use (MU) is the set of standards defined by the Medicare and Medicaid Electronic Health Records (EHR) Incentive Programs that governs the use of EHRs and allows eligible providers and hospitals to earn incentive payments by meeting specific criteria. The goal of MU is to promote the implementation and effective use of EHRs to improve health care in the United States (Smith & Burnes Bolton, 2013). The benefits of the meaningful use of EHRs include:

- *Complete and accurate information.* With EHRs, care providers have the information they need to provide the best possible care.
- *Better access to information.* EHRs facilitate greater access to the information needed to diagnose and treat health problems earlier and improve health outcomes for patients. EHRs allow information to be shared among offices, hospitals, and across health systems, which facilitates care coordination.
- *Patient empowerment.* EHRs can empower patients and families to take a more active role in their health. They can receive electronic copies of their healthcare records and share their health information securely over the Internet with their families and care providers.

In order to achieve MU, eligible providers and hospitals must adopt an EHR that has the technical capabilities to ensure the systems are capable of performing defined required functions. Thereafter, providers and hospitals must use the technology to achieve specific objectives.

The MU objectives and measures evolve over 5 years: Stage 1 is capturing and sharing data via EHRs. Stage 2 is advancing clinical processes with EHRs. Stage 3 is requiring that providers and hospitals use EHRs to demonstrate improved patient outcomes (Table 11-2).

Information Systems Quality and Accreditation

Quality management and measuring patient care efficiency, effectiveness, and outcomes are necessary for accreditation and licensing of healthcare organizations. This is demonstrated by documentation of patient care processes and outcomes. The plan of care outlines what patient care needs to occur, orders are entered to prescribe needed care, and documentation confirms that the care was provided. Computers can capture and aggregate data to demonstrate both the processes of care and the patient outcomes achieved.

The Joint Commission (TJC), an independent, not-for-profit organization, evaluates and provides accreditation and certification to more than 15,000 healthcare organizations and programs in the United States. Accreditation and certification by TJC are recognized nationwide as symbols of an organization's commitment to meeting performance standards focused on improving the quality and safety of patient care.

The *Comprehensive Accreditation Manual for Hospitals* and the manuals for other healthcare programs include a chapter of standards for information management. Planning for information management is the initial focus of the chapter, since a well-planned system meets the internal and external information needs of an organization with efficiency and accuracy. The goals of effective information management are to obtain, manage, and use information to improve patient care processes and patient outcomes, as well as to improve other organizational processes. Planning is also necessary to provide care continuity should an organization's information systems be disrupted or fail. Planning also is necessary to ensure privacy, security, confidentiality, and integrity of data and information.

TABLE 11-2   STAGES OF MEANINGFUL USE

STAGE 1 CRITERIA FOCUS ON:	STAGE 2 CRITERIA FOCUS ON:	STAGE 3 CRITERIA FOCUS ON:
Electronically capturing health information in a standardized format	More rigorous health information exchange (HIE)	Improving quality, safety, and efficiency, leading to improved health outcomes
Using that information to track key clinical conditions	Increased requirements for e-prescribing and incorporating lab results	Decision support for national high-priority conditions
Communicating that information for care coordination processes	Electronic transmission of patient care summaries across multiple settings	Patient access to self-management tools
Initiating the reporting of clinical quality measures and public health information	More patient-controlled data	Access to comprehensive patient data through patient-centered HIE
Using information to engage patients and their families in their care		Improving population health

Source: www.healthit.gov/policy-researchers-implementers/meaningful-use. Nursing leaders can learn more about MU at http://healthit.gov.

In the 2013 TJC accreditation manual chapter "The Record of Care, Treatment and Services," standards and recommendations for the components of a complete medical record are provided. It details documentation requirements that include accuracy, authentication, and thorough, timely documentation. Other standards address the requirements for auditing and retaining records (TJC, 2013b).

All nurses, including nurse leaders, share responsibility to ensure that cost-effective, high-quality patient care is provided. Nursing administrative databases, containing both clinical and management data, support decision making for these purposes. Administrative databases assist in the development of the organization's information infrastructure, which ultimately allows for links between management decisions (e.g., staffing or nurse/patient ratios), costs, and clinical outcomes.

Selection of a clinical information system and software partner may be one of the most important decisions of a chief nursing officer and the nursing leadership team. Nurse leaders and direct care nurses must be members of the selection team, participate actively, and have a voice in the selection decision. Remember, nurses are knowledge workers who require data, information, and knowledge to deliver effective patient care. The information system must make sense to the people who use it and fit effectively with the processes for providing patient care. Box 11-4 identifies key elements of an ideal clinical information system that can guide the decision making necessary for selecting or developing health information software. Before making a selection, visit organizations already using the software to obtain practical and strategic information. Discussions at site visits include both the utility and performance of the software and the customer service and responsiveness of the vendor.

Information Systems Hardware

Placing the power of computers for both entering and retrieving data at the point of patient care is a major thrust in the move toward increased adoption of clinical information systems. Many hospitals and clinics are using a number of computing devices in the clinical setting—desktop, laptop, or, increasingly, tablet computers; and smart phones—as we learn about both the possibilities and limitations of different hardware solutions. Theoretically, nurses may work best with robust mobile technology. Installing computers on mobile carts, also known as *computers on wheels* or *COWs,* may increase work efficiency and save time. However, if the cart is cumbersome to move around or if concern about infection risk is associated with moving the cart from one room to another, some organizations favor keeping one cart stationed in each patient care room or installing hardwired bedside computers.

Wireless Communication

Wireless (WL) communication is an extension of an existing wired network environment and uses radio-based systems to transmit data signals through the air without any physical connections. Telemetry is a clinical use of WL communication. Nurses can communicate with other healthcare team members, departments, and offices and with patients through the use of pagers, smart phones, and wireless computers. Nurses can send and receive e-mail, clinical data, and other text messages. The Internet can be accessed on these devices.

WL systems are used by emergency medical personnel to request authorization for the treatments or drugs needed in emergency situations. Laboratories use WL technology to transmit laboratory results to physicians; patients awaiting organ transplants are provided with WL pagers so that they can be notified if a donor is found; and parents of critically ill

---

BOX 11-4   ELEMENTS OF THE IDEAL HOSPITAL INFORMATION SYSTEM

- Data are standardized and use structured terminology.
- The system is reliable—minimal scheduled or unscheduled downtime.
- Applications are integrated across the system.
- Data are collected at the point of care.
- The database is complete, accurate, and easy to query.
- The infrastructure is interconnected and supports accessibility.
- Data are gathered by instrumentation whenever possible so that only minimal data entry is necessary.
- The system has a rapid response time.
- The system is intuitive and reflective of patient care delivery models.
- The location facilitates functionality, security, and support.
- Screen displays can be configured by user preference.
- The system supports outcomes and an evidence-based approach to care delivery.

children carry WL pagers when they are away from a phone. Visiting nurses using a home monitoring system employ WL technology to enter vital signs and other patient-related information. Inpatient nurses can send messages to the admissions department when a patient is being transferred to another unit without having to wait for someone to answer the telephone. Increasingly, whole hospitals use WL technology to deploy their information systems to the point of patient care.

New hardware for patient information systems has both advantages and disadvantages. Portable devices, such as smart phones and tablet computers, are less expensive than placing a stationary computer in each patient room. In addition, each caregiver on a shift can be equipped with a device. Portable, hand-held devices allow access to information at the point of care, both for retrieval of information and entry of patient data. Disadvantages stem from their size and portability. They have a small display screen, limiting the amount of data that can be viewed on the screen and the size of the font. Portable devices can also be put down and forgotten, dropped and broken, and targeted for theft. Small devices require a convenient and adequate place to store the devices when they are not in use and to charge their batteries, when needed. Finally, WL technology may not operate with the speed necessary to advantage busy healthcare workers in fast-paced environments.

Management of the hardware designed to advantage clinical information system software is important. Nursing leaders must make knowledgeable decisions about the type of hardware to use, the education needed to use it effectively, and the proper care and maintenance of the equipment. Important questions to ask include the following: What data and information do we need to gather? When and where should it be gathered? How difficult is the equipment to use? Has the hardware been tested sufficiently to ensure purchase of a dependable product?

COMMUNICATION TECHNOLOGY

Communication technology is an extension of WL technology that enables hands-free communication among mobile hospital workers. Hospital staff members wear a pendant-like badge around their neck and, by simply pressing a button on the badge, can be connected to the person with whom they wish to speak by stating the name or function of the person.

Voice technology may also enhance the use of computer systems in the future. **Speech recognition (SR)** is also known as *computer speech recognition.* The term *voice recognition* may also be used to refer to speech recognition but is less accurate. SR converts spoken words to machine-readable input. SR applications in everyday life include voice dialing (e.g., "Call home"), call routing (e.g., "I would like to make a collect call"), and simple data entry (e.g., stating a credit card or account number). In health care, preparation of structured documents, such as a radiology report, is possible. In all these examples, the computer gathers, processes, interprets, and executes audible signals by comparing the spoken words with a template in the system. If the patterns match, recognition occurs and a command is executed by the computer. This allows untrained personnel or those whose hands are busy to enter data in an SR environment without touching the computer. Voice technology will also allow quadriplegic and other physically challenged individuals to function more efficiently when using the computer. SR systems recognize a large number of words but are still immature. The speaker must use staccato-like speech, pausing between each clearly spoken word; and these systems must be programmed for each user so that the system recognizes the user's voice patterns.

Automating the healthcare delivery process is not an easy task. Patient care processes are often not standardized across settings, and most software vendors cannot customize software for each organization. Some current versions of the electronic patient record have merely automated the existing schema of the chart rather than considering how computers could permit data to be viewed or used differently from manual methods. The complexity of decision making about health information systems software and hardware has given rise to the science of informatics.

INFORMATICS

Informatics is "a science that combines a domain science, computer science, information science, and cognitive science" (Hunter, 2001, p. 180). The term *nursing informatics* was probably first used and defined by Scholes and Barber in 1980 in their address to the International Medical Informatics

Association (IMIA) at the conference that year in Tokyo. They defined nursing informatics as "the application of computer technology to all fields of nursing—nursing services, nurse education, and nursing research" (p. 73).

Nursing informatics is now a thriving subspecialty of nursing that combines nursing knowledge and skills with computer expertise. Like any knowledge-intensive profession, nursing is greatly affected by the explosive growth of both scientific advances and technology. Nurse informatics specialists manage and communicate nursing data and information to improve decision making by consumers, patients, nurses, and other healthcare providers. Nurse informatics specialists formed the American Nursing Informatics Association (ANIA) in the early 1990s to provide networking, education, and information resources that enrich and strengthen the roles of nurses in the field of informatics, including the domains of clinical information, education, and administration decision support. In addition, nursing informatics is represented in the American Medical Informatics Association (AMIA) and the IMIA by working groups that promote the advancement of nursing informatics within the larger interdisciplinary context of health informatics.

The Nursing Informatics Working Group of AMIA defined their practice specialty as "the science and practice (that) integrates nursing, its information and knowledge, with management of information and communication technologies to promote the health of people, families, and communities worldwide" *(www.AMIA.org/programs/working-groups/ nursing-informatics)*.

Many undergraduate and graduate nursing education programs recognize that it is essential to prepare nurses to practice in a technology-rich environment (National League of Nursing [NLN], 2008; Warren & Connors, 2007). Noting the federal initiatives pushing the adoption of electronic health records throughout all healthcare institutions by the year 2014, the NLN stressed that it is imperative that graduates of today's nursing programs know how to use and advantage "informatics tools to ensure safe and quality care" (NLN, 2008, p. 1). Certification as a nurse informatics specialist by the American Nurses Credentialing Center (ANCC) requires specific coursework and specific experience and/or continuing education.

Informatics is interdisciplinary and in its truest form, it focuses on the care of patients rather than on a specific discipline (Hannah & Ball, 2011). Although specific bodies of knowledge exist for each healthcare profession (e.g., nursing, dentistry, dietetics, pharmacy, medicine), they interface at the patient. Working with integrated clinical information systems demands interdisciplinary collaboration at a high level.

PATIENT SAFETY

The patient care environment is complex and prone to errors. Nurses are the healthcare workers who prevent accidents in patient care and create safety daily (IOM, 2004). In addition to physical challenges, resource challenges, and interruptions characteristic of nursing work, nurses are challenged by inconsistencies and breakdowns in care communication. Communication and information difficulties are among the most common nursing workplace challenges and are frustrating and potentially dangerous for patients.

Information technology is identified as an essential tool for advancing patient safety (Malloch, 2007). Nurses, other health professionals, and patients and families rely increasingly on information technology to communicate, manage information, mitigate error potential, and make informed decisions (Bakken et al., 2004; Marin, 2004). Health information technology has the potential to improve—or obstruct—work performance, communication, and documentation (Ash, Berg, & Coiere, 2004). Because nurses play a central role in patient care, the extent to which information technology supports or detracts from nurses' work performance can be expected to affect patient outcomes (Kossman & Scheidenhelm, 2008).

Nurses identified that the highest percentage of their top 10 challenges are related to systems and technology put in place to accomplish patient care (Krichbaum et al., 2007). Nurses spend up to 40% of their workday meeting ever-increasing demands from the systems in which they work to provide patient care (Ebright, Patterson, Chalko, & Render, 2003). Nurses rank new, excessive, or changing forms and documentation systems number 2 among the variables contributing most to complexity compression. Only inadequate staffing ranks higher (Krichbaum et al., 2007).

Documentation to meet organizational, accreditation, insurance, state, and federal requirements, as well as provide information needed by other healthcare providers, imposes a heavy demand on nurses' time. Documentation requirements lessen nursing time for direct contact with patients and families. Westbrook, Duffield, Li, and Creswick (2011) reported that nurses spent approximately 37% of their time with patients. Reduced nursing availability affects patient safety and care quality. Nurses in acute care settings spend, on average, one quarter to one half of their time documenting patient care (Ammenwerth, Mansmann, Iller, & Eichstadter, 2003; Frankel, Cowie, & Daley, 2003; Korst, Eusebio-Angeja, Chamorro, Aydin, & Gregory, 2003; Kossman & Scheidenhelm, 2008). Finishing documentation is one reason nurses do not complete work on time—it is a form of mandatory overtime (Trossman, 2001).

IMPACT OF CLINICAL INFORMATION SYSTEMS

Clinical information systems that provide access to patient information and provide clinical decision support can reduce errors and inefficiencies (Ball, Weaver, & Abbot, 2003). Patient information in an electronic clinical information system is organized and legible. Nurses see all of the medications prescribed for a patient in one location; doses are written clearly, and drug names are spelled correctly. The patient problem list shows acute and chronic health conditions and complete allergy information. Abnormal findings are highlighted and can be graphed and compared with interventions. Alerts signal nurses that critical information has been entered in the electronic record. For example, critical test results signal the need for provider notification and intervention. An alert that a patient is at risk for falling signals the need for additional monitoring and interventions to ensure safety. Nursing reminders to perform pressure area care reduce the incidence of this important hospital acquired condition.

When standards for care are not being followed, clinical information systems can generate alerts, reminders, or suggestions. Rules remind care providers to perform required care. When documentation is not recorded for medication administration, IV tubing change, or wound care, for example, the system generates a reminder based on rules that have been agreed to by providers. Evidence-based practices are integrated in the process of care as providers are guided to select the most appropriate course of action.

Errors are prevented by eliminating problems stemming from illegible handwriting. Computerized order entry also eliminates the nursing time required for clarification of illegible and incomplete orders. Transcription is no longer required, orders are sent directly to the performing department, and patient care needs are communicated more clearly and quickly to all clinicians. Medication dosing, drug allergy, and drug-drug interaction checking all have significant impact on patient safety (Mekhjian et al., 2002).

Impact on Communication

Integrated information systems allow all members of the interdisciplinary patient care team to see pertinent patient information and plan care based on what is currently happening and what should occur in the future. Everyone knows who is responsible for the patient and who needs to communicate about the patient's care. Clinical information systems provide multiple users with simultaneous, real-time access to patient records. Patient care hand-offs are safer when information is not unavailable or lost in the process. Patient care processes are facilitated, and treatment delays are decreased. The patient's care experience is also improved by decreasing redundant data collection by multiple members of the care team.

Impact on Patient Care Documentation

Nurses spend much time documenting patient care activities. Clinical documentation in an electronic information system improves access to patient information and increases documentation efficiency and organization (Kossman & Scheidenhelm, 2008). In an intensive care setting, automatic downloads of patient vital signs, ventilator settings, and IV intake provide efficiency and are timesaving for nurses (Frankel, Cowie, & Daley, 2003). Redundant documentation is eliminated with an integrated clinical information system, and completeness of nursing documentation has increased with some systems (Larrabee et al., 2001).

Impact on Medication Administration Processes

The *Quantros MEDMARX* database includes annual records of medication errors. In 2006, approximately 25% of errors involved some aspect of computer

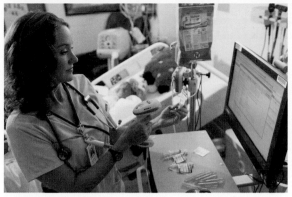

Bar code medication administration "closes the loop" on medication safety by providing a double-check of the five rights of medication administration at the point nurses actually give patients their ordered medications.

technology as at least one cause of the error. Most errors related to technology involved mislabeled bar codes on medications, mistakes at order entry because of confusing computer screens, or other problems with information management (TJC, 2008). Errors also were related to dispensing devices and human factors, such as failure to scan bar codes or overrides of bar-code warnings.

Computerized provider order entry (CPOE) can be an effective mechanism for improving patient safety. Unintended consequences however can occur, and new kinds of errors can be detected (Ash et al., 2007). Safeguards built into clinical information systems can avert an error, but awareness of the potential for new issues is vital.

Automated medication administration systems that use bar-code technology can ensure that the right patient gets the right medication, in the correct dose, by the appropriate route, and at the specified time. However, this new information technology must not impede nurses' care of patients. Faced with urgent or emergent situations with patients, technical difficulties, or poor work re-design, unorthodox and potentially unsafe work-arounds are sometimes invented when the medication administration system is not usable and obstructs patient care (Koppel, Wetterneck, Telles, & Karsh, 2008).

Closed-loop electronic prescribing, dispensing, and bar-code patient identification systems reduce prescribing errors and medication adverse events and increase confirmation of patient identity before administration. However, time spent on medication-related tasks increases for physicians, pharmacists, and nurses (Franklin, O'Grady, Donyai, Jacklin, & Barber, 2007).

SAFELY IMPLEMENTING HEALTH INFORMATION TECHNOLOGY

Despite the promise of positive impact from clinical information systems, success is not a guarantee. Remaining alert to its limitations and risks is crucial, because new technology and increasing automation make work less transparent and create opportunities for new types of errors (Reason, 2002). According to McBride (2005):

> Information technology is not a panacea, and will not fulfill its promise unless it is harnessed in support of foundational values. That is why every nurse cannot afford to be unconnected to this transformation, but must take an active role in ensuring that IT is used in service to our profession's values. After all, nurses are knowledge workers. (p. 188)

The Joint Commission warns that as health information technology is adopted, users must be mindful of the safety risks and preventable adverse events that implementation can create (TJC, 2008). The report notes that any form of technology can adversely affect patient care safety and quality if it is designed or implemented improperly. TJC suggests 13 actions, which are presented in Table 11-3.

A clinical information system's success or failure is related to the system's "fit" with the organizational culture, the information needs of its users, and users' work processes and practices (Kaplan, 2001; Kaplan & Harris-Salamone, 2009). Duke University Medical Center informatics experts wrote that they had learned in 1993 that "ongoing planning, adjusting, fitting the technology to the work, and adapting policy formation were more important than the technology itself" (Stead et al., 1993, p. 225). The same is true today!

Relying too heavily on health information technology for communication can reduce teamwork and may negatively affect patient safety and care quality (Ash et al., 2004). Although improved access and better-organized information can eliminate nurses' locating information for other nurses and physicians,

TABLE 11-3   THE JOINT COMMISSION RECOMMENDATIONS FOR SAFELY IMPLEMENTING HEALTH INFORMATION TECHNOLOGY

	SUGGESTED ACTION
1	Examine work processes and procedures for risks and inefficiencies. Resolve problems identified before technology implementation. Involve representatives of all disciplines—clinical, clerical, and technical—in the examination and resolution of issues.
2	Involve clinicians and staff who will use or be affected by the technology, along with information technology (IT) staff with strong clinical backgrounds, in the planning, selection, design, reassessment, and ongoing quality improvement of technology. Involve pharmacists in planning and implementing any technology that involves medication.
3	Assess your organization's technology needs. Require IT staff to interact with users outside their own facility to learn about real-world capabilities of potential systems from various vendors; conduct field trips; look at integrated systems to minimize the need for interfaces.
4	Continuously monitor for problems during the introduction of new technology and address issues as quickly as possible to avoid workarounds and errors. Consider an emergent issues desk staffed with project experts and champions to help rapidly resolve problems. Use interdisciplinary problem solving to improve system quality and provide vendor feedback.
5	Establish training programs for all clinical and operations staff, designed appropriately for each group and focused on how the technology will benefit staff and patients. Do not allow long delays between training and implementation. Provide frequent refresher courses or updates.
6	Develop and communicate policies delineating staff authorized and responsible for technology implementation, use, oversight, and safety review.
7	Ensure that all order sets and guidelines are developed, tested, and approved by the Pharmacy and Therapeutics Committee (or equivalent) before implementation.
8	Develop a graduated system of safety alerts in the new technology to help clinicians determine urgency and relevancy. Review skipped or rejected alerts. Decide which alerts need to be hard stops in the technology and provide supporting documentation.
9	Develop systems to mitigate potential computerized provider order entry (CPOE) drug errors or adverse events by requiring department and pharmacy review and sign off. Use the Pharmacy and Therapeutics Committee (or equivalent) for oversight and approval of electronic order sets and clinical decision support (CDS) alerts. Ensure proper nomenclature and printed label design, eliminate dangerous abbreviations and dose designations, and ensure electronic medication administration record (e-MAR) acceptance by nurses.
10	Provide environments that protect staff doing data entry from undue distractions when using the technology.
11	Maximize the potential of the technology to maximize safety. Continually reassess and enhance safety effectiveness and error detection. Use error-tracking tools, and evaluate events and near-miss events.
12	Monitor and report errors and near-miss events. Pursue potential system errors or use problems with root cause analysis or other forms of failure-mode analysis. Consider reporting significant issues to external reporting systems.
13	Re-evaluate the applicability of security and confidentiality protocols. Reassess Health Insurance Portability and Accountability Act (HIPAA) compliance periodically to ensure that the addition of technology and the growing responsibilities of IT staff have not introduced new security or compliance risks.

information technology will never eliminate the need for personal communication and teamwork.

Successful development and implementation of nursing information technology depend on nurses working in partnership with organizational leadership, information systems vendors, and systems analysts to create tools that truly benefit nurses. When nurses have the systems and tools needed to provide patient care effectively and efficiently, safety and care quality will follow. Direct-care nurses must work with informatics nurses and information system developers and programmers in system development, implementation, and ongoing improvement. Nurses are key partners in every phase of the clinical information life cycle (Benham-Hutchins, 2009). By combining computer and information science with nursing science, the goals of supporting nursing practice and the delivery of high-quality nursing care can be achieved (Delaney, 2007). The Literature Perspective on p. 203 identifies some recommendations related to health information technology (HIT) successes and failures.

LITERATURE PERSPECTIVE

Technology and Nursing Resource Planning

Resource: Harper, E.M. (2012). Staffing based on evidence: Can health information technology make it possible? *Nursing Economics, 30,* 262-267.

The potential to use health information technology as a tool to manage effective use of nursing resources is a fairly new topic that has only recently been explored by leaders in nursing informatics (Douglas, 2011; Douglas, 2010; Hyun, Bakken, Douglas, & Stone, 2008). It is a significant topic because a clear and compelling case has been demonstrated for the association of nurses, nursing care, and clinical outcomes for patients and financial outcomes for organizations (Aiken, Clark, Sochalski, & Silber, 2002; American Nurses Association, 2010; Douglas, 2010; Eck-Birmingham, 2010). Nonetheless, leaders must balance nursing staffing and care quality against financial constraints in an era of cost containment.

There is little agreement of the best approach to achieve nurse/patient ratios that support safe, high-quality nursing care for all patients. A strict ratio may ignore individual patient care needs; whereas attempts to capture details about care needs or derive a formula that precisely predicts care needs and forecasts required staff requirements are very difficult and have not been broadly agreed upon.

Harper (2012) reported a pilot study that used a clinical information system (CIS) to identify factors that lead to a model that predicts nursing care needs. In the pilot study, a Clinical Demand Index was developed by identifying how nurses spend their time, using the CIS for data mining, and identifying variables most closely related to how nurses spend their time. The pilot demonstrated that clinical data from the electronic health record can be extracted in real time and used to calculate the intensity of nursing care required by patients in a given clinical setting.

Implications for Practice

Can you think of patient care activities that should be included in a measurement of nursing care intensity? Administering medications, monitoring patients following a procedure, and admitting a new patient for an inpatient stay are a few examples. Which of these have you documented electronically during your nursing education? Are there other nursing care activities that you regularly and routinely document? Were you aware of the potential to mine data from the clinical information system? What protections for patient information security need to be in place to ensure confidentiality and personal health information are not jeopardized by an initiative such as this?

the readings. Reviewing the medication list, you note he is receiving hydralazine (Apresoline). Processing the data that you have collected, you implement "falls precautions," send a communication order to monitor his blood pressure and other symptoms frequently, and notify the physician if the situation has not changed.

EXERCISE 11-5

Think about the data that you gather and document every day: vital signs, intake and output, laboratory and test results, and the patient's responses to care. What data did you automatically combine or reorganize to help you make a decision regarding patient care? How did you use this information to improve your patient's outcome? How and with whom did you communicate the data and information? How did technology combine or organize data?

FUTURE TRENDS AND PROFESSIONAL ISSUES

Biomedical Technology

Numerous devices continue to be developed. As an example, twenty-first century IV pumps offer safety features, accuracy, advanced pressure monitoring, ease of use, and versatility.

Information Technology

Health care in the United States is expensive and of variable quality. Recognizing that informatics can play an important role in controlling costs and improving quality, the federal government's economic stimulus

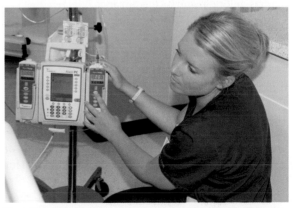

Twenty-first century IV pumps offer safety features, accuracy, advanced pressure monitoring, ease of use, and versatility.

Imagine that a patient you are caring for complains of light-headedness and nausea. When documenting vital signs, you note that the blood pressure measurement is lower than it was the day before. Graphing the values across several days illustrates a steady decline in

plan in 2009 earmarked $20 billion for health information technology. However, the money must be spent wisely, not quickly. One consideration suggested was to use the money to move the health information technology industry toward strong, mandated data standards. Data standards are at the foundation of integrated, interoperable information systems that will permit an emergency department or operating room to transfer data to inpatient hospital units and permit hospitals to send data to a patient's primary care record in the provider's office.

Electronic Patient Care Records

Multiple terms have been used to define electronic patient care records, with overlapping definitions. Both electronic health record (EHR) and electronic medical record (EMR) have gained widespread use, with some health informatics users assigning the term *EHR* to a global concept and *EMR* to a discrete localized record. An EHR refers to an individual patient's medical record in digital format. The EHR is a longitudinal electronic record of patient health information generated across encounters in any care delivery setting. EHR systems coordinate the storage and retrieval of individual records with the aid of computers. The EHR is most often accessed on a computer, often over a network, and may include EMRs from many locations and/or sources. Among the many forms of data often included are patient demographics, health history, progress and procedure notes, health problems, medication and allergy lists (including immunization status), laboratory test results, radiology images and reports, billing records, and advance directives.

Credit card–like devices called smart cards store a limited number of pages of data on a computer chip. The implementation of computer-based health information systems will lead to computer networks that will store health records across local, state, national, and international boundaries. The smart card serves as a bridge between the clinician terminal and the central repository, making patient information available to the caregiver quickly and cheaply at the point of service because the patients bring it with them. This will help coordinate care; improve quality-of-care decisions; and reduce risk, waste, and duplication of effort. Patients are mobile and consult many practitioners, thereby causing their records to be fragmented. With the electronic smart card, patients, providers,

---

BOX 11-5   SMART CARDS

1. Patient demographics/photo identification
2. ICE—in case of emergency—contact and other key information
3. Patient medical history: for example, allergies, medications, immunizations, laboratory results
4. Past care encounter summaries, including surgical procedures
5. Patient record locations and electronic address information
6. Ability to upload or download patient information

---

and notes can be brought together in any combination at any place. Box 11-5 provides examples of the types of data that are recorded on smart cards.

Data Privacy and Security

Data protection, systems' security, and patient privacy are concerns with electronic health records. However, patients' rights to privacy of their data must be maintained whether recorded in a manual or automated system. With computerized data, any person with the proper permission may access the information anywhere in the world and multiple people can do so simultaneously. Data can also be inadvertently sent to the wrong individual or site. Information security and privacy are important concerns as development of electronic health information systems accelerates at the beginning of the twenty-first century.

A firewall protects the information in the central data repository from access by unauthorized users. It is a network security measure that keeps electronic intruders from accessing an organization's data on its private network while allowing members of the organization to reach the Internet. Organizational policies on the use, security, and accuracy of data must be developed and monitored for compliance.

Communication Technology
Telecommunications

Telecommunications and systems technology facilitate clinical oversight of health care via telephone or cable lines, remote monitoring, information links, and the Internet. Telehealth is the use of modern telecommunications and information technologies for the provision of health care to individuals at a distance and the transmission of information to provide that care. This is accomplished using two-way interactive videoconferencing and high-speed telephone lines, fiberoptic cable, and satellite transmissions. Patients sitting in front of the teleconferencing camera can be diagnosed, treated, monitored, and educated by nurses and physicians. EKGs and radiographs can be viewed and transmitted. Sophisticated electronic stethoscopes and dermascopes allow nurses and physicians to hear heart, lung, and bowel sounds and to look closely at wounds, eyes, ears, and skin. Ready access to expert advice and patient information is available no matter where the patient or information is located. Patients in rural areas and prisons especially benefit from this technology.

Telecommunication also supports distance learning, which has been possible for some years, with enhanced opportunities to engage learners in online classrooms. With online or "virtual" classrooms, learners from anywhere in the world with computer access can log into a university's or other group's online learning system via the Internet.

Informatics

In 2011, the Healthcare Information and Management Systems Society (HIMSS) identified that just over 90% of American hospitals had implemented some component of an EMR. The American Nurses Association recognized nursing informatics as a specialty nursing practice in 2001. Although more than 8000 nurses are practicing in informatics, many more are needed to achieve widespread development and adoption of effective health information systems (Sensmeier, 2008).

Many opportunities exist to improve the safety, efficiency, and effectiveness of nursing care. The goal of informatics nurses and nursing leaders is to use information technology to ensure that critical information is available to caregivers at the point of care to make health care safer and more effective while improving efficiency. This requires interconnected and integrated healthcare technology across hospitals, healthcare systems, and geographic regions. Standards for data systems that operate efficiently with one another (termed "interoperability") and attention to data security and patient privacy are necessary.

Nurses are working as leaders in several national initiatives to lay the groundwork and guide progress toward the goal of a nationwide health information network. Every nurse can embrace technology to improve nursing practice. Some strategies to accomplish this include (1) involving nurses in every decision about health IT that affects their workflow, (2) investing in training nurses to effectively use technology in their practice, and (3) leveraging opportunities to use IT to enable quality improvement (Sensmeier, 2008).

Knowledge Technology

Technology has the potential to shorten the many years that currently exist between the development of new knowledge for patient care and the application of that knowledge in real-time practice with patients. Increasingly, patient conditions that are directly influenced by nursing care are part of the Centers for Medicare & Medicaid Services (CMS) pay for performance and The Joint Commission "never events." Having the best knowledge available regarding clinical phenomena is increasingly important. The focus of nursing care includes medication management, activity intolerance, immobility, risk for falls and actual falls, risk for skin impairment and pressure ulcer, anxiety, dementia, sleep, prevention of infection, nutrition, incontinence, dehydration, smoking cessation, pain management, patient and family education, and self-care.

Norma Lang, a nursing informatics leader, has described the challenges of bringing the best evidence for practice to bear against nursing care (Lang, 2008). First, the challenge of synthesizing the knowledge available in a manner that is useful to clinicians is critical. Then, computerized information systems are needed to provide clinical decision support at the point of care. Finally, the computer system must collect good clinical data to promote ongoing knowledge development for nursing care of patients and families. Several "intelligent" clinical information systems are in development. These systems translate nursing knowledge into reference materials that can be accessed at the point of care. Further, computer applications are in development that assist nurses to take action and execute patient care based on the best evidence for practice (Lang, 2008; Lang et al., 2006; Staggers & Brennan, 2007).

Professional, Ethical Nursing Practice and New Technologies

Technology has and will continue to transform the healthcare environment and the practice of nursing. Nurses are professionally obligated to maintain competency with a vast array of technologic devices and systems. Baseline informatics competency is required for all nurses to function in the twenty-first century.

Because of the increasing ability to preserve human life with biomedical technology, questions about living and dying have become conceptually and ethically complex. Conceptually, it becomes more difficult to define extraordinary treatment and human life because technology has changed our concepts of living and dying. A source of ethical dilemmas is the use of invasive technologic treatment to provide patients with extraordinary means and to prolong life for patients with limited or no decision-making capabilities. Nurses are concerned with individual patient welfare and the effects of technologic intervention on the immediate and long-term quality of life for patients and their families. Patient advocacy remains an important function of the professional nurse.

Safeguarding patients' welfare, privacy, and confidentiality is another obligation of nurses. Security measures are available with computerized information systems, but it is the integrity and ethical principles of system end-users that provide the final safeguard for patient privacy. System users must never share the passwords that allow them access to information in computerized clinical information systems. Each password uniquely identifies a user to the system by name and title, gives approval to carry out certain functions, and provides access to data appropriate to the user. When a nurse signs on to a computer, all data and information that are entered or reviewed can be traced to that password. Every nurse is accountable for all actions taken using his or her password.

All nurses must be aware of their responsibilities for the confidentiality and security of the data they gather and for the security of their passwords.

Nurse leaders must promote the existence and use of an ethics committee in their institutions and assign knowledgeable nurses to serve on these committees. Nurse managers must ensure that policies and procedures for collecting and entering data and the use of security measures (e.g., passwords) are established to maintain confidentiality of patient data and information. Nurse managers must also be knowledgeable patient advocates in the use of technology for patient care by referring ethical questions to the organization's ethics committee.

EXERCISE 11-6

Think about the use of the Internet in health care. How do you use it to look up healthcare information? How would you advise a patient to select appropriate sites?

CONCLUSION

Biomedical, information, communication, and knowledge technology will form a bond in the future, linking people and information together in a rapidly changing world of health care. With new technology comes the need for a new set of competencies. Nursing participation in designing this exciting future will ensure that the unique contributions of nurses to patient and family health and illness care are clearly and formally represented.

THE SOLUTION

We successfully implemented BCMA over an 11-month period in all our inpatient, emergency, and same-day surgery areas. A systematic review of the literature related to BCMA informed our teams of the potential for nurses to work around the system when it obstructed the process of getting medications to patients on time. In addition, site visits to organizations that had implemented BCMA confirmed the evidence from the literature.

The literature and site visits also demonstrated that hardware reliability does indeed impact nurses' use of the system. If devices don't work, nurses work around them to meet patient care needs! We presented our findings and recommendations to nursing leaders and direct care nurses and, in order to provide the most reliable hardware, we opted to hardwire computers and attach Bluetooth bar-code scanners at every patient bedside throughout our organization. In addition, patient care areas have a few mobile computers and scanners to use when patients are not in their rooms. Although this was not an inexpensive option, it ensured that hardware would not be a reason for working around recommended processes for BCMA. Finally, we designed training to systematically address recognized deviations from recommended practice and emphasized the work processes that promoted best practice and patient safety.

Information technology is an essential component of our patient safety program. We report area-specific compliance with BCMA every week to nursing, pharmacy, and informatics leaders who share the information with direct care staff. Most areas comply with work process expectations nearly 95% of the time: surpassing our organizational goal of 90%! More importantly, BCMA has lowered the incidence of adverse drug events in our hospitals and clinics.

—*Janis B. Smith*

Would this be a suitable approach for you? Why?

THE EVIDENCE

Health Information Technology and Patient Safety

Health information technology (HIT) has the potential to reduce healthcare costs, improve efficiency, and enhance patient care safety and quality. HIT is rapidly evolving and changing how we deliver care, while healthcare reform is simultaneously reshaping the environment in which care is provided. A committee of experts was convened by the Institutes of Medicine in 2011 to review the evidence about the impact of HIT on patient safety and to recommend actions, based on evidence, that safeguard patients in our contemporary technology-rich healthcare environment.

The committee found that specific types of HIT can improve patient safety under the right conditions, but these right conditions may not be easily replicated in all settings. Potential safety benefits and concerns were documented for computerized provider order entry (CPOE), clinical decision support (CDS), bar code confirmation of patient identity and medications, and patient engagement tools. However if not designed and implemented appropriately, HIT may add a layer of complexity to the already complex delivery of health care and lead to unintended consequences. HIT must be designed, implemented, used, and continuously improved to positively enable healthcare quality and safety.

Safely functioning HIT provides easy entry and unlimited retrieval of data, has simple and intuitive user interfaces, supports the clinical workflow of all end-users, and permits seamless system interoperability.

Implications for Practice

Have you used more than one information system during your academic preparation in nursing? If yes, were there advantages in design and implementation that you could detect in one setting or another?

Have you used the same information system in more than one setting? If so, did you detect differences in how the system was designed and implemented in different settings?

If you were to participate on the HIT selection or implementation planning teams in your role as a registered nurse, are you confident you could identify features in the system with potential to either support or threaten patient safety (IOM, 2012)?

WHAT NEW GRADUATES SAY

- My first position was at a clinic that used a computerized system I'd not used before. I quickly figured out I had to learn it well in order to survive! Take advantage of every opportunity to learn new technology. That way you won't get so far behind. If you have any downtime, practice using equipment and thinking through the principles associated to a particular device.

- As a newer nurse the idea of having technology as a double-check when administering medications, blood products, breast milk, and so on, via a smart pump and bar-coding technology gives me confidence in what I'm doing.
- As I'm learning and caring for my patients, I appreciate that the system helps me work through next steps based on what I enter.

CHAPTER CHECKLIST

Nurses are the key personnel in the healthcare system to mediate the interaction among science, technology, and the patient because of their unique holistic viewpoint and the "24/7" role of vigilant healthcare providers who preserve the patients' humanity, optimal functioning, and promotion of health. The challenge for the profession is to continue to provide patient-centered care in a technologic society that strives for efficiency and cost-effectiveness. Nurse administrators, managers, and staff must provide leadership in managing information and technology to meet the challenge.

- Types of technologies
  - Biomedical technology
    - Physiologic monitoring
    - Diagnostic testing
    - Intravenous fluid and medication administration
    - Therapeutic treatments

- Information technology
- Knowledge technology
- Information systems
  - Meaningful use
  - Information systems quality and accreditation
  - Information systems hardware
  - Wireless communication
- Communication technology
- Informatics
- Patient safety
- Impact of clinical information systems
  - Impact on communication
  - Impact on patient care documentation
- Impact on medication administration processes
- Safely implementing health information technology
- Future trends and professional issues
  - Biomedical technology
  - Information technology
    - Electronic patient care records
    - Data privacy and security
  - Communication technology
    - Telecommunications
  - Informatics
    - Knowledge technology
  - Professional, ethical nursing practice and new technologies

▌ TIPS FOR MANAGING INFORMATION AND TECHNOLOGY

- Create a vision for the future.
- Match your vision to the institution's mission and strategic plan.
- Learn what you need to know to fulfill the vision.
- Join initiatives that are moving in the direction of your vision.
- Be prepared to initiate, implement, and support new technology.
- Use an automated dispensing system.
- Use biometric technology.
- Use bar-coding systems/bar-code technology.
- Never stop learning, or you will always be behind.

REFERENCES

Akre, M., Finkelstein, M., Erickson, M., Liu, M., Vanderbilt, L., & Billman, G. (2010). Sensitivity of the pediatric early warning score to identify patient deterioration. *Pediatrics, 125*, 763–769.

American Association of Colleges of Nursing Strategic Advisory Group for Graduate-Level QSEN Competencies. (2012). *Graduate-level QSEN competencies: Knowledge, skills and attitudes.* Accessed 15.07.13 at, www.aacn.nche.edu/faculty/qsen/competencies.pdf.

Ammenwerth, E., Mansmann, U., Iller, C., & Eichstadter, R. (2003). Factors affecting and affected by user acceptance of computer-based nursing documentation: Results of a two-year study. *Journal of the American Medical Informatics Association: JAMIA, 10*, 69–84.

Ash, J. S., Berg, M., & Coiere, E. (2004). Some unintended consequences of information technology in health care: The nature of patient care information system-related errors. *Journal of the American Medical Informatics Association: JAMIA, 11*, 104–112.

Ash, J. S., Sittig, D. F., Poon, E. G., Guappone, K., Campbell, E., & Dykstra, R. H. (2007). The extent and importance of unintended consequences related to computerized provider order entry. *Journal of the American Medical Informatics Association: JAMIA, 14*(4), 415–423.

Bakken, S., Cook, S., Curtis, L., Desjardins, K., Hyun, S., Jenkins, M., et al. (2004). Promoting patient safety through informatics based nursing education. *International Journal of Medical Informatics, 73*, 581–589.

Ball, M., Weaver, C., & Abbot, P. (2003). Enabling technologies promise to revitalize the role of nursing in an era of patient safety. *International Journal of Medical Informatics, 69*, 29–38.

Benham-Hutchins, M. (2009). Frustrated with HIT? Get involved! *Nursing Management, 40*(1), 17–19.

Bonzheim, K. (2006). *Process and workflow improvements through technology adoption.* Chicago, IL: Healthcare Information and Management Systems Society.

Breslow, M. J. (2007). Remote ICU care programs: Current status. *Journal of Critical Care, 22*, 66–76.

Considine, K., & Botti, V. (2004). Who, when and where? Identification of patients at risk of an in-hospital adverse event: Implications for nursing practice. *International Journal of Nursing Practice, 10*, 21–31.

Cronenwett, L., Sherwood, G., Pohl, J., Barnsteiner, J., Moore, S., Sullivan, D., et al. (2009). Quality and safety education for advanced nursing practice. *Nursing Outlook, 57*, 338–348.

Delaney, C. (2007). Nursing and informatics for the 21st century. *Creative Nursing, 2*, 4–6.

Drucker, P. (1993). *Post-capitalist society.* New York: Harper Business Publishers.

Ebright, P. R., Patterson, E. S., Chalko, B. A., & Render, M. L. (2003). Understanding the complexity of registered nurse work in acute care settings. *Journal of Nursing Administration, 33*, 630–638.

Frankel, D. J., Cowie, M., & Daley, P. (2003). Quality benefits of an intensive care clinical information system. *Critical Care Medicine, 31*, 120–125.

Franklin, B. D., O'Grady, P., Donyai, K., Jacklin, A., & Barber, N. (2007). The impact of a closed-loop electronic prescribing and administration system on prescribing errors, administration errors and staff time: A before-and-after study. *Quality & Safety in Health Care, 16,* 279–284.

Hannah, K. J., & Ball, M. J. (2011). *Introduction to nursing informatics* (4th ed.). London; New York: Springer-Verlag.

Harrison, P. (May 30, 2013). Alarm fatigue still top technology hazard for 2103. *Medscape,* http://www.medscape.com/viewarticle/805050.

HIMSS Analytics Report. (2012). *Quality and safety linked to advanced information technology enabled processes.* Retrieved February 12, 2012 from, www.himss.org/content/files/thomsonreuterswhitepaperfinal0412.pdf.

Hunter, K. M. (2001). Nursing informatics theory. In V. K. Saba & K. A. McCormick (Eds.), *Essentials of computers for nurses: Informatics for the new millennium* (pp. 179–190). New York: McGraw-Hill.

Institute for Safe Medication Practices (ISMP). (2008). ADC survey shows some improvements, but unnecessary risks still exist. *Safety Briefs, 13,* 1–2.

Institute of Medicine (IOM). (2011). *The future of nursing: Leading change, advancing health.* Washington, DC: National Academy Press.

Institute of Medicine (IOM), Committee on Patient Safety. (2000). *To err is human: Building a safer health care system.* Washington, DC: The National Academies Press.

Institute of Medicine (IOM), Committee on Patient Safety and Health Information Technology. (2012). *Health IT and patient safety: Building safer systems for better care.* Washington, DC: The National Academies Press.

Institute of Medicine (IOM), Committee on Quality Health Care in America. (July 2001). *Crossing the quality chasm: A new health system for the 21st century.* Washington, DC: National Academy Press.

Institute of Medicine (IOM), Committee on the Work Environment for Nurses and Patient Safety. (2004). *Keeping patients safe: Transforming the work environment of nurses.* Washington, DC: The National Academies Press.

Kaplan, B. (2001). Evaluating informatics applications: Some alternative approaches. *International Journal of Medical Informatics, 64*(1), 39–56.

Kaplan, B., & Harris-Salamone, K. D. (2009). Health IT success and failure: Recommendations from the literature and an AMIA workshop. *Journal of the American Medical Informatics Association: JAMIA, 16,* 291–299.

Koppel, R., Wetterneck, T., Telles, J. L., & Karsh, B. T. (2008). Workarounds to barcode medication administration systems: Their occurrences, causes, and threats to patient safety. *Journal of the American Medical Informatics Association: JAMIA, 15,* 408–423.

Korst, L., Eusebio-Angeja, A., Chamorro, T., Aydin, C., & Gregory, K. (2003). Nursing documentation time during implementation of an electronic medical record. *Journal of Nursing Administration, 33,* 24–30.

Kossman, S. P., & Scheidenhelm, S. L. (2008). Nurses' perceptions of the impact of electronic health records on work and patient outcomes. *CIN: Computers, Informatics, Nursing, 26,* 69–77.

Krichbaum, K., Diemert, C., Jacox, L., Jones, A., Koenig, P., Mueller, C., et al. (2007). Complexity compression: Nurses under fire. *Nursing Forum, 42,* 86–94.

Lang, N. M. (2008). The promise of simultaneous transformation of practice and research with the use of clinical information systems. *Nursing Outlook, 56,* 232–236.

Lang, N. M., Hook, M. L., Akre, M. E., Kim, T. Y., Berg, K. S., & Lundeen, S. P. (2006). Translating knowledge-based nursing into referential and executable applications in an intelligent clinical information system. In C. Weaver, C. Delaney, P. Webber, & R. Carr (Eds.), *Nursing and informatics for the 21st century* (pp. 291–304). Chicago: Healthcare Information and Management Systems Society (HIMSS).

Larrabee, J. H., Boldreghini, S., Elder-Sorrells, K., Turner, Z. M., Wender, R. G., Hart, J. M., et al. (2001). Evaluation of documentation before and after implementation of a nursing information system in an acute care hospital. *Computers in Nursing, 19,* 56–65.

Laws, D., & Amato, S. (2010). Incorporating bedside reporting into change of shift report. *Rehabilitation Nursing, 35*(2), 70–74.

Malashock, C., Smith-Shull, S., & Gould, D. A. (2004). Effect of smart infusion pumps on medication errors related to infusion device programming. *Hospital Pharmacy, 39*(5), 460–469.

Malbrain, M. L., Chiumello, D., Pelosi, P., Bihari, D., Innes, R., Ranieri, V. M., et al. (2005). Incidence and prognosis of intraabdominal hypertension in a mixed population of critically ill patients: A multiple-center epidemiological study. *Critical Care Medicine, 33,* 315–322.

Malloch, K. (2007). The electronic health record: An essential tool for advancing patient safety. *Nursing Outlook, 55,* 159–161.

Marin, H. (2004). Improving patient safety with technology. *International Journal of Medical Informatics, 73,* 543–546.

McBride, A. (2005). Nursing and the informatics revolution. *Nursing Outlook, 53,* 183–191.

Mekhjian, H. S., Kumar, R. R., Kuehn, L., Bentley, T. D., Teater, P., Thomas, A., et al. (2002). Immediate benefits realized following implementation of physician order entry at an academic medical center. *Journal of the American Medical Informatics Association, 9*(5), 529–539.

Myers, M. A., & Reed, K. D. (2008). The virtual ICU (vICU): A new dimension for critical care nursing practice. *Critical Care Nursing Clinics of North America, 20,* 435–439.

National League for Nursing (NLN). (2008). *Position statement: Preparing the next generation of nurses to practice in a technology-rich environment—An informatics agenda.* Retrieved March 2, 2010 from, www.nln.org.

Parker, P. J. (2005). One nurse informatics specialist views the future technology in the crystal ball. *Nursing Administration Quarterly, 29*(2), 123–124.

Pevtzow, L. (April 16, 2013). New guidelines to reduce alarm fatigue. *Medscape,* http://www.medscape.com/viewarticle/782597.

Reason, J. (2002). Combating omission errors through task analysis and good reminders. *Quality & Safety in Health Care, 11,* 40–44.

Scholes, M., & Barber, B. (1980). Towards nursing informatics. In D. A. D. Lindberg & S. Kaihara (Eds.), *MEDINFO: 1980* (pp. 7–73). Amsterdam, Netherlands: North-Holland.

Sensmeier, J. (2008). Deep impact: Informatics and nursing practice. *Nursing Management IT Solutions Supplement,* 2–6, September.

Smith, J. B., & Burnes Bolton, L. (2013). What is meaningful use and what are the implications for the future of health care. *Nurse Leader, 11,* 20–21.

Snyder-Halpern, R., Corcoran-Perry, S., & Narayan, S. (2001). Developing clinical practice environments supporting the knowledge work of nurses. *Computers in Nursing, 19*(1), 17–23.

Staggers, N., & Brennan, P. F. (2007). Translating knowledge into practice: Passing the hot potato! *Journal of the American Medical Informatics Association: JAMIA, 14*, 684–685.

Stead, W. W., Bird, W. P., Califf, R. M., Elchlepp, J. G., Hammond, W. E., & Kinney, T. R. (1993). The IAIMS at Duke University Medical Center: Transition from model testing to implementation. *MD Computing, 10*, 225–230.

Stead, W. W. & Lin, H. S. (Eds.). (2009). *Computational technology for effective health care: Immediate steps and strategic directions.* Washington, DC: National Academies of Science.

The Joint Commission (TJC). (2008). *Sentinel event alert: Safely implementing health information and converging technologies.* Retrieved September 24, 2009, from, www.jointcommission.org/SentinelEvents/SentinelEventAlert/sea_42.htm.

The Joint Commission (TJC). (2013a). *Sentinel event alert: Medical device alarm safety in hospitals.* Retrieved June 6, 2013 from, www.jointcommission.org/assets/1/18/SEA_50_alarms_4_5_13_FINAL1.PDF.

The Joint Commission (TJC). (2013b). *TJC accreditation manual e-dition.* Retrieved May 21, 2013, from, https://e-dition.jcrinc.com/MainContent.aspx.

The TIGER Initiative. (2010). *Informatics competencies for every practicing nurse.* Retrieved July 14, 2013 from, www.tigersummit.com/uploads/3.Tiger.Report_Competencies_final.pdf.

Trossman, S. (2001). The documentation dilemma: Nurses poised to address paperwork burden. *The American Nurse, 33*, 1, 9,18.

Vidal, M. G., Ruiz Weisser, J., Gonzalez, F., Toro, M. A., Loudet, C., Balasini, C., et al. (2008). Incidence and clinical effects of intra-abdominal hypertension in critically ill patients. *Critical Care Medicine, 36*, 1823–1831.

Warren, J., & Connors, H. (2007). Health information technology can and will transform nursing education. *Nursing Outlook, 55*, 58–60.

Westbrook, J., Duffield, C., Li, L., & Creswick, N. (2011). How much time do nurses have for patients? A longitudinal study quantifying hospital nurses' patterns of task time distribution and interactions with health professionals. *BMC Health Services Research, 11*, 319.

Wood, S. (March 9, 2013). "Alarming" use of unnecessary ECG monitors, ubiquitous. possibly harmful. *Medscape,* http://www.medscape.com/viewarticle/780537.

SUGGESTED READINGS

American Nurses Association. (2008). *Nursing informatics: Practice scope and standards of practice.* Silver Spring, MD: Nursesbooks.org.

Englebardt, S. P., & Nelson, R. (2005). *Health care informatics: An interdisciplinary approach.* St Louis: Mosby.

Hebda, T. L., & Czar, P. (2013). *Handbook of informatics for nurses & healthcare professionals.* Boston: Pearson.

McGonigle, D. (2008). *Nursing informatics.* Boston: Jones & Bartlett Publishing.

Saba, V., & McCormick, K. A. (2011). *Essentials of nursing informatics.* New York: McGraw-Hill Medical.

Weaver, C., Delaney, C., Webber, P., & Carr, R. (2006). *Nursing and informatics for the 21st century.* Chicago: Healthcare Information and Management Systems Society (HIMSS).

ADDITIONAL REFERENCES

Aiken, L., Clark, S., Sochalski, J., & Silber, J. (2002). Hospital nurse staffing and patient mortality, nurse burnout. *JAMA, 288*, 1987–1993.

American Nurses Association. (2010). *Registered Nurse Save Staffing Act of 2010 (S.3491 / H.R.5527).* Retrieved from, http://safestaffingsaveslifes.org/whatisANADoing/FederalLegislation.aspx.

Douglas, K. (2010). The human side of staffing. *Nursing Economic$, 28*, 56–62.

Douglas, K. (2011). What every nurse executive should know about staffing and scheduling technology initiatives. *Nursing Economic$, 29*, 273–275.

Eck-Birmingham, S. (2010). Evidence based staffing: The next step. *Nurse Leader, 8*, 24–35.

Harper, E. M. (2012). Staffing based on evidence: Can health information technology make it possible? *Nursing Economics, 30*, 262–267.

Hyun, S., Bakken, S., Douglas, K., & Stone, P. W. (2008). Evidenced-based staffing: Potential roles for informatics. *Nursing Informatics, 26*, 159–168.

Institute of Medicine. (2012). *Health IT and patient safety: Building safer systems for patient safety.* Washington D.C: The National Academies Press.

Locsin, R. C. (2005). *Technological competency as caring in nursing: A model for practice.* Indianapolis, IN: Sigma Theta Tau International.

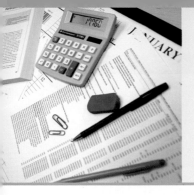

12

Managing Costs and Budgets

Sylvain Trepanier

This chapter focuses on methods of financing health care and specific strategies for managing costs and budgets in patient care settings, something that has become increasingly important as healthcare delivery evolves. Factors that escalate healthcare costs, sources of healthcare financing, reimbursement methods, cost-containment and value-based purchasing as part of The Patient Protection and Affordable Care Act, and implications for nursing practice are discussed. Various budgets and the budgeting process are explained. In addition to clinical competency and caring practices, understanding the cost issues in healthcare delivery and the ethical implications of financial decisions is essential for nurses to contribute fully to the health of patients and populations.

LEARNING OUTCOMES

- Explain several major factors that are escalating the costs of health care.
- Evaluate different reimbursement methods and their incentives to control costs.
- Differentiate costs, charges, and revenue in relation to a specified unit of service, such as a visit, hospital stay, or procedure.
- Value why all healthcare organizations must make a profit.
- Give examples of cost considerations for nurses.
- Discuss the purpose of and relationships among the operating, cash, and capital budgets.
- Explain the budgeting process.
- Identify variances on monthly expense reports.

KEY TERMS

budget	cost-based reimbursement	organized delivery
budgeting process	cost-based system	system (ODS)
capital expenditure budget	cost center	payer mix
capitation	diagnosis-related group (DRG)	payers
case mix	fixed costs	price
cash budget	full-time equivalent (FTE)	productive hours
charges	managed care	productivity
contractual allowance	nonproductive hours	profit
cost	operating budget	prospective payment system

providers	utilization	variance
revenue	value-based purchasing	variance analysis
unit of service	variable costs	

THE CHALLENGE

Marcus Johnson, RN, MSN
Director of Medical-Surgical Services, Central Hospital,
Tempest Health Care System, Detroit, Michigan

Central Hospital (CH) is one of nine acute care hospitals that make up the Tempest Health Care System (THCS). Medical-Surgical Services (MSS) account for 200 of CH's 367 beds. The primary sources of revenue for CH are managed care (42%), Medicare (36%), and self-pay (22%).

The nation has experienced an economic crisis of historic proportion. Locally, three major employers in THCS's market have threatened to file bankruptcy and have laid off thousands of employees.

Revenues for both CH and THCS have declined drastically. Inpatient admissions have decreased, and the payer mix is shifting from managed care to more self-pay. THCS administrators insist that all hospital operations stay budget-neutral. The next fiscally responsible step is to require that variable expenses in hospitals be reduced. Because labor costs are the greatest variable expense in a hospital, such thinking often leads to demands to reduce nursing staff or to substitute lower-paid personnel. As the nurse director of the MSS, my goal is to maintain a high-quality, high-performance work team that adds value for patients. In this situation, what steps can be taken before reducing staff in the MSS? How can I remain budget-neutral during times of economic crisis?

What do you think you would do if you were this nurse?

INTRODUCTION

Healthcare costs in the United States continue to rise at a rate greater than general inflation. In 2011, for example, Americans spent $2.6 trillion for health care—approximately 17% of the gross domestic product (GDP). This equals approximately $8000 per capita. The healthcare cost is projected to equal $4.8 trillion by 2021 (Centers for Medicare & Medicaid Services [CMS], 2011b). Yet millions of uninsured and underinsured Americans do not have access to basic healthcare services. With the exception of South Africa, the United States was the only industrialized nation where health care was viewed as a privilege rather than a right.

Despite our huge expenditures, major indicators reveal significant health problems in the United States, as well as large disparities in health status related to gender, race, and socioeconomic status (*Healthy People 2020*, 2011). Our infant mortality rate is among the highest of all industrialized nations, and black infants die at more than twice the rate of white infants. Average life expectancy is lower than that in most developed countries, and men have a life expectancy that is 6 years less than that of women. One in eight women will develop breast cancer during her lifetime, with black and Native American women experiencing a much higher death rate than white women.

Violence-related injuries are on the rise, and unintentional injuries, such as motor vehicle accidents, are a leading cause of death. Clearly, we are not receiving a high value return for our healthcare dollar.

The large portion of the GDP that is spent on health care poses problems to the economy in other ways, too. Funds are diverted from needed social programs such as childcare, housing, education, transportation, and the environment. The price of goods and services is increased, and therefore the country's ability to compete in the international marketplace is compromised. As the amount of the GDP devoted to healthcare expenses rises, the more vulnerable the healthcare industry is to external influences. This creates a major concern for an industry that already expresses concerns about being overregulated. Nurses must fully understand the cost of health care to ensure the fiscal viability of our healthcare system.

WHAT ESCALATES HEALTHCARE COSTS?

Total healthcare costs are a function of the prices and the utilization rates of healthcare services (Costs = Price × Utilization) (Table 12-1). Price is the rate that healthcare providers set for the services they deliver, such as the hospital rate or physician fee.

TABLE 12-1	RELATIONSHIP OF PRICE AND UTILIZATION RATES TO TOTAL HEALTHCARE COSTS

PRICE	×	UTILIZATION RATE	=	TOTAL COST	% CHANGE
$1.00		100		$100.00	0
$1.08*		100		$108.00	+8.0%
$1.08		105†		$113.40	13.4%
$1.08		110‡		$118.80	18.8%

*8% increase for inflation.
†5% more procedures done.
‡10% more procedures done.

Utilization refers to the quantity or volume of services provided, such as diagnostic tests provided or number of patient visits.

Price inflation and administrative inefficiency are leading contributors to increasing prices for health services. In recent decades, rises in healthcare prices have dramatically outpaced general inflation. Examples of factors that stimulate price inflation are: insurance premiums, medical technology, drug costs, health plan administration, and waste. Administrative inefficiency or waste is primarily a result of the large numbers of clerical personnel whom organizations use to process reimbursement forms from multiple payers. U.S. hospitals spend an average of 20% of their budgets on billing administration alone! This single fact indicates why some hospital administrators advocate for the elimination of multiple payers.

Several interrelated factors contribute to increased use of medical services. These include unnecessary care, consumer attitudes, healthcare financing, pharmaceutical usage, and changing population demographics and disease patterns. Unnecessary care can be defined as care prescribed that does not contribute to the well-being of a patient. An example is additional laboratory tests that are unrelated to the plan of care. Furthermore, there might not be any substantial evidence supporting the additional care. A substantial amount of unnecessary care does not add health benefits for patients.

Our attitudes and behaviors as consumers of health care also contribute to rising costs. In general, we prefer to "be fixed" when something goes wrong rather than to practice prevention. When we need "fixing," expensive high-tech services typically are perceived as the best care. Many of us still believe that the physician knows best, so we do not seek much information related to costs and effectiveness of different healthcare options. When we do seek information, it is not readily available or understandable. Also, we are not accustomed to using other, less costly healthcare providers, such as nurse practitioners.

The way health care is financed contributes to rising costs. When health care is reimbursed by third-party payers, consumers are somewhat insulated from personally experiencing the direct effects of high healthcare costs. In most instances, however, consumers do not have many incentives to consider costs when choosing among providers or using services. In addition, the various methods of reimbursement have implications for how providers price and use services.

Evidence of pharmaceutical usage can be seen in advertisements in magazines and on television. No longer do pharmaceutical companies attempt to influence only the prescribers. They go directly to the consumer, who then goes to the prescriber. Because of some typical drug benefit programs, the consumer often is unaware of the total cost of a medication, which may be a "quick fix" (described previously) or a lifestyle enhancement, such as sexual enhancers or skin conditioning.

Changing population demographics also are increasing the volume of health services needed. For example, chronic health problems increase with age, and the number of older adults in America is rising. The fastest growing population is the group aged 85 years and older, and Baby Boomers are moving into their senior years. Infectious diseases such as acquired immunodeficiency syndrome (AIDS) and tuberculosis, as well as the growing societal problems of obesity, heart disease, homelessness, drug addiction, and violence, increase demands for health services.

HOW IS HEALTH CARE FINANCED?

On March 23, 2010, historic healthcare reform was signed into law (The Patient Protection and Affordable Care Act, also referred to as ObamaCare). This phased-in legislation includes some features that take effect quickly and others that are delayed for several years. Preexisting conditions that often limited an individual's ability to secure health insurance starts with coverage for children. Although the enacted legislation does not cover the entire population, a great majority will be covered. By 2014, an estimated additional 32 million U.S. citizens could have access to health insurance, either from a private insurer or Medicaid, regardless of preexisting conditions. This coverage changes how individuals are insured and thus how they are viewed within the system. Multiple demands for nurses, especially those in advanced practice roles, will continue to emerge over the next several years. As all of these changes unfold, opportunities and challenges exist for the way in which health care will be delivered and paid for, and those changes will alter what nursing does.

Health care is paid for by three major sources: government (Medicare and Medicaid); private health insurance, and out-of-pocket (CMS, 2013). Three fourths of the government funding is at the federal level. Federal programs include Medicare and health services for members of the military, veterans, Native Americans, and federal prisoners. Medicare, the largest federal program, was established in 1965 and pays for care provided to people 65 years of age and older and some disabled individuals. Medicare Part A is an insurance plan for hospital, hospice, home health, and skilled nursing care that is paid for through Social Security taxes. Nursing home care that is mainly custodial is not covered. Medicare Part B is an optional insurance that covers physician services, medical equipment, and diagnostic tests. Part B is funded through federal taxes and monthly premiums paid by the recipients. Medicare does not cover outpatient medications, eye or hearing examinations, or dental services. The drug benefit plan, effective in 2006, has been viewed as beneficial but very difficult to understand.

Medicaid, a state-level program financed by federal and state funds, pays for services provided to persons who are medically indigent, blind, or disabled and to children with disabilities. As of 2011, Medicaid covered nearly 60 million Americans (Kaiser Family Foundation, 2011). The federal government pays between 50% and 83% of total Medicaid costs based on the per capita income of the state. Services funded by Medicaid vary from state to state but must include services provided by hospitals, physicians, laboratories, and radiology departments; prenatal and preventive care; and nursing home and home healthcare services.

Private insurance is the second major source of financing for the healthcare system. Most Americans have private health insurance, which usually is provided by employers through group policies. Individuals can purchase health insurance, but typically the rates are higher and provide minimal coverage. Health insurance that is so intertwined with employment is problematic and contributes to the number of uninsured and underinsured Americans. Many of the uninsured workers are those employed in small businesses that cannot afford to provide group insurance and those that have part-time, seasonal, or service positions.

Individuals also pay directly for health services when they do not have health insurance or when insurance does not cover the service. Costs paid by individuals are called *out-of-pocket expenses* and include deductibles, copayments, and coinsurance. Health insurance benefits often cover limited preventive care and typically do not cover cosmetic surgeries, alternative healthcare therapies, or items such as eyeglasses and nonprescription medications.

HEALTHCARE REIMBURSEMENT

Prices in health care are not set by the same economic equilibrium found in all major industries. For the most part, pricing is highly influenced by the government and the reimbursement plans. For example, both Medicare and Medicaid impose pricing on hospitals and there is no room for negotiation. Health services researchers do not agree on the exact effects of these reimbursement methods on cost and quality. However, considering these effects is important because changes in payment systems have implications for how care is provided in healthcare organizations. In fact, the government offered a reimbursement payment from cost-based system, to prospective payment system, and now a system that pays on performance (pay-for-performance), otherwise known as value-based purchasing.

A **cost-based system** consists of the cost of providing a service plus a markup for **profit.** Third-party payers often put limitations on what they will pay by establishing usual and customary **charges** by surveying all providers in a certain area. Usual and customary charges rise over time as providers continually increase their prices. In **cost-based reimbursement,** all allowable costs are calculated and used as the basis for payment. Each payer (government or insurance company) determines what the allowable costs are for each procedure, visit, or service. Charges and cost-based reimbursement are retrospective payment methods because the amount of payment is determined after services are delivered. When the reimbursed costs are less than the full charge for the service, a **contractual allowance** or discount exists. Charges and cost-based reimbursement were the predominant payment method in the 1960s and 1970s but have been largely supplanted by payer fee schedules determined before service delivery.

The **prospective payment system** is a method in which the third-party payer decides in advance what will be paid for a service or episode of care. If the costs of care are greater than the payment, the provider absorbs the loss. If the costs are less than the payment, the provider makes a profit. In 1983, Medicare implemented a prospective payment system (PPS) for hospital care that uses **diagnosis-related groups (DRGs)** as the basis for payment.

EXERCISE 12-1

What is the contractual allowance when a hospital charges $800 per day to care for a ventilator-dependent patient and an insurance company reimburses the hospital $685 per day? What is the impact on hospital income **(revenue)** if this is the reimbursement for 2500 patient days?

The DRG system is a classification system that groups patients into categories based on the average number of days of hospitalization for specific medical diagnoses, considering factors such as the patient's age, complications, and other illnesses. Payment includes the expected costs for diagnostic tests, various therapies, surgery, and length of stay (LOS). The cost of nursing services is not explicitly calculated. With a few exceptions, DRGs do not adequately reflect the variability of patient intensity or acuity within the DRG. This is problematic for nursing because the amount of resources (nurses and supplies) used to care for patients are directly related to the patient acuity. Therefore many nurses believe that DRGs are not good predictors of nursing care requirements. In past years, Medicare also began reimbursing home health agencies, nursing homes, and ambulatory care providers through a PPS.

In addition to Medicare, some state Medicaid programs and private insurance companies use a DRG payment system. Although DRGs are not currently used for specialty hospitals (pediatric, psychiatric, and oncology), they are a dominant force in hospital payment. Implementation of a PPS with DRGs resulted in increased patient acuity and decreased LOS in hospitals, along with a greater demand for home care. The need for hospital and community-based nurses also increased.

The pay for performance system was introduced in the early 2000s and used a system that reimbursed hospitals and eventually providers based on performance and outcomes and not on the cost associated with providing the care. The premise of this payment system is based on quality outcomes. It is also referred to as **value-based purchasing** offering rewards and incentives to high performing organization. This approach was first used with the passage of the Medicare Prescription Drug, Improvement, and Modernization Act of 2003. (Kaiser Family Foundation, 2004). This law provided incentives to hospitals that voluntarily submitted data on 10 quality measures.

The pay for performance system eventually evolved into the Hospital Value-Based Purchasing Program (HVBPP) established by the Affordable Care Act and became effective October of 2012. The incentives are based on how well a hospital performs on each measure or how much a hospital improves its performance on a measure as compared to its performance at baseline. The overall score includes clinical process of care measures and patient experience of care measures. A summary of hospital outcomes affecting HVBPP is offered in Box 12-1 (CMS, 2011a).

BOX 12-1   HOSPITAL OUTCOMES AFFECTING HVBPP

PATIENT OUTCOMES	HOSPITAL-ACQUIRED CONDITIONS	PATIENT SATISFACTION
AMI, CABG, CHF, pneumonia mortality rate	Retained foreign body	Nurse communication
Post-op hemorrhage or hematoma	Falls	Physician communication
Hip/knee replacement	Stage III and IV pressure ulcers	Staff responsiveness
Physiologic and metabolic derangement	Infections (catheter-associated urinary tract infection, central line bloodstream infection, surgical site)	Pain management
	Poor glycemic control	Communication of medications
		Cleanliness of the environment
		Discharge information
		Hospital overall score

AMI, Acute myocardial infarction; *CABG,* coronary artery bypass graft; *CHF,* chronic heart failure; *HVBPP,* hospital value-based purchasing program.

EXERCISE 12-2

Medicare reimburses a hospice $70 for home visits. For one particular group of patients, it costs the hospice an average of $98 per day to provide care. What are the implications for the hospice? What options should the hospice nurse manager and nurses consider?

EXERCISE 12-3

For each reimbursement method, think about the incentives for healthcare providers (individuals and organizations) regarding their practice patterns. What incentives could change the quantity of services used per patient or the number or types of patients served? Are these incentives efficient? List the incentives. How might each method affect overall healthcare costs? (Think in terms of effect on utilization and price.) What do you think the effect on quality of care might be with each payment method?

THE CHANGING HEALTHCARE ECONOMIC ENVIRONMENT

Health care is a major public concern, and rapid changes are occurring in an attempt to reduce costs and improve the health and wellness of the nation. As shown in Box 12-2, strategies shaping the evolving healthcare delivery system include managed care, organized delivery systems (ODSs), and competition based on price, patient outcomes, and service quality. These strategies affect both the pricing and use of health services.

BOX 12-2   HEALTHCARE DELIVERY REFORM STRATEGIES

STRATEGIES	KEY FEATURES
Managed care	Health plan that includes both service and finance
Organized delivery systems	Networks of organizations; providers and payers
Competition based on price, patient outcomes, and service quality	Basis of cost and quality

Managed care, also known as "managed cost," is a term that brings together the delivery and financing function into one entity, in an attempt to control the consumption of resources (Finkler, Jones, & Kovner, 2013). A major goal of managed care is to decrease unnecessary services, thereby decreasing costs. Managed care also works to ensure timely and appropriate care. Health maintenance organizations (HMOs) are a type of managed care system in which the primary physician serves as a gatekeeper who determines what services the patient uses. Because HMOs are paid on a capitated basis, it is to the HMO's advantage to practice prevention and use ambulatory care rather than more expensive hospital care. In other forms of managed care, a non-physician case manager arranges and authorizes the services provided. Many insurance companies have used case managers for years. Nurses who work in home health and ambulatory settings often communicate with insurance company case managers to plan the care for specific patients. PPOs and point-of-service (POS)

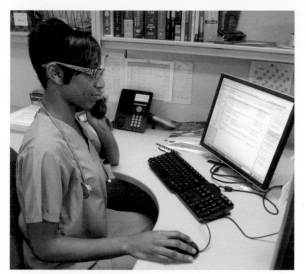

Nurses in ambulatory care settings often work directly with insurance companies to plan patient care.

WHAT DOES THIS MEAN FOR NURSING PRACTICE?

What does the healthcare economic environment mean for the practicing professional nurse? We must value ourselves as providers and think of our practice within a context of organizational viability and quality of care. To do this, we must add "financial thinking" to our repertoire of nursing skills and we must determine whether the services we provide add value for patients. In other words, it is critical to determine and advertise the *value* of nursing care. Services that add value are of high quality, affect health outcomes positively, and minimize costs. The following sections help develop financial thinking skills and ways to consider how nursing practice adds value for patients by minimizing costs.

WHY IS PROFIT NECESSARY?

Private, nongovernmental healthcare organizations may be either for-profit (FP) or not-for-profit (NFP). This designation refers to the tax status of the organization and specifies how the profit can be used. Profit is the excess income left after all expenses have been paid (Revenues − Expenses = Profit). FP organizations pay taxes, and their profits can be distributed to investors and managers. NFP organizations, on the other hand, do not pay taxes and must reinvest all of their profits, commonly called *net income* or *income above expense,* in the organization to better serve the public.

All private healthcare organizations must make a profit to survive. If expenses are greater than revenues, the organization experiences a loss. If revenues equal expenses, the organization breaks even. In both cases, nothing is left over to replace facilities and equipment, expand services, or pay for inflation costs. Some healthcare organizations can survive in the short run without making a profit because they use interest from investments to supplement revenues. The long-term viability of any private healthcare organization, however, depends on consistently making a profit. Box 12-3 presents a simplified example of an income statement from a neighborhood not-for-profit nursing center.

Nurses and nurse managers directly affect an organization's ability to make a profit. Profits can be

plans are other types of managed care plans that give the patient more options than traditional HMOs do for selecting providers and services.

ODSs comprise networks of healthcare organizations, providers, and payers. Typically, this means hospitals, physicians, and insurance companies. The aim of such joint ventures is to develop and market collectively a comprehensive package of healthcare services that will meet most needs of large numbers of consumers. Hospitals, physicians, and payers will share the financial risks of the enterprise. Although hospitals share some risk now with prospective payment, physicians have not generally shared the risk. This risk-sharing is expected to provide incentives to eliminate unnecessary services, use resources more effectively, and improve quality of services.

Competition among healthcare providers increasingly is based on cost and quality outcomes. Decision making regarding price and utilization of services is shifting from physicians and hospitals to payers, who are demanding significant discounts or lower prices. Scientific data that demonstrate positive health outcomes and high-quality services are required. Providers who cannot compete based on price, patient outcomes, and service quality will find it difficult to survive as the system evolves.

BOX 12-3	INCOME STATEMENT OF REVENUES AND EXPENSES FROM A NEIGHBORHOOD NURSING CENTER: FYE DECEMBER 31, 2010		
Revenues			
Patient revenues		$283,200	
Grant income		60,000	
Other operating revenues		24,000	
TOTAL		$367,200	$367,200
Expenses			
Salary costs		$140,400	
Supplies		64,400	
Other operating expenses (e.g., rent, utilities, administrative services)		79,900	
TOTAL		$284,700	$284,700
Excess of revenues over expenses [profit]*			$82,500

FYE, Fiscal year ending.
*Loss would be shown in parentheses ( ) or brackets [ ].

achieved or improved by decreasing costs or increasing revenues. In tight economic times, many managers think only in terms of cutting costs. Although cost-cutting measures are important, especially to keep prices down so that the organization will be competitive, ways to increase revenues also need to be explored.

> **EXERCISE 12-4**
> Obtain a copy of an itemized patient bill from a healthcare organization and review the charges. What was the source and method of payment? How much of these charges was reimbursed? How much was charged for items you regularly use in clinical care?

COST-CONSCIOUS NURSING PRACTICES

Understanding What Is Required to Remain Financially Sound

Understanding what is required for a department or agency to remain financially sound requires that nurses move beyond thinking about costs for individual patients to thinking about income and expenses and numbers of patients needed to make a profit. In a fee-for-service environment, revenue is earned for every service provided. Therefore increasing the volume of services, such as diagnostic tests and patient visits, increases revenues. In a capitated environment

in which one fee is paid for all services provided, increasing the overall number of patients served and decreasing the volume of services used is desirable. With capitation, nurses must strive to accomplish more with each visit to decrease return visits and complications. In today's value-based purchasing environment and reimbursement methodology, nurses need to understand their organization's reimbursement environment, identify how they can influence patient outcomes such as hospital-acquired conditions (HACs), patient satisfaction, and strategy for realizing a profit in its specific circumstances.

Knowing Costs and Reimbursement Practices

As direct caregivers and case managers, nurses are constantly involved in determining the type and quantity of resources used for patients. This includes supplies, personnel, and time. Nurses need to know what costs are generated by their decisions and actions. Nurses also need to know what items cost and how they are paid for in an organization so that they can make cost-effective decisions. For example, nurses need to know per-item costs for supplies so that they can appropriately evaluate lower-cost substitutes.

Case management has become a very important role for all acute care organizations. Nurses must partner with case management in reaching organizational goals. The ideal partnership includes the following contribution by the nursing staff: knowledge of patient goals, expected outcomes, and anticipated discharge date; comprehensive assessment of the patient and family; appropriate and timely interventions when the patient is not progressing as expected; appropriate management of pain, activity, skin integrity, bowel and bladder integrity, and cognition; ongoing patient and family education regarding discharge planning and preventing readmission; and identifying barriers to discharge (Bower, 2013).

In ambulatory and home health settings, nurses must be familiar with the various insurance plans that reimburse the organization. Each plan has different contract rules regarding preauthorization, types of services covered, required vendors, and so on. Although nurses must develop and implement their plans of care with full knowledge of these reimbursement practices, the payer does not totally drive the care. Nurses still advocate for patients in important ways while also working within the cost and contractual constraints. Moreover, when nurses understand the reimbursement practices, they can help patients maximize the resources available to them.

In hospitals, the cost of nursing care usually is not calculated or billed separately to patients; instead, it is part of the general per-diem charge. One major problem with this method is the assumption that all patients consume the same amount of nursing care and the acuity of the patient is not considered. Another problem with bundling the charges for nursing care with the room rate is that nursing as a clinical service is not perceived by management as generating revenue for the hospital. Rather, nursing is perceived predominantly as an expense to the organization. Although this perception may not matter in a capitated setting in which all provider services are considered a cost, accurate nursing care cost data are needed to negotiate managed care contracts. In addition, patients do not see direct charges and so have no way to understand the monetary value of the services they receive.

EXERCISE 12-5
How was nursing care charged on the bill you obtained? What are the implications for nursing in being perceived as an expense rather than being associated with the revenue stream? Why will this perception be less important in a capitated environment?

Capturing All Charges in a Timely Fashion

Nurses also help contain costs by ensuring that all possible charges are captured. Several large hospitals report more than $1 million a year lost from supplies that were not charged. In hospitals, nurses must know which supplies are charged to patients and which ones are charged to the unit. In addition, the procedures and equipment used need to be accurately documented. In ambulatory and community settings, nurses often need to keep abreast of the codes that are used to bill services. These codes change yearly, and sometimes items are bundled together under one charge and sometimes they are broken down into different charges. Turning in charges in a timely manner is also important because delayed billing negatively affects cash flow by extending the time before an organization is paid for services provided. This is particularly significant in smaller organizations.

EXERCISE 12-6
You used three intravenous (IV) catheters to do a particularly difficult venipuncture. Do you charge the patient for all three catheters? What if you accidentally contaminated one by touching the sheet? How is the catheter paid for if not charged to the patient? Who benefits and who loses when patients are not charged for supplies?

Using Time Efficiently

The adage that time is money is fitting in health care and refers to both the nurse's time and the patient's time. When nurses are organized and efficient in their care delivery and in scheduling and coordinating patients' care, the organization will save money. In a value-based purchasing environment, doing as much as possible during each episode of care is particularly important to decrease repeat visits and unnecessary service utilization. Because LOS is the most important predictor of hospital costs (Finkler, Jones, & Kovner 2013), patients who stay extra days cost the hospital a considerable amount. Decreasing LOS also makes room for other patients, thereby potentially increasing patient volume and hospital revenues. Nurses can become more efficient and effective by evaluating their major work processes and eliminating areas of redundancy and rework. Automated clinical information systems that support integrated practice at the point of care will also increase efficiency and improve patient outcomes.

EXERCISE 12-7
The Visiting Nurse Association (VNA) cannot file for reimbursement until all documentation of each visit has been completed. Typically, the paperwork is submitted a week after the visit. When the number of home visits increases rapidly, the paperwork often is not turned in for 2 weeks or more. What are the implications of this routine practice for the agency? Why would the VNA be very vulnerable financially during periods of heavy workload? What are some options for the nurse manager to consider to expedite the paperwork?

Discussing the Cost of Care with Patients

Talking with patients about the cost of care is important, although it may be uncomfortable. Discovering during a clinic visit that a patient cannot afford a specific medication or intervention is preferable to finding out several days later in a follow-up call that the patient has not taken the medication. Such information compels the clinical management team to explore optional treatment plans or to find resources to cover the costs. Talking with patients about costs is important in other ways, too. It involves the patients in the decision-making process and increases the likelihood that treatment plans will be followed. Patients also can make informed choices and better use the resources available to them if they have appropriate information about costs.

EXERCISE 12-8
A new patient visits the clinic and is given prescriptions for three medications that will cost about $120 per month. You check her chart and discover that she has Medicare (but not Part D) and no supplemental insurance. How can you determine whether she has the resources to buy this medicine each month and if she is willing to buy it? If she cannot afford the medications, what are some options?

Evaluating Cost-Effectiveness of New Technologies

Cost-effectiveness is defined as a method to achieve a specific outcome for the least possible cost. The advent of new technologies is presenting dilemmas in managing costs. In the past, if a new piece of equipment was easier to use or benefited the patient in any way, nurses were apt to want to use it for everyone, no matter how much more it cost. Now they are forced to make decisions regarding which patients really need the new equipment and which ones will have good outcomes with the current equipment. Essentially, nurses are analyzing the cost-effectiveness of the new equipment with regard to different types of patients to allocate limited resources. This is a new and sometimes difficult way to think about patient care and at times may not feel like a caring way to make these decisions. However, such decisions conserve resources without jeopardizing patients' health and thus create the possibility of providing additional healthcare services.

EXERCISE 12-9
Last year, a new positive-pressure, needleless system for administering IV antibiotics was introduced. Because the system was so easy to use and convenient for patients, the nurses in the home infusion company where you worked ordered it for everyone. Typically, patients get their IV antibiotics four times each day. The minibags and tubing for the regular procedure cost the agency $22 a day. The new system costs $24 per medication administration, or $96 a day. The agency receives the same per-diem (daily) reimbursement for each patient. Discuss the financial implications for the agency if this practice is continued. Generate some optional courses of action for the nurses to consider. How should these options be evaluated? What secondary costs, such as the cost of treating fewer needle-stick injuries, should be included?

Predicting and Using Nursing Resources Efficiently

Because healthcare organizations are service institutions, the largest part of their operating budget typically is for personnel. For hospitals, in particular, nurses are the largest group of employees and often account for most of the personnel budget. Staffing is the major area nurse managers can affect with respect to managing costs, and supply management is the second area. To understand why this is so, it is helpful to understand the concepts of fixed and variable costs.

The total fixed costs in a unit are those costs that do not change as the volume of patients changes. In other words, with either a high or a low patient census, expenses related to rent, utilities, loan payments, administrative salaries, and salaries of the minimum number of staff to keep a unit open must be paid. Variable costs are costs that vary in direct proportion to patient volume or acuity. Examples include nursing personnel, supplies, and medications. Break-even analysis (BEA) is a tool that uses fixed and variable costs for determining the specific volume of patients needed to just break even (Revenue = Expenses) or to realize a profit or loss. BEA can be calculated using this formula:

$$\text{Break-Even Quantity (N)} = \frac{\text{Fixed Costs (FC)}}{\text{Price (P)} - \text{Variable Cost per Patient (VC)}}$$

In hospitals and community health agencies, patient classification systems are used to help managers predict nursing care requirements (see Chapter 14). These systems differentiate patients according to acuity of illness, functional status, and resource needs. Some nurses do not like these systems because they believe the essence of nursing is not captured. However, we need to remember that these are tools to help managers predict resource needs. Used appropriately, patient classification systems can help evaluate changing practice patterns and patient acuity levels as well as provide information for budgeting processes.

EXERCISE 12-10
Given the definitions for fixed and variable costs, why do you think nurse managers have the greatest influence over costs through management of staffing and supplies?

Managing staffing and decreasing LOS can achieve the most immediate reductions in costs. Hospitals strive to lower costs so that they will attract new contracts and be attractive as partners in provider networks. Therefore staffing methods and patient care delivery models are being closely scrutinized. Work redesign, a process for changing the way to think about and structure the work of patient care, is the predominant strategy for developing systems that better utilize high-cost professionals and improve service quality. Increased staff retention, patient safety, and positive patient outcomes result from effective work redesign processes.

Using Research to Evaluate Standard Nursing Practices

Nurses use research to restructure their work to ensure they add value for patients. In 2005, Koelling, Johnson, Cody, and Aaronson studied the effect of patient education by a nurse educator on the clinical outcomes of patients with heart failure and validated an approach to these patients. In this randomized, controlled trial, one group of patients received standard discharge information and the other group of patients received standard discharge information and 1 hour of one-on-one education from a nurse educator. All subjects were followed by telephone after discharge to collect data concerning post-hospitalization clinical events, symptoms, and self-care practices. Patients who received the additional 1-hour teaching session with the nurse educator showed improved clinical outcomes, increased adherence to self-care management, and reduced costs of care because of a reduction in re-hospitalizations. The costs of care, including the costs associated with the additional education session, resulted in a savings of $2823 per patient in the education group as compared with the control group. The findings from this economic evaluation support the implementation of nursing education programs for patients with chronic heart failure as evidenced by improved patient outcomes and reduced costs. Box 12-4 summarizes some cost-conscious strategies for nursing practice. Further, the Literature Perspective on p. 222 describes the need for a business case related to outcomes.

BOX 12-4 STRATEGIES FOR COST-CONSCIOUS NURSING PRACTICE

1. Understanding what is required to remain financially sound
2. Knowing costs and reimbursement practices
3. Capturing all possible charges in a timely fashion
4. Using time efficiently
5. Discussing the costs of care with patients
6. Partnering with case management in reaching organizational goals
7. Evaluating cost-effectiveness of new technologies
8. Predicting and using nursing resources efficiently
9. Using research to evaluate standard nursing practices

LITERATURE PERSPECTIVE

Resource: Virkstis, K.L., Westheim, J., Boston-Fleischhauer, C., Matsui, P.N., & Jaggi, T. (2009). Safeguarding quality: Building the business case to prevent nursing-sensitive hospital-acquired conditions. *The Journal of Nursing Administration, 39*(7/8), 350-355.

In October 2008, the Centers for Medicare & Medicaid Services (CMS) initiated a program that would negatively affect reimbursement for 11 hospital-acquired patient conditions that were judged reasonably preventable. CMS took the stand that it would decrease reimbursement if these conditions were not documented to be present on admission to the hospital. Four of the 11 conditions (catheter-associated urinary tract infections, falls and trauma, vascular catheter–associated infections, and stages III and IV pressure ulcers) have been identified as nursing-sensitive indicators. This article presents a review of the literature related to two of these nursing-sensitive indicators—patient falls and pressure ulcers. The authors found that the average cost burden for a hospital-acquired pressure ulcer ranged anywhere from $3529 per case to $52,931 per case. The average cost burden for a patient fall in the hospital was $15,418. The article includes tools that nursing leadership can use to estimate potential cost avoidance savings that can be recognized in their individual facilities for falls and pressure ulcers. Through their analysis, these authors found that the strongest business case for nursing leadership is to concentrate their efforts on cost savings through prevention of these two hospital-acquired conditions.

Implications for Practice

The findings from this study show that significant cost savings are associated with the prevention of two nursing-sensitive, hospital-acquired conditions—specifically, falls and pressure ulcers. Thus nurses must employ a comprehensive fall prevention and skin integrity program. Both programs should at a minimum offer a standardized screening process using a valid and reliable tool, an ability to identify those at risk via visual cues (for example, a complete assessment), the ability to consult a subject matter expert, and the development of a patient specific plan of care that will include targeted interventions aimed at mitigating the risk factors.

BUDGETS

The basic financial document in most healthcare organizations is the budget—a detailed financial plan for carrying out the activities an organization wants to accomplish for a certain period. An organizational budget is a formal plan that is stated in terms of dollars and includes proposed income and expenditures. The budgeting process is an ongoing activity in which plans are made and revenues and expenses are managed to meet or exceed the goals of the plan.

The management functions of planning and control are tied together through the budgeting process.

A budget requires managers to plan ahead and to establish explicit program goals and expectations. Changes in medical practices, reimbursement methods, competition, technology, demographics, and regulatory factors must be forecast to anticipate their effects on the organization. Planning encourages evaluation of different options and assists in more cost-effective use of resources.

EXERCISE 12-11

A community nursing organization performs an average of 36 intermittent catheterizations each day. A prepackaged catheterization kit that costs the organization $17 is used. The four items in the kit, when purchased individually, cost the organization a total of $5. What factors should be considered in evaluating the cost-effectiveness of the two sources of supplies?

TYPES OF BUDGETS

Several types of interrelated budgets are used by well-managed organizations. Major budgets that are discussed in this chapter include the operating budget, the capital budget, and the cash budget. The way these budgets complement and support one another is depicted in Figure 12-1. Many organizations also use program, product line, or special purpose budgets.

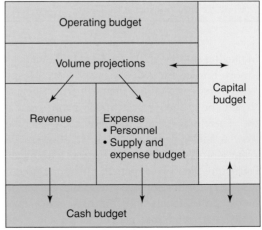

FIGURE 12-1 Interrelationships of the operating, capital, and cash budgets.

Long-range budgets are used to help managers plan for the future. Often, these are referred to as *strategic plans* (Finkler, Jones, & Kovner 2013).

Operating Budget

The operating budget is the financial plan for the day-to-day activities of the organization. The expected revenues and expenses generated from daily operations, given a specified volume of patients, are stated. Preparing and monitoring the operating budget, particularly the expense portion, is often the most time-consuming financial function of nurse managers.

The expense part of the operating budget consists of a personnel budget and a supply and expense budget for each cost center. A cost center is an organizational unit for which costs can be identified and managed. The personnel budget is the largest part of the operating budget for most nursing units. (See The Evidence section on p. 229.)

Before the personnel budget can be established, the volume of work predicted for the budget period must be calculated. A unit of service measure appropriate to the work of the unit is used. Units of service may be, for example, patient days, clinic or home visits, hours of service, admissions, deliveries, or treatments. Another factor needed to calculate the workload is the patient acuity mix. The formula for calculating the workload or the required patient care hours for inpatient units is as follows: Workload volume = Hours of care per patient day × Number of patient days (Table 12-2).

In some organizations, the workload is established by the financial office and given to the nurse manager. In other organizations, nurse managers forecast the volume. In both situations, nurse managers should inform administrators about any factors that might affect the accuracy of the forecast, such as changes in physician practice patterns, new treatment modalities, changes in inpatient versus outpatient treatment practices, and changes in technology or equipment.

The next step in preparing the personnel budget is to determine how many staff members will be needed to provide the care. (This topic is discussed in more detail in Chapter 14.) Because some people work full-time and others work part-time, full-time equivalents (FTEs) are used in this step rather than positions. Generally, one FTE can be equated to working 40 hours per week, 52 weeks per year, for a total of 2080 hours of work paid per year. One half of an FTE (0.5 FTE) equates to 20 hours per week. The number of hours per FTE may vary within an organization in relation to staffing plans, so it is important to check.

The 2080 hours paid to an FTE in a year consists of both productive hours and nonproductive hours. Productive hours are paid time that is worked. Nonproductive hours are paid time that is not worked, such as vacation, holiday, orientation, and sick time. Education may be viewed as either depending on the organization's value for learning. Before the number of FTEs needed for the workload can be calculated, the number of productive hours per FTE is determined by subtracting the total number of nonproductive hours per FTE from total paid hours. Alternatively, payroll reports can be reviewed to determine the percentage of paid hours that are productive for each FTE. Finally, the total number of FTEs needed to provide the care is calculated by dividing

TABLE 12-2 WORKLOAD CALCULATION (TOTAL REQUIRED PATIENT CARE HOURS)

PATIENT ACUITY LEVEL*	HOURS OF CARE PER PATIENT DAY (HPPD)†	×	PATIENT DAYS‡	=	WORKLOAD§
1	3.0		900		2700
2	5.2		3100		16,120
3	8.8		4000		35,200
4	13.0		1600		20,800
5	19.0		400		7600
Total			10,000		82,420

*1, Low; *5*, high.
†High. Number of hours of care needed based on acuity levels and numbers.
‡High. Number of hour 1 patient day.
§Total number of hours of care needed based on acuity levels and numbers of patient days.

BOX 12-5   PRODUCTIVE HOURS CALCULATION

Method 1:   ***Add All Nonproductive Hours/FTE and Subtract from Paid Hours/FTE***

Example:	Vacation	15 days
	Holiday	7 days
	Average sick time	4 days
	Total	26 days

$26 \times 8*$ hours = 208 nonproductive hours/FTE
$2080 - 208 = 1872$ productive hours/FTE

Method 2:   ***Multiply Paid Hours/FTE by Percentage of Productive Hours/FTE***

Example: Productive hours = 90%/FTE
(1872 productive hours of total 2080 = 90%)
$2080 \times 0.90 = 1872$ productive hours/FTE

Total FTE Calculation

Required Patient Care Hours	÷	Productive Hours Per FTE	=	Total FTEs Needed
82,420	÷	1872		= 44 FTEs

FTE, Full-time equivalent.
*Full-time equivalent. FTE pattern.

the total patient care hours required by the number of productive hours per FTE (Box 12-5).

The total number of FTEs calculated by this method represents the number needed to provide care each day of the year. The total FTEs does not reflect the number of positions or the number of people working each day. In fact, the number of positions may be much higher, particularly if many part-time nurses are employed. On any given day, some nurses may be scheduled for their regular day off or vacation and others may be off because of illness. Also, some positions that do not involve direct patient care, such as nurse managers or unit secretaries, may not be replaced during nonproductive time. Only one FTE is budgeted for any position that is not covered with other staff when the employee is off.

EXERCISE 12-12

Change the number of patients at each acuity level listed in Table 12-2, but keep the total number of patients the same. Recalculate the required total workload. Discuss how changes in patient acuity affect nursing resource requirements.

The next step is to prepare a daily staffing plan and to establish positions (see Chapter 14). Once the positions are established, the labor costs that comprise the personnel budget can be calculated. Factors that must

be addressed include straight-time hours, overtime hours, differentials and premium pay, raises, and benefits (Finkler, Jones, & Kovner 2013). Differentials and premiums are extra pay for working specific times, such as evening or night shifts and holidays. Benefits usually include health and life insurance, Social Security payments, and retirement plans. Benefits often cost an additional 25% to 30% of a full-time employee's salary. In other words, about one third of the employee expenses are related to benefits and have to be seriously considered when adding an FTE.

The supply and expense budget is often called the *other-than-personnel services (OTPS) expense budget.*

EXERCISE 12-13

If the percentage of productive hours per FTE is 80%, how many worked or productive hours are there per FTE? If total patient care hours are 82,420, how many FTEs will be needed?

This budget includes a variety of items used in daily unit activities, such as medical and office supplies, minor equipment, and books and journals; it also includes orientation, training, and travel. Although different methods are used to calculate the supply and expense budget, the previous year's expenses usually are used as a baseline. This baseline is adjusted for projected patient volume and specific circumstances known to affect expenses, such as predictable personnel turnover, which increases orientation and training expenses. A percentage factor is also added to adjust for inflation.

The final component of the operating budget is the revenue budget. The revenue budget projects the income that the organization will receive for providing patient care. Historically, nurses have not been directly involved with developing the revenue budget, although this is beginning to change. In most hospitals, the revenue budget is established by the financial office and given to nurse managers. The anticipated revenues are calculated according to the price per patient day. Data about the volume and types of patients and reimbursement sources (i.e., the **case mix** and the **payer mix**) are necessary to project revenues in any healthcare organization. Even when nurse managers do not participate in developing the revenue budget, learning about the organization's revenue base is essential for good decision making.

Capital Expenditure Budget

The **capital expenditure budget** reflects expenses related to the purchase of major capital items such as equipment and physical plant. A capital expenditure must have a useful life of more than 1 year and must exceed a cost level specified by the organization. The minimum cost requirement for capital items in healthcare organizations is usually from $300 to $1000, although some organizations have a much higher level. Anything below that minimum is considered a routine operating cost.

Capital expenses are kept separate from the operating budget because their high cost would make the costs of providing patient care appear too high during the year of purchase. To account for capital expenses, the costs of capital items are depreciated. This means that each year, over the useful life of the equipment, a portion of its cost is allocated to the operating budget as an expense. Therefore capital expenditures are subtracted from revenues and, in turn, affect profits.

Organizations usually set aside a fixed amount of money for capital expenditures each year. Complete well-documented justifications are needed because the competition for limited resources is stiff. Justifications should be developed using the principle of any business case and should include at minimum projected amount of use; services duplicated or replaced; safety considerations; need for space, personnel, or building renovation; effect on operational revenues and expenses; and contribution to the strategic plan.

Cash Budget

The cash budget is the operating plan for monthly cash receipts and disbursements. Organizational survival depends on paying bills on time. Organizations can be making a profit and still run out of cash. In fact, a profitable trend, such as a rapidly growing census, can induce a cash shortage because of increased expenses in the short run. Major capital expenditures can also cause a temporary cash crisis and so must be staggered in a strategic way. Because cash is the lifeblood of any organization, the cash budget is as important as the operating and capital budgets.

The financial officer prepares the cash budget in large organizations. Understanding the cash budget helps nurse managers discern (1) when constraints on spending are necessary, even when the expenditures are budgeted, and (2) the importance of carefully predicting when budgeted items will be needed.

THE BUDGETING PROCESS

The steps in the budgeting process are similar in most healthcare organizations, although the budgeting period, budget timetable, and level of manager and employee participation vary. Budgeting is done annually and in relation to the organization's fiscal year. A fiscal year exists for financial purposes and can begin at any point on the calendar. In the title of some financial reports, a phrase similar to "FYE June 30, 2015" appears and means that this report is for the fiscal year ending on the date stated.

Major steps in the budgeting process include gathering information and planning, developing unit budgets, developing the cash budget, negotiating and revising, and using feedback to control budget results and improve future plans (Finkler & McHugh, 2007). A timetable with specific dates for implementing the budgeting process is developed by each organization. The timetable may be anywhere from 3 to 9 months. The widespread use of computers for budgeting is reducing the time span for budgeting in many organizations. Box 12-6 outlines the budgeting process.

The information-gathering and planning phase provides nurse managers with data essential for

BOX 12-6   OUTLINE OF BUDGETING PROCESS

1. Gathering information and planning
   - Environmental assessment
   - Mission, goals, and objectives
   - Program priorities
   - Financial objectives
   - Assumptions (employee raises, inflation, volume projections)
2. Developing unit and departmental budgets
   - Operating budgets
   - Capital budgets
3. Developing cash budgets
4. Negotiating and revising
5. Evaluating
   - Analysis of variance
   - Critical performance reports

Modified from Finkler, S. A., Kovner, C. T., & Jones, C. (2007). *Financial management for nurse managers and executives* (3rd ed.). St. Louis: Saunders.

developing their individual budgets. This step begins with an environmental assessment that helps the organization understand its position in relation to the entire community. The assessment includes, for example, the changing healthcare needs of the population, influential economic factors such as inflation and unemployment, differences in reimbursement patterns, and patient satisfaction.

Next, the organization's long-term goals and objectives are reassessed in light of the organization's mission and the environmental analysis. This helps all managers situate the budgeting process for their individual units in relation to the whole organization. At this point, programs are prioritized so that resources can be allocated to programs that best help the organization achieve its long-term goals.

Specific, measurable objectives are then established, and the budgets must meet these objectives. The financial objectives might include limiting expenditure increases or making reductions in personnel costs by designated percentages. Nurse managers also set operational objectives for their units that are in concert with the rest of the organization. This is where units or departments interpret what effect the changes in operational activities will have on them. For instance, how will using case managers and care maps for selected patients affect a particular unit? Establishing the unit-level objectives is also a good place for involving direct care nurses in setting the future direction of the unit.

Along with the specific organization and unit-level operating objectives, managers need the organization-wide assumptions that underpin the budgeting process. Explicit assumptions regarding salary increases, inflation factors, and volume projections for the next fiscal year are essential. With this information in hand, nurse managers can develop the operating and capital budgets for their units. These are usually developed in tandem because each affects the other. For instance, purchasing a new monitoring system will have implications for the supplies used, staffing, and staff training.

The cash budget is developed after unit and department operating and capital budgets. Then the negotiation and revision process begins in earnest. This is a complex process because changes in one budget usually require changes in others. Learning to defend and negotiate budgets is an important skill for nurse managers. Nurse managers who successfully negotiate budgets know how costs are allocated and are comfortable speaking about what resources are contained in each budget category. They also can clearly and specifically depict what the effect of not having that resource will be on patient, nurse, or organizational outcomes.

EXERCISE 12-14

If you can interview a nurse manager, ask to review the budgeting process. Ask specifically about the budget timetable, operating objectives, and organizational assumptions. What was the level of involvement for nurse managers and nurses in each step of budget preparation? Is there a budget manual?

The final and ongoing phase of the budgeting process relates to the control function of management. Feedback is obtained regularly so that organizational activities can be adjusted to maintain efficient operations. Variance analysis is the major control process used. A variance is the difference between the projected budget and the actual performance for a particular account. For expenses, a favorable, or positive, variance means that the budgeted amount was greater than the actual amount spent. An unfavorable, or negative, variance means that the budgeted amount was less than the actual amount spent. Positive and negative variances cannot be interpreted as good or bad without further investigation. For example, if fewer supplies were used than were budgeted, this would appear as a positive variance and the unit would save money. This would be good news if it means that supplies were used more efficiently and patient outcomes remained the same or improved. A problem might be suggested, however, if using fewer or less-expensive supplies led to poorer patient outcomes. Or it might mean that exactly the right amount of supplies was used but that the patient census was less than budgeted. To help managers interpret and use variance information better, some institutions use flexible budgets that automatically account for census variances.

EXERCISE 12-15

Examine Table 12-3 and identify major budget variances for the current month. Are they favorable or unfavorable? What additional information would help you explain the variances? What are some possible causes for each variance? Are the causes you identified controllable by the nurse manager? Why or why not? Is a favorable variance on expenses always desirable? Why or why not?

MANAGING THE UNIT-LEVEL BUDGET

How is a unit-based budget managed? At a minimum, nurse managers are responsible for meeting the fiscal goals related to the personnel and the supply and expense part of the operations budget. Typically, monthly reports of operations (Table 12-3) are sent to nurse managers, who then investigate and explain the underlying cause of variances greater than 5%. Many factors can cause budget variances, including patient census, patient acuity, vacation and benefit time, illness, orientation, staff meetings, workshops, employee mix, salaries, and staffing levels. To accurately interpret budget variances, nurse managers need reliable data about patient census, acuity, and LOS; payroll reports; and unit productivity reports.

Nurse managers can control *some* of the factors that cause variances, but not all. After the causes are determined and if they are controllable by the nurse manager, steps are taken to prevent the variance from occurring in the future. However, even uncontrollable variances that increase expenses might require actions of nurse managers. For example, if supply costs rise drastically because a new technology is being used, the nurse manager might have to look for other areas

where the budget can be cut. Information learned from analyzing variances also is used in future budget preparations and management activities.

In addition, nurse managers monitor the productivity of their units. **Productivity** is the ratio of outputs to inputs; that is, productivity equals output/input. In nursing, outputs are nursing services and are measured by hours of care, number of home visits, and so forth. The inputs are the resources used to provide the services such as personnel hours and supplies. Only decreasing the inputs or increasing the outputs can increase productivity. Hospitals often use hours per patient day (HPPD) as one measure of productivity. For example, if the standard of care in a critical care unit is 12 HPPD, then 360 hours of care are required for 30 patients for 1 day. When 320 hours of care are provided, the productivity rating is 113% (360/320 = 1.13), meaning productivity was increased or needed care was not delivered. One must consider the quality component into any productivity model related to care. In home health, the number of visits per day per registered nurse is one measure of productivity. If the standard is 5 visits per day but the weekly average was 4.8 visits per day, then productivity was decreased. Variances in productivity are not inherently favorable or unfavorable and thus require investigation and explanation before judgments can be made about them. For example, an explanation of the variance (4.8 visits per day) might include the fact that one visit took twice the amount of time normally spent on a home visit because of patient needs, thus preventing the nurse from making the standard 5 visits per day. The extra time spent on one patient was productive time but not adequately accounted for by this measure of productivity (visits per day).

Although they do not have a direct accountability for the budget, direct care nurses play an important role in meeting budget expectations. Many nurse managers find that routinely sharing the budget and budget-monitoring activities with the whole team fosters an appreciation of the relationship between cost and the mission to deliver high-quality patient care. Providing the team with access to cost and utilization data allows them to identify patterns and participate in selecting appropriate, cost-effective practice options that work for the staff and patients. Managers and staff who work in partnership to understand that cost versus care is a dilemma to manage rather

TABLE 12-3 STATEMENT OF OPERATIONS SHOWING PROFIT AND LOSS FROM A NEIGHBORHOOD NURSING CENTER: MARCH 31, 2010

CURRENT MONTH				YEAR-TO-DATE		
BUDGET	ACTUAL	VARIANCE	REVENUES	BUDGET	ACTUAL	VARIANCE
Patient Revenues						
21,500	22,050	550	Insurance payment	64,500	66,150	1650
1500	1550	50	Donations	4500	4750	250
23,000	23,600	600	Net Patient Revenues	69,000	70,900	1900
Non-Patient Revenues						
5000	5000	0	Grant income (#138-FG)	15,000	15,000	0
500	500	0	Rent income	1500	1500	0
5500	5500	0	Net Non-patient Revenues	16,500	16,500	0
28,500	29,100	600	Net Revenues	85,500	87,400	1900
Expenses						
PERSONNEL						
7750	8500	(750)	Managerial/ professional	23,250	24,400	(1150)
2000	1800	200	Clerical/ technical	6000	5800	200
9750	10,300	(550)	Net salaries and wages	29,250	30,200	(950)
1200	1400	(200)	Benefits	3600	4000	(400)
10,950	11,700	(750)	Net Personnel	32,850	34,200	(1350)
NON-PERSONNEL						
2500	2500	0	Office operating expenses	7500	7500	0
2000	2100	(100)	Supplies and materials	3000	3050	(50)
300	450	(150)	Travel expenses	900	450	450
4800	5050	(250)	Net Non-personnel	11,400	11,000	400
15,750	16,750	(1000)	Net Expenses	44,250	45,200	(950)
Revenues Over/Under Expenses						
3750	3350	(400)	Net Income	11,250	11,800	550

than a problem to solve will develop innovative, cost-conscious nursing practices that produce good outcomes for patients, nurses, and the organization.

CONCLUSION

Managing costs and understanding budgets are important information for nurses in all positions within the organization. The current emphasis on "value" makes knowing what costs are and how to control them important. Being able to understand the basics of a budget helps nurses at all levels in an organization cite the economic impact of decisions related to care. Considering the paramount influence that nurses have on establishing the value contribution, taking actions at the point of care (such as capturing charges in a timely manner) are as important as actions in the manager's office (such as ensuring proper resource allocation) or actions in the executive suite (such as projecting patient volume or changes in delivery).

In order to further develop the value proposition, the importance of engaging the entire team can't be overstated. Planning significantly impacts the final outcome, which puts nursing in a positive or limited perspective in an organization.

THE SOLUTION

I began by investigating the reasons for our decreased admissions and shift in payer mix. I discovered that one of our highest admitting physicians is now admitting his patients to a competing hospital. I met with him to determine why his admission pattern had changed. Most of his patients are employed in a local industry, and that healthcare provider is Reform Health Insurance (RHI). THCS recently dropped our contract with RHI. His patients are requesting hospitalization at our competitor to stay in-network with their health insurance plan.

In an effort to reduce labor costs without compromising quality patient care, I focused on staffing appropriately to census and patient acuity. During times of low census, staff are now flexed and floated to other MSS units with greater staffing needs. In return, during times of high census, nurses from other units are flexed and floated to our unit.

Our Staff Nurse Council developed an initiative to reduce overtime. The reason for most of our overtime is charting at the end of shift. The overtime reduction initiative emphasizes improved teamwork and concurrent charting to reduce end-of-shift charting.

THCS secured a new contract with RHI, which resulted in an increase in census. Flexing and floating staff continues to be challenging. Nurses prefer to work on their "home" unit but appreciate that their hours are not cut if they float to another MSS unit. The staff-driven initiative regarding overtime has been our biggest success. In an effort to ensure that no nurse has overtime at the end of the shift, the nurses are collaborating, communicating, and supporting each other throughout the shift to facilitate concurrent charting. This effort has improved our financial performance and our employee engagement through a stronger sense of teamwork. Because of the combined efforts of nursing leadership, collaboration with physicians, and innovative initiatives by the frontline staff, we have had no staff reductions, and our financial performance is better than budget.

—*Marcus Johnson*

Would this be a suitable approach for you? Why?

THE EVIDENCE

Anderson and Shelton (2006) share the experiences of two merging hospitals and their use of the same nursing department scheduling system. One hospital used the system for staff scheduling, whereas the other hospital used it for workload measure and management decision making. Staff and leadership personnel were taught the entire content of the system, because information from this system would influence decision making at all levels within the organization. Consistent use of the product produced data that could be drilled down by cost center on FTEs overall, per patient day, overtime, and professional time. This collection of data proved to be invaluable for managers at all levels for both scheduling and overall labor management. Recently, an additional tool included in the system has been instituted to automate shift selections for staff. This feature allows managers to post openings in shifts 6 weeks in advance. Through the computerized system, nurses can easily pick up these additional open shifts. Employee satisfaction has improved as nurses gained more control over their schedules. Full use of the department scheduling system has been linked to improved nurse recruitment and retention. The nurse vacancy rate dropped from 14% to 3%, and nurse turnover dropped to 4% to 5%.

WHAT NEW GRADUATES SAY

- I can see why understanding more about budgets now is so important.
- Because I work part-time while I am enrolled in a graduate program, I can appreciate how the organization's income affects mine.

- Healthcare financing is so complicated. I had no idea that hospitals do not get dollar for dollar what has been billed to payers.
- I think that pay for performance is an excellent way to hold hospitals, nurses, and doctors accountable for the care and services delivered.

- I had no idea how much I can make a difference in my department budget by being careful about the supplies that I use when performing a nursing task.
- I never thought about it this way, but I understand how important it is to determine and advertise the value contribution of nursing services.
- Now I understand why I have to make sure I practice using the latest evidence-based information.

Because this may impact hospital-acquired infection and in turn can affect the reimbursement of my hospital.
- It's very important for me that my patients are always satisfied with my services. It is even more important now that I understand it can also impact the hospital reimbursement.

CHAPTER CHECKLIST

Financial thinking skills are the cornerstone of cost-conscious nursing practice and are essential for all nurses. Nurses must also determine whether the services they provide add value for patients. Services that add value are of high quality, positively affect health outcomes, and minimize costs.

Understanding what constitutes profit and why organizations must make a profit to survive is basic to financial thinking. Knowing what is included in operating, capital, and cash budgets; how they interrelate; and how they are developed, monitored, and controlled is also important. Considering the ethical implications of financial decisions and collectively managing the cost-care dilemma are imperative for cost-conscious nursing practice.

- What escalates healthcare costs?
- How is healthcare financed?
- Healthcare reimbursement
- The changing healthcare economic environment
- What does this mean for nursing practice?

- Why is profit necessary?
- Cost-conscious nursing practices
  - Understanding what is required to remain financially sound
  - Knowing costs and reimbursement practices
  - Capturing all charges in a timely fashion
  - Using time efficiently
  - Discussing the cost of care with patients
  - Evaluating cost-effectiveness of new technologies
  - Predicting and using nursing resources efficiently
  - Using research to evaluate standard nursing practices
- Budgets
- Types of budgets
  - Operating budget
  - Capital expenditure budget
  - Cash budget
- The budgeting process
- Managing the unit-level budget

TIPS FOR MANAGING COSTS AND BUDGETS

- Know the major changes in the organization and how they might affect the organization's budget.
- Analyze the supplies you use in providing care and what is commonly missing as one way to make recommendations about supply needs.
- Evaluate what each of your patients would find most helpful during the time you will be caring for them.
- Decide which of your actions create costs for the patient or the organization.

- Be aware of how changes in patient acuity and patient census affect staffing requirements and the unit budget.
- Know how charges are generated and how the documentation systems relate to billing.
- Be knowledgeable about the anticipated discharge day and discharge plan, and include the patient and the family in the plan upon admission.
- Examine the upsides and downsides of the cost-care polarity thoughtfully.

REFERENCES

Anderson, D. J., & Shelton, W. (2006). Clarify your financial picture with staff management tools. *Nursing Management, 37*(7), 49–51.

Bodenheimer, T., & Grumbach, K. (2009). *Understanding health policy: A clinical approach* (5th ed.). New York: McGraw-Hill.

Bower, K. A. (2013). Managing care: The crucial nursing-case management partnership. *Nurse Leader, 10*(6), 26–29.

Brooks, J. M., Titler, M. G., Ardery, G., & Herr, K. (2009). Effect of evidence-based acute pain management practices on inpatient costs. *Health Services Research, 44*(1), 245–263.

Centers for Medicare & Medicaid Services. (2011a). *Hospital value-based purchasing program.* Retrieved January 20, 2013, from, www.cms.gov/Outreach-and-Education/Medicare-Learning-Network-MLN/MLNProducts/downloads/Hospital_VBPurchasing_Fact_Sheet_ICN907664.pdf.

Centers for Medicare & Medicaid Services (CMS). (2011b). *National health expenditure projections 2011–2021.* Retrieved January 20th 2013, from, www.cms.gov/Research-Statistics-Data-and-Systems/Statistics-Trends-and-Reports/NationalHealthExpendData/Downloads/Proj2011PDF.pdf.

Centers for Medicare & Medicaid Services. (2013). *National health expenditures 2011 highlights.* Retrieved January 21st 2013 from, http://cms.gov/Research-Statistics-Data-and-Systems/Statistics-Trends-and-Reports/NationalHealthExpendData/Downloads/highlights.pdf.

Finkler, S. A., Jones, C., & Kovner, C. T. (2007). *Financial management for nurse managers and executives* (4th ed.). St. Louis: Saunders.

Finkler, S. A., Jones, C. B., & Kovner, C. T. (2013). *Financial management for nurse managers and executives* (5th ed.). St. Louis, Missouri: Saunders.

Finkler, S. A., & McHugh, M. L. (2007). *Budgeting concepts for nurse managers* (4th ed.). St. Louis, Missouri: Saunders.

Healthy people 2020. (2011). Retrieved January 20, 2013, from, www.healthypeople.gov.

Kaiser Family Foundation. (2004). *Prescription drug coverage for medicare beneficiaries: An overview of the medicare prescription drug, improvement, and modernization act of 2003.* Retrieved on January 21, 2013, from, www.kff.org/medicare/upload/Prescription-Drug-Coverage-for-Medicare-Beneficiares-An-Overview-of-the-Medicare-Prescription-Drug-Improvement-Act-2003.pdf.

Kaiser Family Foundation. (2011). *Kaiser Commission on medicaid and the uninsured.* Retrieved January 20, 2013 from, www.kff.org/medicaid/upload/8165.pdf.

Koelling, T. M., Johnson, M. L., Cody, R. J., & Aaronson, K. D. (2005). Discharge education improves clinical outcomes in patients with chronic heart failure. *Circulation, 111,* 179–185.

Virkstis, K. L., Westheim, J., Boston-Fleischhauer, C., Matsui, P. N., & Jaggi, T. (2009). Safeguarding quality: Building the business case to prevent nursing-sensitive hospital-acquired conditions. *The Journal of Nursing Administration, 39*(7/8), 350–355.

SUGGESTED READINGS

Aiken, L. H. (2008). Economics of nursing. *Policy, Politics & Nursing Practice, 9*(2), 73–79.

Birmingham, S. E. (2010). Evidence-based staffing: The next step. *Nurse Leader, 8*(3), 24–26, 35.

Cleverley, W., Cleverley, J. O., & Song, P. H. (2010). *Essentials of health care finance* (7th ed.). Sudbury, MA: Jones & Bartlett Publishers.

Dunham-Taylor, J., & Pinczuk, J. Z. (2010). *Financial management for nurse managers: Merging the heart with the dollar* (2nd ed.). Boston, MA: Jones & Bartlett Publishers.

Finkler, S., Ward, D., & Calabrese, T. (2012). *Accounting fundamentals for health care management* (2nd ed.). Sudbury, MA: Jones & Bartlett Publishers.

Huber, D. (2010). *Leadership & nursing care management* (4th ed.). St. Louis: Saunders.

Kane, R. L., Shamliyan, T. A., Mueller, C., Duval, S., & Wilt, T. J. (2007). The association of registered nurse staffing levels and patient outcomes: Systematic review and meta-analysis. *Medical Care, 45*(12), 1195–1204.

Kovner, A. R., & Knickman, J. R. (2011). *Health care delivery in the United States* (10th ed.). New York: Springer Publishing Company.

Mark, B. A., & Harless, D. W. (2011). Adjusting for patient acuity in measurement of nurse staffing: Two approaches. *Nursing Research, 60*(2), 107–114.

Newbold, D. (2008). The production economics of nursing: A discussion paper. *International Journal of Nursing Studies, 45,* 120–128.

13

Care Delivery Strategies

Susan Sportsman

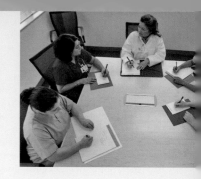

This chapter introduces nursing care delivery models used in healthcare agencies to organize care. The historical development and structure of the case method; functional nursing; team nursing; primary nursing, including hybrid forms of this approach; and nursing case management are presented. The discussion summarizes an overview of key concepts associated with each care delivery model, including the benefits and disadvantages with an explanation of the nurse manager's and direct care nurse's role. In addition, strategies that influence care delivery, such as differentiated practice, "transforming care at the bedside," and transitions models to help patients move through various levels of care are discussed.

LEARNING OUTCOMES

- Differentiate the characteristics of nursing care delivery models used in health care.
- Determine the role of the nurse manager and the direct care nurse in each model.
- Summarize the differentiated nursing practice model and related methods to determine competencies of nurses who deliver care.
- Consider the impact of Transforming Care at the Bedside (TCAB) on the delivery of care in a specific nursing unit.
- Evaluate the effectiveness of transitional care models aimed at reducing unnecessary re-hospitalizations.

KEY TERMS

advanced generalist
associate nurse
case-management model
case manager
case method
charge nurse
clinical nurse leader
critical pathway
differentiated nursing practice
expected outcomes
functional model of nursing

Magnet Recognition Program®
nurse navigator
nursing care delivery model
nursing case management
outcome criteria
patient-focused care
patient outcomes
practice partnership model
primary nurse
primary nursing
staff mix

Synergy Model
team nursing
total patient care
Transforming Care at the Bedside (TCAB)
transitional care models
unlicensed assistive (or nursing) personnel
variances

Jacqueline Ward, RN, BSN
Assistant Director of Nursing, Texas Children's Hospital,
   Houston, Texas

The charge nurses on a newly designed 36-bed hematology-oncology unit were having increased difficulty in making patient assignments because of the layout and design of the 36,000 sq ft unit. In addition, throughout the shift, the nursing staff members were having difficulty remaining engaged with the activities on the unit because of the distance between bedside stations. Also, the layout of the unit made it difficult for a nurse to ask for help when needed.

After occupying the unit for several months and trying diverse methods to enhance teamwork and communication among the staff, it was apparent that a more formal process was needed to resolve these problems. The assistant director of nursing was assigned to coordinate the resolution of the problem. What interdisciplinary resource might provide a helpful analysis or workflow process? What considerations could be made?

What do you think you would do if you were this nurse?

INTRODUCTION

A **nursing care delivery model** is the method used to provide care to patients. Because nursing care is viewed primarily as a cost rather than a source of revenue, institutions evaluate their method of providing patient care for the purpose of saving money, while still providing quality care. In this chapter, various models of nursing care delivery are discussed, including the case method (total patient care), functional nursing, team nursing, primary nursing including hybrid forms, and nursing case management. In addition, the influence of differentiated nursing practice, **Transforming Care at the Bedside,** and **transitional care models** are introduced.

Each nursing care delivery model has advantages and disadvantages, and no single method is ideal. Managers in any organization must examine the organizational goals, the unit objectives, patient population, staff availability, and the budget when selecting a care delivery model. Historical overviews of the common care models are designed to convey the complexity of how care is delivered. This perspective is important because each of these approaches is still used within the broad range of healthcare organizations. In addition, these models often serve as the foundation for new innovative care delivery models.

CASE METHOD (TOTAL PATIENT CARE)

The premise of the **case method** is that one nurse provides total care for one patient during the entire work period. This method was used in the era of Florence Nightingale when patients received total care in the home. Today, **total patient care** is used in critical care settings where one nurse provides total care to one or two critically ill patients. Nurse educators often select this method of care when students are caring for patients. Variations of the case method exist, and it is possible to identify similarities after reviewing other methods of patient care delivery described later in this chapter.

Model Analysis

One advantage for this model of care delivery is that during an 8- or 12-hour shift, the patient receives consistent care from one nurse who is accountable for the continuity of communication with all healthcare providers and implementing the plan of care. The nurse, patient, and family usually trust one another and can work together toward specific goals. Because the nurse is with the patient during most of the shift, even subtle changes in the patient's status are easily noticed (Figure 13-1). Usually, the plan of care is patient-centered, comprehensive, continuous, and holistic. However, if the nurse chooses to deliver this care with a task orientation, it would negate the holistic perspective (Tiedeman & Lookinland, 2004). This model of care should not be confused with nursing case management, which is introduced later in the chapter.

In today's costly healthcare economy, total patient care provided by a registered nurse (RN) is very expensive. Is it realistic to use the highly skilled and extremely knowledgeable professional nurse to provide all the care required in a unit that may have 20 to 30 patients? In times of nursing shortages, there may not be enough resources or nurses to use this model.

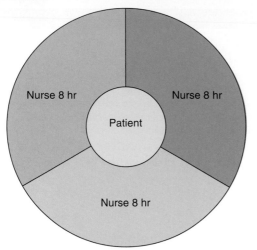

FIGURE 13-1 Case method of patient care for an 8-hour shift.

Nurse Manager's Role

When using the case method of delivery, the manager must consider the expense of the system. He or she must weigh the expense of an RN versus the expense of licensed practical/vocational nurses (LPNs/LVNs) and **unlicensed assistive (or nursing) personnel** (UAPs) in the context of the outcomes required. UAPs are not licensed as healthcare providers. In various healthcare organizations, they may be called technicians, nurse aides, or certified nursing assistants. When the patient requires 24-hour care, the nurse manager must decide whether the patient should have RN care or RN-supervised care provided by LPNs/LVNs or UAPs.

Direct Care Nurse's Role

In the case method, the direct care RN provides holistic care to a group of patients during a defined work time. The physical, emotional, and technical aspects of care are the responsibility of the assigned RN. This model is especially useful in the care of complex patients who need active symptom management provided by an RN, such as the care of the patient in a hospice setting or an intensive care unit. This care delivery model requires the nurse who is assigned to total patient care to complete the complex functions of care, such as assessment and teaching the patient and family, as well as the less complex functional aspects of care, such as personal hygiene. Some nurses find

satisfaction with this model of care because no aspect of nursing care is delegated to another, thus eliminating the need for supervision of others (Tiedeman & Lookinland, 2004).

EXERCISE 13-1

You have recently accepted a position at a home health agency that provides 24-hour care to qualified patients. You are assigned a patient who has care provided by an RN during the day, an LPN/LVN in the evening, and a nursing assistant at night. You are the day RN. You are concerned that the patient is not progressing well, and you suspect that the evening and night shift personnel are not reporting changes in the patient's status. What specific assessments should you make to validate your concerns? How would you justify any change in staffing? What recommendations would you make to the nurse manager, and why?

FUNCTIONAL NURSING

The functional model of nursing care delivery became popular during World War II when there was a severe shortage of nurses in the United States. Many nurses joined the armed forces to care for the soldiers. To provide care to patients at home, hospitals began to increase the number of LPNs/LVNs and UAPs.

The **functional model of nursing** is a method of providing patient care by which each licensed and unlicensed staff member performs specific tasks for a large group of patients. These tasks are in part determined by the scope of practice defined for each type of caregiver. For example, the RN must be responsible for all assessments, although the LPN/LVN and UAPs may collect data that can be used in the assessment. Regarding treatments, an RN may administer all intravenous (IV) medications and do admissions, one LPN/LVN may provide treatments, another LPN/LVN may give all oral medications, one UAP may do all hygiene tasks, and another assistant may take all vital signs (Figure 13-2). This division of aspects of care is similar to the assembly line system used by manufacturing industries. Just as an auto worker becomes an expert in attaching fenders to a new vehicle, the direct care nurse becomes expert in the tasks expected in functional nursing. A **charge nurse** coordinates care and assignments and may ultimately be the only person familiar with all the needs of any individual patient.

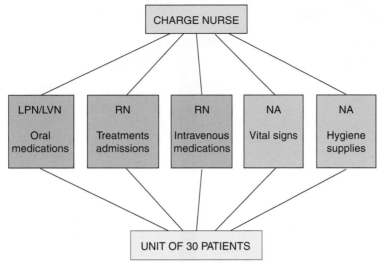

FIGURE 13-2 Functional model of nursing care delivery.

Model Analysis

Several advantages exist for this model of patient care delivery. First, each person becomes efficient at specific tasks, and much work can be done in a short time. Another advantage is that unskilled workers can be trained to perform one or two specific tasks very well. The organization benefits financially from this model because care can be delivered to a large number of patients by mixing staff with a fixed number of RNs and a larger number of UAPs.

Although financial savings may be the impetus for organizations to choose the functional system of delivering care, the disadvantages may outweigh the savings (Figure 13-3). A major disadvantage is the fragmentation of care. The physical and technical aspects of care may be met, but the psychological and spiritual needs may be overlooked. Patients become confused with so many different care providers per shift. These different staff members may be so busy with their assigned tasks that they may not have time to communicate with each other about the patient's progress. Because no one care provider sees patient care from beginning to end, the patient's response to care is difficult to assess. Critical changes in patient status may go unnoticed. Fragmented care and ineffective communication can lead to patient and family dissatisfaction and frustration. Exercise 13-2 provides an opportunity to consider the implications to patient care when the model does not support a holistic patient perspective.

> **EXERCISE 13-2**
> Imagine your mother is a patient at a hospital that uses the functional model of patient care delivery. She just had her knee replaced, and when you ask the nursing assistant for something for pain, she says, "I'll tell the medication nurse." The medication nurse comes to the room and says that your mother's medication is to be administered intravenously and the IV nurse will need to administer it. The IV nurse is busy starting an IV on another patient and cannot give your mother the medication for at least 10 minutes. This whole communication process has taken 40 minutes, and your mother is still in pain. Discuss your perception of the effectiveness of the functional method of patient care in this situation. How effective do you think communication among staff is when a patient has a problem? What could be done to improve this situation?

Nurse Manager's Role

In the functional model of nursing, the nurse manager must be sensitive to the quality of patient care delivered and the institution's budgetary constraints. Because staff members are responsible only for their specific task, the role of achieving **patient outcomes** becomes the nurse manager's responsibility.

Staff members can view this system as autocratic and may become discontented with the lack of opportunity for input. By using effective management and leadership skills, the nurse manager can improve the staff's perception of their lack of independence. The manager can rotate assignments among staff

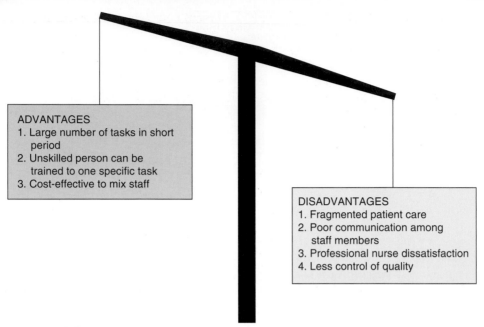

FIGURE 13-3 Advantages and disadvantages of functional nursing.

within legal and organizational contexts to alleviate boredom with repetition. Staff meetings should be conducted frequently. This encourages staff to express concerns and empowers them with the ability to communicate about patient care and unit functions.

Direct Care Nurse's Role

The direct care RN becomes skilled at the tasks that are usually assigned by the charge nurse. Clearly defined policies and procedures are used to complete the physical aspects of care in an efficient and economical manner. However, the functional model of nursing may leave the professional nurse feeling frustrated because of the task-oriented role. Nurses are educated

to care for the patient holistically, and providing only a fragment of care to a patient may result in unmet personal and professional expectations of nurses. As a result, this approach often leads to staff dissatisfaction and, ultimately, unacceptable staff turnover.

The functional method of delivering care works well in emergency and disaster situations. Each care provider knows the expectations of the assigned role and completes the tasks quickly and efficiently. Subacute care agencies, extended care facilities, and ambulatory clinics often use the functional model to deliver care.

TEAM NURSING

After World War II, the nursing shortage continued. Many female nurses who were in the military came home to marry and have children instead of returning to the workforce. Because the functional model received criticism, a new system of team nursing (a modification of functional nursing) was devised to improve patient satisfaction. "Care through others" became the hallmark of team nursing. This type of nursing care delivery remains in use, particularly when reduced reimbursement and nursing shortages have resulted in organizations changing the staff mix and increasing the ratio of unlicensed to licensed personnel.

EXERCISE 13-3

After 6 months of working on a unit that accommodates patients who have had general surgery, you realize that you are bored and frustrated with the functional model of delivering care. You have been administering all the IV medications and pain medications for your assigned patients. You have minimal opportunity to interact with the patients and learn about them, and you cannot be innovative in your care. Discuss strategies you could use to resolve this dissatisfaction with the functional model of nursing care delivery.

In team nursing, a team leader, who is a registered nurse, is responsible for coordinating a group of licensed and unlicensed personnel to provide patient care to a small group of patients. The team leader should be a highly skilled leader, manager, and practitioner, who assigns each member specific responsibilities according to role, licensure, education, ability, competency, and the complexity of the care required. The members of the team report patient progress according to the plan of care directly to the team leader, who then reports to the charge nurse or unit manager (Figure 13-4). There are several teams per unit, and patient assignments are made by each team leader.

Model Analysis

Some advantages of the team method, particularly when compared with the functional approach, are improved patient satisfaction, organizational decision making occurring at lower levels, and cost-effectiveness for the agency. Many institutions and community health agencies currently use the team nursing method. Inpatient facilities may view team nursing as a cost-effective system because it works with an expected ratio of unlicensed to licensed personnel.

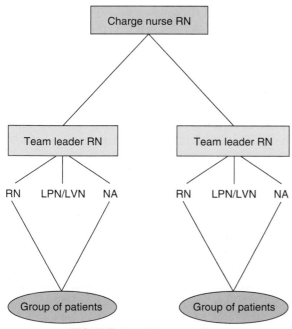

FIGURE 13-4 Team nursing.

Thus the organization has greater numbers of personnel for a designated amount of money.

The team method of patient care delivery has one major disadvantage, which arises if the team leader has poor leadership skills. The team leader must have excellent communication skills, delegation and conflict management abilities, strong clinical skills, and effective decision-making abilities to provide a working "team" environment for the members. The team leader must be sensitive to the needs of the patient and, at the same time, attentive to the needs of the staff providing the direct care (Cioffi & Ferguson, 2009). When the team leader is not prepared for this role, the team method becomes a miniature version of the functional method, and the potential for fragmentation of care is high.

EXERCISE 13-4

Think of a time when you worked with a group of four to six people to achieve a specific goal or accomplish a task (perhaps in school you were grouped together to complete a project). How did your group achieve the goal? Was one person the organizer or leader? How was the leader selected? Who assigned each member a component, or did you each determine what skills you possessed that would most benefit the group? Did you experience any conflict while working on this project? How did the concepts of group dynamics and leadership skills affect how your group achieved its goal? What similarities do you see between the team nursing system of providing patient care and your group involvement to achieve a goal?

Consider the problems that could arise related to equity of patient assignments, continuity of care, or the holistic patient perspectives when team nursing is used. These issues are addressed in the following sections when nurse manager/direct care nurse roles are discussed.

Nurse Manager's Role

The nurse manager, charge nurse, and team leaders must have management skills to effectively implement the team nursing method of patient care delivery. In addition, the nurse manager must determine which RNs are competent and interested in becoming a charge nurse or team leader. Because the basic education of baccalaureate-prepared RNs emphasizes critical thinking, clinical reasoning, and leadership concepts, they are likely candidates for such roles.

The nurse manager should also provide an adequate staff mix and orient team members to the team nursing system by providing continuing education about leadership, management techniques, delegation, and team interaction (see Chapters 1, 3, 4, 18, and 26). By addressing these factors, the manager is aiding the teams to function optimally.

The charge nurse functions as a liaison between the team leaders and other healthcare providers, because nurse managers are often responsible for more than one unit and/or have other managerial responsibilities that take them away from the unit. The charge nurse provides support for the teams on a shift-by-shift basis. Appropriate support requires the charge nurse to encourage each team to solve its problems independently.

The team leader plans the care, delegates the work, and follows up with members to evaluate the quality of care for the patients assigned to their team. In the ideal circumstance, the team leader updates the nursing care plans and facilitates patient care conferences. Time constraints during the shift may prevent scheduling daily patient care conferences or prevent some team members attending those that are held.

The team leader must also face the challenge of changing team membership on a daily basis. Diverse work schedules and nursing staff shortages may result in daily changes in the staff mix of a team and a daily assignment change for team members. The team leader assigns the professional, technical, and ancillary personnel to the type of patient care they are prepared to deliver. Therefore the team leader must be knowledgeable about the legal and organizational limits of each role.

Direct Care Nurse's Role

Team nursing uses the strengths of each caregiver. The direct care nurses, as members of the team, develop expertise in care delivery. Some members become known for their expertise in the psychomotor aspects of care. If one nurse is skilled at starting IVs, she will start all IVs for her team of patients. If a nurse is especially skillful in motivating postoperative patients to ambulate, he should be assigned to the surgical patients. Under the guidance and supervision of the team leader, the collective efforts of the team become greater than the functions of the individual caregivers.

PRIMARY NURSING

A cultural revolution occurred in the United States during the 1960s. The revolution emphasized individual rights and independence from existing societal restrictions. This revolution also influenced the nursing profession, because nurses were becoming dissatisfied with their lack of autonomy. In addition, the hierarchical nature of communication in team nursing caused further frustration. Institutions were also aware of the declining quality of patient care. The search for autonomy and quality care led to the primary nursing system of patient care delivery as a method to increase RN accountability for patient outcomes.

Primary nursing, an adaptation of the case method or total patient care, was developed by Marie Manthey as a method for organizing patient care delivery in which one RN functions autonomously as the patient's primary nurse throughout the hospital stay (Manthey, Ciske, Robertson, & Harris, 1970).

Primary nursing brought the nurse back to direct patient care. The primary nurse is accountable for the patients' care 24 hours a day from admission through discharge. Conceptually, primary nursing care provides the patient and the family with coordinated, comprehensive, continuous care (Tiedeman & Lookinland, 2004). Care is organized, using the nursing process. The primary nurse collaborates, communicates, and coordinates all aspects of patient care with other nurses as well as other disciplines (Tiedeman & Lookinland, 2004). Advocacy and assertiveness are desirable leadership attributes for this care delivery model.

The primary nurse, preferably at least baccalaureate-prepared, is held accountable for meeting outcome criteria and communicating with all other healthcare providers about the patient (Figure 13-5). For example, a patient is admitted to a medical unit with pulmonary edema. His primary nurse admits him and then provides a written plan of care. When his primary nurse is not working, an associate nurse implements the plan. The associate nurse is an RN who has been delegated to provide care to the patient according to the primary nurse's specification. If the patient develops additional complications, the associate nurse notifies the primary nurse, who has 24-hour accountability and responsibility. The associate nurse provides input to the patient's plan of care, and the primary nurse makes the appropriate alterations.

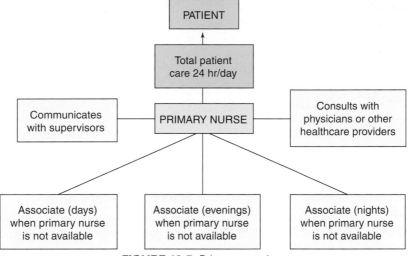

FIGURE 13-5 Primary nursing.

The implications of 24-hour accountability for the primary nurse where compensation is not provided for time apart from scheduled work time are considerable. Those include legal, financial, and professional.

Model Analysis

Tiedeman and Lookinland (2004) cited numerous works that speak to the quality of care and patient satisfaction with primary care. Some studies cited in their work speak to increased quality of care and patient satisfaction, whereas others find no difference in these parameters when compared with team nursing. RNs practicing primary nursing must possess a broad knowledge base and have highly developed nursing skills. In this system of care delivery, professionalism is promoted. Nurses experience job satisfaction because they can use their education to provide holistic and autonomous care for the patient. This high level of accountability for patient outcomes encourages RNs to further their knowledge and refine skills to provide optimal patient care. If the primary nurse is not motivated or feels unqualified to provide holistic care, job satisfaction may decrease.

In primary nursing, patients and families are typically satisfied with the care they receive, because they establish a relationship with the primary nurse and identify the caregiver as "their nurse." Because the patient's primary nurse communicates the plan of care, the patient can move away from the sick role and begin to participate in his or her own recovery.

By considering the sociocultural, psychological, and physical needs of the patient and family, the primary nurse can plan the most appropriate care with and for the patient and family.

A professional advantage to the primary nursing method is a decrease in the number of unlicensed personnel. The ideal primary nursing system requires an all-RN staff. The RN can provide total care to the patient, from bed baths to patient education, even both at the same time! Unlicensed personnel are not qualified to provide this level of inclusive care (Figure 13-6).

A disadvantage of the primary nursing method is that the RN may not have the experience or educational background to provide total care. The agency needs to educate staff for an adequate transition from the previous role to the primary role. One has to ask whether the RN is ready and willing and capable of handling the 24-hour responsibility for patient care. In addition, the nurse practice acts must be evaluated to determine whether primary nurses can be held accountable when they are not physically present.

In times of nursing shortage, primary nursing may not be the model of choice. This model will not be effective if a unit has a large number of part-time RNs who are not available to assume the primary nurse role (24-hour responsibility). In addition, with the arrival of managed care in the 1990s, patients' hospital stays were shorter than in the 1970s, when primary nursing became popular. Expedited stays make it challenging for primary nurses to adequately provide the depth

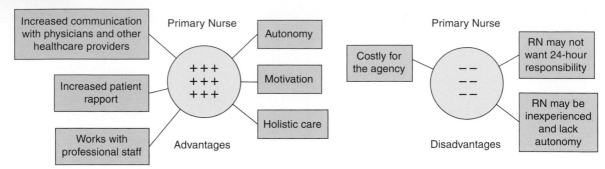

FIGURE 13-6 Advantages and disadvantages of primary nursing.

of care required by primary nursing. If the patient is admitted on Monday and discharged on Wednesday, the primary nurse has a difficult time meeting all patient needs before discharge if he or she is not working on Tuesday. The primary nurse must rely heavily on feedback from associates, which defeats the purpose of primary nursing. In addition, the reduction in reimbursement to hospitals and other organizations associated with managed care caused administrators to consider ways to reduce the cost of care delivery. Because labor costs are the largest expense in care delivery and the nursing staff makes up the largest portion of the labor costs, attention was given to reducing these costs with changes in the model of care delivery.

EXERCISE 13-5

Mr. Faulkner is admitted to the medical unit with exacerbated congestive heart failure. Mike Ross, RN, BSN, is Mr. Faulkner's primary nurse and will provide total care to Mr. Faulkner. Mike notes that this is Mr. Faulkner's third admission in 6 months for congestive heart failure–related symptoms. This is the first admission for which Mr. Faulkner has had a primary nurse. What do you think will be different about this admission with Mike providing primary nursing to Mr. Faulkner? Do you think there will be any difference in continuity of care? How involved do you think Mr. Faulkner will be with his own care in the primary nursing system? What will be the effect on the quality of care provided and the resulting patient outcomes?

EXERCISE 13-6

Imagine you are a primary nurse at an inpatient psychiatric facility. The patients you are assigned to are usually suicidal. How would you feel about the added responsibility for patients even when you were not at work? Is it realistic to expect the nurse to assume the role of the primary nurse with 24-hour responsibility? How would this responsibility affect your personal life? How would you make decisions about the patients and your home life?

Nurse Manager's Role

The primary nursing system can be modified to meet patient, nursing, and budgetary demands while maintaining the positive components that spawned its conception. The nurse manager who implements this care delivery model experiences some benefits. Primary nursing provides the nurse manager an opportunity to demonstrate leadership capabilities, clinical competencies, and teaching abilities to serve as a role model for professional practice. In addition, the roles of budget controller and unit quality manager remain. The traditional roles of delegation and decision making must be relinquished to the autonomous primary nurse. The nurse manager functions as a role model, advocate, coach, and consultant.

Direct Care Nurse's Role

The primary nurse uses many facets of the professional role—caregiver, advocate, decision maker, teacher,

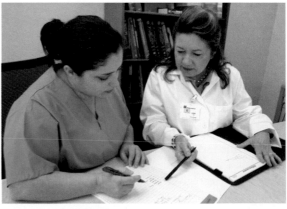

The nurse manager functions as a role model, advocate, coach, and consultant.

collaborator, care coordinator, and manager. Because primary nurses cannot be present 24 hours a day, they must depend on associate nurses to provide care when they are not available. The associate nurse provides care using the plan of care developed by the primary nurse. Changes to the plan of care can be made by the associate nurse in collaboration with the primary nurse. This model provides consistency among nurses and shifts. To function effectively in this setting, direct care nurses will need experience and opportunities to be mentored in this role.

Because it usually is not financially possible for an agency to employ only RNs, true primary nursing rarely exists. Some institutions have modified the primary nursing concept and implemented a partnership model to incorporate their current staff mix.

Primary Nursing Hybrid: Partnership Model

In the practice partnership model (or *co-primary nursing model*) of providing patient care, an RN is paired with a technical assistant. The partner works with the RN consistently. When the partner is unlicensed, the RN allows the assistant to perform basic nursing functions consistent with the state delegation rules. This frees the RN to provide "semi-primary care" to assigned patients. A partnership between an RN and an LPN/LVN allows the LPN/LVN to take more responsibility, because the scope of practice for an LPN/LVN is greater than that of a UAP. In some settings, the partnership is legitimized with an official contract to formalize the relationship. Rehabilitative care settings often use the partnership model to deliver care.

EXERCISE 13-7

You are a primary nurse in a surgical intensive care unit of a small hospital. The unit you work on uses an RN–LPN/LVN partnership to decrease the number of RNs required per shift. You and your partner are assigned four surgical patients. Mr. Jones had a lobectomy 5 hours ago and is on a ventilator; Mrs. Martinez had a quadruple cardiac bypass 14 hours ago; Mr. Wong had a nephrectomy 2 days ago and is receiving continuous peritoneal dialysis; and Mr. Smith has a fractured pelvis and is comatose from a motor vehicle accident 24 hours ago. How would you distribute the staff to provide primary care to these four patients? Do you think it is possible to provide primary care in this situation? What responsibilities would you assume as the primary nurse, and what could you share with the LPN/LVN?

Primary Nursing Hybrid: Patient-Focused or Patient-Centered Care

Another view of primary care is the care delivered in a patient-focused care unit. Developed in the late 1980s, the patient-focused care model integrates principles from business and industry. The goals for this model of care included (1) improving patient satisfaction and other patient outcomes, (2) improving worker job satisfaction, and (3) increasing efficiencies and decreasing costs (Seago, 1999). This model features decentralized, streamlined, and localized care (Graham, 2003). The multidisciplinary team formulates the plan of care after the primary nurse and the physician have assessed the patient.

Patient-focused care units require a change in the physical environment where care is delivered. Services required by patients are decentralized. Satellite laboratories, radiology facilities, pharmacies, and supply rooms are geographically proximate to the patient rooms (Seago, 1999).

Original models of a patient-focused care unit included an RN paired with a cross-trained technician who provided patient-side care, including respiratory therapy, phlebotomy, and electrocardiographs. Modifications in this nurse-managed model include team members who provide direct care activities such as recording vital signs, drawing blood, and bathing patients.

Nurse Management Role

In a patient-focused care unit, the role and scope of the nurse manager expand. No longer is the individual just a manager of nurses. Now the nurse manager assumes the accountability and responsibility to manage nurses and staff from other, traditionally centralized departments. Because the care is focused on the needs of the patient and not the needs of the department, the role of the manager becomes more sophisticated. The nurse manager orchestrates all the care activities required by the patient and family during the hospitalization.

NURSING CASE MANAGEMENT

Another nursing care delivery model that requires a complex set of expectations is the process of nursing case management. Case management is the process of coordinating health care by planning, facilitating, and evaluating interventions across levels of care to achieve measurable cost and quality outcomes. It was first seen in the early 1900s by social workers and public health nurses working in the public sector to identify and obtain resources for the needy. In the 1960s, insurers began to use nursing case management (NCM) as a strategy to manage the needs of complex patients who require coordination over the course of treatment. Acute care hospitals used nurses in this role under the term of *utilization management*, particularly when federal regulations required this service for all Medicare and Medicaid patients (Zander, 2002).

In the mid-1980s, when acute care hospitals began to be reimbursed based upon a certain diagnosis, nursing case management became a popular and effective method to manage shortened lengths of stay for patients while achieving desired patient outcomes and to prevent expensive hospital readmissions. Tufts Medical Center in Boston and Carondelet St. Mary's Hospital in Tucson, Arizona, were leaders in the trend to implement a collaborative system that focuses on comprehensive assessment and intervention and holistic care planning with appropriate referrals to meet the healthcare needs of the patient and the family (Figure 13-7) (Zander, 2002). The nursing case-management process may be "within the walls" of the hospital or "beyond the walls." The success of nursing case-management models has been demonstrated in all healthcare settings, including acute, subacute, and ambulatory settings and long-term care facilities, as well as health insurance companies and the

TABLE 13-1	NURSING CASE-MANAGEMENT SERVICE AREAS
CATEGORY	**SERVICE SETTING**
Acute	Orthopedics, cardiovascular, critical care, high-risk perinatal, oncology, emergency department
Subacute	Skilled nursing centers, rehabilitation units
Ambulatory	Physicians' offices, clinics
Long-term care	Nursing homes, group homes, assisted-living facilities
Insurance companies	Health maintenance organizations (HMOs), preferred provider organizations (PPOs), workers' compensation, Medicaid, Medicare
Community	Nurse-managed centers, home health agencies, urgent care centers, schools, rural settings

Adapted from information presented in Cohen & Cesta (2004); Curtis, Lien, Chan, & Morris (2002); Huber (2010).

community. Table 13-1 identifies some of the service settings using this care delivery model.

The case-management model of patient care delivery maintains quality care while streamlining costs for high-risk, high-volume, high-cost patient populations and seeks the active involvement of the patient, the family, and diverse healthcare professionals. Healthcare organizations have tailored the case-management system to meet their specific needs. The elements of the case-management model are the case manager and the critical pathway.

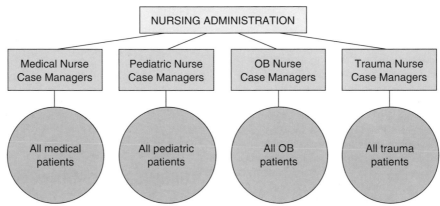

FIGURE 13-7 Nursing case management model in which all patients are assigned to a nurse case manager. *OB,* Obstetric.

Case Manager

The goal of case management is to provide cost-effective care through integration of clinical services in combination with financial services. In addition, the case manager serves as an advocate for the patient and the family. Nurses, social workers, and professionals in other disciplines may work as case managers, bringing with them their discipline-specific skills and knowledge.

The Case Management Society of America (2010) (http://www.acmaweb.org) has identified the standards of practice for case managers. These include:

1. Addressing total individual concerns, including medical, psychosocial, behavioral, and spiritual needs
2. Collaborating to focus upon moving the individual to self-care whenever possible
3. Increasing the involvement of individual and caregivers in the decision-making processes
4. Minimizing fragmentation of care within the healthcare system
5. Using evidence-based guidelines, as available, in the daily practice of case management
6. Focusing on transitions of care, which includes a complete transfer to the next care setting or provider that is effective, safe, timely and complete
7. Improving outcomes by using adherence guidelines, standardized tools, and prevention processes to measure a client's understanding and acceptance of proposed plans, his/her willingness to change and his/her supports to maintain health behaviors
8. Expanding the interdisciplinary team to increase clients and/or their identified support system
9. Moving clients to optimal levels of health and well-being
10. Improving medication reconciliation for a client through collaborative efforts with medical staff
11. Improving adherence to the plan of care for the client, including medical differences

Although inconsistency exists among professional standards about the education for nurse case managers, many organizations prefer master's-prepared clinical nurse specialists who have advanced preparation with the specific populations being served.

Depending on the facility, there may be several case managers to coordinate care for all patients, or a case manager may be assigned to a specific high-risk, high-volume, high-cost population (see Figure 13-7). The case manager may be responsible for coordinating care for up to 20 patients. It is essential that the case manager has frequent interaction with the patient and the healthcare provider to achieve and evaluate expected outcomes.

CRITICAL PATHWAYS

The tool that case managers use to achieve patient outcomes is a clinical pathway. Also referred to as a *multidisciplinary care pathway, integrated care pathway, critical path,* or *collaborative care pathway,* these patient-focused documents describe the clinical standards, necessary interventions, and expected outcomes for the patient throughout the treatment process or hospital stay. These pathways facilitate coordinated and efficient plans to deliver patient care. However, they are not appropriate for all patients and cannot replace professional clinical judgment (D'Entremont, 2009). Pathways are considered useful if the intervention (1) is a structured multidisciplinary plan of care; (2) is used to translate guidelines or evidence into a specific situation; (3) includes steps in a course of treatment or care in a plan, pathway, algorithm, guideline, protocol, or other "inventory of actions"; (4) includes time frames or criteria-based progression; and (5) aims to standardize care for a specific clinical problem, procedure, or episode of health care in a specific population (Kinsman et al., 2010).

If a patient's progress deviates from the normal path, a variance is indicated. A variance is anything that occurs to alter the patient's progress through the normal critical path. The reason(s) for the variance should be analyzed and the care revised to meet the needs of the patients. These reasons may be influenced by patient, provider, or care issues. For example, the symptoms experienced by a patient with a urinary tract infection may not resolve as rapidly as projected because a dose of the antibiotic prescribed was missed in error or because the patient couldn't tolerate the medication prescribed.

Model Analysis

Nursing case management (NCM) is a process for providing comprehensive care for those with complex health problems. Case management provides a well-coordinated care experience that can improve the care outcome, decrease the length of stay, and use multiple disciplines and services efficiently. Families and patients receive care across a continuum of settings, often from diverse institutions. NCMs can often break down invisible institutional barriers for the patient. Nurses receive a sense of satisfaction knowing that the patient and family received coordinated, quality care in a cost-effective manner across the spectrum of the illness or injury. In order to implement this approach effectively, interdisciplinary collaboration and coordination and consensus related to patient outcomes and the time frames proposed must be active.

Nurse Manager's Role

The nurse manager has increased demands when leading a case-management system. Quality improvement is constantly assessed to ensure that the clinical pathway is appropriate for the diagnosis-related group (DRG) and that case managers are adequately managing their caseloads. Reimbursement for the care delivered is tied to effective planning and care delivery within the case-management process. Patient satisfaction is also pertinent to evaluate for quality. If patients are not satisfied with the system, the census may decline.

Communication among all systems must be coordinated. Because the NCM works with all departments within a healthcare organization, the nurse manager may need to facilitate interdepartmental communication. Educating the staff of other departments about the NCM's role and responsibilities will increase the effectiveness of the case-management process.

Direct Care Nurse's Role

The direct care nurse working with a patient who has a case manager as the coordinator of care provides patient care according to the case manager's specifications and must know the extent of the case manager's role. Effective communication to facilitate care is the responsibility of both the case manager and the staff RN.

Navigator Role

A new role, similar in many ways to a case manager, is that of a **nurse navigator.** This role is sometime referred to as a patient navigator, particularly when disciplines other than nurses fulfill the role. In 1990, Dr. Harold Freeman developed the first nurse navigator role at Harlem Hospital in New York in order to facilitate diagnosis and treatment for patients with abnormal breast screening results (Pedersen & Hack, 2010). In 2001, the President's Cancer Panel recommended that funding for community-based programs, such as navigator programs, be increased in order to provide information, screening, treatment, and supportive care. The Patient Navigator Outreach and Chronic Disease Prevention Act of 2005 authorized federal grants to hire and train navigators (from all disciplines) to help patients with cancer and other serious chronic diseases to access screening, diagnosis, treatment, and follow-up care. In 2007, $2.9 million was allocated to this program. Also, in 2006, the Centers for Medicare & Medicaid Services (CMS) funded six demonstration projects to help minority Medicare patients overcome barriers in screening, diagnosis, and treatment (Wells et al., 2008).

Although a number of navigator programs target care of the cancer patient, this role could be implemented when caring for patients with other chronic diseases in a variety of care delivery settings. For example, recent publications reveal that healthcare facilities carry out navigator programs for conditions other than cancer, such as high risk obstetrical care, osteoarthritis, HIV, and asthma. However published articles on cancer-related navigator programs far outnumber those pertaining to other disease states (Wells et al., 2008).

There is no single definition of a navigator. A review of the literature suggests two approaches: (1) the provision of specified services to provide care, and (2) removal of barriers to care (Wells et al., 2008). Wells et al. (2009) suggests that the role of a navigator, regardless of the professional discipline, is operationalized by providing any service that assists patients in overcoming obstacles from screening to treatment, as well as coping with treatment and follow-up. Specifically, navigators are responsible for (1) overcoming health system barriers, (2) providing health education about the disease from prevention to treatment, (3) addressing patient barriers to care, and (4) providing psychosocial support.

The navigator role was conceived to reduce patient barriers to care for vulnerable patients who may cope with delays in access, diagnosis, treatment, and/or fragmented and uncoordinated care. As with many roles in health care, a number of disciplines have skills consistent with the navigator role, including nurses, social workers, health educators, and laypeople.

Wells et al. (2008) acknowledges that the navigator role has much in common with other healthcare professions and other roles aimed at facilitating patient transitions through the care process. The case manager may be oriented toward care for variety of conditions, but a navigator is focused on a single health condition. In addition, a case manager wants to improve the overall health of a patient for the long-term, but a navigator seeks to achieve timely and effective care for the patient for only a defined set of health services. Similarly, patient advocates tend to focus on improving the health care system, but the navigator is tasked with removing specific health system barriers particular to an individual patient.

Although the research thus far is limited, short term, and not highly constructed, initial evaluation of navigator programs suggests that disease screening rates and adherence to diagnostic services after identification of an anomaly have increased. In addition, treatment of patients has improved (Wells et al, 2008). An analysis of evaluations of nurse navigator programs from 2000 to 2010 also identified improved patient satisfaction, induced positive changes in patient attitudes, increased understanding of disease processes, and led to patient perception of a more timely, accessible treatment process (Case, 2011). However, as more patients become eligible for health services as a result of changing reimbursement patterns, a more complete understanding of the role of a navigator and the extent to which they improve the outcome of patients become critical to improving patient care.

DIFFERENTIATED NURSING PRACTICE

One of the factors that makes development and implementation of any nursing care delivery model difficult is the variation in competence of nurses based on education and experience. Over the past 50 years, as multiple entry points in nursing (LPN/LVN, associate degree in nursing [ADN], diploma, bachelor of science in nursing [BSN], and advanced generalist [MSN]) have grown and more is known about the length of time required for a nurse to move from being a novice to competent nurse (Benner, 2001), efforts have been made to document and validate differentiated practice.

Differentiated nursing practice models are models of clinical nursing practice that are defined or differentiated by level of education, expected clinical skills or competencies, job descriptions, pay scales, and participation in decision making (AACN, AONE, & NOADN, 1994): Almost 20 years ago, *A Model for Differentiated Nursing Practice* (AACN, AONE, & NOADN, 1994) proposed that the associate degree nurse (ADN) role functions primarily at the bedside in an institutional setting and in less complex patient care situations. The time frame for care provided by the ADN is defined within a shift or limited period of time, based on activities that provide comfort, physiologic stabilization, or assistance to a peaceful death. The guiding principles of the ADN's work are found in nursing standards, protocols, and pathways.

The BSN role was conceptualized as operating across time from preadmission to post-discharge. The guiding principles of this role are found in the unusual and often unpredictable response of the patient that goes beyond needs addressed in the standards or pathways. Collaborating with other disciplines and agencies, the BSN intervenes to design and facilitate a comprehensive, well-prepared discharge based on the unique needs of the patient and family (AACN, AONE, & NOADN, 1994; AACN, 2009).

The advanced practice registered nurse (APRN) role is based on a master of science in nursing (MSN) or doctorate of nursing practice (DNP) competencies. The APRN perspective is supported by in-depth education in physiology, physical assessment, pharmacology, and a broad healthcare systems perspective. The MSN/DNP creates and defines protocols and pathways and assists with development of standards on emerging new healthcare phenomena. The MSN/DNP role is not bound by setting but, instead, provides a continuum of care across all settings, working with the patient and family throughout wellness or illness or until death (AACN, 2009).

As nursing has evolved and environmental factors have influenced the role of a nurse, conflict over the roles of nurses with varied educational backgrounds and philosophy have erupted. These variations have had a significant impact on the success of the delivery system and the satisfaction of the nurse and the patients. This variation is further complicated by the experience and competence of the nurse in the practice arena. Benner (2001), based on the Dreyfus model of skill acquisition, identified five stages of clinical competence for nurses: novice, advanced beginner, competent, proficient, and expert. She suggests that competence is typified by a nurse who has been on the job in the same or similar situations 2 to 3 years. This would suggest that nurses who are either new graduates or in a new area of clinical practice may require more assistance than those with more experience. A group of nurses who are all at the novice or advanced beginner stage would be less likely than their more experienced counterparts to implement any type of delivery model effectively.

In an effort to clarify the competence level of new graduates, some states, such as Texas, have identified the specific variations in competence among the various educational levels. These competencies can be used by educational programs for curriculum development and evaluation and by employers to determine the specific roles and responsibilities of these graduates. In 1993, the Board of Nurse Examiners and the Board of Vocational Nurse Examiners in Texas adopted the "Essential Competencies of Texas Graduates of Education Programs of Nursing." These competencies identified the knowledge, judgment, skills, and professional values expected of graduates of LVN, diploma/ADN, and BSN programs, varying in complexity, depth, and breadth of the various types of nursing programs. In 2002 and again in 2008, these competencies, including competency statements related to provider of care, coordinator of care, patient advocate, and member of the profession, were revised and educational programs were accountable for demonstrating inclusion of these competencies into their curriculum (Poster et al., 2005; Sportsman et al., 2010).

Role of the Clinical Nurse Leader

In response to a lack of differentiated practice in many worksites and the increased emphasis on patient safety, the American Association of Colleges of Nursing (AACN) developed the clinical nurse leader role in the early 2000s. The clinical nurse leader, which is a protected title for those who successfully complete the clinical nurse leader (CNL) certification examination, is an advanced generalist clinician with education at the master's degree, in contrast to advanced practice registered nurses, whose designation includes clinical nurse specialists, nurse practitioners, nurse midwives, and nurse anesthetists. The CNL oversees the lateral integration of care for a distinct group of patients and may actively provide direct patient care in complex

situations. The CNL uses evidence-based practice to ensure that patients benefit from the latest innovations in care delivery. The CNL collects and evaluates patient outcomes, assesses cohort risk, and has the decision-making authority to change care plans when necessary. This nurse functions as part of the interprofessional team by communicating, planning, and implementing care directly with other healthcare professionals including physicians, pharmacists, social workers, clinical nurse specialists, and nurse practitioners. The CNL is a leader in the healthcare delivery system in all settings in which health care is delivered, and implementation of the role may vary across settings. Box 13-1 outlines the fundamental aspects of the CNL role, as defined by the AACN white paper on the role of the clinical nurse leader (AACN, 2007).

The Synergy Model

Similar to the work of the AACN in developing the CNL, the American Association of Critical-Care

---

BOX 13-1   FUNDAMENTAL ASPECTS OF THE CLINICAL NURSE LEADER (CNL)

- Leadership in the care of the sick in and across all environments
- Design and provision of health-promotion and risk-reduction services for diverse populations
- Provision of evidence-based practice
- Population-appropriate health care to individuals, clinical groups/units, and communities
- Clinical decision making
- Design and implementation of care plans
- Risk anticipation
- Participation in identification and collection of care outcomes
- Accountability for the evaluation and improvement of point-of-care outcomes
- Mass customization of care
- Client and community advocacy
- Education and information management
- Delegation and oversight of care delivery and outcomes
- Team management and collaboration with other health professional team members
- Development and leverage of human, environmental, and material resources
- Management and use of client-care and information technology
- Lateral integration for specified groups of patients

From AACN. (2007). White paper on the role of the clinical nurse leader. Website: www.aacn.nche.edu/Publications/WhitePapers/ClinicalNurseLeader.htm.

Nurses adopted the Synergy Model as the framework for nursing practice as well as for the certification examination for the critical care nurse and the clinical nurse specialist. Some healthcare organizations have adopted this model as their model of care. However, the Synergy Model identifies patient characteristics as "drivers" of the necessary competencies for nurses. When a match between the competencies of the nurse and the characteristics of the patient occurs, the best patient outcomes and safe passage through a hospital stay will be achieved (Brewer, 2006).

The Synergy Model describes the following eight patient characteristics: resiliency, vulnerability, stability, complexity, resource availability, participation in care, participation in decision making, and predictability. The eight nurse competencies are clinical judgment, advocacy and moral agency, caring practices, facilitation of learning, collaboration, systems thinking, response to diversity, and clinical requirement (Brewer, 2006). When the nurse's competency is congruent with the needs exhibited by the patient, synergy is reached and patient care is improved (Kaplow & Reed, 2008). The American Association of Critical-Care Nurses website (*www.aacn.org*) provides information about the Synergy Model and its application in numerous and diverse care settings.

Magnet Recognition Program®

In 1983, the American Academy of Nursing's (AAN) task force on nursing practice in hospitals conducted a study of 163 hospitals to identify and describe variables that created an environment that attracted and retained well-qualified nurses who promoted quality care. Forty-one of these institutions were described as Magnet™ hospitals because of their ability to attract and retain professional nurses. In 1990, the American Nurses Credentialing Center (ANCC), building on the concepts of the 1983 Magnet™ hospital study, developed a program that recognized excellence in the nurses' work environment. Prominent in the designation process is the hospital's documentation of the presence of the Forces of Magnetism.

The Magnet Recognition Program® is designed for hospitals to achieve recognition of excellent nursing care through a self-nominating, self-appraisal process to achieve. The rigorous self-appraisal process is lengthy, often requiring 2 or more years of preparation. The hospital makes application for Magnet™ status, submits documentation to demonstrate its compliance with the Magnet™ standards, and hosts a site visit by Magnet™ appraisers. When the application process is successful, Magnet™ status is awarded for 4 years. For additional information on Magnet™ credentialing, see *www.nursecredentialing.org/magnet/index.html*.

The evidence suggests that hospitals given Magnet™ status are more likely to be hospitals where nurses choose to work. For example, Kramer et al. (2011) studied the perceptions of 12,233 experienced nurses on 717 nursing units in 36 Magnet™ hospitals, using the Essentials of Magnetism II instrument to determine if the characteristics of a healthy productive clinical environment were present on their units. These characteristics include:

• Working with clinical, competent peers
• Collegial/collaborative nurse/physicians relationships
• Clinical autonomy
• Support for education
• Perception of adequate staff
• Supportive nurse managers
• Control of nursing practice
• Transmission and adoption of patient-centered culture

The researchers used the scores on the Essentials of Magnetism II instrument to determine if the nurses felt they were working in a very healthy work environment (VHWE), a healthy work environment (HWE), or an environment that needed improvement. The study found that 82% of nurses on 540 units felt they worked in a healthy or very healthy work environment. Their feelings about the work environment also influenced their perception of the quality of care given to patients (Kramer et al., 2011).

TRANSFORMING CARE AT THE BEDSIDE

The variety of care delivery models and the complexity of patient needs, organizational structures, and technologic advances require individual action to improve practice patterns in specific units. In 2003, the Robert Wood Johnson Foundation and the Institute of Healthcare Improvement joined to create, test, and implement changes to dramatically improve care on medical/surgical units and improve staff satisfaction.

An initiative called Transforming Care at the Bedside (TCAB) was implemented to redesign the work environment of nurses. A group of healthcare experts developed a guiding framework to redesign the work of nurses in medical/surgical units (Viney, Batcheller, Houston, & Belcik, 2006).

The TCAB initiative is based on a set of premises (Box 13-2), which then serve as the underpinnings of four key design themes. These include reliability, vitality and teamwork, patient-centered care, and value-added care processes (Box 13-3). According to Viney et al. (2006),

---

BOX 13-2 TRANSFORMING CARE AT THE BEDSIDE (TCAB) PREMISES

- Patient-centered work redesign can create value-added care processes and result in better clinical outcomes and reduced costs.
- Effective care teams can have a positive impact on patient outcomes.
- Management practices and organizational culture have a significant impact on the work environment.
- Matching staff's knowledge and capabilities with work responsibilities enhances job satisfaction.
- Eliminating inefficiencies through work redesign enhances staff satisfaction and morale.

From Viney, M., Batcheller, J., Houston, S., & Belcik, K. (2006). Transforming care at the bedside: Designing new complex systems in an age of complexity. *Journal of Nursing Care Quality, 21*(2), 143-150.

BOX 13-3 TRANSFORMING CARE AT THE BEDSIDE (TCAB) OBJECTIVE/DESIGN THEMES

- Reliability: The care for moderately sick patients who are hospitalized is safe, reliable, effective, and equitable.
- Vitality: Effective care teams continually strive for excellence within a joyful and supportive environment that nurtures professional formation and career development.
- Patient-centeredness: Patient-centered care on medical/surgical units honors the whole person and family, respects individual values and choices, and ensures continuity of care.
- Increased value: All care processes are free of waste and promote continuous flow.

Adapted from Viney, M., Batcheller, J., Houston, S., & Belcik, K. (2006). Transforming care at the bedside: Designing new complex systems in an age of complexity. *Journal of Nursing Care Quality, 21*(2), 143-150.

---

both the themes and the premises serve as a framework for teams charged with changing care processes.

The TCAB initiative was initially implemented at three pilot hospitals and subsequently moved to other hospitals across the country. Small groups in each hospital came together, first, to learn about the TCAB process and to ask themselves "what do we know" about the work environment related to a particular design theme. The group then was encouraged to tell stories about the work environment consistent with this theme. After the story-telling opportunity, the group participated in a brainstorming session to develop as many innovations as possible that would contribute to the themes they had chosen. Innovations requiring minimal time and resources were then prioritized and selected for a rapid cycle trial.

Critical to practice changes, rapid cycle change is a process that encourages testing creative change on a small scale while determining potential impact. The process involves four stages—plan, do, study, and act (PDSA). During the *plan phase,* the team had to define the objectives and predict how the identified change would contribute to a design, how the change would occur, and what data collection methods were needed. During the *do phase,* the team had to focus on whether the changed occurred as expected and, if not, what interfered with the plan. In the *study phase,* the team had to determine if the innovation worked as predicted and what knowledge was gained. The *act phase* required the team to plan the next actions.

The team and staff participating in the study rated the innovation in terms of adoption, adaptation, or discontinuation. The innovations were implemented for a short period (from a day to several weeks) at least twice during the prototype testing phase and the pilot testing phase. If the outcomes of testing the innovation are positive, the new design can be easily spread to other participating sites.

Transforming Care at the Bedside has been implemented across the world. For example, Chaboyer et al. (2010) reports the significant effects of implementation of 13 TCAB improvement strategies on medication errors and patient falls on 2 nursing units in a hospital in Australia. The results noted that rapid change management cycles can be useful when implementing numerous clinical changes in a short time period.

TRANSITIONAL CARE

As the cost of health care escalates and reimbursement strategies change, hospital stays shorten and patients transition to alternative care, including home, more rapidly than in earlier years. In addition, payers have developed approaches to financially penalize providers for hospital readmissions. A review of a number of studies find there are serious quality and safety problems following discharge from acute care. Patients may not understand their medication instructions or how to care for themselves. They may not know how to recognize warning signs of health problems or how to follow up. Peikes, Lester, Gilman, and Brown (2013) report that 15% to 45% of patients experience health problems or do not receive adequate follow-up care.

In response to the concerns around transitions in care, in 2011 the Centers for Medicare & Medicaid Services (CMS) funded the Community-based Care Transition Program (CCTP) to test promising care interventions for Medicare beneficiaries at high risk for being readmitted after the initial hospitalization (Peikes et al., 2013). Common factors in these programs include comprehensive discharge planning including instruction about medications and warning signs of health problems, contact with a provider following discharge, emphasis on helping patients manage their medications, and assisting with communication between the patient and primary and specialty caregivers. (See the Research Perspective on p. 250 for more details.)

INTERPROFESSIONAL EDUCATION AND COLLABORATION

Most of the care models discussed in this chapter address the organization of nursing care. Apart from case management, the majority of the models do not focus on the impact of interprofessional collaboration on the outcomes of patient care, communication, and collaboration, which is increasingly important as the complexity of health care increases. National and international organizations have called for strategies to improve collaboration among health professions to improve the delivery care system.

To support these recommendations, calls for interprofessional education (IPE) have sounded. For example, in 2003 the Committee on the Health Professions Education Summit from the Institute of Medicine recommended that in order to meet the challenges of the twenty-first century, health professions should work in interdisciplinary teams (IOM, 2003). In 2006 the World Health Organization (WHO) announced the creation of the WHO Study Group on Interprofessional Education and Collaborative Practice to develop a global strategy to implement IPE and collaborative practices worldwide. In 2010, the WHO and their partners reinforced their commitment to interprofessional education (IPE) and interprofessional collaboration IPC, stating that these strategies will improve health care across the world. (Pinto et al, 2012). In 2011, the IOM report, *The Future of Nursing Leading Change, Advancing Health* states that "Nurses should be educated with physicians and other health professions both as students and throughout their careers in lifelong learning opportunities" (p. 2).

CONCLUSION

Each patient care delivery model has identified strengths and weaknesses. No perfect method for delivering nursing care to groups of patients and their families exists. No one model addresses all needs of the wide range of settings and sizes of healthcare organizations. In addition, in times of local or national emergencies, the typical model of care may be replaced with one designed to best fit the emergency. (See Table 13-2 for examples of structure and process in organization that might influence the delivery of care used.)

This chapter describes the traditional patient care delivery models that have been used over the past half century. The complexity of the current healthcare system, the shortage of health professionals, and the pressures to ensure patient safety and cost-effective care have led many organizations to explore alternative models to deliver patient care using interprofessional collaboration, in all levels of care. New models of care are being tested, as demonstrated by the Research Perspective on p. 250 and the Literature Perspective on p. 251.

TABLE 13-2   STANDARDIZED SET OF ORGANIZATIONAL CRITERIA

ORGANIZATIONAL STRUCTURES	ORGANIZATIONAL PROCESSES	PATIENT CARE DESCRIPTORS
Governance	Care planning	Case mix severity
Teaching status	Patient assessment/monitoring	Intensity of service/skills
Aggregated units	Documentation	Length of stay
Technology level	Policies/procedures	Diagnosis-related groups (DRGs)
Case mix	Patient education	
Operating budget	Supplies	
Nursing hours/day	Implementation of physicians' orders	
Skill mix	Patient/family communication	
Nurse:patient ratio	Symptom management	
Use of temporary staff	Staff communication	
Nursing education/experience	Medication administration	
Support for professional development	Standards of care	
Continuing education	Unit activities	
Expert resources		
Support personnel		
Physical layout		

Adapted from Deutschendorf, A. (2003). From past paradigms to future frontiers: Unique care delivery models to facilitate nursing work and quality outcomes. *Journal of Nurse Administration, 33*(1), 51-58.

 RESEARCH PERSPECTIVE

Resource: Peikes, D., Lester, R.S., Gilman, B., & Brown, R. (2013). The effects of transitional care models on re-admissions: A review of the current evidence. *Generations: The Journal of the Western Gerontological Society*, 36(4), 44-55.

This study considered the result of evaluations of transitional programs for patients moving from one level of care to another, based on six models supported by the Centers for Medicare & Medicaid Services (CMS) Community-based Care Transition Program (CCTP). The study found that four of these models had rigorous evidence that they were effective in reducing patients rehospitalization within 30 days. The following chart describes the models that demonstrated such positive results.

MODEL	DESCRIPTION
Transitional Care Model	An Advanced Practice Nurse (APN) provides in-hospital planning and home follow-up care for patients with Congestive Heart Failure, particularly transitional care and medication administration
Care Transitions Intervention	RN/APN coach provides tools and teaches self-management. Home visits and telephone calls, patient-assembled personal health record, follow-up on red flag symptoms, and communication with primary and specialty care providers are emphasized
Project Re-Engineered Discharge (Project RED)	Nurse discharge advocates for and provides patient education, medication reconciliation, instructions about red flags, teach-back learning processes, coordination of physician appointments and follow-up testing, evidence-based written discharge, clinical pharmacist telephone to reinforce.

Implications for Practice

With changing reimbursement models designed to reduce the cost of care by delivering more care in settings other than acute care hospitals, nurses must be knowledgeable of care delivery models that focus on alternative care settings, in addition to acute care hospitals. As the emphasis on transitioning patients through the healthcare delivery system as rapidly as possible becomes the norm, opportunities for nurses to deliver safe, quality care to patients while reducing the cost of care will increase.

LITERATURE PERSPECTIVE

Resource: Burston, S, Chaboyer, W., Wallis, M., & Stanfield, J. (2011). A discussion of approaches to transforming care: Contemporary strategies to improve patient safety. *Journal of Advanced Nursing, 67*(11), pp. 2488-2495.

This article evaluates the effectiveness of three approaches that are used to transform care, changing the way that nurses do their work in order to improve patient safety. These approaches included Transforming Care at the Bedside (TCAB). TCAB, as previously discussed, is a bottom-up approach to improving care. The Productive Ward, primarily implemented in the United Kingdom, has a similar purpose and also is a bottom-up approach. The Studer Group, a top-down approach, focuses on evidence-based leadership principles to improve care through service, quality, people, finance, and growth.

Implications for Practice

Each of these approaches, though different in specific attributes, have similar aims. In addition, they may be combined into a hybrid approach, which can also be effective in making changes to improve patient safety.

THE SOLUTION

As an assistant director of nursing, I am responsible for ensuring the delivery of excellent patient care to patients admitted to our hematology-oncology unit. The nurses on the unit were committed to this approach but were faced with communication challenges. Collaborating with other members of the leadership team, receiving feedback from the staff nurses, and seeking out best practices from my peers in the healthcare community produced a solution. We initiated a sit-down report for all nurses called the "huddle" and established a "nurse buddy" system.

The huddle is conducted at the beginning of the shift after each nurse has obtained report from the nurse on the previous shift and has had the opportunity to review each patient's plan of care. The nurses are paged and notified that the huddle will occur. The huddle is facilitated by the charge nurse, who surveys each nurse on his or her workload and the projected times he or she would need assistance with patient care.

The nurse buddy system was initiated to provide the patient-side nurse with an immediate resource—someone other than the charge nurse. These two nurses provide each other with assistance on an as-needed basis. The buddy is assigned at the time all patient assignments are made and is in close proximity.

The feedback is very positive. The charge nurse has a clearer picture of the status of the patients, families, and staff. Because the staff nurses are more engaged, they state that they are involved with the unit's operational needs for the day. Patient care is planned collaboratively so that each nurse is available to the buddy at times of need. Overall, teamwork and communication have been enhanced.

—Jacqueline Ward

Would this be a suitable approach for you? Why?

THE EVIDENCE

Wolf and Greenhouse (2007) recognize the need for healthcare system change and the importance of a well-developed care delivery model in addressing these changes. They suggest that it is not necessary to "start from scratch" in developing a model; many valuable lessons, learned from experience and scientific evidence, can be incorporated into new models. The authors suggest three factors beyond the experience of the past that should be considered in developing a new model. First, major healthcare trends, such as changes in patients, providers, information technology, and reimbursement, as well as medical advances, must be considered. Second, identifying what patients want and need is important. Some of the patient needs identified by the authors are those traditionally expected, such as a competent provider to meet their physical, emotional, and spiritual needs. However, an identified need that has not always been expected was "someone to help sort through available information for a solution effective for them." Third, Wolf and Greenhouse suggest that developers must make structural (who will do what?), process (how will it get done?), and outcome (what difference will it make?) decisions to ensure that the new model is in strategic alignment with the organization, sustainable over time, and can be replicated. The article provides specific questions that can be helpful in making these structural, process, and outcome decisions.

WHAT NEW GRADUATES SAY

- I had worked only where team nursing was used and was surprised to experience the primary approach shortly after graduation. While it is more rewarding, it is also scarier if you have a patient with multiple demands.

- Our unit uses a clinical nurse leader and she seems to always have the answer I need.
- I work in a clinic and I would say we are truly a team. We do whatever needs to be done, no matter what our title is.

CHAPTER CHECKLIST

The roles of the nurse manager and direct care nurse vary with each nursing care delivery model. Regardless of the model, the nurse manager must have strong leadership and management skills for the model to be effective. Numerous issues must be considered when a care delivery model is implemented. Without a competent manager, none of the discussed models would be effective.

- Case method (total patient care)
  - Model analysis
  - Nurse manager's role
  - Direct care nurse's role
- Functional nursing
  - Model analysis
  - Nurse manager's role
  - Direct care nurse's role
- Team nursing
  - Model analysis
  - Nurse manager's role
  - Direct care nurse's role
- Primary nursing
  - Model analysis

- Nurse manager's role
- Direct care nurse's role
- Primary nursing hybrid: partnership model
- Primary nursing hybrid: patient-focused or patient-centered care
- Nurse management role
- Nursing case management
  - Case manager
- Critical pathways
  - Model analysis
  - Nurse manager's role
  - Direct care nurse's role
  - Navigator role
- Differentiated nursing practice
  - Role of the clinical nurse leader
  - The Synergy Model
  - Magnet Recognition Program®
- Transforming care at the bedside
- Transitional care
- Interprofessional education and collaboration

TIPS FOR SELECTING A CARE DELIVERY MODEL*

- Look at the organization and the population being served when selecting a care delivery model.
- Consider the organizational structure and processes when selecting the care delivery model.
- There are advantages and disadvantages to any model; there is no ideal approach.

- Know that every model has specific expectations for both managers and staff.
- Determine if there are experienced nurses who provide clinical leadership in specific settings.

REFERENCES

AACN. (2007). *White paper on clinical nurse leader*. Retrieved February, 2013, http://www.aacn.nche.edu/publications/white-papers/cnl.

AACN. (2009). *DNP fact sheet*. Retrieved February, 2013, from, www.aacn.nche.edu/media-relations/fact-sheets/dnp.

AACN, AONE, & NOADN. (1994). Differentiated competencies for nursing practice. *Journal of Nursing Administration*, 25(9), 34–35.

Benner, P. (2001). *From novice to expert: Excellence and power in clinical nursing practice*. Upper Saddle River, NJ: Prentice Hall.

* These tips would be useful also for new graduate nurses evaluating employment opportunities.

Brewer, B. (2006). Is patient acuity a proxy for patient characteristics of the AACN Synergy Model for patient care? *Nursing Administration Quarterly*, 30(40), 351–357.

Case, M. A. B. (2011). Oncology nurse navigator. *Clinical Journal of Oncology Nursing*, 15(1), 33–40.

Chaboyer, W., Johnson, J., Hardy, L., Gehrke, T., & Panuwatwanich, K. (2010). Transforming care strategies and nursing-sensitive patient indicators. *Journal of Advanced Nursing*, 65(5), 1111–1119.

Cioffi, J., & Ferguson, L. (2009). Team nursing in acute care settings: Nurses' experiences. *Contemporary Nurse*, 33(1), 2–12.

Cohen, E., & Cesta, T. (2004). *Nursing case management from essentials to advanced practice application* (4th ed.). Mosby.

Curtis, K., Lien, D., Chan, A., & Morris, R. (2002). The impact of trauma. *The Journal of Trauma*, 53(3), 477–482.

D'Entremont, B. (2009). Clinical pathways: The Ottawa Hospital experience. *The Canadian Nurse*, 105(5), 8–9.

Graham, I. (2003). Leading the development of nursing within a nursing development unit: The perspectives of leadership by the team leader and professor of nursing (electronic version). *International Journal of Nursing Practice*, 9(4).

Huber, D. (2010). *Disease management: A guide for case managers.* Elsevier.

IOM. (2003). *Health professions education: A bridge to quality.* April 18. http://www.iom.edu/Reports/2003/Health-Professions-Education-A-Bridge-to-Quality.aspx. Last Accessed April, 2014.

IOM. (2011). *The future of nursing: Leading change, advancing health.* Committee on the Robert Wood Johnson Foundation Initiative on the Future of Nursing at the Institute of Medicine; Institute of Medicine. www.nap.edu/catalog/12956.html, Last accessed, October, 2012.

Kaplow, R., & Reed, M. (2008). The AACN Synergy Model for Patient Care: A nursing model as a Force of Magnetism. *Nursing Economic$*, 2(1), 17–25.

Kinsman, L., Rotter, T., James, E., Snow, P., & Willis, J. (2010). What is a clinical pathway? A definition to inform the debate. *BMC Medicine*, 8(3).

Kramer, M., Maguire, P., & Brewer, B. (2011). Clinical nurses in magnet hospitals confirm productive, healthy unit work environment. *Journal of Nursing Management*, 12, 5–17.

Manthey, M., Ciske, K., Robertson, P., & Harris, I. (1970). Primary nursing: A return to the concept of "my nurse" and "my patient". *Nursing Forum*, 9, 65–83.

Pedersen, A., & Hack, T. F. (2010). Pilots of oncology health care: A concept analysis of the patient navigator role. *Oncology Nursing Forum*, 37, 55–60. Available at: http://ons.metapress.com/index/N6105M6772875248.pdf.

Pinto, A., Lee, S., Lombardo, S., Salama, M., Ellis, S., Kay, T., et al. (2012). The impact of a structured inter-professional education on health care professional students: Perceptions of collaboration in a clinical setting. *Physiotherapy Canada*, 64(2), 145–156.

Poster, E., Adams, P., Clay, C., Garcia, B., Hallman, A., Jackson, B., et al. (2005). The Texas model of differentiated entry-level competencies of graduates of nursing programs. *Nursing Education Perspectives*, 26(1), 18–23.

Seago, J. (1999). Evaluation of a hospital work redesign: Patient-focused care. *Journal of Nursing Administration*, 29(11), 31–38.

Sportsman, S., Poster, E., Curl, E., Walker, P., & Hooper, J. (2010). Differentiated essential competencies: A view from practice. *Journal of Nursing Administration*, 42(1), 59–63.

Tiedeman, M., & Lookinland, S. (2004). Traditional models of care delivery: What have we learned (electronic version)? *Journal of Nursing Administration*, 34(6), 291–297.

Viney, M., Batcheller, J., Houston, S., & Belcik, K. (2006). Transforming care at the bedside: Designing new care systems in an age of complexity. *Journal of Nursing Care Quality*, 21(2), 143–150.

Wells, K. J., Battaglia, T. A., Dudley, D. J., Garcia, R., Greene, A., Calhoun, E., et al. (2008). Patient navigation: State of the art or is it science? *Cancer*, 113(8), 1999–2010.

Wolf, G. A., & Greenhouse, P. K. (2007). Blue print for design: Creating models that direct change. *Journal of Nursing Administration*, 37(9), 381–387.

Zander, K. (2002). Nursing case management in the 21st century: Intervening where margin meets mission. *Nursing Administration Quarterly*, 26(5), 58–67.

SUGGESTED READINGS

Brown, J., Smith, C., Stewart, M., Trim, K., Freeman, T., Beckhoff, C., et al. (2009). Level of acceptance of different models of maternity care. *Canadian Nurse*, 105(1), 19–23.

Hix, C., McKeon, L., & Walters, S. (2009). Clinical nurse leader impact on clinical microsystem outcomes. *Journal of Nursing Administration*, 39(92), 71–76, February.

IOM. (2011). *The future of nursing: Leading change, advancing health.* Committee on the Robert Wood Johnson Foundation Initiative on the Future of Nursing at the Institute of Medicine; Institute of Medicine. www.nap.edu/catalog/12956.html.

Kaplow, R., & Reed, M. (2008b). The AACN Synergy Model for Patient Care: A nursing model as a Force of Magnetism. *Nursing Economic$*, 26(1), 17–25.

Lake, E., Shange, J., Klaus, S., & Dunton, N. (2010). Patient falls: Association with magnet status and nursing unit staffing. *Research in Nursing and Health*, 33, 413–425.

Lookinland, S., Tiedeman, M., & Crosson, A. (2005). Nontraditional models of care delivery: Have they solved the problem? *Journal of Nursing Administration*, 35(2), 74–80.

Peikes, D., Lester, R. S., Gilman, B., & Brown, R. (2013). The effects of transitional care models on re-admissions: A review of the current evidence. *Generations: Journal of American Society on Aging*, 26(4), 44–55.

Tachibana, C., & Nelson-Peterson, D. (2007). Implementing the clinical nurse leader role using the Virginia Mason Production system. *Journal of Nurse Administration*, 37(11), 477–479.

Wells, K. J., Battalion, T. A., Dudley, D. J., Garcia, R., Greene, A., Calhoun, E., et al. (2008). Patient navigation: State of the art or is it science? *Cancer*, 113(8), 1999–2010.

Wiggins, M. (2008). The Partnership Care Delivery Model: An examination of the core concept and the need for a new model of care. *Journal of Nursing Management*, 16, 629–638.

INTERNET RESOURCES

AACN's Healthy workplace initiative. www.aacn.org/WD/HWE/Content/hwehome.content?menu=hwe.

American Association of Colleges of Nursing. *White paper on the role of the clinical nurse leader*. Website: www.aacn.nche.edu/Publications/WhitePapers/ClinicalNurseLeader.htm.

American Case Management Association. Website: www.acmaweb.org.

American Nurses Credentialing Center. *History of the Magnet program*. Website: www.nursecredentialing.org/Magnet/ProgramOverview/HistoryoftheMagnetProgram.aspx.

Case Management Society of America. Website: www.cmsa.org.

Clinical Practice Guidelines Online. Agency for Healthcare Research and Quality (AHRQ). National Guidelines Clearinghouse. http://www.guideline.gov/.

RWJ Foundation launches Transforming Care at the Bedside Virtual Resource Center. Website: www.rwjf.org/pr/product.jsp?id=31512.

Transforming Care at the Bedside (TCAB) Tool Kit. Robert Wood Johnson Foundation. Website: www.rwjf.org/pr/product.jsp?id=30051&c=EMC-CA137.

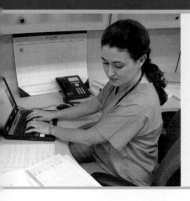

Staffing and Scheduling

Susan Sportsman

This chapter explores research regarding the relationship between nurse staffing and various nurse and patient outcomes. It discusses the interrelationship between the personnel budget and the staffing plan. Measures for evaluating unit productivity and the impact of various staffing and scheduling strategies on overall nursing satisfaction and continuity of patient care are discussed. These key points are critical to nurse managers' ability to deliver safe and effective care in their areas of responsibility while maintaining a high degree of employee satisfaction on the unit. Understanding the impact of nurse-sensitive indicators on patient outcomes helps nurse managers control the unit's labor expenses. Their ability to use this information and communicate about staffing to employees is critical to effectively managing productive services and being a valuable member of the leadership team.

LEARNING OUTCOMES

- Evaluate the impact of patient and hospital factors, nurse characteristics, nurse staffing, and other organizational factors that influence nurse and patient outcomes.
- Integrate current research into principles to effectively manage nurse staffing.
- Analyze activity reports to determine the effectiveness of a unit's productivity.
- Examine personnel scheduling needs in relation to patients' requirements for continuity of care and positive outcomes, as well as the nurse manager's need to create a schedule that is balanced and fair for all team members.
- Relate floating, mandatory overtime, and the use of supplemental agency staff to nurse satisfaction and patient care outcomes.

KEY TERMS

average daily census (ADC)	mandatory overtime	scheduling
average length of stay (ALOS)	nonproductive time	staffing
cost center	nurse outcomes	staffing plan
direct care hours	nurse-sensitive data	staffing regulations
factor evaluation system	nursing productivity	units of service
fixed full-time equivalents (FTEs)	overtime	variable FTEs
forecast	patient outcomes	variance report
full-time equivalents (FTEs)	percentage of occupancy	workload
indirect care hours	productive time	
labor cost per unit of service	prototype evaluation system	

Mary Ellen Bonczek, BSN, RN, MPA, NEA-BC
Senior Vice President and Chief Nurse Executive, New Hanover
Regional Medical Center, Wilmington, North Carolina

The inpatient general surgical units of a large regional medical center has a total of 54 beds, and the surgical trauma intensive care unit (STICU) has 16 beds. The organization was faced with severe capacity constraints as it prepared to begin a master site facility plan that would result in an additional 120 beds over the next 3 years. The lack of a step-down unit for surgical patients was a particular void in service. The coronary care unit (CCU), medical intensive care unit (MICU), and cardiovascular intensive care unit (CVICU) all have step-down units to which they can transfer patients and free up beds for truly critical patients. Beds that were already filled with general surgery patients were targeted to be the step-down unit for the STICU.

The challenge to develop the surgical step-down unit included the identification of the appropriate number of step-down beds needed by considering the volume of patients in STICU that could be transferred to the surgical step-down unit. Admission and discharge criteria for this step-down unit needed to be developed and approved by the medical staff. New equipment needs also had to be identified. The staff competencies necessary to provide appropriate care to these patients had to be considered and education plans developed. In addition, a staffing plan had to be outlined. Communication to the nursing staff was critical—some feared that they would lose their jobs because the critical care staff would assume their positions.

What do you think you would do if you were this nurse?

INTRODUCTION

The passage and implementation of The Patient Protection and Affordable Care Act of 2010 has resulted in uncertainty regarding the number of patients who will be eligible for care when the legislation is fully implemented, the costs to deliver necessary care, and the reimbursement that healthcare organizations will receive for providing services. To manage the potential costs associated with caring for patients new to the system, efforts to reduce cost, while encouraging care in less expensive environments, will continue to be emphasized.

Healthcare organizations, particularly in acute care settings, have recognized that controlling labor costs is critical for overall cost reduction. Because nursing salaries constitute some of the major drivers of labor costs in a healthcare organization, nurse leaders are increasingly challenged to tightly manage both staffing and scheduling within their assigned cost centers. Staffing, which involves planning for hiring and deploying qualified human resources to meet the needs of a group of patients, is a primary responsibility of the nurse manager. It is also a major way in which a nurse in that role can influence quality of care. Scheduling, on the other hand, is a function of implementing the staffing plan by assigning unit personnel to work specific hours and days of the week.

Nurse managers must make skilled staffing and scheduling decisions to ensure that safe and cost-effective care is provided by the appropriate level of caregivers. No matter what the practice setting—acute care, home care, or long-term care—managers have an increasing accountability for establishing and monitoring effective and efficient staffing systems.

THE STAFFING PROCESS

AHRQ Nurse Staffing Model

Over the last decade, a significant amount of research has been done in the United States to evaluate links among nursing staffing, workloads, skills mix, and patient outcomes. An analysis of this research demonstrates that ensuring adequate staffing levels has been shown to:

- Reduce medical and medication errors
- Decrease patient complications
- Decrease mortality
- Improve patient satisfaction
- Reduce nurse fatigue
- Decrease nurse burnout
- Improve nurse retention and job satisfaction (ANA, 2013).

Because of the emphasis on patient safety and positive patient outcomes in health care, research to define the "best practices" of staffing has been a high priority over the last 20 years. Consistently the research suggests that increasing the numbers of registered nurses results in many positive benefits to patients, such as a reduction in hospital-related mortality and failure to rescue, both of which are nurse-sensitive outcomes (Kane, Shamliyan, Mueller, Duval, & Wilt, 2007).

Based upon a meta-analysis of research related to the impact of staffing upon patient safety, Kane et al. (2007) developed the Agency for Healthcare Research and Quality (AHRQ) framework, which continues to direct ongoing research. This framework considers the impact of patient and hospital factors, nurse staffing, nurse characteristics, nurse outcomes, medical care, and organizational factors on patient outcomes. This framework, shown in Figure 14-1, can be useful not only for further research, but also for nurse managers to develop best practices for staffing.

Patient Factors

The acuity or severity of a patient's conditions, influenced by their age, primary diagnosis, co-morbidities, and treatment stage, is a key component in determining the staffing required for safe care. However, the dynamic nature of patient care often makes it difficult to quantify the care needs of patients at any given time. However, it is helpful to consider the patient variables, depicted in Table 14-1, in a specific unit as staffing decisions are made.

TABLE 14-1	PATIENT VARIABLES AFFECTING STAFFING DECISIONS	
Number of patients	Stage of illness	
Range of conditions	Family situation and needs	
Observations and interventions required	Treatment required	
Patients' satisfaction		

Revised from Douglas, K. (2010). Ratios – If only it were that easy. *Nursing Economic$, 28*(2), 119-125.

Patient classification systems used primarily in acute care settings have been developed in an effort to give nurse managers the tools and language to describe the acuity of patients on their unit. More seriously ill patients receive higher classification scores, indicating that more nursing resources are required to provide patient care. Nurse managers use the classification data to adjust the unit's staffing plan for a given time or to quantify acuity trends over longer periods as they forecast their staffing needs during the budget process.

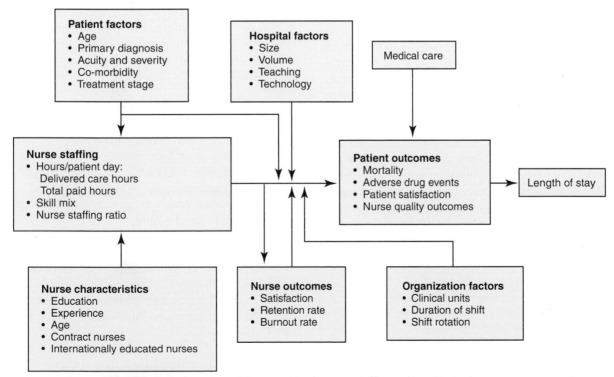

FIGURE 14-1 Conceptual framework of nurse staffing and patient outcomes.

Patient Classification Types

Two basic types of patient classification systems exist: prototype and factor. A prototype evaluation system is considered both subjective and descriptive. It classifies patients into broad categories and uses these categories to predict patient care needs. The relative intensity measures (RIMs) system is a prototype system. This system classifies patient care needs based on their diagnosis-related group (DRG). The data are then fed to an electronic decision support system that integrates clinical and financial information.

A factor evaluation system is considered more objective than a prototype evaluation system. It gives each task, thought process, and patient care activity a time or rating. These associations are then summed to determine the hours of direct care required, or they are weighted for each patient. Each intervention is given a name and a definition and is further specified to incorporate a list of all associated interventional activities. The list of interventions is comprehensive and applicable to inpatient, outpatient, home care, and long-term care patients.

Typically, if these systems are used for staffing decisions, organizations use a combination. Some patient types with a single healthcare focus, such as maternal deliveries or outpatient surgical patients, would be appropriately classified with a prototype system. Patients with more complex care needs and a less predictable disease course, such as those with pneumonia or stroke, are more appropriately evaluated with a factor system.

Numerous potential problems exist with patient classification systems. The issue most often raised by administrators relates to the questionable reliability and validity of the data collected through a self-reporting mechanism. Another concern with patient classification data relates to the inability of the organization to meet the prescribed staffing levels outlined by the patient classification system.

EXERCISE 14-1

Administrators worry that they risk potential liability if they do not follow the staffing recommendations of the patient classification system. If the classification data indicate that six caregivers are needed for the upcoming shift but the organization can provide only five caregivers, what are the potential consequences for the organization if an untoward event occurs?

Concern over the accuracy of biased data and the inability to meet predicted staffing levels outlined by the patient classification systems has caused many healthcare organizations to abandon patient classification as a mechanism for determining appropriate staffing levels. Staff morale is at risk when acuity models indicate one level is necessary and the organization cannot increase staffing to meet those needs. Likewise, staff morale is at risk without acuity models when it is clear to staff that patient needs exceed care capacity.

PRODUCTIVITY MODELS

Forecasting Unit Staffing Requirements

Nurse managers often in concert with the others in nursing administration and financial services, are responsible for determining the number of staff required in every unit for every shift. Recognizing factors, including related research, that influence staffing can inform decisions regarding development of the staffing plan. However, other issues must be considered when determining an appropriate staffing level for a specific unit. The staffing plan for a unit is initiated in concert with the development of the personnel budget. The person(s) responsible for projecting staffing needs of the unit should consider a number of factors when forecasting the unit's workload for the upcoming year, including the following:

1. Projected units of services (UOS)
2. Historical staffing requirements
3. Effectiveness of the current staffing plan
4. Trends in acuity on the unit
5. Anticipated skill mix or other personnel changes
6. Experience and education of staff
7. New physicians, programs, services, or technology anticipated to affect staffing
8. Patient outcomes
9. Need for educational updates driven by changes in patient care guidelines (Upenieks, Akhavan, & Kotlerman, 2008)

Various mathematical formulations were used in the past to create personnel budgets and staffing patterns. However, these formulas were developed when the average length of stay and reimbursement patterns were much different than they are today. The current difficulties related to staffing in health care suggest that current methods used to predict personnel budgets and staffing patterns have become increasingly complex and ineffective. To improve this situation, Fitzpatrick and Brooks (2010) suggest the use of optimization models that rely on computer and logistic sciences to identify the best solution to particular staffing problems

Given the difficulty in measuring the acuity of patients with available patient classification systems, many hospitals use productivity models as a framework for determining the staffing levels of a unit. Productivity in hospitals is defined as the output per unit of input. Input includes both full-time equivalent employees and part-time workers, and the output is adjusted occupied beds (including both the inpatient census and the outcome activities),

Based upon interviews of nurses on a number of nursing units in three Texas hospitals, Hamilton and Campbell (2011) described the use of productivity instruments, sophisticated technologies that calculate the staffing patterns required on a unit. As previously noted, specific unit productivity is based upon assumptions about the number, type, and acuity of patients projected to be admitted on a unit in the context of the organization's financial goals. The result of the calculations is a staffing matrix, which gives the number of patients expected to be on the unit at midnight of each day projected. The matrix also provides the number of personnel (RNs, LVNs/LPNs, unit secretaries, and charge nurses) required to meet the daily demands of the projected number of nurses. The matrix is then used to develop the monthly staffing schedule for the unit.

Every shift provides opportunities to increase or decrease the number of staff on the unit based on available staff, patient census, and patient acuity level. However, the charge nurse and, ultimately, the nurse manager have the responsibility to meet the goals established by the matrix. If the number of staff required on a shift-by-shift basis exceeds the number budgeted in a given month, an equal reduction at some other time within the month must be made in order to meet the productivity necessary to meet the targets (projections). In this way, the availability of staff is dictated by the projections for profitability.

The productivity of a unit is monitored on a shift-by-shift basis. The charge nurse is expected to complete unit reports, sending them electronically to a number of hospital offices, typically the staffing office, payroll, financial officer, and nursing administration. These reports may include such information as:

- Productivity index for the pay period (100% is desirable)
- Amount of overtime
- Amount of supplemental (contract) workers
- Benchmarks against results of peer units
- Actual labor costs (total and per patient day)
- Projected costs (total and per patient day)
- Variance of costs
- Training and orientation costs
- Worked full-time equivalent (FTE) variance compared to target

The nurse manager, and ultimately the nurse executive, are responsible for variances and, as previously discussed, must align the staffing decisions with the financial objectives (Hamilton & Campbell, 2011).

EVALUATION OF EFFECTIVE STAFFING

National Database of Nursing Quality Indicators

The National Database of Nursing Quality Indicators (NDNQI) also provides an opportunity to monitor staffing effectiveness in a specific nursing service or unit. The NDNQI, a program of the American Nurses Association, provides a benchmarking report comparing "like" participating organizations and units around the country. This database is a major national nursing database that provides quarterly and annual reporting of structure, process, and outcome indicators to evaluate "nursing-sensitive" measures at the unit level. Nursing-sensitive measures reflect the structure, process, and outcomes of nursing care (NDNQI, 2013). Collaborative Alliance for Nursing Outcomes (CALNOC), a similar program, is commonly used in California and some other Western states.

The NDNQI database was built upon the 1994 American Nurses Association (ANA) Patient Safety and Quality Initiative. This initiative involved a series of pilot studies across the United States to identify nurse-sensitive indicators to use in evaluating patient care quality. These nurse-sensitive indicators included both structures of care and care processes, which in turn influence care outcomes. Nurse-sensitive indicators are distinct and specific to nursing and different from medical indicators of care quality (NDNQI, 2013)

NDNQI is a comprehensive, national nursing database that provides hospitals with nursing unit level comparison on 18 quality indicators that can be used in quality improvement plans to prevent adverse events. Of particular importance is that these measures include hospital-acquired conditions and adverse events listed in the rules established by the Centers for Medicare & Medicaid Services (CMS) to preclude payment for care resulting from pressure ulcers, falls, and bloodstream infections. In addition, NDNQI measures nursing workforce issues related to quality of care, including staffing levels, turnover, and RN education and certification rates (NDNQI, 2013).

Hospitals can benchmark (or compare) their own data against other similar hospitals and participate in the ongoing research on **nurse-sensitive data**. Table 14-2 on p. 261 outlines the nurse-sensitive indicators included in the NDNQI project. The comparison of like-units is very important, because patient acuity and activity; patient care goals, clinical tasks, role expectation, team relations, and social milieu vary by unit and affect the patient outcomes.

The measures included in the NDNQI database can be important in making staffing decisions when the accumulated evidence underlying these measures are included. For example, research related to hours per patient day (HPPD) required to provide the necessary nursing care for patients on the unit can provide evidence for constructing an effective staffing plan for a unit.

For example, in 2007 Dunton, Gajewski, Klaus, and Pierson studied the relationship between hours per patient days (HPPD) in relation to falls and suggested that:

- Lower falls rates were related to higher total nursing hours (including RN, licensed practical nurse/licensed vocational nurse [LPN/LVN] and unlicensed nursing personnel [UNP]) per patient day and a higher percentage of nursing hours supplied by RNs.
- For every increase of 1 hour in total nursing HPPD, fall rates were 1.9% lower.

- For every increase of 1 percentage point in the nursing hours supplied by RNs, the fall rate was 0.7% lower (Dunton et al., 2007).

Nurse managers may also use clinical or human resource indicators other than those identified by NDNQI to evaluate the effectiveness of the staffing and quality of patient care. Box 14-1 on p. 262 identifies some of these indicators.

In 2013, building upon the results by Dunton et al. (2010), Lake, Shang, Klaus, & Dunton performed a retrospective, cross-sectional study also using 2004 NDNQI data, This study compared the impact of nursing staffing (nursing care hours per patient day) and nurse characteristics (education, national certification, and hospital Magnet™ status) on the fall rates in 108 Magnet™ and 528 non-Magnet™ hospitals.

This study found that:

- The mean fall rates among all hospitals studied was consistent with the findings from Lake, Shang, Klaus and Dunton (2010).
- Falls were 5% lower in Magnet™ hospitals, suggesting that the characteristics required for Magnet™ status may influence positive outcomes.
- One additional RN per patient day was associated with a 3% lower fall rate in ICUs.
- An increase in LPNs/LVNs and UNPs per patient day is associated with a 2% to 4% higher fall rates in non-ICUs.

Registered Nurse Staffing

The recognition that the number of registered nurses providing care to patients is associated with better patient outcomes in acute care leads to a discussion regarding the best model to ensure sufficient staffing. Two major approaches have been put forward. The first requires a specific number of patients cared for by one nurse per shift (mandated nurse-patient ratios). Legislation to mandate specific nurse-patient ratios was initially implemented in California in 1999 and fully implemented in 2004. This law requires that a nurse must care for no more than:

- Six patients in a psychiatric unit
- Five patients in a medical-surgical unit
- Four pediatric patients
- Three patients in a labor and delivery unit
- Two patients in intensive care units

Aiken et al. (2010) examined the effects of California's 2004 minimum nurse-patient staff ratio

TABLE 14-2   NURSE-SENSITIVE INDICATORS INCLUDED IN THE PAIN ASSESSMENT/ INTERVENTION/REASSESSMENT CYCLES COMPLETED

INDICATOR	SUB-INDICATORS	MEASURE(S)
1. Nursing Hours per Patient Day	a. Registered Nurses (RNs) b. Licensed Practical/Vocational Nurses (LPNs/LVNs) c. Unlicensed Nursing Personnel (UNP)	Structure
2. Patient Falls		Process & Outcome
3. Patient Falls with Injury	a. Injury Level	Process & Outcome
4. Pediatric Pain Assessment, Intervention, Reassessment (AIR) Cycle		Process
5. Pediatric Peripheral Intravenous Infiltration Rate		Outcome
6. Pressure Ulcer Prevalence	a. Community Acquired b. Hospital Acquired c. Unit Acquired	Process & Outcome
7. Psychiatric Physical/Sexual Assault Rate		Outcome
8. Restraint Prevalence		Outcome
9. RN Education/Certification		Structure
10. RN Satisfaction Survey Options	a. Job Satisfaction Scales b. Job Satisfaction Scales—Short Form c. Practice Environment Scale (PES)†	Process & Outcome
11. Skill Mix: Percent of total nursing hours supplied by Agency Staff	a. RNs b. LPNs/LVNs c. UNP	Structure
12. Voluntary Nurse Turnover		Structure
13. Nurse Vacancy Rate		Structure
14. Healthcare-Associated Infection a. Urinary catheter–associated urinary tract infection (UTI) b. Central line catheter–associated bloodstream infection (CABSI) c. Ventilator-associated pneumonia (VAP)		Outcome

ANA, About National Database of Nursing Quality Indicators (NDNQI): http://www.nursingquality.org/About-NDNQI

mandate for acute care facilities by comparing patient outcome data and hospital staffing information at hospitals in California, New Jersey and Pennsylvania. Researchers also surveyed 22,236 hospital nurses in the three states. According to the nurse survey, 88% of the California nurses working in a medical-surgical area reported overseeing only 5 patients, as required by the California law. In contrast, 33% of the Pennsylvania nurses surveyed and 19% of those surveyed in New Jersey reported being responsible for 5 or fewer patients. California nurses cared for 2 fewer patients than nurses in New Jersey and 1.7 fewer patients than nurses in Pennsylvania. The analysis suggested that if California's nurse-patient levels had been instituted in Pennsylvania and New Jersey during the time of the study, the states could have achieved 10.6% and 13.0% fewer deaths respectively among general surgical patients. The study also found that California nurses reported higher job satisfaction and the perception that they provided better patient care than did nurses surveyed in Pennsylvania and New Jersey (Aiken et al., 2010).

The second approach for appropriate staffing requires the development of a staffing plan, which holds hospitals accountable for projecting the nursing needs on each unit for a period of time, typically for 6 months or a year. Hospitals are also responsible for monitoring the extent to which actual staffing

BOX 14-1   OTHER INDICATORS OF STAFFING EFFECTIVENESS

Clinical or Service Indicators
- Family complaints
- Patient complaints
- Adverse drug events
- Injuries to patients
- Postoperative infections
- Upper gastrointestinal bleeding
- Shock/cardiac arrest
- Length of stay

Human Resource Indicators
- Overtime
- Staff vacancy rate
- Staff turnover rate
- Understaffing as compared with the hospital's staffing plan
- Nursing care hours per patient day
- Staff injuries on the job
- On-call or per diem use
- Sick time

matches the staffing plans, making revisions as necessary. These plans often require that direct care nurses are part of the nurse staffing committee to ensure that safe nurse-to-patient ratios are based on patient needs and other related criteria. The first legislation mandating such a committee was passed by the Texas state legislature in 2002. As of October 2008, seven states (Connecticut, Illinois, Nevada, Ohio, Oregon, Texas, and Washington) had some sort of legislation requiring a nursing staffing plan in acute care hospitals (ANA, 2013)

The American Nurses Association has opted to support the nurse staffing committee as the approach to insure safe staffing. ANA has supported a number of efforts to pass national legislation, similar to the state laws currently in place. In 2013, as an example, HR 1821: The Registered Nurse Safe Staffing Act was introduced in the U.S. Congress, which requires all acute care hospitals to establish a committee made up of 55% direct care RNs. The plans must:
- Establish upwardly adjustable minimum ratios of direct care to patients for each unit and shift
- Include input from direct care RNs
- Be based on patient numbers and variable intensity of care required

- Take into account:
  - Level of education, training, and experience of RNs providing care
  - Staffing levels and services provided by other healthcare personnel
  - Unit and facility level staffing
  - Quality and patient care and national comparisons, as available
  - Other factors impacting delivery of care, including unit geographic and available technology
- Consider staffing levels recommended by specialty nursing organizations
  - Ensure that RNs are not forced to work on units where they are not trained or experienced (ANA, 2013)

Those who support a specified nurse-patient ratio based on the type of unit (e.g., ICU, medical-surgical) believe this approach will require hospitals to either find sufficient numbers of nurses to meet the ratio or shut down units. Those who prefer the nurse staffing plan approach believe that use of a staffing plan is built on nursing judgment that will allow staffing to be flexible, depending on patient acuity, nurse experience, configuration of the unit, and other factors. The ANA developed a Website (*http://safestaffingsaveslives. org/*) devoted specifically to staffing. This Website, *Safe Staffing Saves Lives*, includes the principles of safe staffing developed by ANA that apply to all clinical care settings (Box 14-2 on p. 263).

24-Hour Staffing

Most of the research regarding safe staffing has been done in acute care hospitals or long-term care facilities. As a result, these findings must be applied to other healthcare settings with some caution. In addition, little research regarding the differences in staffing in any clinical environment has been conducted for off-peak hours (nights and weekends). Despite the fact that hospital activity is at its peak from 7 AM to 7 PM weekdays, when maximum resources are available in the nurses work environment, this time represents only 36% of the time that nurses work in acute care or long-term care. During the remaining 64% of the time, nurses work in off-peak environments with (1) scaled-back ancillary personnel, (2) fewer (often less-experienced) staff, (3) minimal supervision, and (4) strained communication with

Principles

The nine principles identified by the expert panel for nurse staffing and adopted by the ANA Board of Directors on November 24, 1998, are listed below. A discussion of each of the three categories is available through ANA.

I. Patient Care Unit Related

a. Appropriate staffing levels for a patient care unit reflect analysis of individual and aggregate patient needs.

b. There is a critical need to either retire or seriously question the usefulness of the concept of nursing hours per patient day (HPPD).

c. Unit functions necessary to support delivery of quality patient care must also be considered in determining staffing levels.

II. Staff Related

a. The specific needs of various patient populations should determine the appropriate clinical competencies required of the nurse practicing in that area.

b. Registered nurses must have nursing management support and representation at both the operational level and the executive level.

c. Clinical support from experienced RNs should be readily available to those RNs with less proficiency.

III. Institution/Organization Related

a. Organizational policy should reflect an organizational climate that values registered nurses and other employees as strategic assets and exhibit a true commitment to filling budgeted positions in a timely manner.

b. All institutions should have documented competencies for nursing staff, including agency or supplemental and traveling RNs, for those activities that they have been authorized to perform.

c. Organizational policies should recognize the myriad needs of both patients and nursing staff.

on-call healthcare providers (Hamilton, Eschiti, Hernandez, & Neill, 2007).

The problems identified by Hamilton et al. (2007) are corroborated in other studies. Researchers have associated weekends and nights with increased mortality in hospitals for more than 25 diagnoses/patient groups. For example, Becker (2007) found acute myocardial infarction more likely to result in death among Medicaid patients admitted on weekends. Peberdy et al. (2008) found lower survival rates from inpatient cardiology units at nights and on weekends, even after adjusting for potentially confounding factors. Although the reasons for the differences in risk in off-peak hours are under investigation, nurse managers must be cognizant of these differences and staff during off-peak times in a prudent manner to minimize patient risk. Direct care nurses need to be proactive in this knowledge by helping to document differences that exist during these times.

External Factors Influencing Staffing

An important source for guidance in projecting staffing requirements is the licensing regulations of the state, typically through the department of health, which often reflect legislation discussed earlier. Staffing regulations or recommendations can relate to the minimum number of professional nurses required on a unit at a given time or to the amount of minimum staffing in an extended-care facility or prison.

However, note that licensing standards and staffing regulations by state departments of health are not the only regulatory bodies that affect staffing plans. A number of national organizations with missions related to continuous improvement in the safety and quality of health care provided to the public. The Joint Commission (TJC) is an example of this type of organization. TJC works to support performance improvement in healthcare organizations through establishing standards and survey accreditation processes. To comply with the most recent TJC patient care standards related to staffing, for example, an institution must provide an adequate number and mix of staff consistent with the hospital's staffing plan to meet the care, treatment, and service needs of the patients. TJC is not prescriptive as to what constitutes "adequate" staffing. However, in response to increasing public concerns about patient care safety and quality, TJC correlates an organization's clinical outcome data with its staffing patterns to determine the effectiveness of the overall staffing plan.

During the TJC accreditation process, the surveyor reviews the staffing plans developed by the nurse manager for any obvious staffing deficiencies—for example, a shift or series of shifts in which the unit staffing plan is not met. The surveyor also interviews direct care nurses outside of the presence of nurse managers to inquire about their perceptions of the units' staffing adequacy. Surveyors may review the staffing effectiveness data for that unit as it compares with any variations from the staffing plan to identify quality-of-care concerns. Nurse managers are well advised to prepare a balanced staffing plan that supports a unit's unique patient care needs and the scrutiny of the TJC survey process. They also should post this staffing plan and the compliance reports for staff to see on a routine basis. In some states, this posting is required.

Additional regulatory agencies that provide accreditation services similar to those provided by TJC include the American Osteopathic Association (AOA), the Center for Accreditation of Rehabilitation Facilities (CARF), the Accreditation Association for Ambulatory Health Care (AAAHC), the Det Norske Veritas (DNV), the National Committee for Quality Assurance in Behavioral Health, and the Community Health Accreditation Program. Additionally other groups are emerging. Thus, knowing what an organization's accrediting body says about staffing is highly important.

Consumer expectations may also play a role in the development and implementation of the staffing plans. Exceeding the expectations of consumers for care and services is a major strategy for maintaining and improving the long-term viability of any healthcare organization. Recognizing that the patient expects to receive high-quality nursing care that is delivered promptly and efficiently by nurses who are satisfied with their workload has a significant influence on the development of a staffing plan.

Organizational policies and clear expectations communicated to staff are essential to manage high and low volume as well as changes in acuity. Proposed personnel budgets and staffing plans that cannot flex up or down when patient acuity or volumes change put the nurse manager in a position in which patient safety may not be maintained and financial obligations cannot be met. In addition, mechanisms must be in place and internally publicized to allow staff to ask for additional help as needed. Patient, staff, and physician satisfaction; service and care improvement; and patient safety improvement are all outcomes of a solid staffing plan. Nurse managers are obligated to consider these variables when preparing the personnel budget.

Nurse Characteristics

Kane et al. (2007) defined nurse characteristics as the age, experience, and education of the nurse who is providing care. In addition, the use of supplemental (agency/contract) nurses and internationally educated nurses is a variable that influences nurse staffing. Although not specifically identified in the AHRQ conceptual framework, other factors such as the use of float pools and overtime also may affect patient outcomes.

Ridley (2008), in reviewing literature from 1986 to 2006 regarding the relationship between patient safety and nurse education level, found that when studies discriminate between registered nurses and other types of nursing personnel (LPNs/LVNs or UNPs), the evidence shows an increased number of RNs and a larger percentage of RNs relative to other nursing personnel decrease adverse patient outcomes sensitive to nursing care.

Education

In a landmark study in 2003, Aiken, Clarke, Cheung, Sloane, and Silber examined whether the proportion of hospital RNs educated at the baccalaureate level or higher was associated with risk-adjusted 30-day mortality and failure to rescue. Interest in this idea has persisted.

Using Pennsylvania nurse survey and patient discharge data from 1999 and 2006, the researchers found that a 10-point increase in the percentage of nurses holding a baccalaureate degree in nursing within a hospital was associated with an average reduction of 2.12 deaths for every 1000 patients; and for a subset of patients with complications, they found an average reduction of 7.47 deaths per 1000 patients. They estimated that if all 134 hospitals in the study had increased the percentage of their nurses with baccalaureate degrees by 10 points during the study's time period, some 500 deaths among general, orthopedic, and vascular surgery patients might have been prevented. The findings provide support for efforts to increase the production and employment of baccalaureate nurses.

In 2011, the Institute of Medicine (IOM), in partnership with the Robert Wood Johnson Foundation, assessed and responded to the need to transform the nursing profession. One of the recommendations of this study was to increase the proportion of nurses with a baccalaureate degree to 80% by 2020. In making this recommendation, the IOM noted that the level of education required for entry into nursing has been widely debated for more than 40 years. The IOM report recognizes that there is no conclusive evidence of a causal relationship between the academic degree obtained by RNs and patient outcomes, despite the groundbreaking work of Aiken et al. (2003). However, the report cites the work of Estabrooks, Midodzi, Cummings, Ricker, and Giovannetti (2005); Friese et al. (2008); Tourangeau et al. (2007); and Van den Heede et al. (2009) that offer evidence similar to Aiken, Clarke, Cheung, Sloane, Silber, 2003).

Other studies reported in the IOM study suggested that the clinical experience, qualifications before entering a nursing program, and the number of BSN-prepared RNs that received an earlier degree confound the value added through the 4-year period (IOM, 2011). Despite this ongoing debate regarding the value of a BSN, the IOM report suggested that an all-BSN workforce would provide a more uniform foundation for the "reconceptualized roles" of nursing in the future. Although a BSN education is not a panacea for all that is to be expected, it does, according to the report "introduce students to a wider range of competencies in such areas as health policy and health care financing, leadership, quality improvement and systems thinking" (pp. 168–169).

Overtime

Kane et al. (2007) reviewed seven descriptive studies that used survey methodology to find that nurses were working long hours. Because more nurses are choosing to work 12-hour shifts, the risk of working more than 12 hours is high, given that nurses often cannot finish their work by the end of their scheduled shift. Evidence continues to emerge showing that working more than 12 hours and rotating shifts can lead to errors that compromise patient safety (Kane et al., 2007).

In 2012, Stimpfel, Sloane, and Aiken surveyed nurses in four states and found that more than 80% of the nurses were satisfied with scheduling practices at their hospital, despite the fact that the majority work 12 hour shifts. However, as the proportion of hospital nurses working shifts of more than 13 hours increased, patients' dissatisfaction with care increased. Furthermore, nurses working shifts of 10 hours or longer were up to 2.5 times more likely than nurses working shorter shifts to experience burnout and job dissatisfaction and expressed an intent to leave the job. Extended shifts undermine nurses' well-being, may result in expensive job turnover, and can negatively affect patient care.

Building upon the scientific literature that documents adverse physiologic and psychological effects of shift work of all types including disruption to biological rhythm, sleep disorders, health problems, and diminished performance at work, job dissatisfaction, and social isolation, Tzischinsky et al. (2008) investigated health problems and sleep disorders between female and male nurses, between nurses on daytime and other shifts, and between sleep-adjusted and non–sleep-adjusted shift nurses. They also evaluated the relationships between adjustment to shift work and errors, patient incidents, and absenteeism from work. Gender, age, and weight were more significant factors than shift work in determining the well-being of nurses. Shift work by itself was not a risk factor for nurses' health and organizational outcomes. Those nurses who were "non-adaptive" to shift work were found to work as effectively and safely as their colleagues who were adaptive. They had no more absenteeism or involvement in errors or patient incidences.

Despite the somewhat contradictory findings regarding shift work in nursing, fatigue, and nurse performance and satisfaction, the nurse manager should consider the potential risks when scheduling staff.

The type of overtime that is required may influence the outcomes. *Requiring* staff to stay on duty after their shift ends to fill staffing vacancies is called **mandatory overtime**. Mandatory overtime has become a major negotiating point for nurses in unionized settings, and some state nursing associations that use workplace advocacy strategies to improve the work environment in their states have developed legislation that prohibits mandatory overtime. The ANA and other nursing organizations oppose mandatory overtime, because it is seen as a risk to both patients and nurses.

In contrast, *requesting* staff to stay on duty after their shift ends to fill staffing vacancies is called overtime. This differs from mandatory overtime because staff experience no employment consequences. In addition, in a given week, nurses may work in more than one employment setting as a means of increasing their income. Although this practice is an individual decision, tired and overworked nurses are more likely to have compromised decision-making abilities and technical skills because of fatigue.

EXERCISE 14-2

Review a healthcare organization's policies on overtime. Is mandatory overtime covered in the policy? Are the consequences for failing to work mandatory overtime when requested to do so by a supervisor outlined in the policy?

How would you respond to a nurse manager who required you to stay on the job after your shift was over? Develop a list of questions you might ask on a job interview relating to use of overtime in the organization.

What does the state board of nursing in your state allow regarding mandatory overtime? As a nurse manager, how would you respond to a staffing shortage without mandatory overtime as an option? Develop a list of strategies for eliminating mandatory overtime, if such exists.

Supplemental (Agency/Contract) Staff and Float Pools

Many nurses choose to work for staffing agencies. They may be hired by a nursing unit as an independent contractor for a shift, a week, or longer. Advantages of working for an agency are higher hourly rates of pay, diversity in work assignments, exposure to a variety of work teams, and the ability to travel.

Organizations may use supplemental staff to fill temporary staff vacancies. Despite the response to an unexpected vacancy, nurse managers must consider the potential negative aspects of depending on supplemental staff to meet the unit's staffing plan. Patients should be unable to distinguish supplemental staff from unit staff. However, the ability to provide that level of orientation to supplemental agency or contract staff is often difficult.

The evidence regarding the impact of the use of supplemental nurses on patient outcome is mixed. Kane et al. (2007) showed no association between hours worked by contract nurses and the rates of urinary tract infection, pneumonia, pressure ulcers, surgical wound infections, and bloodstream infections. In contrast, the increase in patient falls seemed evident as the number of hours worked by supplemental nurses increased.

Another strategy that may be used to deal with unanticipated staff vacancies involves "floating" nurses from one clinical unit to another to fill the vacancy. Kane et al (2007) found that the use of float nurses was associated with an increased risk of nosocomial infections and rate of bloodstream infections; however, further research is necessary to validate this finding. In practice, the use of float nurses may be effective if the nurses are deployed from a centralized flexible staffing pool and they have the competencies to work on the unit to which they are assigned. Nurses willing to work as float nurses are generally experienced nurses who maintain a broad range of clinical competencies. They often receive added compensation for their willingness to be flexible and to float to a variety of units on short notice.

When an organization does not have the flexibility of a staffing pool, the organization may expect nurses to float across clinical units to fill vacancies. To ensure patient safety and nurse satisfaction, the organization must develop a policy regarding the reassignment of the staff to clinically similar units. If direct care nurses are asked to be reassigned to an area outside of their sphere of clinical competence, they should be asked to support only basic care needs and not assume a complete and independent assignment. This practice should be used only on an emergency basis or with the nurse's agreement, because being required to float is often a "dissatisfier" for nurses and potentially a concern for patient safety.

Hospital Factors

According to the AHRQ conceptual model, hospital factors include the size of the hospital, the volume of patients seen, whether the hospital is a teaching hospital, and the extent to which technology is used in the hospital. Kane et al. (2007) reviewed a study by Seago, Spetz, and Mitchell (2004) that found for-profit hospitals and systems had fewer RN productive hours for medical-surgical nursing. A number of studies have found that the type of unit affected hospital RN staffing. Intensive care, pediatric, and maternity units had significantly higher RN staffing than medical/surgical or gynecologic units. Controlling for size, rural hospitals also had higher RN staffing (Kane et al., 2007).

Studies exploring the relationship between increased RN-to-patient ratios found that the effect of increasing the number of RNs to patients was greater in surgical patients and in ICUs. The evidence of the effect of increased RN-to-patient ratios in medical units is less consistent and needs further investigation (Kane et al., 2007). The nurse surveillance capacity of a hospital (those factors that strengthen or weaken the nurses' ability to observe patients for signs of difficulty) also affects the quality of care given. Nurse surveillance capacity is composed of nurse staffing, education, expertise, and experience, as well as nurse practice environment characteristics. Kutney-Lee, Lake, and Aiken (2009) found that greater nurse surveillance capacity was significantly associated with better quality of care and fewer adverse events. (See the following Literature Perspective.)

Regardless of the characteristics of the hospital, managers must be concerned with the financial health of the institution. As a result, hospital financial officers are often reluctant to increase the number of RN staff because of fear of escalating costs. However, Dall, Chen, Seifert, Maddox, and Hogan (2009) found that for each additional patient care RN employed at 7.8 HPPD, over $60,0000 annually will be saved from reduced medical cost and improved national productivity (accounting for 72% of labor costs). This is only a partial estimate of the economic value of nursing because it omits the intangible benefits of reduced pain and suffering by patients and family members, the reduced risk of rehospitalization, benefits to the hospital such as improved reputation and reduced malpractice claims, and other indirect costs. Unfortunately, from the hospital administrators' perspective, healthcare facilities realize only a portion of the economic value of professional nursing, because under current reimbursement systems, the incentive is for hospitals to staff at levels below where the benefit to society equals the cost to employ an additional nurse (Kane et al., 2007).

Nurse Outcomes

Nurse outcomes include staff vacancy rate, nurse satisfaction, staff turnover rate, retention rate, and nurse burnout rate. Kane et al. (2007) noted that while patient outcomes are the ultimate concern, nurse outcomes can interact with nurse staffing to affect patient outcomes. In addition, patient outcomes will, in turn, affect length of stay (LOS), and greater complication rates may increase the length of stay for patients.

A number of studies evaluated by Kane et al. (2007) focused on the impact of nurse satisfaction on patient outcomes. In a survey of 8760 nurses, Sochalski (2004), as described by Kane et al. (2007), examined the relative risk of adverse events among Medicare patients in relation to perceived quality of care. Nurses responded to the survey question, "In general, how would you describe the quality of nursing care delivered to patients in your unit on your last shift?" A reduction by 16% in the relative risk of patient falls and medication errors corresponded to a 30% increase in nurses satisfied with the care provided. However, Kane et al. (2007) also reviewed a number of studies that did not detect a significant improvement in patient satisfaction in relation to nurse satisfaction.

Kane et al. (2007) reported on the impact of nurse autonomy and nurse turnover in relation to patient outcomes. For example, they cited a study by Seago, Spetz, and Mitchell (2004) that found a 2% increase in nurse autonomy accompanied a 0.5% reduction in pressure ulcer rates.

ORGANIZATIONAL FACTORS THAT AFFECT STAFFING PLANS

Organizational factors described in the AHRQ conceptual framework include issues such as types of clinical units and the duration of the shift nurses

 LITERATURE PERSPECTIVE

Resource: Chutney-Lee, A., Lake, E. T., & Aiken, L. H. (2009). Development of the hospital nurse surveillance capacity profile. *Research in Nursing & Health, 32*(2), 217-228.

Surveillance by nurses is a key component of improved patient care. This article defines, operationalizes, measures, and evaluates **nurse surveillance capacity**, which includes organizational features that enhance or weaken nurse surveillance. Nurse surveillance capacity is composed of nurse staffing, education, expertise, and experience, as well as nurse practice environment characteristics. This study found that greater nurse surveillance capacity was significantly associated with better quality of care and fewer adverse events.

Implications for Practice

Evaluating the nurse surveillance capacity in a particular nursing work environment may assist the nurse manager to improve nurse surveillance and patient outcomes on his or her unit.

work, as well as the extent to which shifts are rotated. These factors are typically addressed in the structure and philosophy of the nursing service department, organizational staffing policies, organizational supports, and services offered.

Structure and Philosophy of the Nursing Services Department

A nursing philosophy statement outlines the vision, values, and beliefs about the practice of nursing and the provision of patient care within the organization. The philosophy statement is used to guide the practice of nursing in the various nursing units on a daily basis. Nurse managers must propose a staffing plan and a personnel budget that allow consistency between the written philosophy statement and the observable practice of nursing on their units. It is demoralizing for nurses to feel that they cannot comply with their nursing philosophy statement or professional values because of problems associated with consistently inadequate staffing.

The philosophy statement also guides the establishment of the overall structure of the nursing service department and the staffing models that are used within the organization. The staffing model adopted by the organization plays a major role in determining the mix of professional and assistive staff needed to provide patient care.

Organizational Staffing Policies

Nurse managers are guided in their development of unit personnel budgets by the organization's staffing policies. For example, the organization develops a policy that identifies the rate at which an employee earns overtime and other benefit time. Therefore nurse managers will be in compliance with these laws if they adhere to their organizational staffing policies.

Organizational Support Systems

A critical variable that affects the development of the nursing personnel budget is the presence, or absence, of organizational systems that support the nurse in providing care. If the organization has recognized the need to keep the professional nurse at the bedside, support systems to allow that to happen will be evident. Examples of support systems that enhance the nurse's ability to remain on the unit and provide direct care to patients include transporter services, clerical support services, and hospitality services.

However, professional nurses often work in organizations that require them to function in the role of a multipurpose worker, particularly in acute or long-term care. Because nurses in these settings are generally scheduled to work 24 hours a day, 7 days a week, they may be required to provide services for other professionals who provide more limited hours of care to patients. Wise nurse managers identify what costs are being incurred in the unit as a result of the absence of adequate organizational support systems and develop strategies to put those systems into place or justify the budget accordingly. Important to this consideration is the seminal study by Upenieks et al. (2008), which found that a number of activities that were not actual direct care activities performed at the patient's bedside were considered value-added activities, because they represented a direct benefit to the patient. (See the following Research Perspective.)

 RESEARCH PERSPECTIVE

Resource: Upenieks, V., Akhavan, J., & Kotlerman, J. (2008). Value-added care: A paradigm shift in patient care delivery. *Nursing Economic$, 6*(5), 294-300.

The purpose of the study was to (1) gain an understanding of how much time direct care RNs spent in value-added care and (2) determine whether increasing the combined level of RNs and unlicensed nursing personnel (UNP) increased the amount of time spent in value-added care compared with time spent in necessary tasks and waste. The study found that a number of activities that were not actual direct-care activities performed at the patient's bedside, including collaborating with team members, reviewing charts, preparing medications, teaching activities, and communicating with family members, were considered value-added activities, because they represented a direct benefit to the patient.

Implications for Practice

This study reflects the work done by the Robert Wood Johnson Foundation's initiative, *Transforming Care at the Bedside*, designed to increase the amount of time nurses spend in value-added activities and to reduce time spent in non–value-added activities to improve workflow efficiency, encourage care processes free of waste, and promote continuous flow of patient activities through the appropriate use of nurses and UNP.

Services Offered

When developing a staffing budget, nurse managers must consider the services offered on the unit, as well as organizational plans to provide new or expanded clinical services. For example, a manager of an inpatient surgical unit must consider the potential effect of offering a new surgical procedure to the community. What projections have been made for this market? What is the expected length of stay for patients undergoing this new procedure? What are the national standards for care for this type of patient? A nurse manager will use this information to project added staff to manage these changes in service.

Conversely, nurse managers must also be aware of any organizational plans to delete an existing service that their unit supports. For example, if a nurse manager in a home care setting knows that reimbursement for a certain procedure in the home has declined to the point that this service must be discontinued, allowances for fewer required staffing resources in the coming year must be made.

The difficulties related to staffing in health care suggest that current methods used to predict personnel budgets and staffing patterns have become increasingly complex and ineffective. Fitzpatrick and Brooks (2010) suggested the use of optimization models that rely on computer and logistic sciences to identify the best solution to particular staffing problems (Fitzpatrick & Brooks, 2010). (See the following Literature Perspective.)

Units of Service

Units of service (UOS) are productivity targets, such as nursing hours per patient day (HPPD) or hours per visit for emergency departments. The UOS multiplied by the volume for a clinical area determines the number of staff needed in a given time period. The formula can be adjusted for total paid staff or just for those required for the delivery of direct patient care.

To develop an adequate personnel budget, the amount of work performed by a nursing unit, or cost center, is referred to as its workload. Workload is measured in terms of the units of service defined by the cost center. Nurse managers must understand the nature of the work in their area of responsibility to define the units of service that will be used as their workload statistic and to forecast, or project, the volume of work that will be performed by their cost center during the upcoming year.

Calculation of Full-Time Equivalents

Nurse managers use the unit's forecasted workload to calculate the number of full-time equivalents (FTEs) that will be needed to construct the unit's overall staffing plan. The distinction between an employee in a position and an FTE is important. Chapter 12 describes FTEs and how they are calculated. To achieve a balanced staffing plan, nurse managers must determine the correct combination of full-time and part-time positions that will be needed.

 LITERATURE PERSPECTIVE

Resource: Fitzpatrick, T.A., & Brooks, B.A, (2010). The nurse leader as logistician: Optimizing human capital. *The Journal of Nursing Administration, 40*(2), 69-74.

Ten-day hospital length of stays, cost-based reimbursements, and unlegislated staffing ratios were common when the mathematical formulas currently used to create personnel budgets and staffing patterns were developed. However, healthcare delivery has become much more dynamic and complex in the twenty-first century and the old formulas, based on averages, are no longer adequate. Because these formulas use a single number, usually an average, to represent uncertain outcomes, the "flaw of averages" tends to promote zero-sum solutions. For example, if the solutions meet financial goals, staff satisfaction is sacrificed. Conversely, if staff satisfaction is achieved, financial targets are not met.

The authors suggest that optimization models, using the power of computer science and logistics science, can simulate solutions for complex staffing problems. These solutions consider myriad constraints and variables and arrange them in such a way to produce the optimal answer solution. For example, the real-world problems are defined as a set of mathematical equations, addressing *objectives* (minimize cost, maximize preferences, and perfect coverage), *variables* (skill and staff mix, demand fluctuation, and cost differentials) and *constraints* (staff availability, union rules) to determine the best solution.

Implications for Practice
Although these modeling tools and techniques have not yet been widely used in health care, they are available. The authors suggest that executive teams should include experts with these modeling and analytical skills. In addition, nurse executives also may want to gain these skills.

Nurse managers must also consider the effect of productive and nonproductive hours when projecting the FTE needs of the unit. Productive time is the paid hours that are actually worked on the unit. Productive hours can be further defined as direct or indirect. Direct care hours are used to pay for the care of patients. Indirect care hours are used to pay for other required unit activities, such as staff meetings or, often, continuing education attendance.

Nonproductive time (see Chapter 12) includes those hours of benefit time that are paid to an employee for vacation, holiday, personal, or sick time and, in some organizations, for an employee attending orientation or continuing education activities. In most practice settings, nurses must be replaced when they are off duty and accessing their paid benefit time off. Managers must be aware of the average benefit hours required for their unit, or they will understate their FTE needs. This requires nurse managers to consider carefully how to allocate their budgeted FTEs into full-time and part-time positions to meet the staffing requirements for the unit when a portion of the staff is taking paid time off. In addition, looking at the number of employees being paid for any specific day may not reflect the number actually providing care. So the nurse manager's role must include competencies in finances, information technology, and automation of staffing and scheduling programs. If healthcare organizations follow the approach of some businesses to increase jobs by creating more part-time positions, major implications for staffing scheduling will need to be considered.

EXERCISE 14-3

Select a hospital-based department and determine the hours of operation. Assess the master scheduling plan and determine how many RNs are needed to ensure that each shift has one RN present. Assuming that a 36-hour work week (three 12-hour shifts) will equal one FTE, convert the required number of registered nurse positions to FTEs. Complete the exercise assuming a 40-hour work week (five 8-hour shifts) and compare the FTE variance.

Distribution of Full-Time Equivalents

Nurse managers must consider a number of variables when they begin the process of distributing FTEs into the unit staffing plan. The staffing plan, which is based on the unit's approved personnel budget AND the projected staffing needs to ensure patient safety, as previously discussed, serves as a guide for creating the unit's schedules for the upcoming year. Variables that must be considered by managers when creating master staffing plans include the following:

1. The hours of operation of the unit
2. The basic shift length for the unit
3. Known activity patterns for the unit at various times of day
4. Maximum work stretch for each employee
5. Shift rotation requirements
6. Weekend requirements
7. Personal and professional requirements and requests for time off (e.g., school schedule, meetings for professional development, and support for models of shared governance)

Each of these variables interrelates with the others, so few "absolutes" are possible. For example, initially one might think that a 24/7 unit might require more staff than a 7 AM TO 6 PM area. If the 24/7 unit, however, is providing basic care all day and few activities at night (e.g., a long-term care facility), fewer staff might be needed than for the 7 AM TO 6 PM area if that were, for example, a day surgery unit.

The master staffing plan must consider the distribution of fixed FTEs in the plan. Fixed FTEs are held by those employees who will be scheduled to work, no matter what the volume of activity. These employees generally hold an exempt or salaried position, meaning their compensation does not depend on the unit's workload. Examples of employees who typically hold a fixed FTE include the nurse manager, the clinical nurse specialist, and the education staff.

The manager then distributes the variable FTEs into the staffing plan. Variable FTEs are held by those employees who are scheduled to work based on the workload of the unit. These employees are considered non-exempt or hourly wage employees, meaning their compensation depends on the actual number of hours worked in a given pay period. Examples of employees who typically hold a variable FTE position include direct care nurses, clerical staff, and other ancillary support staff assigned to the unit.

SCHEDULING

Scheduling is a function of implementing the staffing plan by assigning unit personnel to work specific hours and specific days of the week. The nurse manager is often challenged to take the FTEs that are allotted through the personnel budget, distribute them appropriately, and create a master schedule for the unit that also meets each employee's personal and professional needs. Although completely satisfying each individual staff member is not always possible, a schedule can usually be created that is both fair and balanced from the employee's perspective while still meeting the patient care needs. Creating a flexible schedule with a variety of scheduling options that leads to work schedule stability for each employee is one mechanism likely to retain staff, which is within the control of nurse managers.

Constructing the Schedule

Mechanisms are typically in place within an organization for staff to use in requesting days off and to know when the final schedule will be posted. In addition, most organizations have written policies and procedures that must be followed by nurse managers to ensure compliance with state and federal labor laws relative to scheduling. These policies also aid managers in making scheduling decisions that will be perceived as fair and equitable by all employees.

Schedules are usually constructed for a predetermined block of time based on organizational policy—for example, weekly, biweekly, or monthly, typically using the staffing matrix for each unit. The unit schedule may be prepared in a decentralized fashion by nurse managers or by unit staff through a self-scheduling method. In some organizations, centralized staffing coordinators may oversee all of the schedules prepared for the patient care units. Each method of schedule preparation has pros and cons.

Decentralized Scheduling—Nurse Manager

One decentralized method for preparing the schedule involves nurse managers developing the schedule in isolation from all other units. In this model, the nurse managers approve all schedule changes and actually spend time on a regular basis drafting the staff schedule, considering only the staffing needs of the unit. In other decentralized models, managers do the preliminary work on schedules and then submit them to a centralized staffing office for review and for the addition of any needed supplemental staff. The advantage of this decentralized model is that the accountability

for submitting a schedule in alignment with the established staffing plan rests with managers. These individuals are ultimately the ones responsible for maintaining unit productivity in line with the personnel budget, so the incentive to manage the schedule tightly is strong. The negative aspect of this decentralized method relates to the inability of any individual nurse manager to know the "big picture" related to staffing across multiple patient care units. Requests for time off are approved in isolation from all other units, and a real potential with this model is that each manager will make a decision at the unit level that will be felt in aggregate as a "staffing shortage" across multiple units.

Staff Self-Scheduling

A self-scheduling process has the potential to promote staff autonomy and to increase staff accountability. In addition, team communication, problem-solving, and negotiating skills can be enhanced through the self-scheduling process. Successful self-scheduling is achieved when each individual's personal schedule is balanced with the unit's patient care needs.

Self-scheduling has become more complicated in the wake of care delivery changes and the decentralization of many activities to the individual patient care units. The professional nursing staff cannot work in isolation of other care members when creating a schedule. Assessing the readiness of support staff to participate in this type of initiative is critical as resource utilization and cost containment continue to be major focal points of concern.

Self-scheduling or flexible scheduling needs to be properly managed. Although personal needs of the staff are important to meet, the patient care needs on the unit are the paramount focus for building a schedule. Unit standards for a staffing plan are established, and then a negotiated schedule that results in meeting the needs of staff and patients is the expected and ultimate outcome.

Centralized Scheduling

One benefit to centralized scheduling is that the staffing coordinator is usually aware of the abilities, qualifications, and availability of supplemental personnel who may be needed to complete the schedule. In many organizations, the centralized staffing coordinator is also aware of each unit's personnel budget and any constraints it may impose on the schedule. On the other hand, a disadvantage to centralized staffing is the limited knowledge of the coordinator relative to changing patient acuity needs or other patient-related activities on the unit. Developing a mechanism for the centralized staffing coordinator to share unit-specific knowledge with the respective nurse manager can resolve this disadvantage satisfactorily.

Many organizations have invested in computer software designed to create optimal schedules based on the approved staffing plans for individual units. The centralized staffing coordinator maintains the integrity of the computerized databank for each unit; enters schedule variances daily; generates planning sheets, drafts, and final schedules; and runs any specialized productivity reports requested by nurse managers. Nurse managers review the initial schedule created by the computer, make necessary modifications, and approve the final schedule.

Variables That Affect Staffing Schedules

Nurse managers must consider many variables to create a fair and balanced schedule. Examples of variables nurse managers can anticipate and must consider as they prepare the unit's schedule are found in Box 14-3. Other unanticipated variables can complicate the best-prepared schedule. When faced with call-ins for illness, funeral leaves, jury duty, or an emergent need for a leave of absence (LOA), nurse managers must attempt to fill a shift vacancy on short notice. Requesting staff to add hours over their planned commitment, floating staff from another unit or securing someone from a staffing pool, contracting with agency nursing staff, and seeking overtime are examples of strategies that nurse managers may be compelled to use to ensure safe staffing of their units. However, as discussed, many potential negative consequences are associated with using these strategies.

EXERCISE 14-4

Assume you are going on a job interview. Considering your personal preferred work schedule, what scheduling practices would be most satisfying to you and might lead you to accept employment with the organization? What scheduling practices might cause you to look elsewhere for a job? Develop a list of questions to ask your potential employer regarding scheduling practices in his or her organization.

BOX 14-3   ANTICIPATED SCHEDULING VARIABLES

- Hours of operation
- Shift rotations
- Weekend rotations
- Approved benefit time for the schedule period—for example, vacations and holidays
- Approved leaves of absence/short-term disability
- Approved seminar, orientation, and continuing education time
- Scheduled meetings for the schedule period
- Current filled positions and current staffing vacancies
- Number of part-time employees

EVALUATING UNIT STAFFING AND PRODUCTIVITY

Nurse managers are increasingly pressed to justify their staffing decisions to their staff, senior management, and accrediting agency. The unit activity/production report, which provides a variety of measures of unit workload, can be helpful in such justification. In addition, a review of the extent to which the actual staffing over a specific time period matches the staffing plan, particularly coupled with various outcomes over the same period, gives a picture of the productivity and effectiveness of the unit. Although the format of these reports may vary, the kinds of information typically available to nurse managers in an activity report are included in Box 14-4 on p. 273.

In the inpatient setting, the average daily census (ADC) is one measure considered by nurse managers to project the potential workload of the unit. The ADC is a simple measure of the average number of patients being cared for in the available beds on the unit trended over a specific period. The formula for calculating the ADC is found in Box 14-4. If a unit's ADC is trending upward, the nurse manager should propose additional personnel to manage this increase in patient volume. If the ADC is trending downward, the nurse manager should propose the need for fewer resources to manage this downward census trend. In the acute care setting, a unit's ADC can be extremely volatile based on the patterns of admissions, transfers, and discharges on the unit. In a long-term care setting, however, the unit's ADC may be very stable over prolonged periods. Nurse managers may note census trends based on a particular shift, the day

BOX 14-4 TYPICAL UNIT ACTIVITIES PRODUCTIVITY REPORT INDICATORS

- Volume statistic: number of units of service for the reporting period
- Capacity statistic: number of beds or blocks of time available for providing services
- Percentage of occupancy: number of occupied beds for the reporting period
- Average daily census (ADC): average number of patients cared for per day for the reporting period
- Average length of stay (ALOS): average number of days that a patient remained in an occupied bed

Formulas for Calculating Volume Statistics

Assume that a 20-bed medical-surgical unit *(capacity statistic)* accrued 566 patient days in June *(volume statistic)*. Ninety-eight of these patients were discharged during the month.

Average Daily Census (ADC) on this unit is 18.9:

Formula: patient days for a given time period divided by the number of days in the time period
a. 30 days in June
b. 566 patient days/30 days = ADC of 18.9

Percentage of Occupancy for June is 95%:

Formula: daily patient census (rounded) divided by the number of beds in the unit
    19 patients in a 20-bed unit =
    19 patients/20 beds = 95% occupancy

Average Length of Stay for June is 5.8

Formula: number of patient days divided by the number of discharges
    566 patient days/98 patient discharges = 5.8 (rounded)

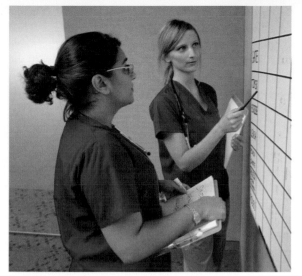

Calculating the percentage of occupancy is essential when developing a unit's staffing plan.

of the week, or the season of the year. The addition of new physicians, the creation of new programs or services, and many other variables may also affect a unit's average daily census. Admissions and discharges increase staffing demands. Nurse managers must maintain a strong grasp on these measures of workload to prepare an adequate staffing plan for their unit.

Another way of assessing a unit's activity level is to calculate the percentage of occupancy. The unit's occupancy rate can be calculated for a specific shift, on a daily basis, or as a monthly or annual statistic. The formula for calculating the percentage of occupancy is also found in Box 14-4. Nurse managers use the percentage of occupancy to develop the unit's staffing plan. Optimal occupancy rates may vary

by practice setting. In a long-term care facility, the organization would desire 100% occupancy rates. However, in an acute care facility, 85% occupancy rates would ensure the best potential for patient throughput.

Another measure of unit activity that may be considered by nurse managers is the average length of stay (ALOS), or the average number of days each patient stays in an occupied bed. As reimbursement dollars have decreased, so have lengths of stay. However, the cost of treating the patient has not decreased as dramatically because patient acuity is greater. Essentially, hospitals need to provide more care in less time for fewer dollars with the same, if not better, outcomes. For this reason, as a unit's ALOs trends downward, the need for staffing resources may not change substantially or it may actually climb. The formula for calculating the average length of stay is also found in Box 14-4.

The measures just mentioned provide the nurse manager with an understanding of the number of patients who have been admitted to the unit over a period of time. The nurse is then charged with matching the needs of these patients with the appropriate number of staff members. Managers have positions and subsequent budgeted nursing salary dollars in the personnel budget based on the estimated units of service that will be provided in the unit. If managers can provide more care to more patients while spending the same or fewer salary dollars, they have increased their unit productivity. Conversely, if the same or more salary dollars are spent to provide less care to fewer patients, managers have decreased their unit productivity.

Nursing productivity is a formula-driven calculation. Unit of service (UOS) multiplied by the volume (patient days or emergency department visits) equals hours available to create direct productive staffing plans. Those hours multiplied by a nonproductive factor (e.g., 1.12) to account for paid time off equals the total hours available for the staffing plan. Getting a ratio of patients to RN is essential. This is then applied to the total hours available, and the support structure (nursing assistants or unit clerks) can be built accordingly. Patient type, scope of service, and acuity and/or classification of the patient are all factors correlated with patient outcomes that drive staffing decisions. Meeting these productivity standards is important to ensure the financial well-being of the organization. However, if the safety needs of the patients are put at risk to achieve this productivity level, the consequences are harmful to patients, staff, and the organization as a whole.

Calculating nursing productivity is challenging for nurse managers because it is difficult to quantify the efficiency and effectiveness of individual nurses providing care to patients. Individual nurses can vary greatly in their critical-thinking abilities, their skill levels, and their ability to make timely and accurate decisions that affect patient outcomes.

Variance Between Projected and Actual Staff

Organizations can use labor cost or a straight FTE model for comparison of actual with projected staff. Labor cost per unit of service is a simple measure that compares budgeted salary costs per budgeted volume of service (productivity target) with actual salary costs per actual volume of service (productivity performance). This measure requires managers to staff according to their staffing plan because the plan reflects the approved personnel budget. Box 14-5 shows an analysis of labor costs per units of service.

BOX 14-5   ANALYSIS OF LABOR COSTS PER UNIT OF SERVICE

1. A manager of a cardiac telemetry unit proposes the following in the personnel budget. These are the unit's productivity targets.
   Total patient days: 5840
   - ADC = 16
   - Staffing plan for ADC of 16:
     - Day shift: 3 RNs and 3 UNP (50% RN skill mix)
     - Evening shift: 3 RNs and 3 UNP (50% RN skill mix)
     - Night shift: 3 RNs and 1 UNP (75% RN skill mix)
   - Direct care labor costs are also projected by the manager based on the average RN and UNP salaries for this unit
   - Target = $139.32 per patient, or $2229.12 per day
2. The manager actually staffs as follows:
   - ADC = 16
   - Actual staffing for ADC of 16:
     - Day shift: 4 RNs and 2 UNP (66% RN skill mix)
     - Evening shift: 4 RNs and 2 UNP (66% RN skill mix)
     - Night shift: 3 RNs (100% RN skill mix)
   - Direct labor costs for this day = $145.44 per patient, or $2327.04 per day
3. The manager has incurred a variance:
   - Exceed target by $6.12 per patient, or $97.92 for the day

ADC, Average daily census; *RN,* registered nurse; *UNP,* unlicensed nursing personnel.

Typically, nurse managers must evaluate and explain changes in productivity resulting in a difference between the projected staffing plan and the actual schedule, using a variance report. If managers compare the two numbers and the actual productivity performance number is higher than the target, they have spent more money for care than they budgeted. A number of variables may cause the labor costs to be higher than anticipated, such as increased overtime, paying bonus pay for regular staff, using costly agency resources, or a higher-than-anticipated amount of indirect education or orientation time.

If managers compare the two numbers and the actual productivity performance number is lower than the target, they have spent less money for care than they budgeted. Managers must also explain this high degree of productivity. One variable that may cause the labor costs to be lower than anticipated is an increased nonprofessional skill mix or consistently understaffing their unit.

Having a productivity performance number that is either higher or lower than that planned does not represent effective management. Assuming that staffing plans were an accurate reflection of the conditions on the specific units, if managers compare the actual productivity performance with their productivity target and the two numbers match, the managers have probably managed effectively. However, given the dynamic nature of patient care, an ongoing evaluation of the conditions on the unit as well as the extent to which proposed staffing levels are reached or exceeded should be monitored on an ongoing basis. Variance reports provide an opportunity for such evaluation.

EXERCISE 14-5

Assume you are working in the charge nurse role. One of the staff assigned to work with you becomes ill and must go home suddenly, leaving his designated patient assignment to be assumed by someone else. As a charge nurse, what factors would you consider as you determine how to reassign this work to other nurses? If you were a co-worker on the shift, instead of the charge nurse, what effective follower behaviors might you demonstrate to support the charge nurse in this situation? Can you identify behaviors of co-workers that would complicate the staffing situation further?

Impact of Leadership on Productivity

Nurse managers must possess staffing and scheduling skills to prepare a staffing plan that balances organizational directives with unit needs for care and services. They must spend time each month evaluating their unit's productivity performance. Yet it is also important that nurse managers improve unit productivity by spending more of their work time coaching and mentoring staff and providing them with clear information and direction related to meeting unit productivity goals. Nurse managers are the chief retention officers and need to perform their duties accordingly.

CONCLUSION

Staffing and scheduling are some of the greatest challenges for a nurse manager. When these functions are performed well, the resulting satisfaction of the unit staff contributes to positive patient outcomes. When they are not performed well, low morale and discontent result. The manager has various data available to help in planning the staffing patterns for the unit. Success, however, depends on the unit staff and the manager working collaboratively to meet the needs for care.

THE SOLUTION

A staff meeting was called to discuss the impact of the transition of a number of beds for surgical trauma ICU (STICU) step-down patients on the inpatient general surgery unit. Information was given to all staff regarding the potential size of the step-down unit and the methods for staffing this unit. Staff members were assured that no jobs would be lost and that appropriate training would be provided to current staff to ensure their competence.

Six beds were determined to be the initial number of step-down beds to be incorporated into the surgical inpatient unit. Staff members were involved in the design of the space from the perspective of identifying which rooms were to be used and what in-room supplies and equipment would be necessary. Continuous pulse oximetry and bedside computers were among the top equipment needs identified.

A staffing plan was established for the step-down unit, and staff members on the general surgery unit were first to be offered the positions. The unit's staffing plan was filled with staff members from the general surgical unit, as well as a related unit. Educational plans were developed and the STICU nursing staff members were open and welcoming when the new step-down staff rotated and

partnered with the STICU staff in the critical care environment. The new step-down staff completed didactic education, and the same STICU nurses provided backup for them when the unit opened.

Continuous discussions were held with the medical staff involved through a champion who was identified within the department of general surgery. Talking points were distributed to the medical staff and the other hospital staff to keep everyone current with the progress. Interdisciplinary teams were developed around the care models and are now engaged in daily patient care conferences to monitor progress of patients.

The unit has been open for 6 months and is a success. We have no vacant positions, critical care beds are more available, medical staff are pleased with the care delivered, patient satisfaction for this unit is very good, and the staff feel accomplished and proud of their contribution to the overall capacity challenge!

—*Mary Ellen Bonczek*

Would this be a suitable approach for you? Why?

THE EVIDENCE

Kane et al. (2007), in a meta-analysis of 94 observational studies done between 1990 and 2006, found consistent evidence that suggests an increase in the number of registered nurses (RNs) relative to the number of patients on a unit was associated with a reduction in hospital-related mortality, failure to rescue, and other nurse-sensitive outcomes. The increased number of nurses also influenced a reduced length of stay after adjustment for patient characteristics is considered. However, none of these studies demonstrated a causal relationship. Kane et al. (2007) noted that hospitals with an overall commitment to high-quality care through sufficient staffing may also invest in other actions that improve quality.

WHAT NEW GRADUATES SAY

- Fortunately I had clinical experiences on various shifts before I graduated. Working evenings was an adjustment but not a hardship.
- I found the greatest challenge in a community clinic was choosing services provided by a staff of one. For example, when our STD (Sexually Transmitted Disease) nurse calls in sick, I'm it!
- I love being able to self schedule. And, if I get overwhelmed, I remind myself I made my own schedule.

CHAPTER CHECKLIST

This chapter addresses the managerial functions of staffing and scheduling and asserts that skills in both functions are needed by the nurse manager to maintain unit productivity and patient and staff satisfaction.

- The staffing process
  - AHRQ nurse staffing model
  - Patient factors
    - Patient classification types
- Productivity models
  - Forecasting unit staffing requirements
- Evaluation of effective staffing
  - National Database of Nursing Quality Indicators
  - Registered nurse staffing
  - 24-hour staffing
  - External factors influencing staffing
  - Nurse characteristics
    - Education
  - Overtime
  - Supplemental (agency/contract) staff and float pools
- Hospital factors
- Nurse outcomes
- Organizational factors that affect staffing plans
  - Structure and philosophy of the nursing services department
  - Organizational staffing policies
  - Organizational support systems
  - Services offered
  - Units of service
  - Calculation of full-time equivalents
  - Distribution of full-time equivalents
- Scheduling
  - Constructing the schedule
    - Decentralized scheduling—nurse manager
    - Staff self-scheduling
    - Centralized scheduling
  - Variables that affect staffing schedules
- Evaluating unit staffing and productivity
  - Variance between projected and actual staff
  - Impact of leadership on productivity

TIPS FOR STAFFING AND SCHEDULING

- Know state laws and voluntary accreditation (professional society and institutional) standards for staffing.
- Integrate ongoing research regarding the impact of various factors on patient outcomes into staffing plans.
- Identify current demands for staff and anticipate externally imposed changes such as services offered and availability of RNs and LPNs/LVNs.
- Value the various responses to short staffing from the manager, staff, and patient perspectives.
- Recognize the complexity of staffing issues and how they relate to staff satisfaction, community perception, budget, and accreditation standards.

REFERENCES

Aiken, L. H., Clarke, S. P., Cheung, R. B., Sloane, D. M., & Silber, J. H. (2003). Educational levels of hospital nurses and surgical patient mortality. *JAMA: The Journal of the American Medical Association, 290*(12), 1617–1623.

Aiken, L., Sloane, D., Cimiotti, J., Clarke, S., Flynn, L., Seago, J., et al. (2010). Implications of the California nurse staffing mandate for other states. *Health Services Research, 45*(4), 904–921, August.

American Nurses Association. (2013). *National Data for Nursing Quality Indicators (NDNI)*. http://www.nursingquality.org. Last accessed, April, 2014.

American Nurses Association (ANA). (2008). *Principles for nurse staffing*. Washington, DC: Author. Retrieved September 28, 2009, from, http://safestaffingsaveslives.org/.

American Nurses Association. (2013). Safe Staffing: The Registered Nurse Safe Staffing Act. HR 876/S. 58. www.nursingworld.org/SafeStaffingFactsheet.aspx. Last accessed, April, 2014

Becker, D. J. (2007). Do hospitals provide lower quality care on weekends? *Health Services Research, 42*(4), 1589–1612.

Dall, T., Chen, Y., Seifert, R., Maddox, P., & Hogan, P. (2009). The economic value of professional nursing. *Medical Care, 47*(1), 97–104.

Dunton, N., Gajewski, B., Klaus, S., & Pierson, B. (2007). The relationship of nursing workforce characteristics to patient outcomes. *Online Journal of Issues in Nursing, 12*(3).

Estabrooks, C. M., Midodzi, W. K., Cummings, C. C., Ricker, K. L., & Giovannetti, P. (2005). The impact of hospital nursing characteristics on 30 day mortality. *Nursing Research, 54*(2), 74–84.

Fitzpatrick, T., & Brooks, B. (2010). The nurse leader as logistician: Optimizing human capital. *Journal of Nursing Administration, 40*(2), 69–74.

Friese, C. R., Lake, F., Aiken, L., Silber, J., & Sochaski, J. (2008). Hospital nurse practice environments and outcomes for surgical oncology patients. *Health Service Research, 43*(4), 1145–1163.

Hamilton, P., & Campbell, M. (2011). Knowledge for re-forming nursing's future: Standpoint makes a difference. *Advances in Nursing Science, 34*(4), 280–296.

Hamilton, P., Eschiti, V. S., Hernandez, K., & Neill, D. (2007). Differences between weekend and weekday nurse work environments and patient outcomes: A focus group approach to model testing. *The Journal of Perinatal & Neonatal Nursing, 21*(4), 331–341.

Institute of Medicine (IOM). (2011). *The future of nursing: Leading change, advancing health*. Washington, DC: The National Academies Press.

Kane, R. L., Shamliyan, T., Mueller, C., Duval, S., & Wilt, T. (2007). *Nursing staffing and quality of patient care: Evidence report/technology assessment No. 151*. (Prepared by the Minnesota Evidence-based Practice Center under Contract No. 290-02-0009.) AHRQ Publication No. 07-E0005, Rockville, MD: Agency for Healthcare Research and Quality.

Kutney-Lee, A., Lake, E. T., & Aiken, L. H. (2009). Development of the hospital nurse surveillance capacity profile. *Research in Nursing & Health, 32*(2), 217–228.

Lake, E., Shang, J., Klaus, S., & Dunton, N. (2010). Patient falls associated with hospital Magnet status in nursing unit staffing. *Research in Nursing and Health, 33*, 415–425.

Peberdy, M. A., Ornato, J. P., Larkin, G. L., Braithwaite, R. S., Kashner, T. M., Carey, S. M., et al. (2008). Survival from in-hospital cardiac arrest during nights and weekends. *JAMA: The Journal of the American Medical Association, 299*(7), 785–792.

Ridley, R. T. (2008). The relationship between nurse education level and patient safety: An integrative review. *Journal of Nursing Education, 47*(4), 149–156.

Seago, J., Spetz, J., & Mitchell, S. (2004). Nurse staffing and hospital ownership in California. *Journal of Nursing Administration, 34*(5), 228–231.

Shreve, J., Van Den Bos, J., Gray, T., Halford, M., Rustagi, K., & Ziemkiewicz, E. (2010). *The economic measurement of medical errors (Milliman)*. Schaumberg, IL: Society of Actuaries' Health Section.

Sochalski, J. (2004). The relationship between nurse staffing and the quality of nursing care in hospitals. *Medical Care, 42*(Suppl. 2), 1167–1173.

Stimpfel, A., Sloane, D., & Aiken, L. (2012). The longer the shifts for hospital nurses, the higher the levels of burnout and patient dissatisfaction. *Health Affairs, 31*(11), 2501–2509.

Tourangeau, A., Doran, D., McGillis Hall, L., O'Brien Pallas, L., Pringle, D., Tu, J., & Cranley, L. (2007). Impact of hospital nursing care on 30-day mortality for acute medical patients. *Journal of Advanced Nursing, 57*(1), 32–44.

Tzischinsky, A., Epstein, O., Here, P., & Lavie, P. (2008). Shift work in nursing: Is it really a risk factor for nurses' health and patients' safety? *Nursing Economics, 26*(4), 250–257.

Upenieks, V., Akhavan, J., & Kotlerman, J. (2008). Value-added care: A paradigm shift in patient care delivery. *Nursing Economic$, 6*(5), 294–300.

Van den Heede, K., Lesaffre, E., Diya, L., Vleugels, A., Clarke, S. P., Aiken, L. H., et al. (2009). The relationship between inpatient cardiac surgery mortality and nurse numbers and educational levels: Analysis of administrative data. *International Journal of Nursing Studies, 46*(6), 796–803.

SUGGESTED READINGS

Boswell, C., Gatson, Z., Baker, D., Vaughn, G., Lyons, B., Chapman, P., et al. (2008). Application of evidence-base practice through a float project. *Nursing Forum, 43*(3), 126–132.

Clarke, S. (2007). Registered nurse staffing and patient outcomes in acute care: Looking back, pushing forward. *Medical Care, 45*(12), 1126–1128.

Garrett, C. (2008). The effect of nurse staffing patterns on medical errors and nurse burnouts. *AORN Journal, 87*(6), 1191–1204.

Hamilton, P., & Campbell, M. (2011). Knowledge for re-forming nursing's future: Standpoint makes a difference. *Advances in Nursing Science, 34*(4), 280–296.

Hofler, L. (2008). Nursing education and transition to the work environment: A synthesis of national reports. *Journal of Nursing Education.*

Institute of Medicine (IOM). (2011). *The future of nursing: Leading change, advancing health.* Washington, DC: The National Academies Press.

Lake, E., Shang, J., Klaus, S., & Dunton, N. (2010). Patient falls associated with hospital magnet status in nursing unit staffing. *Research Nursing and Health, 33,* 415–425.

Mittmann, N., Seung, S., Pusterzu, L., Isogai, S., & Michaels, D. (2008). Nursing workload associated with hospital patient care. *Journal of Advanced Nursing, 16*(1), 53–56.

Pappas, S. (2008). The cost of nurse-sensitive adverse events. *Journal of Nursing Administration, 38*(5), 230–236.

Stimpfel, A., Sloane, D., & Aiken, L. (2012). The longer the shifts for hospital nurses, the higher the levels of burnout and patient dissatisfaction. *Health Affairs, 31*(11), 2501–2509.

Thomas-Hawkins, C., Flynn, L., & Clarke, S. (2008). Relationships between registered nurse staffing, processes of nursing care, and nurse-reported patient outcomes in chronic hemodialysis units. *Nephrology Nursing Journal, 35*(2), 123–145.

Tzischinsky, A., Epstein, O., Here, P., & Lavie, P. (2008). Shift work in nursing: Is it really a risk factor for nurses' health and patients' safety? *Nursing Economics, 26*(4), 250–257, July-August.

Van den Heede, K., Clarke, S., Sermeus, W., Vleugels, A., & Aikens, L. (2007). International experts' perspectives on the state of the nurse staffing and patient outcomes literature. *Journal of Nursing Scholarship, 39*(4), 290–297.

INTERNET RESOURCES

ANA Staffing Principles: http://nursing2015.files.wordpress.com/2008/09/_17ana-principles-on-safe-staffing.

National Database of Nursing Quality Indicators (NDNQI): www.nursingquality.org/data.aspx.

The Joint Commission: www.jointcommission.org/standards_information/npsgs.aspx.

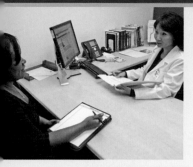

Selecting, Developing, and Evaluating Staff

Diane M. Twedell

Two of the most important functions of a nurse manager are interviewing and hiring employees for an organization. Followers play an important role in interviewing and want to be clear about various role expectations.

Effective communication of roles and role expectations among all members can facilitate improved performance, increased worker satisfaction, and most importantly, improved quality of care delivered. The role of the manager as a coach who empowers employees to grow as followers and develop their leadership skills in a learning environment is explored.

LEARNING OUTCOMES

- Relate concepts of role theory to position descriptions.
- Distinguish key points for the interview of a potential employee.
- Delineate the various performance appraisal processes.
- Examine specific guidelines for performance feedback.

KEY TERMS

coaching	position description	role theory
empowerment	role ambiguity	
performance appraisal	role conflict	

Melissa Bertelson, RN, BSN
Nurse Manager, Mayo Clinic Health System

I have had to face a multitude of challenges since recently accepting the role as the nurse manager of a medical surgical unit and a critical care unit. I also was receiving complaints of poor morale and undesirable behavior in the workplace. It became clear to me that I needed to focus on discovering the causes behind these negative types of behavior and develop techniques to deal with the causes. I also needed to find a way to stay connected to staff despite having considerably less time to spend on the unit.

High anxiety and uncertainty ruled among staff because of a vast number of changes the facility was experiencing including: integrating with another facility of similar size and structure, less than ideal economic conditions, and healthcare legislation changes. The staff was also experiencing change within the unit with electronic medical record upgrades, staffing changes, and a new manager. It was obvious that staff needed to have expectations and accountabilities defined.

What do you think you would do if you were this nurse?

INTRODUCTION

Healthcare delivery systems are businesses that are economically driven. Whether the setting is inpatient or ambulatory, the emphasis is on providing the highest quality of care at an affordable price. The nurse manager is a key individual whose leadership can directly influence many environmental functions. Race and Skees (2010) reported that an effective nurse leader can exemplify the vision and values of an organization and promote a mentoring culture. Other functions begin with the selection of the right person for the right position and having the manager function in the role of coach. As a coach, the nurse manager can assist and encourage employees to perform at their highest levels in an empowered and self-directed manner.

The role of follower cannot be overrated! A strong patient care unit has both effective leaders and team members who understand their role in meeting the goals for quality patient care. Professional healthcare providers must clearly understand what is expected of their performance, including the ramifications of not meeting those expectations. This performance can be achieved only when all members of the organization have clearly defined roles and overall objectives.

ROLE CONCEPTS AND THE POSITION DESCRIPTION

The acquisition of a role requires an individual to assume the personal as well as the formal expectations of a specified role or position. Many individuals function within multiple roles. As discussed in the following Theory Box, role theory provides an appreciable framework for the development and evaluation of staff. Today's professional nurse is often a parent, spouse, and community volunteer and maintains full-time employment outside the home. Many skills are necessary for each role. In addition, the role-taker (i.e., the individual actually performing the role) has specified performance objectives within the social context in which the role is enacted. The social context includes the physical and social environment.

THEORY BOX

THEORY/ CONTRIBUTOR	KEY IDEAS	APPLICATION TO PRACTICES
Dynamics in Organizations Kahn, Wolfe, Quinn, Snoek, & Rosenthal (1964) developed this theory.	Roles within organizations affect an individual's interactions with others. Acquisition of these roles is time-dependent and varies based on individual experiences and value systems. For effective communication to take place, role expectations for performance must be understood by all individuals involved.	The role of the professional nurse is complex. Role acquisition, role clarity, and role performance are enhanced by the use of clear position descriptions and evaluation standards.

Role ambiguity in the workplace creates an environment for misunderstanding and hinders effective communication. Individuals do not have a clear understanding of what is expected of their performance or how they will be evaluated. Role conflict is easier to recognize. Employees know what is expected of them, but they are either unwilling or unable to meet the requirements.

Employees must have clear role expectations and perceive that their contributions are valued. Empowerment and control for certain aspects of the environment have been linked to increased personal health, job satisfaction, and individual performance. They are then more likely to be committed to the organization and to provide a higher level of patient care. These principles are applicable to both managers and staff members. A consistent focus on developing staff creates a learning environment directed toward excellence.

Acquisition of the role is time-dependent; individuals apply their life experiences to each role and interpret the role within their own value system. As roles become more complex, the individual may take longer to assimilate the components of each particular role. Nursing graduates enter the profession with various levels of educational and life experiences. The nurse manager plays an integral role in assisting these individuals in the development and acquisition of the complex role of the professional nurse. Role development evolves over time and considers individual needs. Role acquisition is something that nurses can encounter numerous times during their career. As an example, the RN who completes additional academic education and becomes an advanced practice registered nurse takes on a new role. The staff RN who moves to a new or different specialty acquires a new role.

Position descriptions provide written guidelines detailing the roles and responsibilities of a specific position within the organizational context. The position description reflects functions and obligations of a specific work position. Box 15-1 shows examples of expectations for a nurse in ambulatory care.

EXERCISE 15-1

Obtain a position description for a registered nurse from an ambulatory care clinic and a hospital. Compare them and analyze the general categories. Are specific behaviors outlined? What competencies are different? What competencies are similar?

> **BOX 15-1   EXCERPTS FROM AN AMBULATORY RN DIRECT CARE NURSE JOB DESCRIPTION**
>
> - Assesses comprehensive data including physical, psychosocial, emotional, and spiritual needs of the patient.
> - Involves patient, family, and healthcare team members in formulating a culturally appropriate plan of care.
> - Implements plan of care in partnership with patient, family, and healthcare team.

The position description should reflect current practice guidelines for individuals and may have competency-based requirements. As nursing care models shift to the ambulatory setting, home, and the community, professional nurses must have a clear understanding of the performance that is expected. The nurse is also responsible for clearly understanding the position descriptions of the paraprofessionals to whom care is delegated, such as nursing assistants. Clear and concise position descriptions for all employees are important because they provide the basis for roles within the organization.

SELECTING STAFF

The selection of staff is one of the most important functions that nurse managers complete in their daily routines. The nurse manager wants the most qualified individual for the position who also fits the culture of the organization. Choosing the right individual is the challenge! The goal is to match the person with the position with the intent of recruiting and retaining the right staff (see the Literature Perspective on p. 282). Markey and Tingle (2012) note that the selection of competent nursing staff is important with the level of transparency in healthcare organizations. National quality indicators and Hospital Consumer Assessment of Healthcare Providers and Systems highlight the public accountability for patient care services. Health care is centered on caring for people, and nurses with appropriate people skills are essential for producing satisfied patients and families. For example, if an applicant values that the needs of the patient come first and this value is also articulated via the organization, he or she has similar values related to the work of the organization. The applicant and the manager must agree on what defines quality care and the manner in

LITERATURE PERSPECTIVE

Resource: Mullenbach, K.F. (2010). Senior nursing student's perspectives on the recruitment and retention of medical surgical nurses. *Medsurg Nursing*, 19(6), 341-344.

This article reflects the development of plans by senior baccalaureate nursing students to recruit and retain medical surgical nurses for 5 years. Students did this assignment as part of a leadership course that included readings, lectures, and a literature search.

Student recommendations for recruitment included:
- Shadow opportunities
- Student externships
- Being a "student-friendly" unit
- Opportunities to practice skills
- Residency programs and individualized orientation

Student recommendations for retention included:
- Supportive preceptors
- Supportive manager
- Education, with certification and advanced degrees
- Empowerment and autonomy

Implications for Practice

Nurse managers are chief retention officers and it is vital to implement long-term solutions for keeping staff satisfied.

The manager's focus before and during the interview is to be prepared and have well-thought-out questions. Cohen (2013) notes that recruitment can yield poor results if the interview is not well planned. The environment should be comfortable and provide privacy without interruption. The interview questions can be related to the applicant's experience or be directed to evaluate values and critical-thinking skills. This may be accomplished by asking the applicant to describe his or her reactions to challenging situations previously experienced. Bucholz (2011) highlights that behavioral-based interviewing can be a strong predictor of a future employee. A question related to teamwork in an interview could be, *Tell me about a time when you were working in a group and there were problems with other individuals who were not pulling their weight. What did you do to maintain a team environment?*

Further, knowing what characteristics are important for an area helps focus behavioral questions. The Research Perspective presents an example of what those characteristics might be for perinatal areas.

Technical skills are also important for the work environment and therefore must also be discussed or validated. The applicant may be given a case study to read and discuss with the interviewer. The case study could describe a situation for the unit in which the applicant is being interviewed; the content of the case study may require the applicant to prioritize the care of one patient or a group of patients. Questions from the applicant should be answered honestly. Cohen (2013) notes that a packet of interest can be sent to the applicant ahead of

which it should be delivered. The manager must also decide whether members of the existing staff are to be included in the screening and interview process for new employees. Cohen (2013) reported that including staff members in the interview process recognizes staff and shows their opinion is important. Both the manager and applicant must prepare for the interview in order to truly determine if the individual is a good fit for the organization.

RESEARCH PERSPECTIVE

Resource: Falls, E., & Hensen, D. (2012). Characteristics that perinatal nurse managers desire in new nurse hires. *The Journal of Continuing Education in Nursing*, 43(4), 182-186.

This article focuses on how the Quality and Safety Education for Nurses (QSEN) competencies were used by nurse managers to determine characteristics desired in perinatal nurses.

A descriptive study used a survey design. A convenience sample of perinatal nurse managers was obtained. Managers were asked to list the five most important criteria when hiring a new graduate nurse. Definitions of the QSEN competencies were provided and

managers indicated importance of these competencies on a scale of 4 (very important) to 1 (not at all important).

Managers looked to the QSEN competencies of teamwork and collaboration, safety, and patient-centered care as qualities they desired in a new graduate nurse.

Implications for Practice

The QSEN competencies may be a valuable tool to reflect on when selecting new graduate registered nurses.

time including the nurse manager's business card, information about the specific unit, and the organizational mission and vision statements. A tour of the unit and a review of the position description are helpful to give the applicant information about the expectations of the role. At the conclusion of the interview, it is important for the nurse manager to clarify concrete issues. An indication of follow-up should be more than "don't call us, we'll call you." Applicants should know the time line of when they can expect to hear about their interview result, who will contact them, and how they will be contacted. Thank applicants for the interview, and end interviews on a positive note.

The applicant also has responsibilities in preparation for the employment interview. The applicant must be on time and appropriately dressed. Conservative dress is always acceptable. A uniform is not necessary and usually not even preferable. First impressions may be lasting impressions. Smith (2010) notes that researching the facility and position description will help an applicant gain insight into the organization. The applicant should be prepared to answer questions honestly and thoughtfully. The prospective employee wants to make the right decisions just as much as the employer does. The manager and the applicant must have a clear understanding of the values and organizational goals for nursing care to ensure that the applicant is well-suited for the role. The applicant should focus on the topic and avoid irrelevant conversations. In addition to describing previous situations and how they were handled, the applicant may be asked to describe personal strengths and weaknesses. At the end of the interview, the applicant should thank the manager for his or her time and verify when the selection will be made and how it will be communicated. It is also appropriate to send the manager a brief note of appreciation for the interview. Furthermore, if the manager requested additional information, the applicant should provide that as quickly as possible.

EXERCISE 15-2

Select a job that you have or have had. Reflect on your interview process. Did you know the organization's mission and goals? Briefly describe the mission. Did you understand how your role fit with or helped to meet the mission and goals? Explain in detail.

DEVELOPING STAFF

Once the interview and offer are completed and an applicant has accepted the position, strategies are used to help the individual acclimate to the new organization and/or role. Some organizations use residency programs for new graduates that may last as long as 1 year and are designed to help new graduates transition from the role of student to that of professional nurse. Other strategies that exist in every organization and may vary in amount of time focus on orientation to the organization, department, specialty, and role. Orientation to the organization usually is a structured program that is generally applicable to all new employees. It may include outlining the mission, benefits, safety programs, and other specific topics. Orientation to the work area usually depends on the specialty area involved, the skills that need to be verified, and the environment itself. The orientation period must be used efficiently to benefit both the employee and the organization. Retention of new nursing personnel begins on the day of their hire because costs for replacement and turnover can be substantial. McConnell (2011b, p. 272) noted that "for technical and professional employees, turnover costs climbs with qualifications and salary of position, so for a professional costing $60,000 per year, the cost of turnover can amount to as much as $120,000." Factors related to turnover cost include human resource expenses, temporary replacement costs, lost productivity, training, relocation expenses and terminal pay outs. Although the cost of turnover may be cited differently, the cost of replacement is high.

Orientation can accomplish a variety of things. Orientation is a time for new employees to learn the work environment and the staff. McConnell (2011a) shared that effective appropriate training has a measurable impact on reducing turnover as does complete effective new employee orientation. Many institutions provide preceptors, who are considered to be expert clinicians and resources. Preceptors work with orientees to complete a needs assessment to help direct and guide the orientation of the new employee in the clinical setting. They also attempt to find out how a new employee likes to learn. Various learning style assessment tools are available for preceptors to use. When preceptors understand the learning styles of new employees, a better focus for implementation of the orientation goals is provided. After learning styles have been identified, new employees work with preceptors who understand specifically how to address the individualized learning needs of new employees in a manner that enhances learning.

Continued development of the staff is a unique role for the nurse manager. The challenge is to merge a group of individuals with varying levels of expertise and experience. If the focus is centered on professional socialization and development, a common thread will "weave" itself throughout all employees. That common thread may be a particular philosophy of care delivery, further development of critical-thinking skills for a specific specialty, or political activities in which members are involved. Some units encourage a monthly journal club or a brief presentation by employees to summarize information learned from a conference. One nursing unit could send a staff member to monthly open meetings of the state board of nursing. This staff member then could summarize the report of the meeting for the rest of the staff to keep them informed of the legal aspects of professional nursing.

Empowerment strategies are useful for individual professional development, as well as for overall staff development. Empowerment is a process that acknowledges the values and judgment of individuals and trusts that their decisions will be the correct ones.

For individuals to feel empowered, the environment must be open and they must feel safe to explore and develop their own potential. The organizational environment must encourage individuals to employ the freedom of making decisions while retaining accountability for the consequences of those decisions. Farr-Wharton, Brunetto, and Shacklock (2011, p. 1394) note that empowerment "hinges on supervisors releasing control and encouraging employees to take responsibility for making decisions related to the job, thereby increasing the meaning of work for them and their level of competence." Positive feedback or coaching, achievement recognition, and support for new ideas may enhance employees' feelings of empowerment and their ability to perform effectively. Pellico and Violano (2010, p. 106) stated that "defining professional goals sets the stage for continued growth and development."

One strategy for staff empowerment is providing timely feedback for performance contributions, not simply during the annual performance appraisal. Supporting the implementation of innovative ideas and providing opportunities for mentoring relationships are also valuable approaches for the manager and staff. Many organizations use shared governance as a guide for accountability. A premise of shared governance is that power, control, and decision making can empower staff and enhance individual and group accountability.

PERFORMANCE APPRAISALS

Feedback to employees regarding their performance is one of the strongest rewards an organization can provide. Performance appraisals are individual evaluations of work performance. Ideally, evaluations are conducted on an ongoing basis, not just at the conclusion of a predetermined period. Evaluations, however, are usually done annually and also may be required after a scheduled orientation period for new employees. McConnell (2011a) identifies the following:

The appraisal process is in part intended to encourage improvement in the performance of employees whose work is at the minimum acceptable level or better. The appraisal is also intended to encourage employees with previously outstanding performance to maintain that level. An employee's regular performance appraisal should never be the time when an employee first hears that he or she is performing below a minimum acceptable level.

The process of providing feedback, for either an above-average or a below-average performance, is best received at a time closest to the incidents being evaluated. Addressing both the positive and negative issues related to performance is important. According to McConnell (2011a, p. 192), it is "within the context of the one to one relationship the manager should be cultivating and maintaining with each employee." Many nurse managers perceive the appraisal as a time-consuming process of endless paperwork. Instead, nurse managers should embrace the appraisal process as a key time for assisting with staff development. Appraisals should be designed so that they can be supported in court if the need arises. Court decisions can be made based on the evidence, or lack of evidence, presented in the evaluation instrument. Consider, for example, the individual who has been fired for reasons of poor work performance. The employee must be provided written notice that performance is unsatisfactory, and that notice must specify what the employee must accomplish for satisfactory performance. This simple condition can make the difference for either the employee or the employer to justify the fairness for termination. Performance appraisals can be either formal or informal. Performance appraisals may also include personal and peer evaluations, as well as managerial components.

An informal appraisal might be as simple as immediately praising the individual for performance recognized. A compliment from a family member or patient might be conveyed. Some units have a specific bulletin board for thank-you notes from patients and their families. Sometimes a simple "Thank you for all your hard work today!" can be extended from the manager to the staff. In addition, staff members have a responsibility to show the manager their appreciation and give positive and negative feedback.

The formal performance appraisal involves written documentation according to specific organization guidelines. Whether the evaluation is informal or formal, it does not preclude interim evaluations. The primary reason for an interim evaluation is so that praise or corrections are made as close to an episode as possible.

Brief anecdotal notes entered into the employee's file on a regular basis are important. These anecdotal notes, when accumulated over time, provide a more accurate cumulative appraisal. The anecdotal note describes an occurrence, either favorable or unfavorable, in a brief and concise manner. The purpose is to assist the manager with information throughout an entire rating period.

Example of an Anecdotal Note: Nurse "Johnson"

2/09/13: Patient (Joyce Allen) and family described the wonderful care that she received from Ms. Johnson during this hospitalization. All members of the family noted that when Ms. Johnson was in the room, "We felt like we were the most important people in the world." She made the patient feel "special and not just like another number." Compliment relayed to employee on 2/15/13. (Note in employee's anecdotal record with a signature and date by nurse manager.)

Additional methods may be incorporated into the performance appraisal in the form of competency assessment. Kubin and Fogg (2010, p. 28) identified that "competency combines skills, knowledge, and behaviors to properly perform in a variety of patient care situations." Integration of relevant competency assessment data into the evaluation process further enhances the individual employee's sense of empowerment, as well as accountability for the evaluation process.

Coaching

The overall evaluative process can be enhanced if the manager employs the technique of coaching. Coaching is a process that involves the development of individuals within an organization. This coaching process is a personal approach in which the manager and the employee interact on a frequent and regular basis with the ultimate outcome that the employee performs at an optimal level. Coaching can be individual or may involve a team approach. When implemented in a planned and organized manner, it can promote team building and optimal performance of the employees. Coaching is a learned behavior for the nurse manager and takes time and effort to be developed. The rewards for both the employee and the nurse manager are significant; communication is enhanced, and the performance appraisal process is an active one between the employee and the manager.

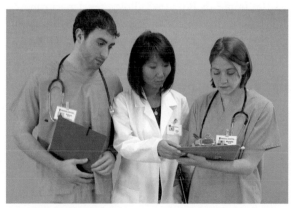

Coaching can promote team building and optimal performance of the employees.

The formal performance appraisal usually involves the use of a standard form or method developed by the organization to measure employee performance. The commonly used appraisal methods and forms are displayed in Box 15-2. New employees must have a clear understanding of the performance standards are and what good performance looks like. Giving a new employee a job performance appraisal form provides a basis for how their performance will be measured. The example in Box 15-3 illustrates a performance appraisal form in which a nurse manager can evaluate a direct care nurse related to health teaching and promotion.

PERFORMANCE APPRAISAL METHODS

Measuring performance can occur in various ways. See Box 15-2 for a listing of methods. Each method will be delineated in the following paragraphs.

Critical Incidents Method

The critical incidents type is a performance appraisal method in which a manager keeps a written record of positive and negative performance of employees throughout a designated time period. No standard form is use; however, a list of documented incidents is kept for employment and legal purposes.

Management by Objectives

Management by objectives (MBO) was popularized by Peter Drucker (1954). MBO is a process in which manager and employee jointly set goals for the employee, periodically evaluate performance, and reward according to results. During the performance appraisal, the employee and manager address the goals and objectives. Box 15-4 shows an example of goals and accomplishments used in MBO.

Narrative Method

The narrative method requires a manager to write a statement about the employee's performance. This can be done in the form of a written letter/document and is based on the manager's writing style and content.

Graphic Rating Scale Form

The graphic rating scale form is a performance appraisal checklist on which a manager rates employee performance on a continuum, such as excellent, good, average, and poor. The continuum usually includes a numerical scale from 1(low) to 5 (high). See Box 15-5 for an example of a graphic rating scale for employee performance.

Behaviorally Anchored Rating Scales

The behaviorally anchored rating scale (BARS) method is a performance appraisal that provides a description of every assessment along a continuum. BARS describes the employee's performance both

---

BOX 15-5   GRAPHIC RATING SCALE

CRITERIA	ALMOST NEVER 1	2	3	4	ALWAYS EXCEEDS 5
1. Completes nursing care in a professional and competent manner					
2. Is reliable; comes to work on time					
3. Is absent from work					

BOX 15-6   EXAMPLES OF A BEHAVIORALLY ANCHORED SCALE

Emergency department (ED) direct care nurse responsibilities for patient admitted with chest pain: (ED records evaluated per protocol; minimum 10/rating period). Met/Unmet

1. Vital signs recorded within 5 min of admission _____
2. Cardiac monitor, IV, lab tests, and EKG done within 15 min _____
3. If sublingual nitroglycerin given, vital signs recorded every 5 min for 30 min _____
   a. Chest pain changes evaluated per protocol _____
   b. Post–chest pain 12-lead EKG documented _____

---

quantitatively and qualitatively. Box 15-6 provides an overview of how established nursing standards can be incorporated into the appraisal of performance using peer review.

What Method is the Best?

Which instrument/method of appraisal is best? The mission and goals of the organization determine the methods used. A combination of several methods is probably superior to any one method. The primary success of any performance appraisal lies in the skills and communication abilities of the manager. The manager has the responsibility to educate employees about the process and tools for performance appraisals. Role ambiguity and uncertainty of standards of practice and methods for evaluation are significant contributors to decreased work satisfaction. The best-designed instrument will fail if the manager is ineffective and cannot communicate with the employee. Finally, some linkage of the outcomes of the appraisal process to salary and benefits conveys a reinforcement of the process of appraising and its importance for individual professional development.

PERFORMANCE APPRAISAL ENVIRONMENT

The appraisal instrument is not the only factor in the evaluation process. The appraisal should be conducted professionally and in a positive manner. It is an ideal time for communication between the employee and the manager. Preventing interruptions is paramount. This time is important for clarification of employee and organizational goals. Evaluation of employee performance should be objective and unemotional. The evaluation instruments should be clearly completed, and time should be allowed for discussion. Goals may be established. The manager and the employee should sign the appraisal forms, and each should be provided a copy. The effectiveness of the entire appraisal method relies on the manner in which the manager uses the tools and the feedback that the employee receives. Effective communication between the manager and employees can prevent potential performance problems on a unit. Specific behaviors by the manager enhance the actual appraisal process (Box 15-7).

BOX 15-7   KEY BEHAVIORS FOR THE PERFORMANCE APPRAISAL SESSION

- Provide a quiet, controlled environment, without interruptions.
- Maintain a relaxed but professional atmosphere.
- Put the employee at ease; the overall objective is for the best job to be done.
- Review specific examples for both positive and negative behavior (keep an anecdotal file for each employee).
- Allow the employee to express opinions, orally and in writing.
- Write future plans, training needs and goals.
- Set follow-up date as necessary to monitor improvements, if cited.
- Show the employee confidence in his or her performance.
- Be sincere and constructive in both praise and criticism.

CONCLUSION

For staff and managers, selecting new members of their team is critical to success. Hiring someone who is a less than desirable fit for the team can be expensive and lead to team dissatisfaction. Selecting the right people makes their development and evaluation more productive.

THE SOLUTION

I decided to work on communication and trust building to combat the uncertainty. I started by spending short periods of time on the unit most days of the week to foster communication and open dialogue. I practiced active listening skills, asked open-ended questions, and discussed any issues the staff encountered during their shift. I implemented an open-door policy; the staff were welcome to bring me any questions, concerns, or comments at any time. I started communicating with staff by sending weekly updates by e-mail. This weekly e-mail highlighted six or seven items that occurred over the week, or a concern or question that I have an answer for or an update about. I also included a positive accomplishment or compliment each week to promote a more positive environment.

I changed the style of staff meetings. I decided that though I had definite issues and process changes to cover, the staff's concerns and voices were just as important to include on the agenda. I left ample time to raise concerns, discuss issues, and, in appropriate instances, discuss solutions to those issues. This technique has allowed staff to take responsibility to correct the problems on their own by developing a plan of action, an acceptable time frame to work on the issue, and a plan to report findings or results.

I chose to conduct all the recent staff performance evaluations that were due over the last 6 months; previously, various supervisory staff assisted the manager with these evaluations. At each staff member's review I discussed some basic expectations about attitude, behavior, teamwork, and accountability. This was to create consistency, incite a ripple effect of positive energies, and set the tone for the unit for the years ahead.

Though I have only been at this for less than a year, improvement is occurring. Many staff are openly communicating their concerns, and often before they even finish voicing their issue, they want to discuss what their idea of a solution is and how they think we could implement and measure the possible solution. The staff is also taking a more active role in staff meetings, and I have heard some compliments from them about these specific changes. Aligning expectations and accountabilities has been critical for educating staff and helping promote a positive base of teamwork to work from.

—*Melissa Bertelson*

Would this be a suitable approach for you? Why?

THE EVIDENCE

Recruitment and retention of nurses is one of the most important functions that a nurse manager performs. The nurse manager sets the tone for the unit and new employees. An atmosphere of mutual respect, trust, and empowerment is key to nurse retention.

Coaching staff is a critical method to develop a high performance nursing staff. Clear communication, expectations, and accountabilities based on role theory is pivotal to role clarity of new employees.

WHAT NEW GRADUATES SAY

- Clear expectations and direct communication from a nurse manager ease some of the stress of starting a new job.

- The support of a positive preceptor made all the difference for me during my transition from oriented to novice nurse.

CHAPTER CHECKLIST

The manager plays a key role in the selection and development of staff. As a role model, the manager is also key in the establishment of the type of work environment that exists. Managers must be supportive and develop their staff to their highest potential. They must have accurate position descriptions and tools for evaluation of employee performance. These are integral to role development and professional socialization. Managers must also use various communication methods to empower their employees. Coaching and implementation of empowerment strategies positively contribute to overall staff performance as well.

- Role concepts and the position description
- Selecting staff
- Developing staff
- Performance appraisals
  - Coaching
- Performance appraisal methods
  - Critical incidents method

- Management by objectives
- Narrative method
- Graphic rating scale form
- Behaviorally anchored rating scales
- What method is best?
- Performance appraisal environment

TIPS FOR CONDUCTING AN INTERVIEW

- Prescreen the applicant, and schedule a time for the interview.
- Prepare questions in advance. Be concise but thorough.
- Control the environment for noise and interruptions.

- Explain and clarify the role for which the applicant is interviewing.
- Be a good listener.
- Answer questions honestly.
- Inform the applicant when he or she will be informed of the decision.

REFERENCES

Bucholz, L. (2011). Hiring the right person for the job. *Plastic Surgical Nursing, 31*(3), 124–125.

Cohen, S. (2013). Recruitment and retention: How to get them and how to keep them. *Nursing Management, 44*(4), 11–14.

Drucker, P. F. (1954). *The practice of management* (1st ed.). New York: Harper.

Falls, E., & Hensen, D. (2012). Characteristics that perinatal nurse managers desire in new nurse hires. *The Journal of Continuing Education in Nursing, 43*(4), 182–186.

Farr-Wharton, R., Brunetto, Y., & Shacklock, K. (2011). The impact of intuition and supervisory-nurse relationships on empowerment and affective commitment by generation. *Journal of Advanced Nursing, 68*(6), 1391–1401.

Kahn, R. L., Wolfe, D. M., Quinn, R. P., Snoek, J. D., & Rosenthal, R. A. (1964). *Occupational stress: Studies in role conflict and ambiguity.* New York: Wiley.

Kubin, L., & Fogg, N. (2010). Back to basics boot camp: An innovative approach to competency assessment. *Journal of Pediatric Nursing, 25,* 28–32.

Markey, L., & Tingle, C. (2012). Screening RNs: A change in hiring practice. *Nursing Management, 43*(2), 13–15.

McConnell, C. R. (2011a). Addressing problems of employee performance. *The Health Care Manager, 30*(2), 185–192.

McConnell, C. R. (2011b). Addressing employee turnover and retention: Keeping your valued performers. *The Health Care Manager, 30*(3), 271–283.

Mullenbach, K. F. (2010). Senior nursing student's perspectives on the recruitment and retention of medical-surgical nurses. *Medsurg Nursing: Official Journal of the Academy of Medical-Surgical Nurses, 19*(6), 341–344.

Pellico, L. H., & Violano, P. (2010). Creating a room of our own. *Journal for Nurses in Staff Development, 26*(3), 104–107.

Race, T. K., & Skees, N. (2010). Changing tides: Improving outcomes through mentorship on all levels of nursing. *Critical Care Nursing Quarterly, 33*(2), 163–174.

Smith, L. (2010). Are you ready for your job interview? *Nursing, 40*(4), 52–54.

SUGGESTED READINGS

Batson, V. D., & Yoder, L. H. (2012). Managerial coaching: A concept analysis. *Journal of Advanced Nursing, 68*(7), 1658–1669.

Crater, M. R., & Tourangeau, A. E. (2012). Staying in nursing: What factors determine whether nurses intend to stay employed? *Journal of Advanced Nursing, 68*(7), 1589–1600.

Wong, C. A., & Laschinger, H. K. S. (2013). Authentic leadership, performance, and job satisfaction: The mediating role of empowerment. *Journal of Advanced Nursing, 69*(4), 947–959.

Changing the Status Quo

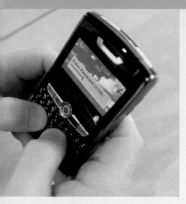

16

Strategic Planning, Goal-Setting, and Marketing

Mary Ellen Clyne

This chapter discusses the actualization of several organizational elements of planning for the future, with a focus on the strategic planning process, goal-setting, management by objectives, and marketing. Specific examples of planning and marketing strategies as used in healthcare organizations are presented when appropriate.

LEARNING OUTCOMES

- Articulate the value and importance of conducting an environmental assessment.
- Explore the planning process.
- Review the purpose of a mission statement, a philosophy, and established goals and objectives.
- Apply goal-setting and strategic planning.
- Explain the process of strategic planning in establishing a product line in an acute care hospital setting.
- Determine the value of marketing plans in health care.

KEY TERMS

marketing   strategic planning

THE CHALLENGE

Lea Rodriguez, MAS, RN
Vice President of Patient Care Services, Clara Maass Medical
Center, Belleville, New Jersey

In an effort to prevent hospital-acquired conditions (HACs), nurse managers were focused on the prevention of central line–associated bloodstream infections (CLABSIs) in the intensive care units (ICUs). Specifically, the unit nurses wanted to ensure that their patients would not be subjected to CLABSIs while in the ICU. The nurse

managers and the unit nurses wanted to bring their vision of preventing CLABSIs to reality. The team is aware that failure to actualize this vision will result in decreased reimbursement from Medicare for the enterprise. Bringing the vision to reality was a challenge.

What do you think you would do if you were this nurse?

INTRODUCTION

Given the turbulent times we face in health care, as well as the aging population in our society, now, more than ever, healthcare organizations are under enormous pressure to reduce expenses and contain costs. With the implementation of the Affordable Care Act, major reforms are required, and the healthcare system has responded by restructuring the following imperatives:

- Empowering patients
- Ensuring care across the continuum that is both coordinated and comprehensive
- Securing appropriate use of resources, advanced technology, and work force
- Focusing on health promotion and wellness

Nurses are instrumental in the development of planning and executing new strategies for the future and thus in influencing the direction of health care. As technology advances, for example, nurses must be at the forefront of this paradigm shift. This paradigm shift will require nurses to embrace, apply, and evaluate the use of such new technology. By demonstrating our ability to adopt and use new technology, we will be able to provide nursing with the expertise and earn the credibility to serve as advisors, directors, and influencers of technology. Thus by our active participation and expertise, we can ensure that technology will be used to meet nursing's information needs, to advance nursing practice, and to ensure nursing's continued viability. According to Waneka and Spetz (2010) information technology has positively impacted both nursing and patient satisfaction.

The operational definition of *proactive* is simply "aggressive planning." It provides direction for one's efforts and toward which others must then react. Thus greater control is possible so that one's vision becomes a probability, not just a possibility. The importance of proactive, thoughtful, deliberate planning in the face of uncertainties cannot be overestimated. *Proactive* means that everyone in the organization manages his or her work and professional life and how he or she relates to the organization's goals and missions.

STRATEGIC PLANNING

Strategic planning is a process by which the guiding members of the organization envision their future and develop the necessary and appropriate procedures and operations to actualize that future. Focus is designed to encompass the organization's emphasis on mission statements, strategic action plans, changes in policies and procedures, environmental factors affecting the organization, and the development and execution of new services.

The strategic planning process shown in Figure 16-1 consists of the following series of steps:

- Search the external, internal, and organizational environment to determine those forces or changes that may affect the work of the organization or that may be crucial to its survival.
- Analyze the organization's **s**trengths, **w**eaknesses, **o**pportunities, **t**hreats (SWOT analysis) and its potential for dealing with change.
- Develop and evaluate the various strategies available to the organization to meet these opportunities and threats.
- Revise organizational mission, philosophy, goals, and objectives based on the information acquired during the previous steps.

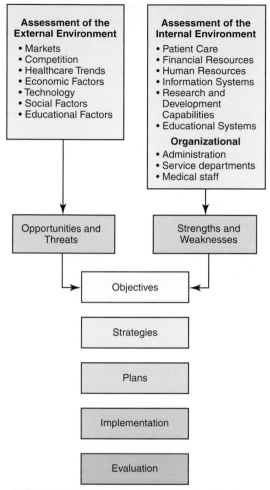

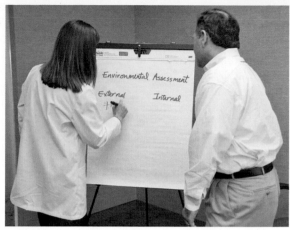

A strong and dynamic strategic plan results in efficient and effective use of resources.

FIGURE 16-1 Key steps in strategic planning.

- Select the best strategic option that balances the organization's potential with the challenges of changing conditions, taking into account the values of its management and its social responsibilities.
- Prepare the strategy.
- Execute and evaluate the strategy.

Reasons for Planning

In today's healthcare environment, which is marked by healthcare reform along with extreme turbulence and complexity, strategic planning for healthcare organizations must be more than an outline of a business plan. Therefore, to survive the ongoing change and restructuring of the healthcare system, the strategic plan becomes the fundamental tool for creating and sustaining the organizational vision for the future. This process leads to achievement of goals and objectives, gives meaning to work life, and provides direction and improvement for operational activities of the organization. Furthermore, a strong and dynamic strategic plan, if used, results in efficient and effective use of resources and reflects the organizational culture and customer focus. Numerous reasons exist for nurse leaders to plan in a proactive, systematic manner, including: (1) knowledge regarding philosophy, goals, and external and internal operations of the organization is necessary; and (2) an understanding of the planning process is paramount.

Phases of the Strategic Planning Process

Strategic planning is a proactive process which is vision-directed, action-oriented, creative, outside the box, innovative, and oriented toward positive change for growth while embracing chaos (Guillien and Garcia-Canal, 2012). A successful strategic plan will incorporate the creation of a business plan; this plan is integrated with a financial plan so that resources can be allocated and time can be allotted for implementation. The capital resources required for its realization must also be determined (Guillien and Garcia-Canal, 2012). According to Guillien and Garcia-Canal (2012), execution of the strategic plan is paramount for organizations; failure to be focused on execution will paralyze the organization. A strong and dynamic strategic plan results in efficient and effective use of resources.

The term *strategic planning process* is the development of a plan of action covering 3 to 5 years. The initial phase is the most difficult.

According to Schoemaker, Krupp, and Howland (2013), an *adaptive strategic leader* is someone who is resolute and flexible, and resilient when setbacks transpire. Six core competencies comprise the strategic leader: anticipate, challenge, interpret, decide, align, and learn (Schoemaker, Krupp, & Howland, 2013). The strategic leader needs to assess his or her weaknesses within the six core competencies and then rectify them to be effective (Schoemaker et al., 2013). The strategic leader searches for a new path through a vigorous dialog with various constituents, both internally and externally. Although strategic planning is often achieved at the executive level of an organization, staff and managers provide a valuable perspective.

Phase 1: Assessment of the External, Internal, and Organizational Environment

External Environmental Assessment. Assessment of the external environment is the initial phase in the strategic planning process. The economic, demographic, technologic, social-cultural, educational, and political-legal factors are assessed in terms of their impact on opportunities and threats within the environment. Healthcare leaders can assess the effect of competitors on their environment, thus plan and monitor their own operations, and develop other creative and visionary programs as they work within the framework of their institutional mission and goals. Schoemaker et al. (2013) suggested that a strategic leader of an organization must anticipate how competitors may respond to the strategic plan. Once that is realized, the response can be incorporated into the plan. An example appears in Box 16-1.

EXERCISE 16-1

What is your opinion about the demographic situation in the city in which you live or work? What is the cultural makeup of the area? What is the gap between the real needs and services provided to patients in your organization?

Internal Environmental Assessment. The internal assessment of the environment relates to the institution of health care and includes a review of the effectiveness of the structure, size, programs, financial resources, human resources, information systems, and

---

BOX 16-1   AN EXAMPLE OF ENVIRONMENTAL ASSESSMENT

A community-based acute care hospital is undertaking a study to examine accessibility, availability, quality, and effectiveness of developing an Orthopedic Center of Excellence. One of the initial steps is to conduct an environmental scan. The factors considered are the following:

- Economic forces and the escalating rates of healthcare costs
- The numbers and types of health professionals, including board-certified orthopedic physicians who are specializing in innovative joint replacement, operating room (OR) orthopedic nurses and OR orthopedic surgical technicians (certified), orthopedic direct care nurses (certified), case managers, social workers, physical and occupational therapists, and pain management specialists
- Cost of orthopedic implants and reimbursement
- The social, political, and regulatory forces, including strategic priorities of the government in health promotion and disease prevention
- The diagnostic services available, including magnetic resonance imaging (MRI) and nuclear diagnostic imaging
- Community outreach and educational opportunities

Patient Trends

- Demographic and population trends (population, employment, socioeconomic indicators, education, ethnicity, and lifestyle issues, with particular emphasis on minority groups)
- Trends in health care (increased emphasis on wellness programs and enhanced technologies)
- Prospective users' input about current and future services

---

research and development capabilities of the organization. In addition, education and training of staff and public demands are reviewed. The management team involves all levels of staff in this process and focuses on the purpose of the organization; the mission and goals; the capabilities, skills, and relationships of various professional and related staff; and the weaknesses and strengths of staff in such areas as leadership, planning, coordination, research, and staff development.

Organizational Environmental Assessment. The organizational environment assessment relates to the hospital administration, service departments, and medical staff. The process is considered an informal evaluation of relationships that define the organizational boundaries to assess for structure and loyalties that may affect the achievement of work. Also, the organizational climate must be assessed because it can shape the strategic direction of the organization.

Phase 2: Review of Mission Statement, Philosophy, Goals, and Objectives

Mission Statement. A mission statement reflects the purpose and direction of the healthcare organization or a department within it. A statement of philosophy provides direction for the organization and/or department within it. The content usually specifies organizational beliefs regarding the rights of individuals, beliefs regarding health and nursing, expectations of practitioners, and commitment of the organization to professionalism, education, evaluation, and research. The importance of the mission statement cannot be overstated, yet it is questionable how many individuals in an organization, when questioned directly, can articulate their mission statement or the philosophy.

Covey (1990) identified that the mission statement is vital to the success of an organization and believes that everyone should participate in the development of the mission statement: "The involvement process is as important as the written product and is the key to its use" (p. 139). "An organizational mission statement, one that truly reflects the deep shared vision and values of everyone within that organization, creates a unity and tremendous commitment" (p. 143).

EXERCISE 16-2

Select a healthcare organization with which you have been affiliated. How effective is the organizational structure (i.e., is the organization operating effectively and efficiently)? Is the mission visible in the actual care delivered? What overall human resources are present (e.g., table of organization, various titles, and numbers of people)? What information systems are used? Critique these questions as they apply to the nursing component only.

An example of a mission statement for a newly developed joint replacement program might be to provide quality, to be integrated, and to use the patient-focused healthcare model.

Goal-Setting. Goal-setting is the process of developing, negotiating, and formalizing the targets or objectives of an organization. Organizational goals must be appropriate for the organization. If the goals are not appropriate and not executed, then the plan will most likely fail, which carries negative implications for the organization (Guillien & Garcia-Canal, 2012).

Using the example from Box 16-1, the joint replacement program might have five goals:
1. Provide comprehensive patient/family education across the continuum of care.
2. Develop protocols for standardized patient care programs in terms of activities of daily living, physical and occupational therapy, recreational exercise, and pain management.
3. Incorporate a multidisciplinary approach to patient care through the use of physicians, nurse practitioners, nurses, case managers, social workers, physical and occupational therapists, dietitians, home care personnel, and clergy.
4. Enhance community support programs for arthritic patients.
5. Ensure that the Website is current, with information and services available to patients.

EXERCISE 16-3

Obtain and review a healthcare organization's mission statement. Based on what it says and means to you, create a goal statement that fits.

Practical insights from these studies that are critical to nurse administrators are that specific goals are more likely to lead to higher performance than are vague or very general goals, such as "try to do your best." Feedback, or knowledge of results, is more likely to motivate individuals toward higher performance levels and commitment to goal achievements. For example, as organizations have become more focused on their data related to care, they have been able to focus on specific goals and behaviors that result in better care.

Four key steps in implementing a goal-setting program are as follows:
1. Set goals that are specific and adhere to a deadline.
2. Promote goal commitment by providing instructions and support to employees and managers.
3. Support the achievement of goals with appropriate feedback as soon as possible.
4. Monitor performance at appropriate intervals.

Objectives. The ability to write clear and concise objectives is an important aspect of nursing leadership. Effective objectives are known as *S.M.A.R.T. objectives* and include the following:

Specific The objective statement is properly constructed and describes exactly what is to be accomplished.
- It begins with the word *to,* followed by an action verb.
- It specifies a single result to be achieved.
- It specifies a target date for its attainment.

Measurable The objectives are measurable.
- They provide the level of accomplishment of the end result.
- They leave no question as to what is expected.

Agreed On The objectives are agreed on by all parties.
- Mutual agreement is reached by all parties who will be responsible for execution and monitoring.

Realistic The objectives must be created within the realm of possibility and a challenge.
- The objectives should not be unrealistic or unattainable.
- They must be written in the span of control for the specific team working toward the goals.
- The team has to be accountable for follow-through.

Time Bound The objectives should establish a time frame for which the activity or improvement must be achieved.
- Time lines and deadlines are adhered to.
- The time line must be well-defined by avoiding statements such as "in the future."

Phase 3: Identification of Strategies

The third phase of the strategic planning process involves identifying major issues, establishing goals, and developing strategies to meet the goals. The term *strategy* can be defined as an organized and innovative plan that assists an organization to achieve its objectives. All departmental managers are involved in this process and are responsible for preparing a detailed plan of action, which may include the following: development of short-term and long-term objectives, formulation of annual department objectives, allocation of resources, and preparation of the budget. Table 16-1 identifies an action plan for creating, implementing, and evaluating an orthopedic center of excellence based on the environmental assessment in Box 16-1 on p. 294.

TABLE 16-1   STRATEGIC PLAN OF ACTION FOR THE DEVELOPMENT, IMPLEMENTATION, AND EVALUATION OF AN ORTHOPEDIC CENTER OF EXCELLENCE

OBJECTIVE	ACTIVITIES	RESPONSIBLE COUNCIL	TIME FRAME
1. To develop an Orthopedic Center of Excellence	1.1 To conduct a needs assessment • Primary and secondary service area • Demographic review • Out migration	Director of Nursing Orthopedic product line manager Strategic planning and marketing director	January 2016
	1.2 To conduct a literature review related to each of these topics: • Orthopedic product lines • Innovative orthopedic joint replacement procedures • Programs related to the orthopedics evidence-based practices for joint replacement	Orthopedic product line manager Operating room (OR) director Vice president of medical affairs Director of rehabilitative services Nurse practitioner Direct care nurse	January 2016
	1.3 To form an advisory committee comprising community representatives to oversee the development and implementation of the center	Patient satisfaction director Physician champion Vice president of patient care services Orthopedic staff across the continuum of care Director of rehabilitation services Vice president of medical affairs	February 2016

TABLE 16-1	STRATEGIC PLAN OF ACTION FOR THE DEVELOPMENT, IMPLEMENTATION, AND EVALUATION OF AN ORTHOPEDIC CENTER OF EXCELLENCE—cont'd		
OBJECTIVE	**ACTIVITIES**	**RESPONSIBLE COUNCIL**	**TIME FRAME**
	1.4 To develop the organizational structure, mission statement, philosophy, and objectives, and revise accordingly	All parties	March 2016
	1.5 To develop policy and procedure manuals for staff in all areas	Orthopedic staff across the continuum of care Medical staff Standards staff Nurse practitioners Director of education Direct care nurses	Ongoing
	1.6 To determine the business structure of the organization (i.e., legalities regarding partnerships, corporations, and proprietorship)	Nurse practitioners Medical staff Vice president of medical affairs Orthopedic product line manager Vice president of patient care services Assistant vice president of patient care services Office of general counsel	Ongoing
	1.7 To develop a budget	Assistant vice president of patient care services Orthopedic product line manager/ nurse manager	March 2016 Ongoing
	1.8 To develop a business site for the organization: • All renovations • Equipment • Supplies	Consultants and orthopedic product line manager	April 2016
	1.9 To develop a marketing program (newspapers, telephone, signs, and direct mailings)	Nurse practitioners Orthopedic product line manager Director of strategic planning and marketing Medical staff Direct care nurses	February 2016 Ongoing
2. To implement and evaluate the effectiveness and efficiency of these programs	2.1 To develop patient questionnaires related to satisfaction regarding care provided	Nurse practitioners Orthopedic product line managers Director of patient satisfaction Orthopedic frontline staff across the continuum Direct care nurses	April 2016
	2.2 To develop cost-effective analysis studies to evaluate each of the programs being provided	Orthopedic product line manager	Ongoing
	2.3 To collect and collate data related to use of services by orthopedic patients	Nurse practitioners Staff across the continuum of care Pharmacists Medical staff Orthopedic product line manager Quality director	Ongoing

Phase 4: Implementation

The fourth phase of strategic planning is that the specific plan for action is executed in order of priority. This entails open communication with staff (this is paramount) regarding the priorities for the next year and subsequent periods; development of revised policies and procedures regarding the changes; and the creation of area and individual objectives related to the plan. The specific plan needs to be focused on marketing, programs, operations, budget, and human resource.

Phase 5: Evaluation

On a consistent basis, at regular intervals, the strategic plan is reviewed at all levels to determine whether the execution of goals, objectives, and activities is on target. As stated, a sense of flexibility regarding the objectives is important to consider, and objectives may change as a result of legislation, budget changes, and change in structure or other environmental factors. Therefore alternative activities may need to be adapted to the situation. For example, one agency was informed that the budget had to be decreased by $250,000 over the next 3 months. The staff became involved in the development of creative methods for ensuring that the necessary changes occurred. Savings were realized with restructuring, reducing expenses, and, when appropriate, converting intravenous (IV) to oral (PO) medication administration.

EXERCISE 16-4

You are a direct care nurse in a healthcare organization and the Chair of the Professional Practice Committee has assigned you to work on a planning committee. The purpose of the committee is to devise long-term and short-term departmental goals for nursing.

The population of the town is 55,000, and the population is aging. The senior population probably will increase over the next 5 years. Many in the community are seeking assistance for arthritis complications such as building better bones and exercise programs, physical therapy opportunities, and community education.

The hospital has both inpatient and an outpatient rehabilitation programs with a specialized orthopedic unit; the unit is staffed with nurses who are nationally certified in orthopedics and with world-renowned, board certified orthopedic surgeons. Additionally, the organization achieved disease-specific certification by The Joint Commission for total knee replacement and hip replacement.

Considering the concepts of this strategic planning situation, in what direction should this nursing department consider moving during the next 5 years? How will you identify long-term and short-term plans? What additional information will your committee need to plan realistically for the next 5 months and the next 5 years?

MARKETING

Marketing is about identifying and meeting both human and social needs (Kotler & Keller, 2009). Marketing allows an organization to remain relevant to its customers in order to develop and execute services to meet those needs by establishing a niche, or specially focused market. The benefits of marketing include increased customer satisfaction, the potential to become the hospital of choice for both patients and employees, improved resource attraction, and improved operational efficiency. The underlying assumption is that marketing helps manage the exchange of goods and services in a more efficient manner. Marketing consists of many forms, including the advertisements in newspapers and, more recently, on websites. The Literature Perspective identifies broad examples of using Websites. Marketing can also use surveys (see the Research Perspective).

Strategic Marketing Planning Process

The strategic marketing planning process is similar to the strategic planning process and the nursing

---

 LITERATURE PERSPECTIVE

Resource: Spoerl, B. (2012). 6 Trends in an era of consumer-driven healthcare. Becker's Hospital Review. Retrieved June 13, 2013, from www.beckershospitalreview.com/strategicplanning/6-trends-in-an-era-of-consumer-driven-healthcare.html.

Marketing for health care was established later compared to other fields. Healthcare marketing is known for disseminating messages about services and product lines that could be complex and expensive. With the birth of social media, many healthcare organizations are becoming savvy in creating their own Websites. Healthcare organizations have developed Websites that list services available and locations for such services. Healthcare consumers can now research information that could assist them in their decision to seek health care or to glean more information about available services. Websites developed by healthcare organization focus their marketing effort to retain their patient population and market share. Specifically, consumer-driven marketing involves: interactive Websites, podcasts, and even blogs. Understanding new trends in marketing and social media helps nurses and others to be competitive in their communication.

Implications for Practice

Nurses have the opportunity to program Websites or at least to convey information about what patients are seeking as supports for their care.

RESEARCH PERSPECTIVE

Resource: Clyne, M., Dilligard, R., Langish, R., Ruddy, K., & Vega, D. (2009). Knowledge, attitudes, beliefs and practices regarding breast cancer screening in female health care workers in an acute care hospital in Northern New Jersey. Unpublished researched—Sigma Theta Tau Poster Session, Seton Hall University, South Orange, NJ.

A convenience sample of female healthcare workers (n = 411) in an acute care hospital setting was used for this study to examine the knowledge, attitudes, beliefs, and practices regarding breast cancer screening. For this descriptive study, a 12-item, 5-point Likert questionnaire was distributed to all female healthcare workers as a paycheck attachment in October (Breast Cancer Awareness Month).

Half of the respondents had a family history of cancer, 80% performed a self-examination of the breast, 79% indicated their

physician encouraged them to have a mammogram, and 95% had insurance. Perceptions about receiving a recommendation for a mammogram tended to be positive, and mammogram was believed to be more effective than examination by self or the physician.

Implications for Practice

This study has specific implications for designing marketing strategies, including the authors' recommendations about developing educational programs regarding the importance of screening, prevention, and early detection of breast cancer. Furthermore, nurses need to advocate for the availability of searchable databases so patients can find important information.

---

process. Figure 16-2 on p. 300 offers a comparative chart outlining the steps in the process.

The steps of the strategic marketing planning are as follows:

- Analyze the organization-wide mission, objectives, goals, and culture to which the marketing strategy must contribute.
- Assess organizational strengths, weaknesses, opportunities, and threats (SWOT analysis) presented by the external environment.
- Analyze the future environment the marketer is likely to face with respect to the public served; competition; and the social-cultural, political, technologic, and economic environment.
- Determine the marketing mission, objectives, and specific goals for the relevant planning period.
- Formulate the core marketing strategy to achieve the specified goals.
- Implement the necessary organizational structure and the systems within the marketing function to ensure proper follow-through of the designed strategy.
- Establish detailed programs and tactics to carry out the core strategy for the planning period, including a timetable of activities and the assignment of specific responsibilities.
- Establish benchmarks to measure interim and final achievements of the program.
- Execute the planned program.
- Monitor performance, and adjust the core strategy, tactical details, or both as needed.

Although healthcare organizations have marketing departments, nurses are involved in the process because of their direct involvement with the users of service—the patients.

Assessment

Determining Organization-Level Mission, Objectives, and Goals

A marketing plan is developed by the executive leaders of the organization and advisory board to do the following:

1. Determine the organization-level long-term culture, mission, objectives, and goals.
2. Assess the organization's potential future external environment.
3. Assess the organization's current and potential strengths, weaknesses, opportunities, and threats.

Analyzing Organizational Strengths and Weaknesses

In the marketing process, an environmental assessment is conducted to identify and research the target market. An example of this is conducting a needs assessment of the services currently provided by an organization to develop new services or promotional activities to meet the needs of the population being served.

Focus groups may consist of interviews with key staff; review of documents; observation of staff; visits to competitors; and overview of advertisements, brochures, and other documents as deemed appropriate. Nurses often have great insight about needs because patients convey their desires and lack of services during care delivery.

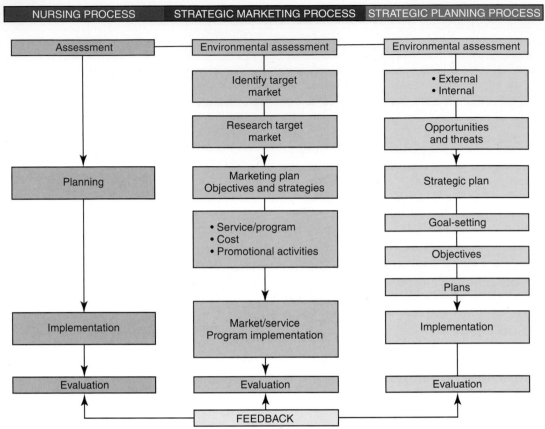

FIGURE 16-2 Marketing framework as compared to using the nursing process and strategic planning.

Analyzing External Threats and Opportunities

The three components of the external environment are (1) the public environment, which consists of groups and organizations that affect the organization (e.g., public, media, regulatory agencies); (2) the competitive environment, which consists of other organizations that vie for the attention and loyalty of customers; and (3) the macro-environment, which consists of demographic, economic, technologic, political, and social forces to which the organization must adapt.

Setting Marketing Mission, Objectives, and Goals

The marketing mission, objectives, and goals must align with the organizational mission, objectives, and goals. The marketing focus is geared to changing market conditions, much as a financial advisor evaluates changing investment market conditions. The market,

comprising both external and internal markets, influences the way an organization moves toward its vision.

Planning

The environmental assessment is followed by the development of a marketing plan. This plan outlines the service or program to be provided, includes a detailed budget-cost analysis, and describes the promotional activities designed to promote the program. "Predicting the future" is difficult in turbulent times. To anticipate problems and plan for the future, forecasting involves considering multiple factors that could occur. The process requires several components:
- Assessing the current and potential future situation
- Identifying the strengths, weaknesses, opportunities, and threats
- Defining the driving forces in the environment
- Developing optional scenarios

- Identifying the preferred action
- Developing a plan of action
- Executing the plan of action
- Evaluating and monitoring the plan

Forecasts should be estimates of how accurately a situation can provide optional futures and learning experiences and be considered for their influence in convincing managers of the need for change, be cost-effective, and be used for their ritualistic purpose. Rather than using the "shooting at a target" metaphor, it may be more appropriate to think of forecasters as art teachers, helping line (and clinical) managers paint updated pictures of their future. For example, in forecasting the number of patients who will need orthopedic services in a community, a manager needs to consider an environmental scan comprising the aging population and morbidity and mortality related to inactivity underlying orthopedic problems.

Implementation and Execution

The implementation, or execution, phase includes the establishment of the program and promotional activities designed to communicate benefits of the service or program to patients. Forms of promotion may include media releases, brochures, pamphlets, newsletters, and "word-of-mouth" advertising. Pamphlets and brochures are promotional materials that inform individuals about the benefits of a healthcare agency's programs and services.

Evaluation and Monitoring

The evaluation may incorporate customer satisfaction surveys, interviews with customers, and further research studies designed to assess reasons that customers are using or not using a service, program, or product. Feedback is an essential component of the marketing process.

Box 16-2 represents steps in the strategic marketing planning process in relation to the delivery of breast cancer screening services to female healthcare workers in an acute care community hospital in a suburban area of northern New Jersey.

CONCLUSION

Nurses can play an active role and be given responsibilities relating to planning, goal-setting, and marketing. Each of us has some sense of what is important today and sustainable for tomorrow in the context of our cultural perspective. Most of us sense the difference between fads and trends and how each affects us personally and professionally. Nursing leaders are

---

BOX 16-2 MISSION STATEMENT, GOALS, AND OBJECTIVES OF A NORTHERN NEW JERSEY BREAST CANCER SCREENING PROGRAM

Mission Statement

To reduce the leading cause of cancer deaths in women by delivering a comprehensive, organized, and evaluated breast cancer screening program for female healthcare workers in northern New Jersey. The Breast Cancer Screening Program is committed to delivering a program that is sensitive to women's needs, builds on health-promoting behaviors, and fosters partnerships with interest groups in the healthcare community.

Overall Goals

To integrate health promotion strategies and medical practice to reduce mortality from breast cancer by having 100% of eligible female healthcare workers participate in annual mammography screening.

Objectives

- To detect breast cancer earlier than would occur if organized screening was not available
- To develop and implement a hospital mobilization plan for the program

- To develop and implement a social marketing plan, including a health education component for the program
- To articulate protocols and standards for healthcare professionals associated with the program
- To establish protocols for the interaction of the target population with the program
- To develop and implement training and technical assistance for those associated with the delivery of the program
- To develop a partnership with healthcare professionals that will facilitate program delivery
- To establish a regional breast screening service so that all women in the target population have equal access to breast screening
- To document the follow-up of all women in whom an abnormality has been detected
- To provide screening that is sensitive and acceptable to the target population
- To evaluate the program on a continual basis, including needs assessment and measurement of process, economic, and outcome variables

accountable for setting goals, including their followers in those activities, and aligning tasks with the mission and goals of the organization. As nursing leaders represent the profession, organization, or community, they are marketing each of those elements. Nurse

leaders can positively contribute to formal marketing strategies through various activities such as focus groups or evaluating responses to marketing materials. However, the focus should be on how nurse leaders' actions contribute to future quality.

THE SOLUTION

Trying to find common ground to achieve the vision of preventing HACs, specifically CLABSIs, for the nursing staff and the nursing management team was of utmost importance. Given the fact that we had developed a Professional Practice Council and Nursing Research Council, I thought this might be a great starting place for the staff to develop a creative way to bring their vision to actuality. Specifically, we have unit-based councils and a representative from the unit-based council reports into the Professional Practice Council and the Nursing Research Council to review the evidenced-based practices. This is truly an empowered group with decision-making capacity for nursing staff.

1. The literature for CLABSIs was reviewed and disseminated among the members of the unit-based councils. Dialog ensued, and staff members were very interested in the research findings and how they could actualize it for their unit.
2. The unit nurses were enthusiastic about such an opportunity. They gladly participated because the results would undoubtedly have a profound impact on preventing CLABSIs, which would enhance patient care, quality, and safety.
3. The findings and implications of preventing CLABSIs were reviewed and discussed with the Professional Practice Council. Final decision making about how we were going to embrace this newly found evidenced-based practice and decision making was conducted by the council members.

4. Wanting this to be a win-win moment for the staff, I made sure they had all the appropriate resources available to them in making changes to our policies and procedures. I ensured that all potential barriers were removed for success in making their vision come true.
5. The staff members felt a strong sense of ownership to this vision and were instrumental in the success of the changes.

The utilization of our Professional Practice Council and Nursing Research Council provides the nurses with a paradigm shift that they can make a difference in the care they deliver each and every day. Additionally, the nurses can be recognized for the value of their expertise to resolve/prevent any potential HACs or patient safety issues. The nurses are an empowered group of professionals who turned their vision into a reality based on nursing research and best practices. The council members take great pride in their accomplishments and I am just as proud of them! The nurses are fantastic role models and mentors to others. I am in awe of their commitment to excellence in patient care, and their efforts do not go unnoticed; I am honored to work with them.

—Lea Rodriguez

Would this be a suitable approach for you? Why?

■ THE EVIDENCE

According to Twibell et al. (2012), nursing leaders must focus on retaining their novice nurses because we can expect a shortage of 260,000 nurses by 2025. It costs an organization approximately $82,000 when a nurse resigns (Twibell et al., 2012). Additionally, Twibell et al. (2012) conducted a literature review and applied the SWOT analysis to assess why novice nurses were resigning from healthcare organization and noted that 30% of them resigned within the first year of employment.

Several nursing leaders were faced with high nursing turnover rates in their organization. The vision of

these nursing leaders was to retain their novice nurses. The nurse managers decided to conduct focus groups and exit interviews with the direct care nurses to elicit feedback. From the feedback, a new strategic plan was executed.

The plan was designed to establish connections, provide individualized orientation, and use a check-in process with educators and managers. In addition to a decreased turnover rate, the organization realized significant cost savings by retaining the new nursing staff, and nurse satisfaction increased for both the new nursing staff members and the nursing leaders.

WHAT NEW GRADUATES SAY

- I always heard about organizations having a mission, vision, and value statement. I was surprised to learn that my healthcare organization had one. More interesting was that it was easy to understand and the employees lived by it!
- I am so proud to work with nurses who provide such high quality care. We have been nation-ally recognized for our quality outcomes such as achieving an A rating for our Leapfrog scores. Now the organization can create a marketing plan to let the community and other stakeholders know what a great quality organization we are!

CHAPTER CHECKLIST

The operational effectiveness of any organization depends on its strategic planning. Nurse leaders/managers must be knowledgeable of the critical elements to facilitate the process. Setting goals and defining marketing strategies for product line development are part of the role of professional nurses to achieve effective organizational results in creating a niche market in healthcare services.

- Strategic planning
  - Reasons for planning
  - Phases of the strategic planning process
    - Phase 1: Assessment of the external, internal, and organizational environment
      - External environmental assessment
      - Internal environmental assessment
      - Organizational environmental assessment
    - Phase 2: Review of mission statement, philosophy, goals, and objectives
      - Mission statement
      - Goal-setting
      - Objectives
    - Phase 3: Identification of strategies
    - Phase 4: Implementation
    - Phase 5: Evaluation
- Marketing
  - Strategic marketing planning process
  - Assessment
    - Determining organization-level mission, objectives, and goals
    - Analyzing organizational strengths and weaknesses
    - Analyzing external threats and opportunities
    - Setting marketing mission, objectives, and goals
  - Planning
  - Implementation and execution
  - Evaluation and monitoring

TIPS FOR PLANNING, GOAL-SETTING, AND MARKETING

- Be clear about the organization's mission and vision; ensure they meet the needs of those you serve, and stay true to them.
- Read and listen to wide sources of data to determine what is happening and what trends could affect you and your organization, and be flexible if changes are imminent.
- Be clear about your role in the organization and its success. Actively participate in the process.
- Think about what messages others need to hear about you and the services you provide.

REFERENCES

Clyne, M., Dilligard, R., Langish, R., Ruddy, K., & Vega, D. (2009). *Knowledge, attitudes, beliefs and practices regarding breast cancer screening in female health care workers in an acute care hospital in Northern New Jersey.* Unpublished researched—Sigma Theta Tau Poster Session, South Orange, NJ: Seton Hall University.

Covey, S. (1990). *The seven habits of highly effective people.* Toronto: Simon & Schuster.

Guillien, M., & Garcia-Canal, E. (2012). Execution as a strategy. *Harvard Business Review, 90*(10), 103–107.

Kotler, P., & Keller, K. (2009). *Marketing management.* Upper Saddle River, NJ: Prentice Hall.

Schoemaker, P., Krupp, S., & Howland, S. (2013). Strategic leadership: The essential skills. *Harvard Business Review, 91*(1/2), 131–134.

Spoerl, B. (2012). 6 Trends in an era of consumer driven health care. *Becker's Review,* Retrieved June 13, 2013, from www.beckershospitalreview.com/strategicplanning/6-trends-in-an-era-of-consumer-driven-healthcare.htlm.

Twibell, R., St. Pierre, J., Johnson, D., Barton, D., Davis, C., Kidd, M., et al. (2012). Why new nurses don't stay. *The American Nurse, 7*(6), 1–6.

Waneka, R., & Spetz, J. (2010). Hospital information technology systems' impact on nurses and nursing care. *Journal of Nursing Administration, 40*(12), 509–514.

SUGGESTED READINGS

Galunic, C., & Hermreck, I. (2012). How to help employees get strategy. *Harvard Business Review, 90*(12), 24.

Groysberg, B., & Slind, M. (2012). Leadership is a conversation: How to improve employee engagement and alignment in today's flatter, more networked organizations. *Harvard Business Review, 99*(6), 76–84.

Lafley, A., Martin, R., Rivikin, J., & Siggelkow, N. (2012). Bringing science to the art of strategy. *Harvard Business Review, 90*(9), 56–66.

Luther, K., & Resar, R. (2013). Tapping front line knowledge: Identifying problems as they occur helps enhance patient safety. *Healthcare Executive, 26*(1), 84–87.

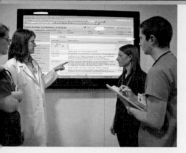

Leading Change

Elaine S. Scott

This chapter highlights the increasing changes in health care and describes how all nurses must be change agents. The nature of change and the elements of the change process are reviewed. The theories, conceptual frameworks, and human responses to change are considered in an effort to understand the magnitude of managing the change experience. The roles of both the direct care nurse and the nurse manager in navigating change in the healthcare system are explored. Direct care nurses support change by remaining open to and engaging in new models of care, evidence-based practices, and requirements for ensuring safe and effective patient care. Nurse managers and leaders work to facilitate change. Nurse leaders must anticipate, prepare for, oversee, and sustain change to achieve improved outcomes and professional and organizational goals. Avenues for promoting staff empowerment and engagement are examined as proactive change management strategies leaders can use to facilitate rapid, efficient, and almost continuous change.

LEARNING OUTCOMES

- Analyze the nature and types of change in the healthcare system.
- Evaluate theories and conceptual frameworks for understanding and navigating change.
- Examine the use of select functions, principles, and strategies for initiating and managing change.
- Formulate desirable qualities of both direct care nurses and nurse leaders who are effective change agents.
- Explore methods for sustaining change.

KEY TERMS

barriers	chaos theory	learning organization
change agents	complexity theories	planned change
change leaders	facilitators	second-order change
change process	first-order change	unplanned change

THE CHALLENGE

Sharon McEvoy, RN
Nurse Manager, Clara Maass Medical Center, Belleville, New
*   Jersey*

As a nurse manager on a large medical/surgical unit, I often noticed that our nursing assistants did a lot of running around in and out of patients' rooms. They often answered call bells for the same things over and over, all day long. In addition, I saw that the professional nursing staff could not always locate the nursing assistants because they were so spread out over the geographic layout of the unit. Around the same time, patient satisfaction and staff satisfaction had either reached a plateau or remained low. I heard a presentation about hourly rounding and then found some articles explaining how the practice had been introduced in many hospitals across the country. I brought the articles to my staff and introduced the concept to them. The challenge, I told them, is to anticipate patients' needs rather than respond to them as we all had been doing for years. How could I make hourly rounding work on our unit without resistance? Would our patient and staff satisfaction increase? How would the staff adjust to the change?

What do you think you would do if you were this nurse?

INTRODUCTION

At no time in history have nurses experienced the amount of change that exists in the current healthcare environment. Advances in technology, modifications in best practices, emergent research, and healthcare regulation and reimbursement are in a state of constant flux. Understanding the nature of change and how to navigate through change is an essential skill for the contemporary nurse. Unless nurses know how to promote changes in behavior, patients continue to manage their health in less than desirable ways. Nurses at the bedside, in clinics, and in patients' homes not only support patients in changing their behavior, but also must now foster innovation and promote change in the workplace that advances patient safety and improves patient outcomes.

Nurse leaders must also be excellent change managers. Nurse leaders play the roles of both coach and coordinator, facilitating the changes needed at a system, unit, or team level (Salmela, Eriksson, & Fagerstrom, 2011). During change, nurse leaders keep the delivery of safe and effective care at the center of their attention to ensure that the disruption and chaos of change do not impact patients. By supporting a transparent and evidence-based environment, the nurse leader ensures a culture that will support both patients and staff during the change process (Salmela et al., 2011). So all nurses are change agents in all their roles; that means they prepare for, implement, and sustain change.

THE NATURE OF CHANGE

The concept of change is founded on the belief that individuals and organizations are open systems that can be influenced by internal and external variables. Change involves altering the current state of things. Merriam-Webster's definition of *change* is "to give a different position, course, or direction; to make a shift from one to another" (http://www.merriam-webster.com/dictionary/change). Change can be planned, or it can occur in response to external or internal requirements. For example, as reimbursement methods have changed in health care, health systems have reorganized service delivery, implemented new technology, and created new initiatives such as patient-centered care and transitional care programs. In today's world, change is constant, unavoidable, and pervasive.

Change can happen on a personal level or on an organizational level. Change can be initiated by the individual or the system, or it can be imposed upon either. A patient may decide to lose weight and exercise to maintain health. This is an example of a planned change at a personal level. In contrast, when a federal law changes the reimbursement rates for Medicare patients, healthcare organizations may have to alter service delivery to prevent financial losses. This is an example of an organizational change. When a disaster occurs, an unplanned event disrupts both individual and organizational plans. Almost all organizational changes require personal changes for the individuals employed by the organization.

Types of change can be characterized in several ways based on both intensity and cause. Historically, change was thought of as planned change and unplanned change (Lewin, 1951). **Planned change** is deliberate and organized and has the goal of improvement. **Unplanned change** is disconcerting, unanticipated, and adaptive. These were also referred to as first-order change and second-order change (Weick & Quinn, 1999). **First-order change** is called *kaizen,* a Japanese term meaning "small, steady steps" (Maurer, 2004). First-order change is evolutionary, and in healthcare systems, it is often referenced as continuous improvement. Most quality improvement programs in healthcare systems are illustrations of first-order change. In this type of change, small, ongoing steps are taken to make things better. First-order change is change that is usually in harmony with the values of persons or systems and thus makes sense to the people involved. Second-order change is revolutionary and episodic and is a large part of what healthcare systems are experiencing today. Second-order change requires radical adjustments in a person or in the structure of a system. This type of change may be unanticipated or expected, but in either case, demonstrative change is required for sustainability.

All changes, whether perceived as positive or negative, large-scale or simple, are scary and generate fear. Some individuals embrace change more readily, whereas others resist even the most minuscule change. Although all change requires interventions for successful implementation, the different types of change necessitate different strategies for successful navigation. Hence the **change process** is varied when a change is planned versus unplanned. As change agents, nurses and nurse leaders must understand and be equipped to manage these respective processes.

THE CHANGE PROCESS

Knowledge about the change process is essential for learning to manage it. Central to understanding how to effectively navigate changes in ourselves, patients, and healthcare organizations is the concept of systems. A system is a group of interacting, interrelated, or interdependent elements forming a more complex whole (http://www.merriam-webster.com/dictionary/system). All systems, which can be intricate or simple, have inputs that are collected and processed to develop outputs, or the accomplishment of the goals of the system. Systems have subsystems. For example, an individual is comprised of subsystems such as gastrointestinal, cardiovascular, and pulmonary subsystems. A hospital—one example of a healthcare system—includes subsystems such as nursing, dietary, engineering, medicine, and radiology. Systems theory asserts that if one

part of the system is changed, then it impacts the overall system.

Open systems that function effectively continually exchange feedback among all of the parts to ascertain if the subsystems are healthy and contributing to the goals of the system. If vulnerabilities or weaknesses are present, the system will accommodate to remain stable. Open systems are also influenced by the external environment. Thus healthcare systems and the nurses who work within them are affected by internal factors such as the availability and quality of resources, the levels of staffing, and the processes used to manage patient care. Additionally, external factors such as disease and lifestyle patterns in the community population, healthcare regulation and reimbursement, and the supply of healthcare workers also impact the system. Changes to a system may be anticipated and planned, or they may be sudden and unexpected.

Planned, First-Order Change

Lewin (1947) was one of the first theorists and scholars to study and illuminate the process of planned change. He postulated that change involves a three-stage process that begins by helping a person, group, or organization release a current behavior or process, move toward the new desired reality, and then sustain that new status. These three steps—unfreezing, moving, and refreezing—can be used to analyze almost any type of change. Sometimes unfreezing involves overcoming inertia, the desire to keep things the same. A patient may realize the need to adopt a low-salt diet after being diagnosed with hypertension, or an organization may acknowledge a need to alter the mix of registered nurses and assistants on a unit to lower the cost of care delivery. This begins the change process, but it takes considerably more effort to actually make the change. Examples of forces of change that are facilitators and barriers are shown in Figure 17-1. Unfreezing is the step during which individuals and organizations recognize the need to change and begin to get ready to make that change. This is a time of evaluating the benefits and the costs that the change will entail. This evaluation affects the motivation level generated to make the change.

Lewin (1951) called this evaluation Force Field Analysis. He described it as the forces or influences that impact whether change occurs. If more forces favor change—**facilitators**—then change will be more likely

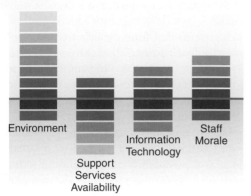

FIGURE 17-1 Examples of forces of change: facilitators and barriers.

to occur. In contrast, if during this analysis more forces are against the change—barriers—then the change will be less likely to occur. Lewin's Force Field Analysis is simple yet robust in helping nurses understand what it takes to make and sustain a change. This theory is particularly relevant when implementing planned change. Change agents need to know whether individuals see the need to unfreeze. This involves listening and assessing to determine if all participants in the change have a shared vision for the change. Organizational change is accomplished through individual change, so understanding the power of the "status quo" is essential. Unless individuals perceive the change will make things better, the resisting forces will limit the success of the change. As in The Challenge (p. 306), changes in how patients' needs were anticipated on an hourly basis on one unit brought about unfreezing. Unfreezing is a critical step in planned change. It is during this phase of change that we realize what people fear and how we can address those fears.

In the second stage, the moving or changing stage of Lewin's theory, planned interventions and strategies are executed to support the implementation of the change. Commonly used methods include education about the need for the change, vision building to conceptualize and bring life to the change, involving individuals in the process of planning and making the change, and implementing small steps toward the change. Information gained during the analysis of the forces for and against the transition can be used to guide the change agent in making a plan and developing strategies to ensure effective

implementation of the change goal. Remembering that a practical first step must be clear can determine the success of a planned change.

The final stage—refreezing—focuses on sustaining the change over a longer period of time. During this time, the change agent works to reinforce the new, desired behaviors and processes by praising, rewarding, and providing feedback. This phase is commonly undermanaged. Nurse managers must implement systems to ensure that changed behaviors or processes continue, measure the impact of the changes, and provide staff with progress reports and evidence of success. Every nurse has to monitor behaviors during this phase because slipping back into routines and more comfortable patterns of performance can easily happen without diligence and dedication to the change initiative.

EXERCISE 17-1

Using Lewin's Force Field Analysis concept, identify the facilitators and barriers in the following situation. Using a scale of 1 to 5, rate the potential strength of each in hindering or expediting attainment of the change. Use "+5" for the highest positive strength toward change occurring and "+1" for the weakest. Use "−5" for the greatest negative strength against the change and "−1" for the weakest.

The inpatient psychiatric unit is about to convert 12 of its 20 voluntary beds into short-term care facility (STCF) beds for patients who are involuntarily committed. These beds would coexist with the voluntary beds that are already on the unit. The involuntary beds were transferred from the license of a nearby facility. The talent and the expertise of the former facility were highly desirable to help with the transition to a unit with a higher acuity with sicker patients; therefore 12 of the former facility's nursing staff members were hired. So far, staff's reaction to the merger has been mixed. Individuals from the former facility, while welcomed enthusiastically by the staff from the present unit, were less than enthusiastic. Added to the change was the news that the former facility filed for bankruptcy, leaving the former employees without their retirement pensions and other benefits.

Lewin's work has been the foundation for many change theorists. Lippitt, Watson, and Westley (1958) further developed Lewin's work by considering more of the human factors that are involved in change. In particular, Lippit et al. created three aspects of the moving phase that further defined what happened to foster change: pushing back on and really clarifying the problem that is requiring the change, examining all of the possible ways to address the problem, developing commitment to one of those plans, and moving individuals from intending to change to actually changing behaviors and processes. Additionally, Lippit et al. also studied what contributed to the effectiveness of change agents in soliciting change. They found that the relationship the change agent had with the group made a demonstrative difference in accomplishing the change.

Unplanned, Second-Order Change

Though Lewin's theory was designed to describe planned or first-order changes, many scholars think the theory is too simplistic to address how unplanned or second-order change occurs (Burnes, 2004). Planned change initiatives are still useful in stable situations; however, the magnitude of change in the world today has led to evolution in the thinking about systems ultimately contributing to the development of complexity theories. These theories address the vast array of nonlinear and unpredictable events that occur in the world. Complexity theories alter the traditional systems thinking approach by asserting that system behavior is unpredictable. This theory views change as emergent and highly influenced by all individuals and subsystems in an organization.

Three elements make up the framework for understanding complexity theories: chaos as order, the ideal of operating on the edge of chaos, and order-generating rules (Burnes, 2004). In complexity theories, chaos is viewed as order beneath randomness. While things may appear chaotic, organizing elements are still beneath them. Operating on the edge of chaos describes the state within which a system holds a careful balance between order and disorder. Finally, order-generating rules as a concept theorize that complex systems function by following simple guidelines that can be redesigned when they no longer work for sustaining or optimizing the system.

Complexity theories suggest that change is not episodic but rather an ongoing experience through which a system adjusts and realigns, recreating itself continuously. This perspective shifts the change experience from a top-down model where leaders design the future and impose it on the system to one where change is systemic, emerging throughout the system, across departments and professions as an adaptive response fostered by decentralized decision making and collaboration.

Some of the more recent thinking about healthcare systems is framed using complexity theory (Dattee & Barlow, 2010; Paley & Eva, 2011; Weberg, 2012). One particularly important illustration of how complex healthcare systems can organize and develop can be seen in the Magnet™ movement in the United States (Abraham, Jerome-D'Emilia, & Begun, 2011; Sanders, 2010). Abraham et al. (2011) characterize this movement as an "organizational innovation" that fosters "decentralized decision making, relatively flat organizational structures, a participative management culture, and empowered middle managers" (p. 306). Because Magnet™ mobilizes an operational framework reflective of the principles derived from complexity theory, it supports a healthcare system in developing and diffusing new ideas, building collective energy to support implementing needed change, and engaging all the nursing subsystems in an organization.

Whether change is planned or unplanned, some researchers have estimated that nearly 70% of all change strategies in organizations fail (Judge & Douglas, 2009). Organizations and individuals can have well-conceptualized visions and plans for change and still fail to be successful. Central to the effective accomplishment of change is engaging the people affected by the change. This is the major task of the nurse manager functioning as a change agent in the healthcare system. In addition, examining personal resistance against change, poor motivation to adopt new technologies, and evidence-based practice strategies is a critical change management skill all nurses must possess. Many things impact how people react to change. The degree to which the change does not conflict with personal values, the context through which change is brokered in the organization, and the amount of substantive changes individuals must make in their behavior all influence change outcomes.

PEOPLE AND CHANGE

Change, whether proactively initiated at the point of change or imposed from external sources, affects people. Change can be mandated by higher administration, it can originate in any department or unit, or it may begin at the level of care delivery. Responses to all or part of the change process by individuals and groups may vary from full acceptance and willing participation to outright rejection or even rebellion.

The initial responses to change may be reluctance and resistance. Reluctance and resistance are common when the change threatens personal security. For example, changes in the structure of an organization can result in changes of position for personnel. Eliminating a critical care nurse position and referring that nurse to the only open position as a home health nurse can certainly result in the nurse feeling angry, displaced, and even temporarily incompetent and isolated.

The innovation-decision process (Rogers, 2003) describes the choice of an individual, over time, to accept or reject a new idea for use in practice (see the Theory Box). According to Rogers, the individual's decision-making actions pass through five sequential stages. The decision to not accept the new idea may

THEORY BOX

Theories for Planned Change

KEY CONTRIBUTORS	KEY IDEA	APPLICATION TO PRACTICE
Six Phases of Planned Change* Havelock (1973) is credited with this planned change model.	Change can be planned, implemented, and evaluated in six sequential stages. The model is advocated for the development of effective change agents and used as a rational problem-solving process. The six stages are as follows: 1. Building a relationship 2. Diagnosing the problem 3. Acquiring relevant resources 4. Choosing the solution 5. Gaining acceptance 6. Stabilizing the innovation and generating self-renewal	Useful for low-level, low-complexity change
Seven Phases of Planned Change[†] Lippitt, Watson, and Westley (1958) are credited with this planned change model.	Change can be planned, implemented, and evaluated in seven sequential phases. Ongoing sensitivity to forces in the change process is essential. The seven phases are as follows: 1. The client system becomes aware of the need for change. 2. The relationship is developed between the client system and change agent. 3. The change problem is defined. 4. The change goals are set and options for achievement are explored. 5. The plan for change is implemented. 6. The change is accepted and stabilized. 7. The change entities redefine their relationships.	Useful for low-level, low-complexity change
Innovation-Decision Process[‡] Rogers (2003) is credited with formulating this process.	Change for an individual occurs over five phases when choosing to accept or reject an innovation/idea. Decisions to not accept the new idea may occur at any of the five stages. The change agent can promote acceptance by providing information about benefits and disadvantages and encouragement. The five stages are as follows: 1. Knowledge 2. Persuasion 3. Decision 4. Implementation 5. Confirmation	Useful for individual change

*Adapted from Havelock, R.G. (1973). *The change agent's guide to innovation in education.* Englewood Cliffs, NJ: Educational Technology Publications.
[†]Adapted from Lippitt, R., Watson, J., & Westley, B. (1958). *The dynamics of planned change.* New York: Harcourt Brace.
[‡]Adapted from Rogers, E.M. (1995). *Diffusion of innovations* (4th ed.). New York: The Free Press.

occur at any stage. However, peer change agents and formal change managers can facilitate movement through these stages by encouraging the use of the idea and providing information about its benefits and disadvantages.

Ideal and common patterns of an individual's behavioral responses to change can facilitate an effective change as described in Rogers's classic work (1995). These responses and brief descriptions are as follows:

- *Innovators* thrive on change, which may be disruptive to the unit stability.
- *Early adopters* are respected by their peers and thus are sought out for advice and information about innovations/changes.
- *Early majority* prefer doing what has been done in the past but eventually will accept new ideas.
- *Late majority* are openly negative and agree to the change only after most others have accepted the change.
- *Laggards* prefer keeping traditions and openly express their resistance to new ideas.
- *Rejectors* oppose change actively, and may even use sabotage, which can interfere with the overall success of a change process.

One might assume that innovators are the ideal nurse change agent, but all of these perspectives are needed to implement effective change. Often the late majority and laggards have a real reason for rejecting the change. Listening to all the perspectives about change is critical for moving change forward.

Ideally, each of these types of nurses can be used to support needed change processes. Innovators can be used to "test" new ideas in a restricted pilot program so that they are not disruptive to others who continue to follow the current process. In this very important sense, the work of the Institute for Healthcare Improvement (IHI) has benefited organizations in using this approach. The focus of IHI is to accelerate rapid, small tests of change, often at the point of care (*www.ihi.org/*). Unit-based decision making to change processes and policies revolves around the staff members working on the unit and depends highly on their ongoing adaptation to evolving realities.

For example, one direct care nurse champion of change expressed to her colleagues her frustration with the many interruptions that occurred while preparing and administering medications. The nurse thought this led to an increased likelihood for error. Discussing the problem resulted in the trial of a possible solution: wearing a prominently colored vest that said, "Do not disturb! Medication administration in process." This idea eventually was spread to all of the units and resulted in demonstrated reductions in medication errors.

All nurses have the capacity to be change agents. Box 17-1 illustrates seven attributes found to characterize what all change agents possess (Katzenbach et al., 1996). Change agents help others transform by advocating for openness and improvement. Nurses who act as change agents understand the change process and are committed to growth. These nurses are optimists, have influence with colleagues, know how to build networks, and facilitate communication. The literature often refers to these individuals as change "champions." In a study on organizational readiness for evidence-based practice (Gale & Schaffer, 2009), essential characteristics of a champion for change were drive and enthusiasm, knowledge about the area of change, good communication skills, and referent power. Nurses who function as positive change agents within the healthcare system are willing to try new things, stay abreast of new evidence about best practices, and are open to change. Nurses who

BOX 17-1	**ATTRIBUTES CHARACTERIZING CHANGE AGENTS**	
ATTRIBUTE	**KEY POINTS**
Commitment to a better way	Excited about designing a better future
Courage to challenge power bases and norms	Closest to the work
Go beyond role, take initiative, think outside the box	Assurance of change happening
Persona	Self-motivated, generate enthusiasm
Caring	Commitment to patients and their welfare
Humility	About the change, not about "me"
Sense of humor	Self-support through challenges

Source: Katzenbach, J.R., Beckett, F., Dichter, S., Feigen, M., Gagnon, C., Hope, Q., & Ling, T. (1996). *Real change leaders.* New York, NY: Random House.

become change agents are lifelong learners who seed new ideas and share innovative practices with other nurses.

Assessment of organizational culture and the readiness of staff and others to engage in making or participating in a change, whether minor or extensive, set the stage for the selection and use of change strategies. The Research Perspective illustrates an example of cultural change in nursing homes. An example of the readiness of staff is found in Exercise 17-2. The willingness of the two nurses to learn new skills and the combined talents of the nursing, clinical education, and administrative managerial staff to work together successfully helped achieve the very different nursing and organizational skills required by the new infusion center.

 RESEARCH PERSPECTIVE

Resource: Mueller, C. (October 27-28, 2008). *Research in culture change in nursing homes.* Hartford Institute for Geriatric Nursing. New York University College of Nursing. Retrieved October 9, 2009, from http://hartfordign.org/uploads/File/issue_culture_change/Culture_Change_Background_Mueller.pdf.

Nursing home culture change is defined as the promotion of a resident-directed environment in which there is empowerment and control over one's living arrangements and day-to-day decision making. In this article, staff, resident, and organizational outcomes were reviewed over the past 20 years to understand the following:

1. How far has nursing home culture change penetrated current U.S. nursing homes?
2. Are there valid and reliable measures of nursing home culture change?
3. What evidence is there that nursing home culture change improves resident, staff, and organizational outcomes?
4. What is the extent of research on nursing homes and nursing home culture change?

Implications for Practice
The conclusion is that the change from the traditional, regulatory-oriented model of a nursing home to a more homelike residence where people may thrive in a manner consistent with their life path is slow. The author summarized the existing literature on nursing home culture change in this country and found that quality of life is improved, staff demonstrates increased work-related satisfaction, and organizations do not suffer more financially as a result of the culture change.

EXERCISE 17-2
From the perspective of a manager applying these functions to a change process, consider the manager's and clinical educator's responsibility to orient two nurses to staff a new infusion center for a small community hospital and identify the appropriate functions.

Both nurses were long-term employees; one was from the medical/surgical float pool, and the other was the bed coordinator whose position was eliminated because of budget reductions. Ideally, the manager, the clinical educator, and the assistant vice president with oversight for this area will map out in writing (1) the goals of the program, (2) the activities for meeting orientation goals, and (3) a schedule for accomplishing them. The nurse manager and the clinical educator agree to check in with each other daily, as well as to meet weekly for a more formal review of the team's progress. Part of this plan includes the option to alter the plan based on unexpected changes. The two nurses will begin the position in 4 weeks and put the prearranged outline of activities into action. The nurse manager's responsibility will be to guide and support the education of the nurses. Unexpected occurrences, such as the nurse manager extending her medical leave of absence by a few days, will require modifying the goal, activities, or time frame of the orientation plan (dynamic quality of process). New information (feedback) guides the overall process.

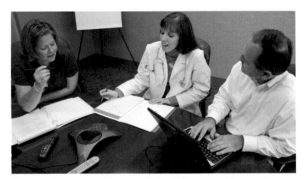
Converting to an electronic health record has to be an inclusive process to be successful.

Answering the self-assessment questions in Table 17-1 can help determine how receptive one is to change and innovation. See Exercise 17-3.

EXERCISE 17-3
Answer the self-assessment questions in Table 17-1 to determine how receptive you are to change.

TABLE 17-1 SELF-ASSESSMENT: HOW RECEPTIVE ARE YOU TO CHANGE AND INNOVATION?

Read the following items. Circle the answer that most closely matches your attitude toward creating and accepting new or different ways.

1. I enjoy learning about new ideas and approaches.	Yes	Depends	No
2. Once I learn about a new idea or approach, I begin to try it right away.	Yes	Depends	No
3. I like to discuss different ways of accomplishing a goal or end result.	Yes	Depends	No
4. I continually seek better ways to improve what I do.	Yes	Depends	No
5. I commonly recognize improved ways of doing things.	Yes	Depends	No
6. I talk over my ideas for change with my peers.	Yes	Depends	No
7. I communicate my ideas for change with my manager.	Yes	Depends	No
8. I discuss my ideas for change with my family.	Yes	Depends	No
9. I volunteer to be at meetings when changes are being discussed.	Yes	Depends	No
10. I encourage others to try new ideas and approaches.	Yes	Depends	No

If you answered "yes" to 8 to 10 of the items, you are probably receptive to creating and experiencing new and different ways of doing things. If you answered "depends" to 5 to 10 of the items, you are probably receptive to change conditionally based on the fit of the change with your preferred ways of doing things. If you answered "no" to 4 to 10 of the items, you are probably not receptive, at least initially, to new ways of doing things. If you answered "yes," "no," and "depends" an approximately equal number of times, you are probably mixed in your receptivity to change based on individual situations.

We do know that the more rapidly change can be incorporated, the more effective the organization is at remaining relevant. Connecting early adopters, such as the unit-based champions, to new ideas and to innovators, such as national peers of an IHI Web-based learning community, keeps them at the cutting edge. When these two groups are supported, an early majority can occur. If as a nurse you realize you are usually a laggard, look to be sure that rejection of new ideas is about some concern with the idea, not with just resisting change. Insight can be gained by using Exercise 17-4.

EXERCISE 17-4

Recall a work or personal situation in which a particular individual tried to get you or a group to do something. What rationale supported the decision of whether to cooperate? Was the idea worthwhile from your perception? Was the person making the suggestions known, understood, and trusted? Was the person making the suggestions aware of the real situation—an essential part of carrying out the idea—or had he or she not received official sanctioning to influence activities? Can you see that change agents need specific qualities and abilities to be trusted by others?

CONTEXT AND CHANGE

Although the people who make up an organization have a great impact on change processes, so too does the culture of the organization. Organizational culture consistently emerges as a fundamental variable in determining the success of efforts to implement change (Latta, 2009). Organizations that are open and aware of community realities and the larger industry context in which they operate are more viable, fluid, and responsive to change. Organizations with proactive cultures that promote employee engagement and participation generate environments that embrace change. Today, nursing organizations that achieve the designation of Magnet™ status are typically those that are flexible, adaptive, and innovative. They can lead change by instituting programs that capitalize on rapid change and thus improve patient safety and nurses' work environments and achieve quality outcomes.

Senge (2006) first characterized learning organizations as those entities that emphasize flexibility and responsiveness. Today's complex healthcare entities can best respond and adapt when the organization values learning and development and when members of the organization complete their work with others using a learning approach. Senge, Kleiner, Roberts, Ross, and Smith (1994, p. 11) explained, "If there is one single thing a learning organization does well, it is helping people embrace change. People in learning organizations react more quickly when their environment changes because they know how to anticipate changes that are going to occur … and how to create the kinds of changes they want. Change and learning may not exactly be synonymous, but they are inextricably linked."

BOX 17-2 FIVE ORGANIZATIONAL DISCIPLINES TO SUPPORT CHANGE AND EVOLUTION

1. Shared vision—the process of creating a common view about where the organization is going
2. Mental models—the practice of helping individuals become aware of how they think, what they value, and how that impacts organizational performance
3. Personal mastery—the fostering of openness in the face of change by maintaining self-awareness and using reflection
4. Team learning—the promotion of teams thinking together, collaborating, and sharing ideas, knowledge, and perspective
5. Systems thinking—the development of frameworks that see the organization as a complex entity whose many parts impact outcomes

Source: Senge, P. (2006). *The fifth discipline*. New York, NY: Doubleday.

These organizations have a culture that is open to change and evolution. Senge (2006) described the five disciplines that these organizations value (Box 17-2).

Systems thinking views the world as a set of multiple visible and invisible parts that interact constantly (Senge, 2006). When the organization values and facilitates development of the deeper aspirations of its members in addition to professional proficiency, it successfully matches organizational learning and personal growth.

How much a change initiative deviates from the norms of a culture impacts the adoption of the change. Higgs and Rowland (2010, p. 369) focused on the "broader contextual factors involved in the change process" and found these are largely ignored by change agents. Context includes both internal and external factors that impact an organization and its ability to change. External factors such as evidence-based practice, new reimbursement patterns that include deductions for negative patient outcomes, and healthcare reform are examples of context variables (Aarons, Hurlbut, & Horwitz, 2011; Packard, 2013). Internal factors such as staffing, nurse education level, and leader competency also must be considered when implementing change. Research has shown that several internal factors impact nurses' ability to participate in change and improvement efforts (Draper et al., 2008). These include education that did not

emphasize continuous improvement, inadequate staff, increased administrative burdens, and duplicate endeavors for change. Additionally, how engaged and empowered nurses feel, both of which are impacted by context, critically influences the effectiveness of change programs (Kitson, 2008).

LEADERSHIP AND CHANGE

In the national bestselling book, *Change Anything*, the authors review the science of change and outline six essential elements that contribute to change effectiveness (Patterson, Grenny, Maxfield, McMillan, and Switzler, 2011). Box 17-3 identifies those elements. First, individuals must be personally motivated to change. While leaders can certainly inspire people to change, ultimately the individual must decide that the change matters. For leaders to inspire change, they must have intimate knowledge of what matters to the people they manage. Kotter (2012) characterizes this as establishing a sense of urgency, and this involves overcoming complacency. This is especially hard when there doesn't seem to be any visible crisis, or the crisis seems irrelevant to the people being asked to change (Kotter, 2012).

To understand what matters to staff, leaders must listen, establish connection, and build trust. Dialogue is a method that helps accomplish this goal. Dialogue is a special kind of discourse that allows individuals with different perspectives to come together and find common goals. To promote dialogue, leaders must serve as facilitators, promoting the sharing of ideas, fears, and honest reactions to the change proposal.

BOX 17-3 CHANGE SUPPORT STRATEGIES

Promote acceptance of the change by viewing the change as a positive experience.
Develop skills essential for supporting the change.
Reduce negative influences and behaviors in the group experiencing the change.
Mobilize positive peer support for the change.
Create financial incentives that reward change agents.
Make structure and process modifications to support the change initiative.

Adapted from Patterson, K., Grenny, J., Maxfield, D., McMillan, R., & Switzler, A. (2011). *Change Anything*. Hatchette Book Group: New York

The purpose of dialogue is to understand and learn from one another. Unlike debate, dialogue is not about winning. Its purpose is to discover what has to be understood and considered to give voice to the whole group.

Dialogue can reveal areas where individuals feel inept or overwhelmed, providing the leader with an understanding of what programs need to be developed to increase personal ability to change and what educational initiatives need to be implemented to support change. Patterson et al. (2011) note that big changes often require staff to learn new skills, end old habits, and increase competency in different areas.

In addition to these personal dimensions that must be addressed to change anything, leaders also need to look at how social systems avert or support change efforts (Patterson et al., 2011). Having a group of change agents and innovators on board to champion an idea builds what Patterson et al. call "social motivation" and "social ability." This group can help staff who are less adept at change and also alert the leader to issues that need to be considered as the change is implemented.

Finally, leaders must create structural motivation and ability within the system so that there are rewards for supporting the changes needed (Patterson et al., 2011). Many times change is about altering the environment, not just motivating the people. For example,

as early as 2008, Hendrich and Chow reviewed structural issues that impact care innovations, including physical redesign of space to reduce walking time, improve lighting, reduce noise, and maximize supply access.

Kotter (2012) makes it clear that change management and change leadership are different. He notes that change management is about keeping the effort to change under control, while change leadership is about creating a vision and fostering major organizational transformation. Box 17-4 shows the essence of Kotter's eight-step change model. This model provides an overview of what leaders need to do to foster change. Each step, carefully executed, mobilizes an organization's accomplishment of change (Kotter, 2012).

Formal leaders in nursing must be effective change leaders. In an increasingly uncertain world, managers and leaders in our profession are challenged to be skilled in using change theory, serving as change agents, and supporting staff during times of change. According to the American Organization of Nurse Executives (AONE) (2005), managers and leaders need to do the following:

- Use change theory to plan for the implementation of organizational change.
- Serve as a change agent, assisting others in understanding the importance, necessity, and processes of change.

BOX 17-4 KOTTER'S EIGHT-STEP MODEL

ATTRIBUTE	PRINCIPLES
Create urgency	Generate open dialogue about external and internal realities impacting the need to change.
Form a powerful coalition	Develop a core group of change advocates that will help build momentum and support individuals through the change experience.
Create a vision for change	Change may involve lots of small alterations, but these must always be connected to a larger, inspiring vision.
Communicate the change vision	People tend to pay attention to what is reinforced, so communicating regularly and consistently is paramount to sustaining the effort.
Remove obstacles	Keep alert for barriers in structure and processes that limit the ability to change; remove them when you find them.
Create short-term wins	Success motivates future success, so create short-term targets and celebrate accomplishing them.
Build on the change	Change is ongoing, so create a culture where continuous improvement is the norm.
Anchor the changes in the culture	Recognize when the change is working, report on the difference it is making, and honor the people who helped make it happen.

- Support staff during times of difficult transitions.
- Recognize one's own reaction to change, and strive to remain open to new ideas and approaches.
- Adapt leadership style to situational needs.

The emergence of complex healthcare systems necessitates changing leadership practices that can mobilize the parts without having to direct every activity. This means perceiving leadership as facilitation and support, not just command and control. Bevan (2011, p. 11) says the leadership efforts that are needed to mobilize change are simple: "be clear about purpose and process; listen to and involve stakeholders; provide needed resources; align systems and processes to support the change; lead with clarity and involvement; communicate relentlessly; track progress; follow up; and course-correct." Each of these functions is easily understood, but accomplishing them in the midst of chaos, staff shortages, and patient emergencies is not easy. Table 17-2 outlines seven factors that Bevan (2011) notes are necessary for successful change. Another effective strategy is the use of leadership rounding tools like those developed by the Studer Group®. The following are examples of actions the leaders are encouraged to practice weekly (Studer, 2009):

- Establish and maintain a human rapport with staff. *(How are your children? What was your vacation like last week?)*
- Ask what is working well for the staff as they perform their daily functions. *(Can you tell me something that is working well for you today?)*
- Ask what is not working well. *(Can you tell me something that is a barrier for you today?)*
- Ask if there is someone whom they would like to especially recognize as a contributor to outstanding patient care.
- Answer any tough questions. *(Is there anything you've been thinking about asking me that you'd like to know?)*

Today's dynamic environment also means that leaders will have less time to plan and that plans must be constantly updated and amended. Nurses are key players in healthcare delivery, and formal leaders must advocate for their inclusion in change planning and implementation. As partners with multiple care providers and pivotal players in open-systems organizations, nurses must become adept at interprofessional collaboration and negotiation to ensure nursing's perspective in change processes. In their classic work, Begun and White (1995) said that nurses had to consider the discipline's dominant logic as a source of structural inertia. Using **chaos theory** components, they suggested that nursing in certain organizations is too "stuck" and thus too unresponsive and unable to adapt to the influences of rapid change. One way the nurse leader can alter the dominant logic is shown in Box 17-5. Using this methodology, the manager becomes adept at addressing an emergent approach to change that takes place over a long period rather than sporadic and episodic reactions to change (Shanley, 2007). Scenario planning (i.e., raising multiple "what if" questions with many possible alternative answers) is an example of the flexibility and creativity urgently needed in nursing today.

TABLE 17-2   BEVAN'S SEVEN CHANGE FACTORS

ATTRIBUTE	PRINCIPLES
Clarity	Clearly state the purpose of the change and the methods that will be used to implement it.
Engagement	Involve and include the people affected by the change and build a sense of commitment around the initiative.
Resources	Provide the resources that are essential for making the change happen.
Alignment	Evaluate all the subsystems that impact and are impacted by the change, and then make sure they support the change endeavor.
Leadership	Equip every leader and every change agent with the skills and abilities needed to mobilize the change.
Communication	Keep a two-way information path that clarifies issues, answers questions, and remains responsive to challenges in accomplishing the change.
Tracking	Monitor and measure to be sure that the goals that lead to the change are being accomplished.

Source: Bevan, R. (2011). *Changemaking.* Seattle, WA: ChangeStart Press.

BOX 17-5   GUIDELINES FOR ALTERING THE DOMINANT LOGIC

DECREASE	INCREASE
• Long-term forecasting	• Short-term forecasting
• Preplanned strategies	• Emergent strategies
• Emphasis on past successes	• Search for new opportunities
• One future vision	• Multiple scenarios
• Rigid, permanent structures	• Self-organizing, temporary structures
• Structural isolation in the workplace	• Structural interdependence in the workplace
• Stability of leadership	• Leadership turnover
• Standardization	• Innovation, experimentation, diversity
• Insulation from other professions and marketplace	• Cooperation and competition
• Marketplace "passivity"	• Marketplace "aggression"
• Expectation of job security	• Self-learning

Source: Begun, J.W., & White, K.R. (1995). Altering nursing's dominant logic: Guidelines from complex adaptive systems theory. *Complexity and Chaos in Nursing*, *2*(1), 10. Used with permission of Angela E. Vicenzi, Editor, *Complexity and Chaos in Nursing*.

Based on a qualitative study, Salmela et al. (2011) proposed a three-dimensional model of the tasks a nurse leader must manage during the change process. These are leading relationships, leading culture, and leading processes. At the core of this model is the patient, a reminder that all change must be managed without harm to the patient experience. These researchers assert that as leaders nurses must enable change while retaining the discipline's ethos of caring. Classic elements of effective change implementation can be found in Box 17-6.

Leading Relationships

Nurse leaders must be able to build relationships with the team and must be aware of the many interdependencies that exist within complex healthcare organizations (Dattee & Barlow, 2010). In this role, a leader serves as a coach, a guide, and a resource. According to Weberg (2012, p. 271), "Leaders must engage in the behavior and work of complexity leadership with an understanding that interconnectedness and change are normal operating conditions." To lead effectively, the leader must be in a relationship with the team, a relationship that fosters trust and promotes openness.

Leading Processes

Past leadership theories place the leader at the helm, in command of the ship. However, new, emergent leadership theories emphasize collective leadership

BOX 17-6   CLASSIC PRINCIPLES CHARACTERIZING EFFECTIVE CHANGE IMPLEMENTATION

- Change agents within healthcare organizations use personal, professional, and managerial knowledge and skills to lead change.
- The recipients of change believe they own the change.
- Administrators and other key personnel support the proposed change.
- The recipients of change anticipate benefit from the change.
- The recipients of change participate in identifying the problem warranting a change.
- The change holds interest for the change recipients and other participants.
- Agreement exists within the work group about the benefit of the change.
- The change agents and recipients of change perceive a compatibility of values.
- Trust and empathy exist among the participants of the change process.
- Revision of the change goal and process is negotiable.
- The change process is designed to provide regular feedback to its participants.

Adapted from Harper, C.L. (2007). *Exploring social change* (5th ed.). Englewood Cliffs, NJ: Prentice Hall.

whereby the person in a formal administrative role serves as a facilitator or a conductor (Salmela et al., 2011; Weberg, 2012). Today's leader must work to solve process problems with the team and must make process changes as they emerge.

Leading a Culture

Leaders determine the culture by deciding what behaviors will be endorsed and what actions will be considered unacceptable. Today's healthcare culture must be one that promotes accountability and rewards best practices. Nurse leaders who empower staff to be continuous learners and risk takers build a culture of curiosity and change. Nurse leaders who keep patient care at the center of every decision will advance the ethos of nursing and connect change to something that matters to nurses.

CONCLUSION

In nursing, we have often bemoaned our lack of singularity and vision, perhaps believing that we should mimic the prevailing world view and seek to become a spider-like or flexible organization. Nursing leadership might mean that we celebrate more innovation and diversity, decide to "break the rules" whenever possible, and embrace the contributions of everyone.

THE SOLUTION

The practice of hourly rounding was introduced to the staff—to both the nursing assistants and the professional nurses. We all developed an hourly rounding log, and it was decided that the unit secretary would announce on the hour for the staff to begin hourly rounding. The nursing staff took to it immediately; the difficulty was coaching the nursing assistants in how to approach patients and anticipate their needs, using a prewritten script. My goal was to make it fun, so I involved other nurse managers to play the role of the patient so the staff could practice. Much focused staff education in the form of didactic lecture material was provided as well. After several months, the change was visible and had an immediate impact on patients and their families. In fact, the chief executive officer of our system, along with the chief nursing officer, visited and thought at first that no patients were on the unit because of the peace and quiet. There were simply no more call bells ringing and no more intercom interruptions. My goal in managing this change was to maintain visibility, never lose sight of the goal and its associated requirements, and constantly praise staff for doing a good job of rounding on the patients. Most of my change

management strategies had to do with sitting down and asking the staff on all shifts about what worked and what didn't, being approachable, and addressing individual issues of concern before they became unit issues. I also draw the line when needed and have welcomed my assistant vice president when she rounds with one of my staff to coach him or her. If one of the staff is still not performing the essential elements of hourly rounding after 3 to 6 months of intensive education and focus, then I will resort to the discipline process. Overall, I respect the work that the staff do every day, and they know that about me. I think my strategy worked because I introduced hourly rounding first as a philosophy that would make the staff happy and more efficient. In fact, I made it a point not to tell them that hourly rounding was for patient satisfaction specifically, though it certainly has increased since we embraced it.

—*Sharon McEvoy*

Would this be a suitable approach for you? Why?

THE EVIDENCE

A huge part of change in today's healthcare organizations is promoting the adoption of evidence-based practice. Lusardi (2012) speaks to changing practice at the bedside by reviewing the following common elements of all evidence-based practice models:

1. Identifying a clinical issue
2. Researching the best practices and evidence about that clinical issue
3. Determining the strength of the evidence
4. Developing a proposal for changing clinical practice
5. Implementing the change
6. Evaluating the impact of the change

Lusardi outlines essential elements for success in implementing evidence-based practice initiatives. There must be adequate resources, strong unit clinical support, administrative directives that reinforce the change, and systems to offer feedback and mentorship of clinical staff during the change.

WHAT NEW GRADUATES SAY

- I remember reading about how rapidly change was occurring, but I had no idea how quickly things change. In part that is because so many things happen simultaneously.
- I thought I liked change. Now that I experience it every day, I am less fond of it. I know we have to, but some days it is just too much.

- I am so excited about the number of things that are changing because I can see what is possible.
- I am not wild about the current experience, but I remember that you have to work through things to make them better.

CHAPTER CHECKLIST

Change is an unavoidable constant in the rapidly transforming healthcare delivery system, requiring all nurses to be change agents. As a result, uncertainty is an element in most healthcare institutions. Creating and leading change rather than merely reacting can promote overall organizational effectiveness.
- The nature of change
- The change process

- Planned, first-order change
- Unplanned, second-order change
- People and change
- Context and change
- Leadership and change
  - Leading relationships
  - Leading processes
  - Leading a culture

TIPS FOR LEADING CHANGE

- Whether involved in planned (low-complexity) or nonlinear (high-complexity) change, create a group of outcome/goal scenarios with prospective actions to achieve.
- People cope and adapt better when they assume the role of continuous learner during accelerated change.
- People involved in change may assume the roles of followers or leaders and may emerge from both informal and formal or internal and external sources.

- Creating a detailed plan and rigidly adhering to it reduce opportunities to moderate the inevitable and changing aspects of a change process, especially in an accelerated change environment.
- Building ambiguity and flexibility into a plan and how it is managed promotes responsiveness and movement toward desired outcomes.

REFERENCES

Aarons, G., Hurlburt, M., & Horwitz, S. (2011). Advancing a conceptual model of evidence-based practice implementation in public service sectors. *Administration and Policy in Mental Health and Mental Health Services Research*, 38(1), 4–23.

Abraham, J., Jerome-D'Emilia, B., & Begun, J. W. (2011). The diffusion of Magnet hospital recognition. *Health Care Manage Rev*, 36(4), 306–314.

American Organization of Nurse Executives (AONE). (2005). *AONE nurse competencies assessment tool*. Retrieved February 2014, from, http://www.aone.org/resources/leadership%20 tools/nursecomp.shtml.

Begun, J. W., & White, K. R. (1995). Altering nursing's dominant logic: Guidelines from complex adaptive systems theory. *Complexity and Chaos in Nursing*, 2(1), 5–15.

Bevan, R. (2011). *Changemaking*. Seattle, WA: ChangeStart Press.

Burnes, B. (2004). Kurt Lewin and complexity theories: Back to the future? *Journal of Change Management*, 4(4), 309–325.

Change. 2013. In Merriam-Webster.com. Retrieved February 8, 2013, from www.merriam-webster.com/dictionary/change.

Dattee, B., & Barlow, B. (2010). Complexity and whole-system change programmes. *J Health Serv Res Policy*, 15(Supp. 2), 19–25.

Draper, D. A., Felland, L., Liebhaber, A., & Melichar, L. (2008). The role of nurse in hospital quality improvement. *Research Brief*, Retrieved 2/3/13 from, www.hschange.com/ CONTENT/972/972.pdf.

Gale, B., & Schaffer, M. (2009). Organizational readiness for evidence-based practice. *Journal of Nursing Administration*, 39(2), 91–97.

Havelock, R. (1973). *Change agents guide to innovation in education*. Englewood Cliffs, NJ: Educational Technology Publications.

Hendrich, A., & Chow, M. (2008). *Maximizing the impact of nursing care quality: A closer look at the hospital work environment and the nurse's impact on patient care quality*. Retrieved February 1, 2013 from, www.healthdesign.org/sites/default/files/HCLeadership%20 4_%20Maximizing%20Impact%20of%20Nursing.pdf.

Higgs, M., & Rowland, D. (2010). Emperors with clothes on: The role of self-awareness in developing effective change leadership. *Journal of Change Management, 10*(4), 369–385.

Judge, W., & Douglas, T. (2009). Organizational change capacity: The systematic development of a scale. *Journal of Organizational Change Management, 22*(6), 635–649.

Katzenbach, J. R., Beckett, F., Dichter, S., Feigen, M., Gagnon, C., Hope, Q., et al. (1996). *Real change leaders*. New York: Random House.

Kitson, A. L. (2008). The need for systems change: Reflections on knowledge translation and organizational change. *J Adv Nurs, 65*(1), 217–228.

Kotter, J. P. (2012). *Leading change*. Boston, MA: Harvard Business Review Press.

Latta, G. F. (2009). A process model of organizational change in cultural context (OC3 Model). *Journal of Leadership and Organizational Studies, 15*(1), 19–37.

Lewin, K. (1947). Frontiers in group dynamics: Concept, method, and reality in social science, social equilibria and social change. *Human Relations, 1*(1), 5–41.

Lewin, K. (1951). *Field theory in social science*. New York: Harper Torchbooks.

Lippitt, R., Watson, J., & Westley, B. (1958). *The dynamics of planned change*. New York: Harcourt Brace.

Lusardi, P. (2012). So you want to change practice: Recognizing practice issues and channeling those ideas. *Crit Care Nurse, 32*(2), 55–64.

Maurer, R. (2004). *One small step can change your life: The Kaizen way*. New York, NY: Workman Publishing Co.

Mueller, C. (October 27–28, 2008). *Research in culture change in nursing homes*. Hartford Institute for Geriatric Nursing. New York University College of Nursing. Retrieved October 9, 2009, from, http://hartfordign.org/uploads/File/issue_culture_ change/Culture_Change_Background_Mueller.pdf.

Packard, T. (2013). Organizational change: A conceptual framework to advance the evidence base. *Journal of Human Behavior in the Social Environment, 23*, 75–90.

Paley, J., & Eva, G. (2011). Complexity theory as an approach to explanation in healthcare: A critical discussion. *Int J Nurs Stud, 48*, 269–279.

Patterson, K., Grenny, J., Maxfield, D., McMillan, R., & Switzler, A. (2011). *Change anything*. New York: Hatchette Book Group.

Rogers, E. M. (1995). *Diffusion of innovations* (4th ed.). New York: The Free Press.

Rogers, E. M. (2003). *Diffusion of innovations* (5th ed.). New York: The Free Press.

Salmela, S., Eriksson, K., & Fagerstrom, L. (2011). Leading change: A three-dimensional model of nurse leaders' main tasks and roles during a change process. *J Adv Nurs, 68*(2), 423–433.

Sanders, T. J. (2010). Propositions for investigating adoption and diffusion of the Magnet hospital concept through the lenses of organization theory. *Journal of Management and Marketing Research, 4*, 1–19.

Senge, P. (2006). *The fifth discipline*. New York: Doubleday.

Senge, P., Kleiner, A., Roberts, C., Ross, R., & Smith, B. (1994). *The 5th discipline fieldbook: Strategies and tools for building a learning organization*. New York: Crown Business.

Shanley, C. (2007). Management of change for nurses: Lessons from the discipline of organizational studies. *Journal of Nursing Management, 15*(5), 538–546.

Studer, Q. (2009). *Hardwiring excellence*. Gulf Breeze, FL: Fire Starter Publishing.

Weberg, D. (2012). Complexity leadership: A healthcare imperative. *Nurs Forum, 47*(4), 268–277.

Weick, K., & Quinn, R. (1999). Organizational change and development. *Annu Rev Psychol, 50*, 361–386.

SUGGESTED READINGS

Chambers, C., & Ryder, E. (2011). Excellence in compassionate nursing care: Leading the change. *Journal of Holistic Healthcare, 8*(3), 46–49.

Mitchell, G. (2013). Selecting the best theory to implement planned change. *Nursing Management—UK, 20*(1), 32–37.

Needleman, J. (2010). Transforming care at the bedside. *PaceSetters, 7*(3), 10–13.

Nickitas, D. M. (2010). A vision for future health care: Where nurses lead the change. *Nursing economic$, 28*(6), 361–385.

Rantz, M., Zwygart-Stauffacher, M., Flesner, M., Hicks, L., Mehr, D., Russell, T., et al. (2012). Challenges of using quality improvement methods in nursing homes that need improvement. *J Am Med Dir Assoc, 13*(8), 732–738.

Roussel, L., Dearmon, V., Buckner, E., Pomrenke, B., Salas, S., Mosley, A., et al. (2012). Change can be good. *Nurs Adm Q, 36*(3), 203–209.

Williams, L. (2011). Organizational readiness for innovation in health care: Some lessons from the recent literature. *Health Serv Manage Res, 24*(4), 213–218.

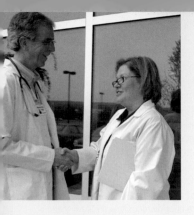

18

Building Teams Through Communication and Partnerships

Karren Kowalski

This chapter explains major concepts and presents tools with which to create and maintain a smoothly functioning team. Life requires that we work together in a smooth and efficient manner, communicate effectively, and develop relationships that produce partnerships. Many important team efforts occur in the work setting. Teams are critical to patient safety because they encourage frequent and ongoing communication and create a safety net, a system in which safeguards and support are a part of the routine functioning of each team member. Such teams often include members with various backgrounds and educational preparation (e.g., physicians, nurses, administrators, allied health professionals, and support staff such as housekeeping and dietary staff members). Each team member has something valuable to contribute and deserves to be treated honorably and with respect. When teams are not working effectively, all team members must change how they communicate and interact within the team.

LEARNING OUTCOMES

- Evaluate the differences between a group and a team.
- Value four key concepts of teams.
- Demonstrate an effective communication interaction.
- Identify at least five communication pitfalls.
- Apply the guidelines for acknowledgment to a situation in your clinical setting.
- Compare a setting that uses agreements with your current clinical setting.
- Develop an example of a team that functions synergistically, including the results such a team would produce.
- Discuss the importance of team to patient safety and quality.

KEY TERMS

acknowledgment	dualism	synergy
active listening	effective communication	team
commitment	group	

THE CHALLENGE

Diane Gallagher, RN, MS
Director, Women's and Children's Services, Rush-Presbyterian–
St. Luke's Medical Center, Chicago, Illinois

An extensive "team" of people works together to care for the neonate in a neonatal intensive care unit (NICU). The team includes physicians, registered nurses, respiratory therapists, physical therapists, social workers, neonatal nurse practitioners, and ancillary staff. Occasionally, specialists are consulted for specific cardiac, neurologic, or gastrointestinal problems. These are intermittent "team" members who play a crucial role in the baby's care.

Recently, a new group of specialists joined our team. They were identified as a top-notch group who would, by virtue of their expertise and reputation, increase the census and revenues for the hospital. Our team was excited to have this opportunity to grow in an area in which we had infrequent experience. However, integration of these new team members did not go smoothly. There were clinical disagreements, communication breakdowns, and interpersonal conflicts. The experience evolved into mutual distrust and control issues.

As disagreements, insults, and complaints escalated on both sides, the situation came to a defining moment when the director of the specialty group said, "I'm never bringing any of our patients here. I'm sending them to the PICU." The response from the NICU team was, "Fine with us; we don't need you, your patients, or the hassle." It seemed reasonable to not work together because, in fact, functionally we were already not working together. This response was in direct conflict with our belief that we could provide a valuable service and make a difference for both the patients and their families. This posed a dilemma for the staff, but everyone felt the situation was hopeless.

No one believed we could function as a team, and therefore further efforts to work together were futile. We had tried and failed. Let's just cut our losses and move on. How does one create a team when no one believes it is possible and some believe it is not even necessary?

What do you think you would do if you were this nurse?

INTRODUCTION

As we experience changes such as cost-cutting and quality and safety issues in health care, teamwork becomes critical. The adage "If we do not all hang together we will all hang separately" was never more true than now as we move through an era in which nursing is accountable for patient outcomes that affect reimbursement for care and the institutional financial bottom line. To create finely tuned teams, communication skills must improve. Each team member must focus on improving his or her own skills, as well as supporting other team members, to grow in effective communication. These skills will be increasingly important as teams negotiate an evolving healthcare system that includes accountable care organizations—an outcome of the 2010 Patient Protection and Affordable Care Act.

In our society, in which so much emphasis is placed on the individual and individual achievement, teamwork is the quintessential contradiction. In other words, with all the focus on individuals, we still need individuals to work together in groups to accomplish goals and keep patients safe. Today's children are educated to be individual achievers and then they are thrust into the work world and expected to be team players. To make this transition requires support and encouragement to learn about the value of teams and their effects on others.

GROUPS AND TEAMS

The definition of group is a number of individuals assembled together or having some unifying relationship. Groups could be all the parents in an elementary school, all the members of a specific church, or all the students in a school of nursing, because the members of these various groups are related in some way to one another by definition of their involvement in a certain endeavor. A team, on the other hand, is a number of persons associated together in specific work or activity. Not every group is a team, and not every team is effective.

A group of people does not constitute a team. From Lencioni's perspective (2012), a team is a group of people with a high degree of interdependence geared toward the achievement of a goal or a task. Often, we can recognize intuitively when the so-called team is not functioning effectively. We say things such as, "We need to be more like a team" or "I'd like to see more team players around here." Consequently, in the process of defining *team*, effective versus ineffective teams should be considered. Teams are groups that have defined objectives, ongoing positive relationships, effective respectful communication, and a supportive environment. Teams are focused on accomplishing a specific task and are essential in providing cost-effective, high-quality health care. As resources are expended more prudently, patient care teams must develop clearly defined goals, use creative problem solving, and demonstrate mutual respect and support. Facilities with ineffective teams will find themselves out of business (Charney, 2011).

EXERCISE 18-1

Think of the last team or group of which you were a part. Think about what went on in that team or group. Specifically think about what worked for you and what did not work. Use the "Team Assessment Exercise" in Table 18-1 to assess specific aspects of your team. Address each of the identified areas and discover how well your team or group functioned. Think about roles, activities, relationships, and general environment. Consider examples of shared decision making, shared leadership, shared accountability, and shared problem solving. These are the concepts that can be used to evaluate the functioning of almost any team of which you are a member.

When a team functions effectively, a significant difference is evident in the entire work atmosphere, the way in which discussions progress, the level of understanding of the team-specific goals and tasks, the willingness of members to listen, the manner in which disagreements are handled, the use of consensus, and the way in which feedback is given and received. The original work done by McGregor (1960) sheds light on some of these significant differences, which are summarized in Table 18-2.

Ineffective teams are often dominated by a few members, leaving others bored, resentful, or uninvolved. Leadership tends to be autocratic and rigid, and the team's communication style may be overly stiff and formal. Members tend to be uncomfortable with conflict or disagreement, avoiding and suppressing it rather than using it as a catalyst for change. When criticism is offered, it may be destructive, personal, and hurtful rather than constructive and problem-centered. Team members may begin to hide their feelings of resentment or disagreement, sensing that they are "dangerous." This creates the potential for later eruptions and discord. Similarly, the team avoids examining its own inner workings, or members may wait until after meetings to voice their thoughts and feelings about what went wrong and why.

TABLE 18-1   TEAM ASSESSMENT EXERCISE

Are We a Team?

Directions: Select a team with which you work. Place a checkmark beside each item that is true of your team. If the statement is not true, place no mark beside the item.
1. The language we use focuses on "we" rather than "you" or "I."
2. When one of us is busy, others try to help.
3. I know I can ask for help from others.
4. Most of us on the team could say what we are trying to accomplish.
5. What we are trying to accomplish on any given work day relates to the mission and vision of nursing and the organization.
6. We treat each other fairly, not necessarily the same.
7. We capitalize on people's strengths to meet the goals of our work.
8. The process for changing policies, procedures, equipment is clear.
9. Meetings are focused on the goals we are trying to achieve.
10. Our outcomes reflect our attention to goals and efforts.
11. Acknowledgment is individual and goal-oriented.
12. Innovation is supported by the team and management.
13. The group makes commitments to each other to ensure goal attainment.
14. Promises are kept.
15. Kindness in communication is evident, especially when bad news is delivered.
16. Individuals can describe their role in the overall work of the group.
17. Other members of the team are seen as trustworthy and valued.
18. The group is cost-effective and time-effective in attaining goals.
19. No member is excluded from the process of decision making.
20. Individuals can speak highly of their team members.

Tally the number of checkmarks and multiply that number by 5. The resultant number is an assessment of how well your team is functioning. The higher the score, the better the functioning.

©The Wise Group, 2007, Lubbock, Texas.

In contrast, the effective team is characterized by its clarity of purpose, informality and congeniality, **commitment,** and high level of participation. The members' ability to listen respectfully to each other and communicate openly helps them handle disagreements in a civilized manner and work through them rather than suppress them. Through ample discussion of issues, they reach decisions by consensus. Roles and work assignments are clear, and members

TABLE 18-2 ATTRIBUTES OF EFFECTIVE AND INEFFECTIVE TEAMS

ATTRIBUTE	EFFECTIVE TEAM	INEFFECTIVE TEAM
Working environment	Informal, comfortable, relaxed	Indifferent, bored, tense, stiff
Discussion	Focused	Frequently unfocused
	Shared by almost everyone	Dominated by a few
Objectives	Well understood and accepted	Unclear, or many personal agendas
Listening	Respectful—encourages participation	Judgmental—much interruption and "grandstanding"
Ability to handle conflict	Comfortable with disagreement	Uncomfortable with disagreement
	Open discussion of conflicts	Disagreement usually suppressed, or one group aggressively dominates
Decision making	Usually reached by consensus	Often occurs prematurely
	Formal voting kept to a minimum	Formal voting occurs frequently
	General agreement is necessary for action; dissenters are free to voice	Simple majority is sufficient for action; minority is expected to go along with opinion
Criticism	Frequent, frank, relatively comfortable, constructive	Embarrassing and tension-producing; destructive
	Directed toward removing obstacle	Directed personally at others
Leadership	Shared; shifts from time to time	Autocratic; remains clearly with committee chairperson
Assignments	Clearly stated	Unclear
	Accepted by all despite disagreements	Resented by dissenting members
Feelings	Freely expressed; open for discussion	Hidden; considered "explosive" and inappropriate for discussion
Self-regulation	Frequent and ongoing; focused on solutions	Infrequent, or occurs outside meetings

Adapted from McGregor, D. (1960). *The human side of enterprise*. New York: McGraw-Hill.

share the leadership role, recognizing that each person brings his or her own unique strengths to the group effort. This diversity of styles helps the team adapt to changes and challenges, as does the team's ability and willingness to assess its own strengths and weaknesses and respond to them appropriately.

The challenges encountered in today's healthcare systems are prodigious. Patient safety issues are at the forefront. Ongoing rounds of downsizing, budget cuts, declining patient days, reduced payments, and staff layoffs abound. Effective teams participate in effective problem solving, increased creativity, and improved health care. The effects of smoothly functioning teams on patient safety and the creation of a just culture are critically important, and one tool set to address these issues, including communication, can be found in the Literature Perspective on p. 325.

GENERATIONAL DIFFERENCES

Team members today may represent four different generations of workers: Veterans, Baby Boomers, Generation X, and Generation Y. Because the workforce is aging, a preponderance of Baby Boomers and Generation Xers might exist in a work setting. Each generation, traditionally interpreted as a span of 20 years, grew up in a different era and was influenced by different historical events and cultural developments (Weingarten, 2009). For example, Veterans live by the rules and do not question authority. Boomers lived through the Cold War and were influenced by the assassinations of President Kennedy, Senator Robert Kennedy, and Martin Luther King, Jr., the Civil Rights movement; and the Women's Rights movement. Generation X nurses were often the latchkey kids because both parents worked outside the home. Divorce was common, and job stability was no longer guaranteed. Generation Y nurses are the future of the profession and have grown up with massive amounts of information and technology. They have experienced terrorism and natural disasters. They are culturally diverse and view education as the key to success. Efforts to understand and bridge these differences can be the difference between

LITERATURE PERSPECTIVE

Resource: Kouzes, J.M., & Posner, B.Z. (2012). *The leadership challenge* (5th ed.). San Francisco: Jossey-Bass, John Wiley & Sons.

This model focuses on how leaders in all walks of life and all aspects of the workplace mobilize people to get extraordinary things done. Ordinary people such as novice nurses can guide others along pioneering journeys to phenomenal accomplishments. The research and work that Kouzes and Posner have done establish relationships as the core of leading any change or initiative. Five key aspects of establishing and maintaining relationships constitute the heart of this leadership model:

- **Model the Way**—Credibility is the foundation of leadership. It is established by consistently *Doing What You Say You Will Do* or by *Setting the Example* for the other team members.
- **Inspire a Shared Vision**—Imagine exciting and ennobling possibilities, and enlist others in these dreams through positive attitude, excitement, and hard work.
- **Challenge the Process**—Seek innovative ways to change, grow, and improve—experiment and take risks.
- **Enable Others to Act**—Foster collaboration by promoting cooperation and building trust. Create a sense of reciprocity or give and take. Establish a sense of "We're all in this together."
- **Encourage the Heart**—Novice leaders encourage their constituents to carry on. They keep hope and determination alive, recognize contributions, and celebrate victories.

Implications for Practice

When nurses use this model to approach leadership, they can strengthen their skills. Each of the examples above provides a way for new, emerging, and established leaders to remain committed to the team with which they work.

---

a dysfunctional and an effective team. Chapter 3 provides more detail about these differences.

COMMUNICATING EFFECTIVELY

Communication in the work environment is not only important to good working conditions that retain nurses but also critical to reduction of medical errors (Maxfield, Grenny, Lavandero, & Groah, 2013). Because of such issues, new graduates go through a facility orientation, which emphasizes communication skills. Many nurses view this as a waste of time that could be used to further technical skills; however, at evaluation time, communication skills are often seen as a significant area for improvement.

The only thing human beings do more often than communicate is breathe. Communication is the most important component of daily activities. It is essential to clinical practice, to building teams, and to leadership. A person cannot *not* communicate. Because communication consists of both verbal and nonverbal signals, humans are continuously communicating thoughts, ideas, opinions, feelings, and emotions. Once the message is sent, it cannot be retracted; it can be amended; the first impression of the communication usually is lasting. However, as important as this initial impression is, it is often an unconscious response or reaction.

How we communicate is also a reflection of self-worth: Once a human being has arrived on this earth, communication is the largest single factor determining what kinds of relationships she or he makes with others and what happens to each in the world (Satir, 1988). Self-worth is a major influence in all communication. Stress results whenever self-worth is threatened, and this can lead to an angry reaction rather than thoughtful conversation.

Communication is learned from watching others. A host of poor examples can be seen in movies and television. Poor communication leads to relationship breakdowns, misunderstandings, high levels of emotion, judgment, and an excess of drama. Nursing programs teach therapeutic communications with patients and their families. However, little focus is placed on effective communication in the workplace, although positive, thoughtful communication is essential to building and maintaining smoothly functioning teams.

A basic model of communication patterns between the sender and the receiver is found in Figure 18-1. Effective communication develops a rhythm in which messages are sent and received in a productive, respectful, and supportive manner (Nemeth, 2008). Communication begins to break down as the rhythm is disrupted. The sender-receiver pattern disintegrates into a nonrhythmic event, as described in Figure 18-1. When nonrhythmic patterns develop, the participants may feel disrespected, upset, and even fearful.

Stress

In her classic work, Satir (1988) identified the connection between stress and self-worth that can evolve as a result of a breakdown in communication. She defined stress as a threat to positive self-worth. Human beings tend to feel stress or anxiety whenever they

Communication Rhythm

Sender ———— Receiver

Sender sends a message.   Receiver actively listens and receives.

Communication Non-rhythm

Sender ———— Sender

Both parties send simultaneously. Neither party is receiving.

Sender ———— No Receiver

Sender sends a message.   The receiver is preoccupied with another matter and is not attending.

No Sender ———— Receiver

The receiver awaits a message or response. The sender "clams up," refusing to speak or send a message.

Receiver ———— Receiver

When both parties are striving to receive and neither party sends a message (e.g., teacher questions what students know and gets no response), silence reigns.

FIGURE 18-1 Potential communication rhythms.

experience an unconscious linking of feelings, behaviors, or comments from others to a lowering of self-esteem or an attack on self-worth. A conscious effort ought to be made to relieve stress through activities such as ensuring specific/scheduled quiet time, requesting peer support, keeping a journal, treating yourself to something special, or going for a walk (Smith & Segal, 2013).

Stress Response Model

When this threat is identified, the receiver often reacts using one of the five communication patterns: attribution of blame, placation, constrained cool-headedness, immaterial irrelevance, or congruence (Balzer-Riley, 2011; Satir, 1988). Each pattern interaction and the source of the interaction are described with examples of each pattern in Table 18-3.

The pattern that produces effective communication, the one to strive for, is congruence. Congruent communication occurs when both the verbal and nonverbal actions fit the inner feelings of the sender and are appropriate to the context of the message. This communication pattern creates the kind of connection between the sender and the receiver that fosters respect, support, and the creation of relationship.

Communication Barriers

In today's busy world, many interruptions and interferences to clear, focused, effective communication create breakdowns. According to Olen's classic work (1993), to be aware of these potential problems allows both sender and receiver to be prepared to minimize such barriers.

- *Distractions:* Distractions most commonly come through sensory perceptions, such as poor lighting or background noise, including music, talking, ringing phones, and interruptions by others. Papers, reports, and heavy workloads can also be distracting.
- *Inadequate knowledge:* The sender and receiver may be at different levels of knowledge, particularly in this time of highly specialized and technical knowledge bases. For multiple reasons, one person may not seek clarity from the other.
- *Poor planning:* The process of organizing, planning, and clearly thinking through what needs to be communicated is very helpful. If the interaction is more spontaneous, it can more easily fall into a nonrhythmic pattern.
- *Differences in perception:* Both the sender and the receiver have their individual mental filters—the way in which they see the world. Because of this individuality, no two filters are the same. Thus the same message is interpreted differently. Add to this, for example, sociocultural, ethnic, and educational differences, and it is easy to see how these differences can occur.
- *Emotions and personality:* Someone who is experiencing distress may not be able to receive another message or may have difficulty keeping his or her emotions out of an unrelated message. Most humans, at some point, bring distress or problems from home to the workplace. If these remain unconscious, they can influence the work setting in a negative or nonproductive way.

TABLE 18-3   COMMUNICATION PATTERNS

PATTERN	INTERACTION	SOURCE	EXAMPLE
Attribution of blame	Sender blames receiver	Fault-finder dictator acts superior as camouflage for fear and low self-esteem	Mostly "you" messages; for example, "You really blew it!"
Placation	Sender placates receiver	Sender's low self-worth: puts herself/himself down	"I was wrong. I'm sorry. It's all my fault."
Constrained cool-headedness	Sender is correct and very reasonable without feeling or emotion	Feelings of vulnerability covered by cool analytical thinking	"Studies have shown that in 75% of cases, the patient is correct. I decided to use research data in coming to a solution."
Irrelevant	Sender is avoiding the issue, ignoring own feelings and feelings of the receiver	Fear, loneliness, and purposelessness	"Wait a minute. Let me tell you about …" (changes the subject)
Congruence	Sender's words and actions are congruent; inner feelings match the message	Any tension is decreased, and self-worth is at a high level	"For now, I feel concerned about the anger and hostility exhibited by Dr. X. I'm wondering what approach would de-escalate him."

Adapted from Satir, V. (1988). *The new peoplemaking.* Mountain View, CA: Science & Behavior Books; and Bradley, J., & Edinberg, M. (1990). *Communication in the nursing context* (3rd ed.). Norwalk, CT: Appleton & Lange.

Communication Pitfalls

Effective communication suggests that the interaction is a rhythmic pattern that is respectful and clear, promotes trust, and encourages the expression of feelings and viewpoints. On the other hand, pitfalls in communication comprise actions, behaviors, and words that create distrust, are dishonoring, and decrease the feelings of self-worth in the receiver. Box 18-1 lists the major pitfalls of communication. These pitfalls lead to communication breakdowns that affect not only the team but also the quality of care to patients.

Communication Guidelines

Effective guidelines can be used when communicating. Such tools as SBAR are often used when conveying clinical information from one caregiver to another (Box 18-2). Most of these tools are used to facilitate a positive outcome and to create an environment in which the communicator can achieve the desired outcome. Unconscious use of any of the pitfalls will most likely result in thwarting the desired outcome. Box 18-3 on p. 329 lists effective guidelines for communication.

> **EXERCISE 18-2**
> In pairs or small groups, compare the effective guidelines for communication with the communication pitfalls. Give examples of each from your own recent personal experience. Hypothesize how you could have changed the pitfalls into a positive interaction.

KEY CONCEPTS OF TEAMS

In rare instances, a team may produce teamwork spontaneously, like kids in a schoolyard at recess. However, most management teams learn about teamwork because they need and want to work together. This kind of working together requires that they observe how they are together in a group and that they unlearn ingrained self-limiting assumptions about the glory of individual effort and authority that are contrary to cooperation and teamwork. Keys to the concept of team include the following:

- Conflict resolution
- Singleness of mission
- Willingness to cooperate
- Commitment

BOX 18-1   COMMUNICATION PITFALLS

1. Giving Advice

It is so tempting to give advice when a co-worker comes with an is-sue or problem. *Don't!* Most often what the person wants is to work through the issue by talking out loud. Just listen.

2. Making Others Wrong

When telling others "our" story of distress, the adversary is always "wrong." The telling of the story to a third party only reinforces how right "I" am and how wrong, bad, or terrible the other person is. If you have an issue or problem, take the problem to the person with whom you are upset. "Take the mail to the correct address." Don't gossip!

3. Being Defensive

Defensiveness occurs when you do not listen, are hostile or aggres-sive, or respond as if attacked when there was no attack. Look for a physiologic signal in your body so that you can identify your own dis-tress. Stop. Breathe. Acknowledge that the message did not come out the way you intended, and begin again.

Also, defensiveness can occur when met with hostile, aggres-sive behavior from another. Rather than choose an emotional re-sponse or react to the attack, know that the other person's behavior has nothing to do with you personally but is the response chosen by that person in a moment of stress. Any one of a dozen other responses could have been chosen. Understand that the person is motivated by fear or hurt.

4. Judging the Other Person

Evaluating another person as "good" or "bad," as someone you like or do not like, or judging their actions or behavior as "stupid" or "crazy" or "inappropriate" is a reflection of how you judge yourself. Who is the hardest person on you? Of course, you are. Know that you can have feelings about situations or behaviors without judging the other person in a negative way. Rather, you can feel compassion for his or her stress and fear, which often drives behavior. This is true particularly when a supervisor or physician is reprimanding you.

5. Patronizing

Speaking to others as though they are less than human or in need of custodial care fails to honor them as human beings. You do not have to be condescending or seek to humiliate in an overly sweet voice. These are merely other versions of judging or making the person wrong. Another approach is to question what is at issue for them in the moment.

6. Giving False Reassurance

One of the great temptations of nurses is to "fix" things and make them better, to rescue the situation or the person involved. To ac-complish this goal, sometimes we reassure inappropriately. Know that you do not have to fix every situation. You can support people to work through situations themselves.

7. Asking "Why" Questions

When working in the team, refrain from asking "why" questions. These tend to create a defensive response in the other person. Instead, ask "What makes you think …"

8. Blaming Others

Saying things such as "You make me so angry" is blaming the other person for your feelings, which you choose at any given time. In nearly every situation, the responsibility for communication break-down is a joint responsibility. You can always choose your response, even if that response is to say, "I can't discuss this with you now. I would like to talk about this later when I am calmer."

BOX 18-2   SBAR COMMUNICATION

Miscommunication is the most commonly occurring cause of senti-nel events and "near misses" in patient care. One of the most popu-lar structured communication systems, created by professionals in the California Kaiser Permanente system, focuses on a method to provide information that honors the system in which practitioners and medical providers learn to glean information and apply it to de-cision-making trees. SBAR is the system that honors the structured transfer of information.

Situation. The nurse identifies the patient, the physician, the diagnosis, and the location of the patient. The nurse describes the patient situation that has instituted this SBAR communication.

Background. Next the nurse provides background information, which could include information relevant to the current situation, mental status, current vital signs (all of them), chief complaint, pain level, and physical assessment of the patient.

Assessment. The nurse offers an assessment of the chief problem and describes the seriousness of the situation. Any specific changes in the patient's condition should be described.

Recommendation. The nurse can make a request of the phy-sician or suggest specific action such as a medication, laboratory work, or an x-ray examination. The nurse could also request that the physician come and evaluate the patient.

www.ihi.org/resources/Pages/Tools/SBARTechniqueforCommunicationASituationalBriefingModel.aspx. (Retrieved July 8, 2013.)

Conflict Resolution

When thinking about conflict, realizing that conflict is fundamental to the human experience can be help-ful. Conflict is an integral part of all human interac-tion (Porter-O'Grady & Malloch, 2010). Therefore the challenge is to recognize the breakdown in the com-munication process and to deal appropriately with it (Porter-O'Grady & Malloch, 2010). Conflicts are usu-ally based on attempts to protect a person's self-esteem or to alter perceived inequities in power, because most human beings believe that other people have greater power, and thus these human beings are unlikely to achieve their objectives (Sportsman, 2005). For example, when a nurse recognizes upset and reaction between two nursing assistants with whom he or she is working, the following steps can be helpful (Sportsman, 2005):

- Identify the triggering event.
- Discover the historical context for each person.
- Assess how interdependent they are on each other.
- Identify the issues, goals, and resources involved in the situation.
- Uncover any previously considered solution.

Assessing the level of working relationship between the conflicted parties is essential, particularly if they work together on a regular basis.

The word *team* is usually reserved for a special type of working together. This working together requires communication in which the members understand how to conduct interpersonal relationships with their peers in thoughtful, supportive, and meaningful ways. Working together requires that team members be able to resolve conflicts among themselves and to do so in ways that enhance rather than inhibit their working together. In addition, team members must be able to trust that they will receive what they need while being able to count on one another to complete tasks related to team functioning and outcomes. To communicate effectively, people must be willing to confront issues and to express openly their ideas and feelings—to use interactive skills to accomplish tasks. In nursing, constructive confrontation has not been a well-used skill. Consequently, if communication patterns are to improve, the onus is on each of us as individuals to change communication patterns. In essence, for things to change, each of us must change.

Singleness of Mission

Every team must have a purpose—that is, a plan, aim, or intention (see the Research Perspective on p. 339). However, the most successful teams have a mission—some special work or service to which the team is 100% committed. The sense of mission and purpose must be clearly understood and agreed to by all (Lencioni, 2012). The more powerful and visionary the mission is, the more energizing it will be to the team. The more energy and excitement are engendered, the more motivated all members will be to do the necessary work.

Willingness to Cooperate

Just because a group of people has a regular reporting relationship within an organizational chart does not mean the members are a team. Boxes and arrows are not in any way related to the technical and interpersonal coordination or the emotional investment required of a true team. In effective teams, members are required to work together in a respectful, civil manner. Most of us have been involved in organizations in which people could accomplish assigned tasks but were not successful in their interpersonal relationships. In essence, these employees received a salary for not getting along with a certain person or persons. Some of these employees have not worked cooperatively for years! Organizations can no longer afford to pay people to not work together. Personal friendship or socialization is not required, but cooperation is a necessity. Traditionally, these interpersonal skills were considered "soft" skills and were difficult to coach people on or to hold them accountable. That is no longer the case. In most organizations, employees can now be terminated for a lack of willingness to work cooperatively with team members.

Commitment

Commitment is a state of being emotionally impelled and is demonstrated when a sense of passion and dedication to a project or event—a mission exists. Often, this passion looks a little crazy. In other words, people go the extra mile because of their commitment. They do whatever it takes to accomplish the goals or see the project through to completion. An example of commitment is discussed by Charles Garfield when he talks about being a part of the team that created the lunar landing module for the first man to walk on the moon. People did all kinds of things that looked crazy, including working extended hours and shifts, calling in to see how the project was progressing, and sleeping over at their work station so as not to be separated from the project—all because everybody knew that he or she was a part of something that was much bigger than himself or herself. They were a part of sending a man to the moon, something that human beings had been dreaming about for thousands of years. It was a historical moment, and people were intensely committed to making it happen.

Many people go through their entire lives hating every single day of work. Needless to say, most of them are not committed. Because we spend an extensive amount of time in the work setting, we must enjoy what we do. for both physical and mental well-being. If this is not the case for you, then try to find a different job or profession—one you might love. Life is too short to do something that you hate doing every day. While you are moving into whatever you decide you love doing, commit to yourself to do your best at whatever you are now doing. Be 100% present wherever you are. Do the best work you are capable of doing. This honors you as a human being, and it honors your co-workers and patients.

EXERCISE 18-3

Box 18-4 contains eight questions. Spend at least 20 minutes in a quiet place thinking about and writing answers to these eight questions. Pay particular notice to question 7.

Many examples of commitment aren't well-known, such as that of Jan Skaggs, the Vietnam veteran who was the driving force behind the building of the Vietnam Veterans Memorial. He was a clerk in the Washington, DC, bureaucracy who attended a veterans' meeting and decided a memorial to those who lost their lives in Vietnam was needed—a memorial that had all 58,000 names inscribed on it. He had only a high school diploma and did not even own a suit, but 5 years and $7 million later, the wall was dedicated (Lopes, 1987). This demonstrates that one

---

BOX 18-4   EXPLORING COMMITMENT

The key to finding your compelling mission/passion that will lead you to success and peak performance is to ask yourself the right questions. Your answers to these questions will help you understand what you need to know about yourself. Read each question, then think carefully for a few minutes, and answer each question honestly. Do not censor or edit out anything, even if it seems impossible or unrealistic—allow yourself to be surprised. Let your imagination soar.

1. Am I deriving any satisfaction out of the work I am now doing?
2. If they did not reward (praise or pay) me to do what I now do, would I still do it?
3. What is it that I really love to do?
4. What do I want to pursue with my time and energy that is worthwhile?
5. What motivates me to reach out and do my best to excel?
6. What is it that only I can say to the world? What needs to be done that can best be done only by me?
7. If I won $40 million in the lottery tomorrow, how would I live? What would I do each day and for the rest of my life?
8. If I were to write my own obituary right now, what would be my most significant accomplishment? Is that enough?

Repeating this exercise often will give you additional insights and information about what you really want and love to do. If taken seriously, the exercise should help you have an understanding of why you selected this profession and whether you have the stamina to do whatever it takes to make a contribution and to make a difference in the practice of nursing.

---

does not have to have a college degree to be committed. Sometimes a college degree can inhibit people from accomplishing their goals because they become diverted from a purpose, from a mission, or from life goals by, for example, good grades. Rather than understanding grades as a tool of measurement, they see them as an end in themselves.

Almost anyone can be taught the technical aspects of what needs to be done in most patient care settings. Teaching people to love what they do or to care about patients and their families—even the most difficult and unique patients and families—is far more difficult.

TOOLS AND ISSUES THAT SUPPORT TEAMS

When individuals come together in a group, they spend considerable time in group process or social dynamics, which allows the group to advance toward becoming a team and c   g a goal. Each person within the group strug   three key questions that must continually be reevaluated and renegotiated. These three questions, according to Weisburg's classic work (1988), are as follows:

1. Am I in or out?
2. Do I have any power or control?
3. Can I use, develop, and be appreciated for my skills and resources?

"In" Groups and "Out" Groups

Most of us want to be valued and recognized by others as a part of the group, one who "knows" or understands. Most people want to be at the core of decision making, power, and influence. In other words, they want to be part of the "in" group, and researchers have demonstrated that those who feel "in" cooperate more, work harder and more effectively, and bring enthusiasm to the group. The more we feel we are not a part of the key group, the more "out" we feel and the more we withdraw, work alone, daydream, and engage in self-defeating behaviors. Often, intergroup conflict results when individuals who feel they are "out" and want to be "in" create a schism or a division that prohibits the team from accomplishing its goals.

Power and Control

Everybody wants at least some power, and everybody wants to feel he or she is in control. When faced with changes that we cannot influence, we feel impotent and experience a loss of self-esteem. Consequently, all of us want to feel that we are in control of our immediate environment and that we have enough power and influence to get our needs met. When a situation or an event arises that we cannot handle, we attempt to compensate for it in some way; most of these ways are not productive to smoothly functioning teams.

EXERCISE 18-4

Think about a time when you and a small group of classmates or co-workers wanted to change something, such as a scheduled time (a class or meeting), an assignment, or an outcome measure (grading curve of a test or a performance evaluation criterion), and the faculty or administration adamantly refused. How did you feel? What was the response? Did you engage in gossip to make others appear wrong? You may have been "right," but the sense of a loss of control or power is very uncomfortable, sometimes resulting in stress and fear. Mature behavior is required to maintain a positive, problem-solving approach.

Use, Develop, and Be Appreciated for My Skills and Resources

Each member of the team has unique skills and resources to bring to the goals and tasks to be accomplished by the team. The Gallup research is quite clear, in its evaluation of the work environment, that one of the most powerful indicators of a successful, supportive work environment can be predicted by the scores from the question "At work, do you have the opportunity to do what you do best every day?" When the score is low in this area, team members clearly do not believe their skills are recognized, well used, or appreciated. To accomplish the goal of having each team member believe that his or her skills are recognized, encouraged, and used and his or her growth is encouraged requires a strong, knowledgeable *team leader*. Fewer than 20% of employees feel their strengths are used every day (Wagner & Harter, 2006). When nurses do not believe their skills are used, they are more prone to be in the "out group." This leads to being unengaged and even disengaged in the workplace. This is not supportive of a positive, creative work environment.

POSITIVE COMMUNICATION MODEL

Whenever human beings are in distress, unengaged, or disengaged or have emotional reaction to a situation or the actions of another, a conditioned response is to move into one or all of the following: *blame, judgment,* or *demand.* These are depicted in the awareness model found in Figure 18-2. With effort and practice, it is possible to create a communication interaction that produces a significantly improved outcome.

When an individual is reacting at the feeling level, he or she tends to move unconsciously to blame. By taking accountability for these feelings, one can move out of blame and own one's feelings by stating, "I feel ..."

Likewise, when an individual is trapped in distress or reaction at the thinking level, he or she most often turns to judgment. By thinking compassionately, one can dismantle the judgment and state what one thinks in a compassionate way: "I think ..."

Finally, when in distress, we make demands that are often unreasonable. By calming yourself, you can find respect for the other human being and make a request for what you want for yourself in a given situation: "I want an effective professional relationship." Wanting the other person to change is

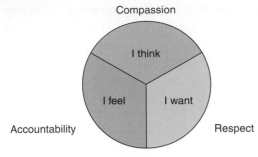

Conscious Reflective Response

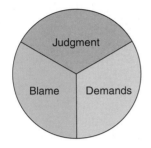

Unconscious Reactive Response

FIGURE   18-2 Awareness model: differentiating between conscious and unconscious responses.

pointless because it is unlikely to happen and you don't control the other person.

Most broken relationships are stuck in blame, judgment, and demand. Being accountable, compassionate, and respectful helps clarify what goes on inside each of us.

Everyone needs to feel as though his or her skills, tools, and contributions are needed and valued and that he or she is respected for what personal contributions are offered to the workplace, team, or group. Everyone has weaknesses, and there is no need to emphasize these or to spend time in ongoing correction. Rather, focus should be placed on people's strengths, specifically, acknowledging and emphasizing what people do well.

Part of focusing on people's strengths is being willing to acknowledge peers, faculty, and the other significant people in one's life (Yu, Harter, & Agrawal, 2013). In contrast, many role models focus on correction. Consequently, many of us spend a large portion of our time correcting others rather than appreciating them for all the wonderful things they are. Focusing on strengths rather than on weaknesses is far more productive and leads to excellence. With all the energy and attention that can be paid, weakness will never be more than average

or mediocre (Rath, 2007). If the focus is on improving our strengths, it is much easier to excel and then to be acknowledged for what we do well. Unfortunately, focusing on weaknesses tends to decrease the appreciation and thus the acknowledgments. Furthermore, we seem to believe that a finite number of available acknowledgments exist and we must not give out too many of them because they must be held in reserve for very important events. In addition, we do not always give acknowledgments in a way they can be received and valued. Box 18-5 can serve as a guide for giving acknowledgment.

To deal with the three personal issues discussed in this section, team members must learn how to state openly what is on their minds and be responsive and respectful as other members of the team do the same. In other words, team members must give and receive feedback constructively.

EXERCISE 18-5

Within the next 3 days, find three opportunities to acknowledge a peer or acquaintance using the five guidelines for acknowledgment shown in Box 18-5. In addition, use these same guidelines to acknowledge yourself for something you have done well.

BOX 18-5   GUIDELINES FOR ACKNOWLEDGMENT

1. Acknowledgments must be specific. The specific behavior or action that is appreciated must be identified in the acknowledgment; for example, "Thank you for taking notes for me when I had to go to the dentist. You identified three key points that appeared on the test."
2. Acknowledgments must be "eye to eye," or personal. Look the person in the eye when you thank him or her. Do not run down the hall and say "Thanks" over your shoulder. Written appreciation also qualifies as "eye to eye."
3. Acknowledgments must be sincere, that is, from the heart. Each of us recognizes insincerity. If you do not truly appreciate a behavior or action, do not say anything. Insincerity often makes people angry or upset, thus defeating the goal.
4. Acknowledgments are more powerful when they are given in public. Most people receive pleasure from public acknowledgment and remember these occasions for a long time. For people who are shy and may prefer no public acknowledgment, this is an opportunity to work on a personal growth issue with them. Public acknowledgment is an opportunity to communicate what is valued.
5. Acknowledgments need to be timely. The less time that elapses between the event and the acknowledgment, the more powerful and effective it is and the more the acknowledgment is appreciated by the recipient.

Group Agreements

One of the most helpful tools available is to have the team members come to an agreement about the ground rules concerning their relationships with one another (Yoder-Wise & Kowalski, 2012). This can take place in various ways. Multiple types of guidelines can even be used to set the context for how people relate. Many hospitals and facilities have service agreements that new employees accept when they are first hired. These are often in the employee handbook and must be used to hold people accountable for behaviors. One example of a set of guidelines comes from the Colorado Center for Nursing Excellence, the nursing workforce center for the state (Box 18-6). These are called the "Commitment to My Team Members." They have gone through multiple transitions and redesigns, but the basic tenets are essentially the same. People must agree on the goals and mission with which they are involved. They have to reach some understanding of how they will exist together. Tenets or agreements such as "I will respectfully speak promptly with any team member with whom I have a problem" go a long way to avoid gossiping, backbiting, bickering, and misinterpreting others. As you review these team agreements either monthly or quarterly, keep in mind that a part of this process is the willingness of members of the team to be accountable for upholding the agreements and to give feedback when the agreements have been violated. Without agreement, people have implicit permission to behave in any manner they choose toward one another, including angry, hostile, hurtful, and acting-out behavior.

Trust

Trust is the basis by which leaders/managers facilitate the activities and the progress of the team. Kouzes and Posner (2012) conducted research on personal best leadership practices that mobilize others to get extraordinary things done. They focused on how leaders build high-performance teams through five key behaviors: modeling the way, inspiring a shared vision, challenging the process, enabling others to act, and encouraging the heart. Poorly performing teams show little evidence of these relational behaviors and, consequently, trust is low for the leader and for each other.

BOX 18-6   COMMITMENT TO MY TEAM MEMBERS

The staff at Colorado Center for Nursing Excellence developed these agreements in 2010. The staff included both professional and support personnel. These agreements are reviewed at each monthly "all staff meeting." This review serves as a reminder of our agreements and each person considers these agreements integral to the smooth functioning of the Team.

- I accept responsibility for establishing and maintaining healthy interpersonal relationships with every member of this team. I recognize that the words, actions and attitudes of each of us individually reflect on the whole of the Colorado Center for Nursing Excellence.
- I will respectfully speak promptly with any team member with whom I am having a problem. The only time I will discuss it with another person is when I need assistance in reaching a satisfactory resolution. The goal of a conversation with a trusted colleague is not to complain or triangulate but to gain insight into resolution. I will always remember to "take the mail to the correct address."
- I will establish and maintain a relationship of trust with every member of this team. My relationships with each of you will be equally respectful, regardless of job title, level of educational preparation, or any other differences that may exist.
- I will accept each team member as they are today, forgiving past problems and asking each person to do the same with me.

- I will remember that no one is perfect and that our errors will be accepted as opportunities for forgiveness, growth and learning.
- Since all members of our team are leaders and followers, we are committed to finding solutions to problems and embracing accountability for the success of the whole organization.

   Different projects have different team members as the leader and the remainder are followers. Sometimes the leader of a specific project is a support person and the followers, both professional staff and support staff, take direction from that person.
- My words, actions and attitudes make my team members feel appreciated, included, and valued. I will have fun and keep a sense of humor at work.
- As leaders we practice what The Center teaches.

   The Center delivers educational offerings on leadership, teaching, quality and safe patient care and presentations. The common threads exemplified in the above agreements are taught and each member of the team is expected to demonstrate the behaviors we teach to participants.
- I expect and accept if at any time I do not comply with the above statements my team members will have a confidential conversation with me directly in order to raise awareness and accountability to the above commitments.

From http://www.coloradonursingcenter.org/center-staff. (Retrieved February 25, 2014.)

Trust is also a major issue among group members, and one of the first questions to come up in the group concerns is whom one can trust or not trust. In the early days of organizational development, McGregor (1967) defined *trust* in the following way:

> Trust means: "I know that you will not—deliberately or accidentally, consciously or unconsciously—take unfair advantage of me." It means, "I can put my situation at the moment, my status and self-esteem in this group, relationship, my job, my career, even my life, in your hands with complete confidence." (p. 163)

One can see from this description how critical trust is within a team (Lencioni, 2012). The leader models trust through behaviors such as facilitating the establishment of ground rules/agreements by which the team will function and holding team members accountable for adhering to the agreements. Trust is probably the most delicate aspect within relationships and is influenced far more by actions than by words. Therefore what people do is more powerful than what they say. Trust is a fragile thread that can be severed by one act. Once destroyed, trust is more difficult to reestablish than its initial creation.

QUALITIES OF A TEAM PLAYER

As early as nursing school, working in teams becomes an important strategy for accomplishing work. Understanding what is required of a strong teammate becomes clear as students are assigned teams for various projects. Most people have participated in teams that did not work and in those that worked very well. Maxwell (2002) identified 17 characteristics that make a good team player:

1. **Adaptable**—Inflexibility does not work in teams. Being rigid in thinking or behavior is destructive to both the individual and to the team.
2. **Collaborative**—Collaboration is more than cooperation. It means each person brings something to the project that adds value to the team and supports the creation of synergy.
3. **Committed**—Commitment is a passion in the face of adversity to take action and make things happen. It is the passion to do whatever it takes to accomplish the team objectives.
4. **Communicative**—Communication should happen early and often. Frequency of interaction

with other team members, talking with them and sharing thoughts, ideas, and experiences—these are the activities that support teamwork.

5. **Competent**—Competence translates as someone who is quite capable and highly qualified and does the job well.
6. **Dependable**—Team members who are dependable follow through and do what they have agreed to do well, without prodding or delay.
7. **Disciplined**—Discipline is doing what you really do not want to do so you can accomplish the goals you really want and includes paying attention to the details in thinking, in emotions, and in the actions you take.
8. **Enlarging**—Helping a teammate advance or grow into a better person or team player; helping teammates advance the team; believing in your teammates before they believe in themselves are examples of value-added contributions.
9. **Enthusiastic**—Enthusiasm focuses on becoming a highly energetic team member who has a positive attitude and believes that the team, together, can be better than anyone dreamed they could.
10. **Intentional**—The team and its members have a purpose for themselves and for the team. Every action counts and is meaningful. The focus is on doing the right things in each moment and following through with these actions to their logical conclusion.
11. **Mission Conscious**—Each team member has a sense of purpose and mission that drives all thoughts, ideas, and actions to do what is best for their team and their cause.
12. **Prepared**—Being prepared translates as preparation for every meeting and event and begins with a thorough assessment of what is needed, aligning the appropriate work with the appropriate effort, addressing the mental aspects of the right attitude, and being ready to take action.
13. **Relational**—The ability to be connected to other members of the team, to be in a relationship with them, is the core of being relationship-oriented. These relationships and the mutual respect upon which they are built create cohesiveness on the team.
14. **Self-Improving**—As a team member, you strive to continually grow and reflect, both routinely and periodically, on how well each venture of

assignment went and what you could have done better. This is a process of self-reflection.

15. **Selfless**—Putting others on the team ahead of yourself through being generous to team members, avoiding "playing politics," showing loyalty toward team members, and valuing interdependence among team members over the American value of being independent are all examples of selflessness.

16. **Solution-Oriented**—Do not be consumed with all of the problems associated with the endeavor; rather, focus on finding the solutions; think about what is possible.

17. **Tenacious**—Being tenacious means giving your all, with determination, and refusing to stop until the goal has been accomplished.

EXERCISE 18-6

Think about the last team project in which you participated. What worked about the team? What did not work about the team? Was there a member who did not carry his or her share of the work? Was there a team member who was a "know it all"? How did you handle the situation? Was there a person on the team who took the lead? How many of the qualities of a good team player do you possess? Be honest. What are areas in which you could improve? What are your strengths; that is, where do you shine?

CREATING SYNERGY

Teams function with varying levels of effectiveness. The interesting part of this is that effectiveness can be created systematically. Truly effective teams are ones in which people work together to produce extraordinary results that could not have been achieved by any one individual (Fuller, 1975). This phenomenon is often described as synergy. In the physical sciences, synergy is found in metal alloys. Bronze, the first alloy, was a combination of copper and tin and was found to be much harder and stronger than either copper or tin separately; the tensile strength of bronze cannot be predicted by merely adding the tensile strength of tin and of copper. It is far greater than simple addition.

We see the same properties of synergy in human endeavors; an example is the 1980 U.S. Olympic hockey team. People who remember the hockey game know the Americans defeated the Russians. The American team consisted of a group of college kids, none of whom could establish a celebrated successful career

in the National Hockey League. However, for 2 weeks they were the best hockey team in the world—and they were the best because they knew how to work together to produce extraordinary results. Working cooperatively, an effective team produces extraordinary results that no one team member could have achieved alone. To create synergy consistently, certain basic rules must be followed:

* Establish a clear purpose.
* Use active listening.
* Be compassionate.
* Tell the truth.
* Be flexible.
* Commit to resolution.

Establish a Clear Purpose

Creative synergy requires a clear purpose. Each member of the team must understand the reason the team is together, determine what he or she wishes to accomplish (as delineated by defined goals and objectives), and express his or her belief in both the value and feasibility of the goals and tasks. Teams function best when the members cannot only tell others about their purpose but also define and operationalize succinctly the meaning and value of this purpose.

Use Active Listening

Active listening means that you are completely focused on the individual who is speaking. It means listening without judgment. It means listening to the essence of the conversation so that you can actually repeat to the speaker most of the speaker's intended meaning. It means being 100% present in the communication. (For guidelines for active listening, see Box 18-7.)

Developing a defensive response or argument in your head while the other person is still speaking is not active listening. To listen actively, a person must be absorbing words, posture, tone of voice, and all the clues accompanying the message so that the intent of the communication can be received. Specific purposes used in active listening, including examples, are found in Table 18-4.

Be Compassionate

To be compassionate means to have a sympathetic consciousness of another's distress and a desire to alleviate the distress. Consequently, it is inappropriate to focus

BOX 18-7   GUIDELINES FOR ACTIVE LISTENING

1. Slow down your internal processes and seek data. Do not interrupt the speaker.
2. The more information you acquire through listening, the less interpretation you do (making up the missing pieces or motivations). The less information you have, the more interpretation you do.
3. Realize that the first words from the other person are not necessarily representative of inner thoughts and feelings. Be patient.
4. When listening, suspend your own beliefs and views and judgments, at least temporarily. Attempt to understand the perspective of the other person, particularly if it is different from yours.
5. Realize that any judgments or "labels" strongly influence the manner in which you listen to the other person.
6. Appreciate the difference between understanding other people's perspective and agreeing with them. First strive to understand. Then you may agree or disagree.
7. Effective listening is based on an inner desire to learn about another's unique experience of the world.

Adapted from Olen, D. (1993). *Communicating: Speaking and listening to end misunderstanding and promote friendship.* Germantown, WI: JODA Communications.

TABLE 18-4   ACTIVE LISTENING

USE OF ACTIVE LISTENING	EXAMPLES
To convey interest in what the other person is saying	I see! I get it. I hear what you're saying.
To encourage the individual to expand further on his or her thinking	Yes, go on. Tell us more.
To help the individual clarify the problem in his or her own thinking	Then the problem as you see it is …
To get the individual to hear what he or she has said in the way it sounded to others	This is your decision, then, and the reasons are … If I understand you correctly, you are saying that we should …
To pull out the key ideas from a long statement or discussion	Your major point is … You feel that we should …
To respond to a person's feelings more than to his or her words	You feel strongly that … You do not believe that …
To summarize specific points of agreement and disagreement as a basis for further discussion	We seem to be agreed on the following points … But we seem to need further clarification on these points …
To express a consensus of group feeling	As a result of this discussion, we as a group seem to feel that …

time and energy on making the other person wrong, especially when your perspective differs from his or hers. It means listening from a caring perspective—one that is focused on understanding the viewpoint of the other person rather than insisting on the "rightness" of one's own point of view.

Tell the Truth

To tell the truth means to speak clearly to personal points and perspectives while acknowledging that they are, merely, personal perspectives. If an observation is made about the tone or behavior of a speaker that affects the ability of others to hear the message, feedback can be provided in a way that does not make the speaker wrong. This is accomplished in an objective rather than subjective manner using neither a cynical nor a critical tone of voice. To be effective, one must own, or be responsible for, personal opinions and attitudes.

Be Flexible

Flexibility and openness to another person's viewpoint are critical for a team to work well together. No single person has all the right answers. Therefore acknowledging that each person has something to contribute and must be heard is important. Flexibility reflects a willingness to hear another team member's point of view rather than being committed to the "rightness" of a personal point of view.

Commit to Resolution

To commit to resolution means that one can agree to disagree with someone even when that perspective is different. Rather than assuming the person is wrong, this is a commitment to hear his or her perspective, listen to the real message, identify differences, and creatively seek solutions to resolve the areas of differences so a common understanding and shared commitment to the issue can be reached. Both parties need to then agree that they feel heard and agree to the resolution. This differs greatly from compromise and majority vote seen in the democratic process. When compromise exists, acquiescence or relinquishing of a significant portion of

TABLE 18-5 ASPECTS OF CONFLICT	
DESTRUCTIVE	**CONSTRUCTIVE**
• Diverts energy from more important activities and issues • Destroys the morale of people or reinforces poor self-concepts • Polarizes groups so they increase internal cohesiveness and reduce intergroup cooperation • Deepens differences in values • Produces irresponsible and regrettable behavior such as name-calling and fighting	• Opens up issues of importance, resulting in their clarification • Results in the solution of problems • Increases the involvement of individuals in issues of importance to them • Causes authentic communication to occur • Serves as a release for pent-up emotion, anxiety, and stress • Helps build cohesiveness among people sharing the conflict, celebrating in its settlement, and learning more about each other • Helps individuals grow personally and apply what they learn to future situations

Adapted from Hart, L.B. (1980). *Learning from conflict*. Reading, MA: Addison-Wesley.

what was desired likely occurred. This generally leaves both parties feeling negative about themselves or the agreement. Consequently, most compromises must be reworked at some future date. Working on conflict and its resolution (Table 18-5) is time-consuming but essential to effectively functioning teams (Lencioni, 2012). Commitment to resolution is integral to the needs of the team. One team member may disagree with another team member, but the successful work of the team is at stake in this conflict. Without commitment to resolution for the sake of the team, individuals often have less impetus to seek a common ground or to agree to disagree.

Synergy cannot occur when one team member becomes a self-proclaimed expert who has the "right" answer. Nor can synergy occur when people refuse to speak. Each team member has good ideas, and these need to be shared. They are not shared, however, when someone feels uncomfortable in the team. It is difficult to speak up and appear wrong or inadequate. The challenge each person faces is to push through discomfort and become a full participant in problem identification and resolution for the overall benefit of the team.

Our society tends to be dualistic in nature. **Dualism** means that most situations are viewed as right or wrong, black or white. Answers to questions are often reduced to "yes" or "no." As a result, we sometimes forget a broad spectrum of possibilities actually exists. Exercising creativity and exploring numerous possibilities are important. This allows the team to operate at its optimal level.

We have all known people who were self-proclaimed experts, to whom it was critically important that they be right and acknowledged as right and who become judgmental of others whose perspectives and opinions differ from theirs. Consequently, being able to tell the truth to one's synergistic team and to encourage team members to stretch and look at different ways of functioning is vital. This requires strong skills in good negotiation and conflict resolution, something for which few of us have been trained. If self-proclaimed experts think we are judging them, they will not hear the questions, the observations, or the "truth" because the message seems to be making them wrong rather than originating from compassion. The most valuable contribution an individual can make to an organization is a passionate commitment to the creation of synergistic teams.

INTERDISCIPLINARY/ INTERPROFESSIONAL TEAMS

Interprofessional teams are essential to quality patient care. Nurses, physicians, dietitians, social workers, case managers, pharmacists, and physical therapists, to name but a few, must work together to achieve cost-effective care while achieving the highest quality of care in the healthcare setting. This means efforts must be expended to understand the various roles and backgrounds of each discipline. At the same time, nurses are frequently leading teams comprising licensed practical/vocational nurses and technicians or assistants of various kinds. Here again, it is critical to understand everyone's role and job description as well as his or her background and who he or she is as an individual and human being. In addition, the collaboration needed in interprofessional teams cannot be created without mutual trust and respect among the members (Maxfield, Grenny, Lavandero, & Groah, 2013).

Several additional aspects of interprofessional work are crucial to creating and maintaining these teams. Coyne (2005) emphasized *the importance of understanding each situation,* which includes clarifying misperceptions and inaccurate information about others within the team including any assumptions that one professional group is favored over another. *Noticing professional expectations and unwritten processes* and cultures of the various professions within the team is also critical to working together seamlessly. It is helpful for nurses to note how other groups talk and behave and to note the special language they use. *Encourage the different disciplines to learn* from each other. For example, in comparing the different codes of ethics, the many similarities, as opposed to the differences, can create commonalities. Most are focused on the patient. The team leader must *set a positive tone.* If the leadership expects interprofessional teamwork and verbalizes and models positive and upbeat attitudes, the various disciplines will work together smoothly.

Frequency of interaction of the team members can create ongoing interactions and familiarity with one another. Team members who are in a professional relationship with one another are more apt to work together smoothly. As an example, a weekly patient care meeting in which patients with significant needs or problems are reviewed allows each profession to address issues from a specific area of expertise. *Keep communication open* includes telling the truth in a way that it can be heard and understood. If an aspect of care is governed by regulations, it is helpful when a knowledgeable member of the team speaks to the issue or regulation, always remembering to phrase the information in a way that facilitates hearing and understanding. At all times the interprofessional team must *focus on the patient.* When the deliberations are focused on the delivery of best patient care for the specific patient, mutual respect can be developed and open sharing of ideas and problem solving occurs.

THE VALUE OF TEAM-BUILDING

The value of team-building is to enhance functioning in any one or all of the following processes (Castner, Foltz-Ramos, Schwartz, & Ceravolo, 2012):
- The establishment of goals and objectives
- The allocation of the work to be performed

- The manner in which a group works: its processes, norms, decision making, and communication patterns
- The relationships among the people doing the work

When things are not going well in an organization and problems need to be resolved, the first intervention people think of is "team-building." Naturally, for teams (a collection of people relying on each other) to be effective, they must function smoothly and communicate effectively to create the best possible work environment. The difficulty is that when organizations are feeling stress and facing difficulties, they generally do not have teams whose members function well together. Team-building can address any one of the aforementioned activities, depending on the available time and other resources. A team-building consultant can teach a team how to set goals and priorities; help a team analyze the distribution of the workload using various team members' strengths (Rath & Conchie, 2009); examine a team's process, norms, decision-making processes, and communication patterns; and promote resolution of interpersonal conflicts or problems within the team.

Regardless of which areas are problematic, appropriate assessment of the team is essential. The problems may be in priority or goal-setting, allocation of the work, team decision making, or interpersonal relationships among the members (see the Research Perspective on p. 339). The success of the team depends on its members and its leadership.

Lencioni (2012) builds a strong case for dealing constructively with building an underlying foundation for teams. He believes that three major components of smoothly functioning teams must be created:
- Mutual trust among the members
- A strong sense of team identity (that the team is unique and worthwhile)
- A sense of team efficacy (that the team performs well and its members are synergistic in their manner of working together)

At the heart of these components are the emotions we often work so hard to keep out of the workplace. However, as human beings, we function in the same way in both work and personal lives. Mutual trust can be developed only when each team member tells the truth about feelings, thoughts, and wants and listens and supports other members of the team to do

RESEARCH PERSPECTIVE

Resource: Klein, C., Granados, D., Salas, E., Huy Le, C., Burke, S., Lyons, R., & Goodwin, G. (2009). Does team building work? *Small Group Research, 40*(2), 181-222.

This classic article reports an extensive meta-analysis of team-building research that focuses on four specific components of teams: goal-setting, interpersonal relationships, problem solving, and role clarification. This analysis includes 103 articles published between 1950 and 2007 and expands the original work of this same group and the analysis conducted in 1999. Previous team-building reviews are also summarized. The outcomes that were measured were cognitive, affective, process, and performance based. The results suggest that team-building activities have a moderately positive effect across all team outcomes, whereas the strongest effect existed for goal-setting and role clarification. The size of the team can also be important, and teams of 10 or fewer members seem to have more success.

This means that most work teams need to be limited in size (fewer than 10 members per group) and that the focus when forming the team is on clarifying the goals of the team and the role of each team member.

Implications for Practice

The Institute of Medicine has set the expectation that all healthcare providers function as a patient-centered team, yet not all curricula prepare practitioners to do so. Using the knowledge about the outcomes of these key components helps practitioners perform more effectively in teams.

BOX 18-8   INTERVIEW QUESTIONS FOR TEAM-BUILDING

1. What do you see as the problems currently facing your team?
2. What are the current strengths of your institution or work group? What are you currently doing well?
3. Does your boss do anything that prevents you from being as effective as you would like to be?
4. Does anybody else in this group do anything that prevents you from being as effective as you would like to be?
5. What would you like to accomplish at your upcoming team-building session? What changes would you be willing to make that would facilitate a smoother-functioning team and accomplishment of the team goals?

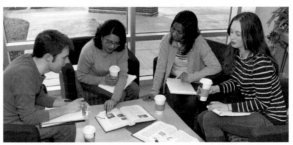

Teams can form strong relationships external to the work environment.

MANAGING EMOTIONS

Probably one of the greatest fears in team-building exercises is that people will become emotional, that they will lose control of themselves or the environment, or that they will appear weakened or vulnerable. Although many people acknowledge that we are all thinking and feeling persons, management/leadership is usually more willing to deal with the "thinking" side than the "feeling" side of individuals within the team.

Because people spend such a large percentage of their time in the work setting, it would be unrealistic to believe that they continually appear in an unemotional and controlled state. Human beings simply do not function that way. What is observed are people's aspirations, their achievements, their hopes, and their social consciousness; they are observed falling in love; falling in hate and anger; winning and losing; and being excited, sad, fearful, anxious, and jealous. Consequently, these "feelings" are important components of organizational life and do much to undermine work effectiveness. Most of us know of situations in which,

---

likewise. Every person yearns to be a part of something bigger than himself or herself—to do something important that makes a difference. Well-functioning teams allow this to happen. Developing such teams can increase nursing job satisfaction and group cohesiveness, decrease nurse turnover rates, and promote patient safety and quality outcomes.

Understandable anxiety exists concerning the safety of being vulnerable and exposed if personal issues are revealed. That is why it is helpful for the team-building facilitator to make a thorough assessment of major issues and the willingness on the part of members to work on issues. One approach is to interview members of the team individually to discover what the critical issues are. The types of questions that might be asked are found in Box 18-8. This kind of tool gives the facilitator some sense of what the major issues are within the group so that he or she has a better understanding of how to work with the group.

because of an emotional disagreement, two individuals have avoided each other for years. Because of the power of emotions and the inevitability of their presence, their effect on interpersonal relationships, and their influence on productivity, the quality of work, and the safety of patients, emotions should be a high priority when examining the functioning of the team. Fortunately, research addresses the importance of emphasizing the "emotional intelligence" of individuals and teams when working in teams (Goleman, 2011). Those teams that address these issues are much more successful and create a positive work environment.

According to Bocialetti's classic work (1988), people are sensitive to what happens when emotions are revealed. When people yell or get angry or upset and when goals, objectives, and tasks are disputed, employees see the following:

- A member intimidating and frightening others within the group
- Embarrassment
- A member overstating or exaggerating another's view to appear right
- Provocation of defensive and hostile responses
- Over-concern with oneself—self-absorption
- Gossip
- Loss of control
- A member distracting others from "real work"
- Disruption or termination of relationships within a group

These are behaviors that destroy any hope of creating a smoothly functioning team, one that supports its members to grow and learn and provide quality patient care. On the other hand, the cost of suppressing emotions or "feelings" includes the following:

- Physical and psychological stress
- Withdrawal from participation
- Loss of energy and depression
- Reduction of learning
- Hiding of important data because of fear
- Festering problems and emotions
- Prevention of others from being acknowledged
- Decreased motivation
- Weakening of the ability to receive constructive feedback
- The loss of one's influence

These types of outcomes lead to the conclusion that suppressing emotions at work is neither healthy nor constructive for team members.

When emotions are handled appropriately within the team, several positive outcomes are possible for the work setting. One creates a sense of internal comfort with the workings of the team and the organization. When stress is lowered and kept at lower levels on average, problems are much more easily resolved. This phenomenon is similar to releasing steam slowly with a steam valve rather than having the gasket blow. Interpersonal relationships on the team are more stable, and people have a sense of closer ties and collegiality when emotions are addressed. Fewer negative relationships or interactions develop, which results in more effective and pleasant working relationships all around.

Work group effectiveness improves when the team is functioning smoothly and emotions and "feelings" are being addressed on a routine basis rather than waiting for a volcanic eruption. It is the daily routines of frustration and boredom and retreat from the group that are likely to undo a team. People who are engaged and have leaders who help them achieve goals are more effective. The skills and tools previously discussed (e.g., speaking supportively) are the basic tools one needs to handle the emotional aspects of the team. Choosing to cope with emotional upset must be a conscious choice, one that requires practice to improve the skill.

REFLECTIVE PRACTICE

The process of reflective practice consists of the active, careful consideration of a belief or knowledge and can derive from "learning from experience." It is an internal learning process in which an issue of concern is closely examined (Freshwater, Taylor, & Sherwood, 2008). Through this reflective process, the nurse may come to see the world differently and, as a result of these new insights, see the work world differently, which can translate to acting differently. Thus, upon reflection of how an interaction progressed with a complex patient, the nurse can examine how this event unfolded compared with how he or she might have wanted the event to occur. This is an opportunity to learn experientially from what works and what does not work so well. Many of us think about what happened during our shift or day as we travel home. The major area for growth is when we identify specific behaviors to exhibit, differently, make a commitment, and take action in changing the behavior. Bringing issues to the conscious level is the first step in personal/professional growth.

THE ROLE OF LEADERSHIP

Teams usually have a leader. In addition, teams function within large organizations that have leaders. Without the approval and the support of the leader, team-building, which can be a costly endeavor in terms of consultation fees as well as work time and resources of the team, is difficult to undertake and of questionable effectiveness. Although very strong teams may be able to educate themselves regarding some of the issues, such as establishing goals and priorities or clarifying their own team process, addressing any kind of relationship issue among team members without a more objective outside party facilitating the process is exceedingly difficult.

Because leadership is such a pivotal part of smoothly functioning teams, it is illuminating to examine leaders more carefully. Truly progressive leaders understand that leadership and followership are not necessarily a set of skills; rather, these are qualities of character. On speaking specifically to leadership, we are not talking about "putting on a role." In actuality, leaders realize their capacity for influence, risk taking, and decision making more fully. Leadership, and to some degree followership, is as much about character and development as it is about education. According to the classic work of Peter Vaill (1991), leadership is concerned with bringing out the best in people. For a leader who believes this, team-building is a natural outgrowth. This type of leader understands that the best in a person is tied intimately to the individual's deepest sense of himself or herself—to one's spirit. The efforts of leaders must touch the spiritual aspect in themselves and others. Warren Bennis (2009) once said that leaders simply care about more people. Consequently, this caring manifests itself in doing whatever it takes to improve team functioning. This may imply involving oneself in team-building with the team. The risk in such an endeavor is that the team leader is open to being vulnerable, to being judged by others, and to being wrong. However, if the leader has been a role model for the team agreement and has held people accountable to these statements,

the team-building exercise will not degenerate into judging and placing blame.

If true leadership is about character development as much as anything, then character development is also beneficial for followers—that is, members of the team. The areas of character development often addressed include communication, particularly those aspects of speaking supportively that avoid placing blame and justifying and enhance understanding the other person's message. Box 18-9 highlights an example of character development from personal experience.

Leaders understand the multiple aspects of the issue of control. They take control of their lives rather than being at the mercy of others—rather than being victims. They have clarity regarding their own control issues. They focus time and energy primarily and almost exclusively on those issues, events, and behaviors over which they have control. Their activities are thus focused primarily on areas relating directly to them—not on world events or other happenings over which they have neither influence nor control.

Confidence, which loosely translates as faith or belief that one will act in a correct and effective way, is a key aspect of character. Thus it follows that confidence in oneself can be closely tied to self-esteem, which is satisfaction with oneself. The greatest deterrent to self-esteem and self-confidence is fear. Fear is described by some as "false evidence appearing real." Susan Jeffers (2006) said the core fear—the one that rules our lives—is one of "I can't handle it." So, the core of our fears is "I can't handle it," and it is exactly the opposite of being confident or holding oneself in high esteem. Working on self-confidence requires an attitude of belief, of confidence, of I "CAN DO" whatever is required (see Box 18-9).

> **F**alse
> **E**vidence
> **A**ppearing
> **R**eal

Simply caring about more people translates into a willingness to focus time and energy on members of the team. From one perspective, caring is risking being with someone and sharing both suffering and joy. Healing often emerges from caring. Behaviors that demonstrate caring include giving of oneself in terms of warmth and

BOX 18-9   THE "CAN DO" BRIGADE: AN ARMY NURSE'S STUDY IN CHARACTER DEVELOPMENT

As life events are reviewed, important or pivotal learning can be identified. One life event that significantly affected me was the year I spent as an Army Nurse Corps officer in South Vietnam. This was the first time I remember an awareness and understanding of confidence in the face of incredible obstacles. I had spent the first 10 months of my nursing career in labor and delivery at Indiana University before volunteering for a guaranteed assignment to Vietnam. I went to Fort Sam Houston for 6 weeks of basic training, where they taught me really important things like how to salute, how to march, and how many men are in a battalion. No one ever asked me if I could start an IV or draw a tube of blood. This was important because Indiana University had the largest medical school class in the United States at that time and nurses did nothing that interfered with medical education. Therefore I had never started an IV or drawn blood. When I arrived in Saigon, they put me in a sedan with another nurse and sent me up to the Third Surgical Hospital, one not unlike the one in *M*A*S*H*. We even had a Major Burns—that was not his name but it was his function. Surgical hospitals receive only battle casualties; their purpose is to stabilize and to transport.

The Third Surgical Hospital was located in the middle of the 173rd Airborne Brigade, whose job it was to defend the Bien Hoa Air Base, where all the sorties in the south were flown during the war. We were stopped at the gate by an MP who stepped up and saluted very snappily. He knew that a staff car must contain either a very-high-ranking officer or, if it was his lucky day, females.

When I was in Vietnam, 500 American women and 500,000 American men were there. The MP looked in the window, saluted snappily, and said "Afternoon, ma'am!" He wanted to know where we were going; he talked to us for a few minutes and assured us that if there was anything he could do for us, we should just give him a call. He saluted us and said, "CAN DO." I didn't understand because I did not know that there are units with very high esprit de corps who attach snappy little sayings at the end of things like salutes, phone conversations, memos, and so forth. The 173rd was the "CAN DO" brigade.

When we got to the hospital and met the chief nurse, she took us down to the mess hall and introduced us to all the doctors and nurses. We were sitting and having coffee when the field phone rang in the kitchen and the mess sergeant yelled out, "Incoming wounded." Everybody got up and started to leave for the preop area. I just sat there until the chief nurse said, "Come on." I said, "You don't understand, I deliver babies." She was not impressed! She took me by the arm and led me to preop.

When we got there, we discovered there were not just a few incoming wounded, there were more than 30, and some were very seriously injured. She immediately told the sergeant to call headquarters battalion of the 173rd Airborne and tell them that the Third Surg needed blood. She turned to me and said, "Lieutenant, you are responsible for drawing 50 units of fresh whole blood." I was shocked! I had never drawn a tube of blood, but I found in the back section of preop a Specialist 4th class who was already setting up "saw horses" and stretchers, putting up IV poles, and hanging plastic blood sets. I started to help, and soon I heard trucks out back. I opened the door and looked outside. There were two huge Army trucks, and kids—17, 18, 19, and 20 years old—were jumping out. They were covered with red mud from the bottom of their boots to the tops of their helmets. I looked at them, and I looked at the clean cement floor, and in an instant, my mother came to me. I put my hand on my hip and said, "Where have you boys been?" One PFC stepped forward and saluted me very snappily and said, "Ma'am, we just came in this afternoon from 30 days in the field, we have been out in the rice paddies chasing the Viet Cong, we have not had a hot meal, and we've not had a shower but Sergeant Major said the Third Surg needs blood!" He saluted smartly and said, "CAN DO!" They were very clear. After 30 days of chasing and being chased by the Viet Cong, giving a unit of blood was easy. "CAN DO!" They were confident. They were kids who had looked into the face of death. At that moment, I knew if they CAN DO, I Can Do! Life requires confidence. With confidence, you can make your dreams come true!

love and particularly giving one's time. The second aspect of caring is truly listening to team members and hearing and understanding them. The third aspect includes being 100% present for them. The fourth is to honor the other person—to see his or her wholeness, possibilities, hopes, and dreams.

Leading the team is clearly not the easiest thing to do, but neither is being an active, fully participating member of the team. Both require taking risks, including being in a relationship. Being in a team-building experience and hearing those things that have not worked for people in their interactions with peers and

the leader can be scary but worthwhile. It requires a focus on personal and professional growth. It requires building character.

CONCLUSION

Whether a nurse is a leader, a manager, or a follower, effective performance requires excellent communication skills. Clear communication builds strong teams and promotes patient safety. Forging new relationships and strengthening old ones are typically facilitated by purposeful communication.

THE SOLUTION

The first question that needed to be asked was, "Were we committed to providing the most optimal care for the neonate?" In other words, why would teamwork be important in this situation? What's the vision or mission? After achieving agreement among the NICU team, we strategized on how to create a "team" with the specialists. Making our intent clear was very important. A meeting with the director of the specialty team, the NICU medical director, and nursing leadership was arranged. We discovered that we shared a common goal: to provide the best care possible for the baby. Keeping that goal as the focus, we then identified areas of mutual respect. From there, both sides were willing to listen to each other's concerns. Care guidelines could be identified, as well as areas of responsibility. Ideas on how to improve the communication process were also discussed. A plan based on patient needs, complete with agreements, was implemented.

Were we a team yet? The answer is "no." There was still a little skepticism and reserve. Everyone seemed to have a "wait-and-see" attitude. The first big chance was identified when the specialty group insisted that a patient of theirs be admitted to the NICU because they believed it was the best place for the baby to be. Another measurable outcome was having the agreements honored. This reinforced to everyone that his or her concerns had been heard and respected. Mutual trust was building, and a collegial relationship began. A year later, it is hard to imagine that this situation ever occurred. There is enthusiasm for this specialty's physicians and their patients. It is certainly a change in attitude.

There are many components to team-building, but the most important component is to be clear about your mission and intentions when working with potential team members. The intention to provide the best care possible assisted each one of us to be more open, creative, and trusting. These are all necessary components of team-building. Remember, teams are made up of individuals. Ask yourself if you are willing to accept responsibility for your response and actions. Be the change that you want to see.

—*Diane Gallagher*

Would this be a suitable approach for you? Why?

THE EVIDENCE

TeamSTEPPS is an integrated program created through the auspices of the U.S. Department of Health & Human Services Agency for Healthcare Research and Quality (AHRQ) and the U.S. Department of Defense (DOD) Healthcare Team Coordination Program; it stresses teamwork and communication among physicians, nurses, and other healthcare personnel to increase patient safety (Castner et al., 2012). Multiple projects and evidence have been accrued regarding the use and implementation of TeamSTEPPS, as well as the outcomes produced from this program. The goal is to produce highly effective interdisciplinary teams that achieve the best outcomes for patients. The tools and strategies used include leadership that coordinates the team and initiates planning, problem solving, and process improvement. Also, situation monitoring is employed. This tool focuses on the ability of the nurse to actively scan behaviors and actions of co-workers; it also fosters mutual respect and team accountability, which creates a safety net for the team and patient. Specific skills are taught that increase the ability of each team member to support other team members by accurately assessing their workload and helping them. These skills protect the team from work overload that might reduce effectiveness and increase risk to patients. The last skill set focuses on communication that highlights clear, accurate information exchange among team members including SBAR, Call-out, and Handoff. The TeamSTEPPS teaching manual, including PowerPoint presentations and teaching videos, is available from the DOD Patient Safety Program for minimal cost.

WHAT NEW GRADUATES SAY

- Everything I do is in teams. If you don't have team skills, you're lost. When therapeutic communication was discussed, I had no idea how often I would use it with my team. Communication really is critical.

- I've worked in two settings this year. My first position was in a place where team work was a set of words, not actions. Now I work where I feel valued and we say little about teams because we simply are one!

CHAPTER CHECKLIST

Nurse managers must help build teams. Although the manager does not have to lead the team, he or she must ensure that the group can function effectively as a team. The team members must be able to communicate with each other effectively, share a single mission, be willing to cooperate with each other, and be committed to achieving their objectives. Successful teamwork requires leadership, trust, and willingness to take risks.

- Groups and teams
- Generational differences
- Communicating effectively
  - Stress
  - Stress response model
  - Communication barriers
  - Communication pitfalls
  - Communication guidelines
- Key concepts of teams
  - Conflict resolution
  - Singleness of mission
  - Willingness to cooperate
  - Commitment
- Tools and issues that support teams
  - "In" groups and "out" groups
  - Power and control
  - Use, develop, and be appreciated for my skills and resources
- Positive communication model
  - Group agreements
  - Trust
- Qualities of a team player
- Creating synergy
  - Establish a clear purpose
  - Use active listening
  - Be compassionate
  - Tell the truth
  - Be flexible
  - Commit to resolution
- Interdisciplinary/interprofessional teams
- The value of team-building
- Managing emotions
- Reflective practice
- The role of leadership

TIPS FOR TEAM-BUILDING

- Commit to the purpose of the team.
- Develop team relationships of mutual respect.
- Communicate effectively, and actively listen.
- Create and adhere to team agreements concerning function and process.
- Build trust.

REFERENCES

Balzer-Riley, J. (2011). *Communication in nursing* (7th ed.). St. Louis, MO: Elsevier.

Bennis, W. (2009). *On becoming a leader*. Reading, MA: Addison-Wesley.

Bocialetti, G. (1988). Teams and management of emotion. In W.B. Reddy & K. Jamison (Eds.), *Team Building blueprints for productivity and satisfaction* (pp. 62–71). Alexandria, VA: NtL Institute for Applied Behavioral Sciences; and San Diego, CA: University Associates.

Castner, J., Foltz-Ramos, K., Schwartz, D., & Ceravolo, D. (October 2012). A leadership challenge: Staff nurse perceptions after an organizational TeamSTEPPS initiative. *Journal of Nursing Administration*, 42(10), 467–472.

Charney, C. (October 2011). Making a team of experts into an expert team. *Advances in Neonatal Care*, 11(5), 334–339.

Coyne, C. (2005). Strength in numbers: How team building is improving care in a variety of settings. *PT Magazine of Physical Therapy*, 13(6), 40–51.

Freshwater, D., Taylor, B., & Sherwood, G. (2008). *Reflective practice in nursing*. Chichester, UK: Blackwell Publishing.

Fuller, B. (1975). *Synergistics: Explorations in the geometry of thinking*. New York: Macmillan.

Goleman, D. (2011). *The brain & emotional intelligence: New insights*. Northampton, MA: More Than Sound.

Jeffers, S. (2006). *Feel the FEAR and DO IT anyway*. New York: Ballantine Books.

Klein, C., Granados, D., Salas, E., Huy Le, C., Burke, S., Lyons, R., et al. (2009). Does team building work? *Small Group Research*, 40(2), 181–222.

Kouzes, J. M., & Posner, B. Z. (2012). *The leadership challenge* (5th ed.). San Francisco: Jossey-Bass, John Wiley & Sons.

Lencioni, P. (2012). *The advantage: Why organizational health trumps everything else in business*. San Francisco, CA: Jossey-Bass.

Lopes, S. (1987). *The wall*. New York: Collins.

Maxfield, D., Grenny, J., Lavandero, R., & Groah, L. (April 29, 2014). *Why safety tools and checklists aren't enough to save lives.* Retrieved from http://www.aacn.org/wd/hwe/docs/the-silent-treatment.pdf.

Maxwell, J. (2002). *The 17 essential qualities of a team player.* Nashville, TN: Thomas Nelson Publishers.

McGregor, D. (1960). *The human side of enterprise.* New York: McGraw-Hill.

McGregor, D. (1967). *The professional manager.* New York: McGraw-Hill.

Nemeth, C. P. (2008). *Improving healthcare team communication: Building on lessons from aviation and aerospace.* Aldershot, UK: Ashgate Publishing.

Olen, D. (1993). *Communicating: Speaking and listening to end misunderstanding and promote friendship.* Germantown, WI: JODA Communications.

Porter-O'Grady, T., & Malloch, K. (2010). *Quantum leadership: A resource for health care innovation* (3rd ed.). Sudbury, MA: Jones & Bartlett.

Rath, T. (2007). *Strengths finder 2.0.* New York, NY: Gallup Press.

Rath, T., & Conchie, B. (2009). *Strengths based leadership: Great leaders, teams, and why people follow.* New York, NY: Gallup Press.

Satir, V. (1988). *The new peoplemaking.* Mountain View, CA: Science & Behavior Books.

Smith, M., & Segal, R. (June 2013). *Stress management: How to reduce, prevent, and cope with stress.* HELPGUIDE.org. Retrieved from, www.helpguide.org/mental/stress_management_relief_coping.htm.

Sportsman, S. (2005). Build a framework for conflict assessment. *Nursing Management, 36*(4), 12–40.

Vaill, P. (1991). *Managing as a performing art.* San Francisco: Jossey-Bass.

Wagner, R., & Harter, J. (2006). *12: The elements of great managing.* New York: Gallup Press.

Weingarten, R. (2009). Four generations, one workplace: A Gen X-Y staff nurse's view of team building in the emergency department. *Journal of Emergency Nursing, 35*(1), 27–30.

Weisburg, M. (1988). Team work: Building productive relationships. In W. B. Reddy & K. Jamison (Eds.), *Team building blueprints for productivity and satisfaction.* Alexandria, VA: NTL Institute for Applied Behavioral Sciences, and San Diego: University Associates.

Yoder-Wise, P. S., & Kowalski, K. (2012). *Fast facts for the classroom nursing instructor: Classroom teaching in a nutshell.* New York, NY: Springer.

Yu, D., Harter, J., & Agrawal, S. (April 2013). U.S. managers boast best work engagement. *Gallup Economy.* Retrieved from, www.gallup.com/poll/162062/managers-boast-best-work-engagement.aspx?utm_source=alert&utm_medium=email&utm_campaign=syndication&utm_content=morelink&utm_term=all%20gallup%20headlines.

SUGGESTED READINGS

Dyer, W. (1994). *Team building issues and alternatives.* Reading, MA: Addison-Wesley.

Francis, D., & Young, D. (1979). *Improving work groups: A practical manual for team building.* San Diego: University Associates.

Hughes, R., Ginnett, R., & Curphy, G. (2009). *Leadership: Enhancing the lessons of experience* (6th ed.). Boston: McGraw-Hill.

Jeffers, S. (1992). *Dare to connect: Reaching out in romance, friendship and the workplace.* Columbia, NY: Fawcett.

Nanus, B. (1995). *Visionary leadership.* San Francisco: Jossey-Bass.

Rosenstein, A., & O'Daniel, M. (2005). Disruptive behavior and clinical outcomes: Perceptions of nurses and physicians. *American Journal of Nursing, 105*(1), 54–64.

Schmieding, N. J. (1993). Nurse empowerment through context structure and process. *Journal of Professional Nursing, 9,* 239–245.

Sculli, G., Fore, A., West, P., Neily, J., Mills, P., & Paull, D. (March 2013). Nursing crew resource management: A follow-up report from the veteran's health administration. *Journal of Nursing Administration, 43*(3), 122–126.

Sibbet, D., & O'Hara-Devereaux, M. (1991). The language of teamwork. *Healthcare Forum Journal, 34,* 27–30.

Smith, M., & Segaal, R. (2013). *Stress management.* Retrieved June 23, 2013 http://www.helpguide.org/mental/stress_management_relief_coping.htm#top.

Thurber, M. (1973). *Rules of the game.* San Francisco: Hawthorne-Stone Real Estate.

19

Workforce Engagement and Collective Action

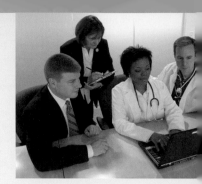

Richard G. Cuming, David Zambrana

Today's nurses expect and, in some situations, demand a greater voice in decisions involving their work life. These decisions involve both the context and the content of their work. Policy, education, and experience influence professional nurses to actively participate in decision making about work environment issues. Specifically, participation in decisions regarding practice is an appropriate expectation of a professional nurse. Collective action is one mechanism available to achieve that participation. Understanding collective action is critical if nurses' efforts to shape the practice environment are to be successful. The manager can capitalize on collective action to accomplish positive outcomes.

LEARNING OUTCOMES

- Distinguish the differences between the role of leaders and followers and the role followership has in collective action.
- Evaluate how key characteristics of selected collective action strategies apply in the workplace through shared governance, workplace advocacy, and collective bargaining.
- Distinguish between the rights of individuals included in collective bargaining contracts and the rights of at-will employees.
- Compare traditional bargaining practices with the contemporary approach, interest-based problem solving (IBPS).
- Evaluate decision-making strategies for their effectiveness within diverse workplace environments.
- Evaluate how participation of direct care nurses in decision making relates to job satisfaction and improved patient outcomes.
- Analyze the influence of culture on the selection of a governance model or model of care delivery.

KEY TERMS

at-will employee	followership	right to work
collective action	governance	role model
collective bargaining	interest-based problem solving	shared governance
culture	Institute for Healthcare	subculture
empowerment	Improvement (IHI)	whistleblower
engagement	mentor	workplace advocacy

THE CHALLENGE

Violet Rhagnanan-Kramer, MSN, RN, NE-BC
Nurse Manager, Neuroscience Intensive Care Unit, Jackson
    Memorial Hospital, Miami, Florida

Rising to the nurse manager position from a frontline role had both advantages and challenges. Adjusting to the role, building relationships, and setting expectations were top priorities. Gaining trust, support, and engagement from the staff was important for me to create the necessary changes in the unit. Among the many challenges were pressure ulcer rates above the national average. I needed to implement a plan to improve the quality of care and decrease unit-acquired pressure ulcers in a neuroscience intensive care unit. Holding staff accountable to high-quality patient care was a goal I had to accomplish as a new nurse manager. I had to decide how to go about this.

What do you think you would do if you were this nurse?

INTRODUCTION

The excitement of beginning a career in nursing or assuming the position of a manager is balanced by events taking place in health care and the effect of these events on nursing, nurses, and health systems. The knowledge gained in the nursing profession provides a background for considering issues within health care and factors that promote or inhibit the achievement of professional nursing practice.

Nurses are deeply involved in the complex clinical problems of individuals, families, and communities because nursing practice requires the acquisition, synthesis, and retrieval of knowledge to provide competent nursing care. Having the time and resources to engage in high-level preparation for quality and competent care can be achieved through the collective actions of nurses.

COLLECTIVE ACTION

Collective action is defined as activities that are undertaken by a group of people who have common interests. Collective action is a benign phrase; it refers to many aspects of daily life, including work. When parishioners contribute to a mission, that is the result of collective action. When nurses work to achieve Magnet™ status, that is the result of collective action. When patient care is delivered in hospitals 24 hours per day, that is the result of the collective action of shifts of nurses. Collective action aids nurses in advocating for patients, families, and communities in the healthcare and political arenas.

The collective action of nurses requires a level of independence during the shift and interdependence among shifts and with other healthcare professionals. Nurses learn quickly to rely on their colleagues but have been less comfortable with formal collectives than some other occupational groups. Several factors may contribute to this discomfort. Chief among those factors are gender, career focus, and view of power. Women have had less experience in working and playing within a team structure than have men. Before Title IX (before 1972), few girls participated in competitive team sports. In addition, historically, many women, including nurses, viewed employment as a job rather than a career. For those individuals, the time to work with others to achieve common goals deprived them of personal time.

Understanding power and learning how to use it are essential for nurses to influence practice, their work environments, and public policies that affect health. Historically, nursing was characterized as an "oppressed group" (Roberts, 2000). The "good" nurse was considered obedient. The Nightingale Pledge reinforced obedience: "With loyalty will I endeavor to aid the physician in his work ..." (Dock & Stewart, 1920). This obedience or acquiescence to authority appears to have been transferred to other authority figures, including but not limited to hospital administrators.

Historically, Minarik and Catramabone (1998) described four main purposes of collective participation for nurses: (1) promote the practice of professional nursing, (2) establish and maintain standards of care, (3) allocate resources effectively and efficiently, and (4) create satisfaction and support in the practice environment. Collective action helps define and sustain individual nurses in achieving these purposes. In the absence of collective action, the average individual has limited influence in achieving his or her purpose. Many children learned the strength and value of collective action early in life as siblings banded together to make a request to their parents. The same strategy has probably served in an organization when, together, a group of peers makes a point or pleads a case. Nurses have identified practice concerns and have joined together to bring about change in numerous practice settings.

Collective action can result in an empowered workforce made up of engaged employees. When large numbers of nurses in a common setting are engaged in the practice environment, the results are impressive: improved work life, reduced nurse turnover, an improved relationship with management, improved patient care, and increased patient satisfaction (McDowell et al., 2010). Nurse managers should actively work toward creating practice environments that promote staff engagement. This is accomplished by leader behaviors that encourage participative decision making, display confidence in employees, and promote autonomy (Hauck, Quinn Griffin, & Fitzpatrick, 2011).

The strategies for developing networks, creating a collective voice, and cultivating a collective require strong leaders and a broad followership. Leaders and followers have separate and distinct roles. Those roles are complementary—each requires the other. The relationship is interdependent. Followers and leaders also share many characteristics. Successful people move easily between the roles of follower and leader.

Though the knowledge and skills of followers may differ from those of the leader, they are not less. Leaders and followers are knowledgeable of the context and content of their practice. Followers are active, involved participants committed to an agreed-upon agenda. They are loyal and supportive to the individual who is setting the pace and the agenda. Good leaders will need good followers to accomplish goals. The nurse who becomes a leader finds that the absence of followers is personally painful.

EXERCISE 19-1

Identify two groups in which you have been a leader (e.g., school, church, sports, clubs, and work). Identify two groups in which you have been a follower. How did your role as a leader differ from your role as a follower? List the skills you used in each role.

Changes in an initiative or an agenda may result in today's leader being tomorrow's follower. The opposite may also be applicable: today's follower may be tomorrow's leader. The change may result from the context of the situation. In the operating room, the surgeon is the acknowledged leader and the anesthesiologist follows that lead with respect to the extent of the anesthesia. If the patient's condition changes, the anesthesiologist becomes the leader and the surgeon may simply step away from the table, an overt act that demonstrates a change in leadership. As healthcare consumers and participants, we salute the clarity.

Informed followers are not submissive participants blindly following a cultist personality. They are effective group members, not "groupies." They are skilled in group dynamics and accountable for their actions. They are willing and able to question, debate, compromise, collaborate, and act. Box 19-1 lists the traits of a good follower.

BOX 19-1   TRAITS OF A GOOD FOLLOWER

- Trustworthy
- Dependable
- Excellent Communicator and Listener
- Team Player
- Courage of Convictions
- Collaborator
- Questioner

From Kouzes, J.M., & Posner, B.Z. (2012). *The leadership challenge* (5th ed.). San Francisco, CA: Jossey-Bass.

Collective action provides a mechanism for achieving professional practice through greater participation in decision making. Porter-O'Grady (2013, p. vii) stated, "Preparation for the leadership role in nursing cannot simply be a unilateral process. Nurses must, in good measure, join in a common effort to advance the profession keeping in mind the best interests of those they serve." The governance structure provides the framework for participation. Participation in decision making regarding one's practice is an appropriate expectation for professional nurses, provides for greater autonomy and authority over practice decisions, contributes to supporting the professional nurse, and is a major component of job satisfaction (Kramer et al., 2008; Pittman, 2007). The privilege and the obligation to participate are inherent in the discipline of nursing. Consistent with the *Code of Ethics for Nurses* (American Nurses Association [ANA], 2010), members of the discipline participate based on their competence. Although nurses are expected to be informed, active participants, not all nurses wish to participate in decisions. For these nurses, going to work and doing their assigned job may fulfill their expectations. They may not perceive themselves as being in a subordinate position, or if they do, it is not a concern for them. Their orientation is to serve the care recipient and to be loyal to the organization. For these individuals, asserting the right and responsibility to participate in decisions may be considered disrespectful to the organization's policies or to the physician, or they may be energy-draining. However, for the professional nurse, participation in practice-related decisions is critical to quality patient care, is expected by society, and is essential to autonomy for nursing. Today's healthcare environment demands that nurses exercise the four key historical concepts identified by Lewis and Batey (1982): responsibility, authority, autonomy, and accountability.

Responsibility

The history of nursing provides evidence of nurses accepting responsibility or the "charge to act." Historically, this charge took the form of unquestioningly and meticulously following the physician's orders and hospital procedures. The "good" nurse rendered disclosure at the convenience of the physician and management. Today, healthcare organizations achieving Magnet™ recognition are characterized by the control of nursing practice by nurses. Nursing and individual nurses must have the power to control practice. The recognition of credentialing, especially certification, has contributed to the exercise of expert power by nurses.

Authority

Authority based on preparation and experience suggests a departure from the tradition of delegating authority to individual nurses based on the physician's or nurse manager's knowledge of the nurse—knowledge that too often was based on personal characteristics, not clinical competence. That statement does not denigrate the collegial relationship between and among nurses and physicians, relationships that are based on mutual respect and trust. Patient care improves when these relationships exist. Authority suggests that nurses use the power of their professional status to act in behalf of the best interest of patients.

Autonomy

Autonomy, the freedom to make independent decisions is critical to the control of nursing practice. To maximize the clinical effectiveness of registered nurses (RNs), they must have autonomy consistent with their scope of practice. Multiple studies demonstrate that a healthcare organization that provides a climate in which nurses have authority and autonomy has better patient outcomes, retains nurses at a higher rate, is more cost-effective, and has evidence of greater patient satisfaction than an organization in which such a climate does not exist (Aiken, Clarke, Sloane, Sochalski, & Silber, 2002; Dunton, Gajewski, Klaus, & Pierson, 2007). Nurse involvement in decision making contributes to higher levels of job satisfaction for the nurse and higher levels of satisfaction with care for the patient and positively influences health outcomes. When nurses share their individual decisions with each other, they help others move toward more expert practice either through acquiring new knowledge or through challenging the decisions made.

Autonomy encourages innovation and increases productivity. Nurse managers have influence in this area of working with staff. Historically, Mrayyan (2004) found that nurses in an international study reported that the three most important variables in increasing nurse autonomy were supportive management, education, and experience. Specific managerial actions were defined as elements of interactions with others, especially when conflict was involved. Helping nurses communicate and supporting them in dealing with conflict aid nurses to describe themselves as having more autonomy.

The Future of Nursing: Leading Change, Advancing Health (Institute of Medicine [IOM], 2011) recommended that nurses practice to the full extent of their scope. In the past, nurses have not availed themselves of their potential for autonomy. Using the research that backed this IOM report, nurses are poised to expend their autonomy rapidly. The timing couldn't be better! The United States is interested in reshaping how care is delivered and in creating new, cost-effective strategies. The work of the **Institute for Healthcare Improvement,** through Transforming Care at the Bedside (TCAB), has shown how sincerely nurses work to create new and improved ways to provide best decisions for patient care.

By supporting unit-level change without complex organizational structure approvals, change occurred more quickly and efficiently and patients benefited. "Stopping the line," a concept from automobile manufacturing, translates to time-outs in health care. Being able to stop activities to be clear about what action is best is an example of autonomous decision making to prevent harm. Leaders, managers, and followers must work together to ensure an environment that supports this action.

Accountability

Accountability focuses the organization and all its members on the purposes and the outcomes of their collective activities. Accountability requires ownership. Although Porter-O'Grady and Malloch (2010) made many points about accountability, the following are six critical considerations in shared governance:

- Defined by the person in the role
- Defined by role, not job or task
- Based on outcomes
- Set in advance
- Linked to results
- Has observable processes

The value of process is determined by the extent to which individuals observe a particular protocol while accomplishing a goal. Accountability focuses on the achievement of the specified outcome. This shift in thinking has had a tremendous effect on healthcare

reimbursement. An example of the shift is evident in patient education. Initialing a form to indicate that patient teaching has occurred is no longer acceptable. The criteria now expect that the patient's behavior has changed. Outcomes have overtaken process in providing evidence! To achieve positive outcomes within an organization, shared accountability is critical. "When responsible adults refuse to share accountability, it poisons human relationships, corrupts professions, and makes self-esteem impossible" (Kupperschmidt, 2004, p. 115).

EXERCISE 19-2

Review the American Nurses Association's (ANA) position statement on "Take Action on Safe Staffing," at *www.nursingworld. org*. From the perspective of a direct care nurse, how do you feel about your professional organization's call to action regarding safe staffing? As a nurse manager, would you have the same perspective? Why or why not?

GOVERNANCE

Nursing **governance** is the methodology or system by which a department of nursing controls and directs the formulation and the administration of nursing policy. Organizational structure provides a framework for fulfilling the organization's mission. Organizational charts show the relationship among and between roles. The structure of the organization and the relationship among the components of the structure are influenced by the individuals selected to interpret and implement the organization's philosophy. A particular form of governance evolves from the mission and values of the organization and the relationships among and between its components. Thus managers and leaders who enact the mission and values on a daily basis support nursing more openly. To paraphrase an adage, behavior speaks louder and has more clout than organizational charts.

Nurses have multiple strategies at their disposal to achieve collective action; three prevalent ones are shared governance, workplace advocacy, and collective bargaining. These strategies are not mutually exclusive. As noted, governance is influenced by the context within which the organizational culture is embedded. Often the culture itself dictates the avenue of collective action.

The **culture** of the geographic area influences the organizational culture and the selected governance structure. For example, in **right-to-work** states, collective bargaining may be tolerated more than supported by nurses and administration. Although mobility and the mass media have diluted the "purity" of geographic cultures, it is prudent to acknowledge how deeply embedded these cultural influences are within the fabric of American society.

When a **subculture** is clearly rooted in the mission of the organization (e.g., delivery of quality care in a cost-effective environment), the possibility of genuine negotiation or problem solving is enhanced. A subculture has its own unique and distinctive features, even as other features overlap with those of the larger culture. Members may adhere to values that are specific to their group while espousing values of the larger society. The presence of congruent subcultures supports healthy relationships. Healthy relationships are an important variable in the development of a strong internal governance structure capable of supporting a professional practice environment that works well for everyone involved.

Nurses and administrators are often members of separate subcultures. This phenomenon should not be given a negative connotation. Several factors may increase the distinct ideologies of the two groups, including the existence of a distant corporate structure and the presence of a union. Both factors may be considered external tensions. By tradition, decision making in the United States has been centralized at the top administrative level. The tendency is to increase the concentration of decision making during economic downturns and the pressures inherent in maintaining a healthy "bottom line." Actions are taken to avoid risk. However, history shows that broader input, not less, is important during these times.

When efforts have been made to address nurses' perceptions about job satisfaction, the relationship between nursing and the top administration of a hospital has been affected. Work environment factors that have a direct impact on nurses' job satisfaction and the ability to influence patient care include supervisory support in patient care decisions and the provision of adequate staffing to provide quality care, positive working relationships with physicians and nurses, and a clear philosophy of nursing; all of these factors are influenced by the relationship between nurses and

administration (Cummings et al., 2008; Manojlovich, 2005; Mrayyan, 2004).

> **EXERCISE 19-3**
>
> Identify four factors in your practice (experience) that contribute to job satisfaction. Compare your responses with those of three practicing nurses who are not supervisors and three practicing nurses who are supervisors. Are your factors similar to the responses of others? Are you surprised by the responses?

In today's work environment, nurses expect a motivating, satisfying work environment that includes support for decision making. Many nurses today are unwilling to remain outside the decision-making loop. Work redesign efforts to increase productivity and lower costs have contributed to increased tension regarding the role of nursing and nurses in decision making. Evolving or creating a system that incorporates others in the decision-making process may be difficult for many individuals in upper-management positions. High-performing organizations that provide quality health care create climates that provide for participation by all stakeholders. Each stakeholder shares responsibility and risk, and that requires optimism and trust.

Contractual models allow nurses to form an organization and contract with the healthcare organization to provide nursing services. A contractual model can be characterized as a self-governance model as opposed to shared governance. Nurses become contract providers instead of employees. Historically, nurses were direct contractors as private-duty nurses before becoming hospital employees.

Shared Governance

Shared governance is described as a democratic, egalitarian concept; it is a dynamic process resulting from shared decision making and accountability (Porter-O'Grady, 2009). According to Porter-O'Grady, Hawkins, and Parker (1997), basic principles of shared governance include partnerships, equity, accountability, and ownership. It is more accurate to say that shared governance *demands* participation in decision making rather than provides for participation. Characteristics of self-governance that empowered nurses were career ladders, access to power, participation in decision making, recognition of accomplishments, and evidence-based practice (Kramer et al., 2008) (see the Research Perspective on p. 352).

RESEARCH PERSPECTIVE

Resource: Barden, A.M., Quinn Griffin, M.T., Donahue. M., & Fitzpatrick, J.J. (2011). Shared governance and empowerment in registered nurses working in a hospital setting. *Nursing Administration Quarterly, 35*(3), 212-218.

This study was conducted in a tertiary care hospital where 348 nurses working across 13 units were invited to participate. Shared governance was in place. The purpose of the study was to determine relationships between how governance was seen and if nurses believed they were empowered. This was a descriptive, correlational study. The sample was 158 RNS. As expected, most were female, in staff positions, and working full-time. The findings indicated a significant relationship existed between perceptions of shared governance and empowerment. Specifically, "access to opportunity" was rated highest, followed by information, support, and resources.

Implications for Practice

Shared governance is critical to a professional practice environment. When nurses experienced shared governance, they described themselves as empowered. In fact, as the view of shared governance increased, so did the perception of empowerment. Nurse leaders would be proactive to assist with empowerment through instituting and supporting shared governance.

Before direct care nurses can be fully engaged, nurse managers need to feel empowered to lead. Nurse administrators can help empower nurse managers by displaying support, improving communication, and providing necessary resources (Regan & Rodriguez, 2011). Once managers are fully engaged, direct care nurses are provided an environment where they are more likely to engage themselves. Consequently, patients benefit from the positive effects of an engaged workforce (Trus, Razbadauskas, Doran, & Suominen, 2012).

Through numerous reports and stories about organizations that have experienced the Magnet™ journey, direct care nurses have praised the quality of their direct involvement through shared governance. In addition, nurses favor work and learning (consistent with the IOM report [2003]) that is interdisciplinary and patient focused.

Some organizations mislabel their governance structures. Although structures may be called "shared governance," they possess few of the characteristics outlined by those who are recognized as experts on the topic. In addition, many organizations have developed thinly veiled mechanisms designed to preclude

nurses from participating in collective action. In today's competitive environment, nurses must be aware of potential implications of various approaches. Professional-practice climates recognize individual and team performance. Increasingly, nurses are seeking organizations that provide professional-practice climates, ones that have effective activities, not just effective documents. Thus, when filling any new, non-entry position external to nursing, wise decision makers include nurses among those being considered.

Workplace Advocacy

Workplace advocacy is an umbrella term encompassing activities within the practice setting. The choice of advocacy to reflect the framework in which nurses control the practice of nursing is consistent with the goals of the profession. Workplace advocacy includes an array of activities undertaken to address the challenges faced by nurses in their practice settings. The focus of these activities is on career development, employment opportunities, terms and conditions of employment, employment rights and protections, control of practice, labor-management relations, occupational health and safety, and employee assistance. The objective of workplace advocacy is to equip nurses to practice in a rapidly changing environment. Advocacy occurs within a framework of mutuality, facilitation, protection, and coordination.

Workplace advocacy must be practiced by both staff and leaders to be effective. For example, healthy workplaces don't just happen. They require active participation of all members of the work unit to create conditions where it is safe to speak up, where hazards can be addressed quickly, where incivility is not tolerated, and where the diversity of staff is supported rather than tolerated. Just as the manager needs to be aware of when a staff member is too tired to work, so too must the staff member acknowledge that condition and make the decision to decline additional work, as an example. Another example of workplace advocacy that might seem to be more of a budget function than a workplace advocacy issue is when a team of nurses explores the best equipment, strategies, and approaches for managing such functions as turning, transferring, and lifting obese patients. Proactively (or at least as quickly as possible) addressing such issues improves the workplace and supports nurses. In turn, patients benefit.

Providing Support for Making and Implementing Decisions

The support needed to make and implement decisions is achieved through role models, mentors, and empowerment. Role models may include the nurse who has excellent clinical skills in assessment. Similarly, observing someone who is skilled in assertive communication, transforming an explosive situation into a positive interaction, is impressive. The implementation of a primary mentorship program for nurses may contribute to the development of these and other skills. Mentoring is a relationship between two individuals, usually with one being more experienced than the other. A mentoring relationship is an ongoing "hands-on" process. Individuals who have experienced a successful mentorship have identified positive, frequently occurring behaviors that characterized their mentor. These behaviors include trust and the opportunity to make decisions that derive from that trust. The value to the organization is in the outcome: the individual will make better decisions that will well serve the organization, the nurse, and the patient.

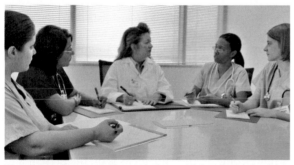

The support needed to make and implement decisions is achieved through role models, mentors, and empowerment.

EXERCISE 19-4

List the characteristics that you would want a mentor to possess. If you have identified a person you would want as a mentor, ask if he or she is willing to mentor you. Identify factors that are contributors and barriers to your seeking a mentorship relationship with the individual. Consider ways that you can address these factors.

Empowerment, or supporting other nurses, is a complex process. Nurses generally want to work hard, continue to learn, perform well, and be involved in the decision-making process. Managers and administrators who support these efforts are empowering nurses and enhancing professionalism and autonomy. An example of empowering nurses involves the act of documenting an unsafe assignment. Accepting an unsafe assignment or refusing an assignment is difficult for nurses—both those nurses at the beginning of their careers and those who are experienced. Critical elements to note are date, unit, assignment, staff available, rationale for objections, and documentation of notification of supervisor. Accurate, concise, and clear documentation can assist the nurse manager by providing a source of data necessary to support the preparation of their budgets and to support the documenters of such occurrences. Many assignments are classified as unsafe because of a lack of personnel and a lack of training of the existing personnel; therefore nurses need to be prepared to respond when an assignment is inappropriate (see the Research Perspective).

 RESEARCH PERSPECTIVE

Resource: Armstrong, K., Laschinger, H., & Wong, C. (2009). Workplace empowerment and Magnet™ hospital characteristics as predictors of patient safety climate. *Journal of Nursing Care Quality, 24*(1), 55-62.

This study was conducted to examine the variables of workplace empowerment and Magnet™ hospital characteristics as predictors of patient safety climate. The framework used to guide the study was Kanter's theoretical model of workplace empowerment in nursing that has linked empowerment in nursing to control over practice, job satisfaction, work productivity, burnout, and organizational commitment. Three hundred randomly selected registered nurses employed in acute care hospital organizations were surveyed about conditions of work effectiveness, practice environment, and safety climate. Results showed moderate to strong correlations between empowerment and Magnet™ hospital characteristics, empowerment and patient safety climate, and Magnet™ characteristics and patient safety climate. The findings support the Kanter theoretical model of workplace empowerment in nursing and suggest that nurses who feel empowered in their workplace will perceive the patient safety climate as positive.

Implications for Practice
Nurses who feel empowered to make decisions and implement patient care strategies may feel that the care environment on the unit is safer and more effective and have higher ratings of job satisfaction. Nurse managers should support nurses to make decisions over their practice and include nursing staff in unit-based plans and activities that affect the work and practice environment.

Empowering nurses is important. Yet, in reality no one person empowers another. What "empowerment" does is create the conditions where a person feels safe to take appropriate risks. Powerless nurses feel more depersonalization in the work environment and are less satisfied with their jobs (Laschinger, Finegan, Shamian, & Wilk, 2004; Leiter & Laschinger, 2006).

COLLECTIVE BARGAINING

Collective bargaining is the performance of the mutual obligation of the employer and representatives of the employees to meet at reasonable times and confer in good faith with respect to wages, hours, and other terms and conditions of employment or the negotiation of any agreement or any question arising from

those terms and conditions. The purpose of collective bargaining or unionization by nurses (Box 19-2) is to secure reasonable and satisfactory conditions of employment, including the right to participate in decisions regarding their practice. Although it is possible to bargain collectively without a union, the union model is commonly used.

The bargaining process has historically been conducted through a series of group-specific positions that did not take into account the opposing party in any way. In 2003, Kaiser Permanente (KP) and the Coalition of Kaiser Permanente Unions (CKPU) underwent a process to transform their labor management process. They adopted the use of interest-based problem solving (IBPS) as the basis for its collective bargaining negotiations. Interest-based negotiations require an understanding of the mutual interests of both parties and use problem-solving tools to prevent positional conflicts and to ultimately achieve better outcomes for all interested parties (Fonstand, McKersie, & Eaton, 2004). Unlike traditional bargaining processes, where each "side" presents demands, IBPS starts with the goal of identifying problems and the related interests. For example, if specific staffing patterns are proposed, they are generally met with resistance. Yet both management and unions are interested in safe care. Focusing on mutual gains rather than differences reframes the discussion. Additionally, because the focus is on "we have a problem we need to solve" rather than "I have a demand you must meet," issues can be addressed in greater depth so that various views are explored. A key strategy of using the past to make examples of the other party being wrong is unwelcome. Rather, the focus is on the present and how to move forward.

Changes in labor law have had a direct impact on the level of union activity in the healthcare sector. The federal role in labor relations is a dynamic, evolving one. The 1935 Wagner Act (National Labor Relations Act) established election procedures for employees to be able to choose their collective bargaining representatives freely. Two years later, the ANA included provisions for improving nurses' work and professional lives. The 1947 Taft-Hartley Act placed curbs on some union activity and excluded employees of not-for-profit hospitals from coverage. The Labor Management Reporting and Disclosure Act of 1959, also known as the Landrum-Griffin Act, provides greater internal democracy within unions. The 1974

BOX 19-2   UNIONIZATION

In non-healthcare industries, unionization is acknowledged as a usual and expected business practice. Improved communication and goodwill cannot eliminate the gap between labor and management. Cooperation between management and labor will remain an illusion unless or until there is sharing of responsibility, power, and profits (Levitan & Johnson, 1983). If cooperation and trust exist between the union and the company, the members of the union will understand when the company is experiencing financial difficulties and management will understand when members of the union experience difficulties. In 1996, the Malden Mills continued to assist employees from company funds when the company could not produce popular Polartec items because of a fire. In 2001, unions representing 1200 workers voted to accept a reduction in pay and benefits in an effort to keep Freightliner in Portland, Oregon (Hunsberger, 2001).

Heckscher (1996) suggested that the union model is outdated because of trends that have made the public policy framework of unionization less useful. In nursing, Porter-O'Grady (2001) takes a much different perspective by identifying it is simply a different reality. Through partnering, the formal union contract "advances the practice of managing well and maintains the foundation of good management" (p. 32). Union activity in nursing and in health care has grown in the past 30 years and has been stimulated by healthcare reorganization, work redesign, and changes in patient care delivery models. Some of the major issues that have led to increased union activity in nursing are as follows:

- Lack of professional autonomy and professional practice models
- Inadequate staffing and unqualified caregivers
- The absence of procedures for reporting of unsafe work environments and poor quality care
- Mandatory overtime and work overload
- Low wages and poor benefits

amendments to the Taft-Hartley Act removed the exemption of not-for-profit hospitals, and employees of these types of organizations have the same rights as industrial workers to join together and form labor unions. The removal of the exemption for not-for-profit hospitals created a frenzy of activity as traditional industrial unions targeted healthcare facilities. The National Labor Relations Board (NLRB) administers the National Labor Relations Act. State laws further define labor law.

Why has an increase in organizing nurses and other healthcare professionals occurred? Health care is a "hot" topic at the state and federal levels. Pittman (2007) found that nurses, both represented by collective bargaining and not represented, were generally satisfied with their work, but represented nurses were more satisfied with regard to compensation (see the following related Literature Perspective). The morning newspaper, nightly news, and a continuous parade

of news magazines have featured countless articles related to health and illness. One may paraphrase Willie Sutton when he was asked why he robbed banks: "That is where the money is." Why organize nurses and other healthcare workers? Because that is where potential members are.

As technology replaces unskilled workers, a smaller pool of workers is available for trade-union organizing. Declining union membership has been the catalyst for unions to explore other membership bases. For example, according to the U.S. Bureau of Labor Statistics (2014), the number of wage and salary workers belonging to a union is approximately 11.3%, down from 11.8% the year before. With numerous groups seeking to represent nurses, nurses seeking collective bargaining should carefully consider the representing agent. (See Box 19-3 for suggested screening criteria.)

Traditional industrial unions are increasingly seeking opportunities to represent nurses for the purpose of collective bargaining and to speak for nursing with boards of nursing, regulatory agencies, and legislatures. Organizing nurses and other healthcare workers for the purpose of collective bargaining is very attractive because of the large numbers of people involved and the decrease in organizing in other sectors. In addition, nurses and other healthcare workers have a low rate of unionization. According to the Bureau of Labor Statistics (2014) (*www.bls.gov/news.release/pdf/union2.pdf*), approximately 12.5% of healthcare occupations were unionized.

Historically, nurses were reluctant to be identified with unions; however, that view has changed. Working together in a cooperative, collaborative manner is important for the safety and quality of care, especially when strain occurs between management and nurses.

 LITERATURE PERSPECTIVE

Resource: Porter, C.A., Kolcaba, K., McNulty, R., & Fitzpatrick, J.J. (2010). The effect of a nursing labor management partnership on nurse turnover and satisfaction. *Journal of Nursing Administration, 40(5)*, 205-210.

This study examined the effect of a hospital-based nursing labor management partnership (NLMP) on nurse turnover and satisfaction. Although these variables have been correlated to work environment, they had never been empirically correlated to an NLMP until this study was published. This study used a quantitative, quasi-experimental design in a large Magnet™-designated urban academic medical center in the Northeastern United States. The organization's nursing workforce consisted of 2200 RNs, of which 2107 were members of the nursing union. The nursing management and union leadership identified that by working together they were able to have a positive effect on both groups, leaving more time to focus on patient care and mutual goals. The results of the study revealed a 3.1% reduction in RN turnover, from 9.9% in 2005 to 6.8% in 2008; and a *T* score improvement in satisfaction of 3.9 from 57.9 in 2005 to 61.77 in 2008.

Implications for Practice
The development of an NLMP is an approach that can be used in most professional nursing environments. The belief is that effective leadership and an engaged nursing workforce can affect outcomes. This process recognizes nurses as leaders on all levels and provides formal and informal mechanisms for professional nurses to work together to achieve shared goals through collaboration and shared decision making or decentralized decision making (both terms can be used interchangeably).

BOX 19-3 SUGGESTED CRITERIA FOR SELECTING A BARGAINING UNIT

- A strong commitment to nursing practice, legislation, regulation, and education
- A well-prepared practice, policy, and labor staff; a minimum of a bachelor's degree in nursing
- Representative of those the bargaining unit represents in both gender and ethnic makeup
- National scope and local implementation
- Control by individual members over bargaining unit activities

Nurses have a legal right to bargain. The American Hospital Association has spent millions of dollars challenging the appropriateness of all-RN bargaining units or a unit separate from other organized employees. In a 1991 unanimous opinion, the Supreme Court of the United States upheld the NLRB's ruling that provides for RN-only units. This decision was critical for nursing. At stake was the ability of nurses to control nursing practice and the quality of patient care. Employees, including nurses, must be accorded workplace rights and the protection that allows them to practice. Nurses must have the freedom to do what the profession and their licensure status require them to do.

Labeling all RNs as supervisors is a second challenge to the right of nurses to organize. RNs monitor and assess patients as a part of their professional practice, not as a statutory supervisor within the definition of the National Labor Relations Act. A 1996 NLRB ruling held that RNs were not statutory supervisors and were protected by federal labor law; the decision was upheld in 1997 by the U.S. Court of Appeals for the Ninth Circuit (Nguyen, 1997). However, a 2001 Supreme Court decision (*National Labor Relations Board v. Kentucky River Community Care, Inc.*, 2001) upheld a lower court's decision to classify RNs as supervisors, though this decision was later appealed.

Nurses as Knowledge Workers

The change from producing a product to providing a service has many implications for management and labor. In the past, employees in manufacturing were treated like interchangeable cogs: when a cog was broken, it was replaced. A large pool of unskilled workers was available to step forward in the steel mill, the coal mine, and the shop floor. The move from an industrial model in society requires a "knowledge worker." The unskilled worker of yesterday did not have a high school diploma. Today, knowledge workers may have multiple college degrees and certifications. When knowledge workers unionize, they develop organizations that are more similar to associations than traditional industrial unions. They become involved in activities such as lobbying and coalition building. Based on nurses' current roles and the expectations we have for what nurses do, nurses are knowledge workers. As the knowledge content of the work increases, the practice of the worker (nurse) is guided more by science than by procedure. Porter-O'Grady (2012) suggested that shared governance is a reframing of knowledge work.

The healthcare system is becoming increasingly complex, and healthcare consumers and payers are demanding high-quality care and best-in-class patient outcomes. All of this requires important and meaningful changes to the current system of nursing education. In the landmark report, *The Future of Nursing: Leading Change, Advancing Health,* the IOM (2011) called for America's nurses to achieve higher levels of education and training in an improved system that facilitates seamless academic progression. The committee responsible for the report recommended that by the year 2020, 80% of U.S. nurses be prepared at the BSN level (currently 50%). This recommendation reflects the expectation that nurses are knowledge workers.

Union or At-Will

The fear of arbitrary discipline and dismissal may be the catalyst for nurses to seek ways to protect themselves from what are perceived to be arbitrary actions. Nurses are seeking assistance from external sources in an effort to balance the assistance available to the organization's administrative personnel. A collective bargaining contract typically alters a balance of power. The discipline structure provided by contract

---

BOX 19-4   WHISTLEBLOWER PROTECTION

Whistleblowing *"refers to a warning issued by a current or former employee of an* organization to the public about a serious wrongdoing or danger created or concealed within the organization" (Hunt, 1995, p. 155). The 1989 Whistleblower Protection Act protects federal workers. The law does not cover the private sector. Some states have specific laws. Whistleblowers need to understand the consequences of action, and inaction, as the shield is an imperfect one (Solomon, 2004). Whistleblowing can result when the people in the administrative structure within an organization fail to hear and respond to issues employees deem as unsafe or illegal.

treats all employees in the same manner and may decrease the manager's flexibility in designing or selecting discipline. Although whistleblower legislation exists (Box 19-4), the current environment in health care places the at-will employee who voices concern about the quality of care in a vulnerable position. Managers of at-will employees have greater latitude in selecting disciplinary measures for specific infractions. State and federal laws do provide a level of protection; however, an at-will employee may be terminated at any time for any reason except discrimination. At-will employees, in essence, work at the will of the employer. Nurses in these positions need to know their rights and accountability.

Union contract language requires management to follow "due process" for represented employees. That is, management must provide a written statement outlining disciplinary charges, the penalty, and the reasons for the penalty. Management is required to maintain a record of attempts to counsel the employee. Employees have the right to defend themselves against charges and the opportunity to settle disagreements in a formal grievance hearing. They have the right to have their representative with them during the process. Management must prove that the employee is wrong or in error. Management maintains the record of counseling. The commitment to nursing requires the manager to be clear about the charge. Although all disciplinary charges are important, those directly related to patient care have a more critical dimension. Clarity in describing the situation is important because it affects patient care, the individual nurse, and nurse colleagues. In a nonunion environment, the burden of proof is generally on the employee.

Many nurses continue to be intimidated by those individuals who charge that "unions are unprofessional." A labor contract, a collective bargaining agreement/union contract, is unrelated to being professional. Sociologists have characterized the responsibilities of the professional as a respect for the duty to perform, respect for the duty to learn, respect for the public interest, and preservation and enhancement of the image (Moore, 1970). Many physicians and many faculty members have collective bargaining contracts. Why? They want to have greater control of

their practice, improve working conditions, and influence their compensation; and the culture of the organization and area support unionization as a strategy to meet those expectations. Contracts are a usual part of our current environment. It is ironic that a contract between an employer and employee is considered unusual. Replacing the adversarial system should be the goal of efforts to redesign the workplace. A new social order in the workplace must be based on a spirit of genuine cooperation between management and nurses.

EXERCISE 19-5

If you practice in a setting with a collective bargaining agreement, secure a copy. Identify the articles of this contract. Are they practice issues or economic issues? What is the relationship between the two? If you work in a setting that does not have a collective bargaining agreement, secure dispute resolution policies. Identify the areas that may be disputed. Are they practice issues or economic issues? What is the relationship between the two?

CONCLUSION

Nurses practice in multiple settings; some have collective bargaining (union) contracts, and others do not. Collective bargaining and non–collective bargaining environments espouse safe, quality care. Both environments exist within the context of state and federal laws. Professional practice models may exist in both environments. Nurses may feel valued in both environments, but there is a critical difference. A contract requires the employer to negotiate within a legally binding framework. Non–collective bargaining environments do not provide that structure.

The future may hold new relationships, and public policy may continue to include provisions that were formally negotiated through contracts. Nurses practice in highly competitive environments. Decision making is at the core of nursing practice. Nurse involvement in decision making contributes to higher levels of job satisfaction for the nurse and higher satisfaction with care for the patient, and it also has a positive influence on health outcomes. Nurses and those they serve benefit from collective action that uses a wide range of strategies.

THE SOLUTION

Using a collaborative approach to engage and empower the staff, pressure ulcer rates were shared with the team. The goal was to decrease our rates below the national benchmark. Armed with data, and recognizing that preventing hospital acquired pressure ulcers is nursing's responsibility, staff willingly participated in creating a corrective action plan. Several staff members became skin champions serving as experts on pressure ulcer prevention. A nurse donated a "Hotlist" board to the unit. The board was used to identify patients at high risk of developing pressure ulcers and interventions to prevent skin breakdown. Having the information and being encouraged to participate in correcting the problem was empowering for the staff. Staff were involved in setting the unit's goal. Sharing information was vital to achieving the successful outcome of near zero incidence

of pressure ulcers within 6 months, which has been sustained in the 4 years since then. Effective communication and articulating clear expectations helped guide the staff and empowered them to act and take responsibility for their nursing interventions. Having an engaged team resulted in high-quality outcomes, and patient and nurse satisfaction. Recognizing and celebrating their efforts communicated that their contributions are valued. The neuroscience ICU has maintained high-quality outcomes (near zero hospital-acquired pressure ulcers) over a 4-year period.

—*Violet Rhagnanan-Kramer*

Would this be a suitable approach for you? Why?

THE EVIDENCE

Collective action requires communication and commitment to the outcomes. Collective action by nurses in organizations seeking Magnet™ designation has been demonstrated effectively.

Collective action encompasses numerous strategies. Nurses involved in unions (a form of collective action) in their organizations describe their gains as positive and their losses as minimal.

Nurses who experience a sense of empowerment in the workplace perceive their organizations as providing safer care than those who do not experience this sense. Empowerment often derives from successful use of collective action.

WHAT NEW GRADUATES SAY

• Selecting the right place to work is critical. You want to have a voice in decisions about nursing; and you want to feel supported when you speak up.

• When a new policy is being considered, we [nurses] are asked for input. Sometimes we're even asked to propose the policy!

CHAPTER CHECKLIST

Collectively, nurses possess the knowledge, skills, abilities, and numbers to influence decisions. Collective action may take many forms. Geographic and organizational contexts influence the formal and informal structures in which nurses participate. An organization's structure establishes the parameters for participation in decision making. Managers establish the context for participation. The decision to organize for the purpose of collective bargaining is important for nurses and for the organization in which they practice. A level of tension exists when an external group becomes a part of an organization's decision-making processes. External groups may enter as a new management consultant, as a part of a merger, as a new owner, or as a union representing registered nurses. The acceptance and appreciation of the external

group are influenced by understanding the rationale for the group's entry and by the respect between the constituencies.

• Collective action
  • Responsibility
  • Authority
  • Autonomy
  • Accountability
• Governance
  • Shared governance
  • Workplace advocacy
  • Providing support for making and implementing decisions
• Collective bargaining
  • Nurses as knowledge workers
  • Union or at-will

TIPS FOR COLLECTIVE ACTION

- Direct care nurses and managers both need to be cognizant of the issues related to collective action and collective bargaining for both the individuals involved and the organization.
- Some states have laws that are more supportive of whistleblowing than others.
- Nurses interested in collective bargaining at their organizations need to be fully aware of what each union organization brings to the bargaining table

and how aware each union organization may or may not be of workplace issues for nurses.
- An understanding of the culture and the organization's approach to any collective action strategy is important for managers and staff.
- Where collective bargaining is the appropriate strategy, develop criteria for the selection of the appropriate collective bargaining agent.

REFERENCES

Aiken, L. H., Clarke, S. P., Sloane, D. M., Sochalski, J., & Silber, J. H. (2002). Hospital nursing staffing and patient mortality, nurse burnout and job dissatisfaction. *Journal of American Medical Association, 288*, 1987–1993.

American Nurses Association (ANA). (2010). *The code of ethics for nurses with interpretive statements*. Washington, DC: Author.

Armstrong, K., Laschinger, H., & Wong, C. (2009). Workplace empowerment and Magnet hospital characteristics as predictors of patient safety climate. *Journal of Nursing Care Quality, 24*(1), 55–62.

Barden, A. M., Quinn Griffin, M. T., Donahue, M., & Fitzpatrick, J. J. (2011). Shared governance and empowerment in registered nurses working in a hospital setting. *Nursing Administration Quarterly, 35*(3), 212–218.

Cummings, G. G., Olson, K., Hayduk, L., Bakker, D., Fitch, M., Green, E., et al. (2008). The relationship between nursing leadership and nurses' job satisfaction in Canadian oncology work environments. *Journal of Nursing Management, 16*, 508–518.

Dock, L., & Stewart, A. (1920). *A short history of nursing*. New York: Putnam & Sons.

Dunton, N., Gajewski, B., Klaus, S., & Pierson, B. (2007). The relationship of nursing workforce characteristics to patient outcomes. *OJIN: The Online Journal of Issues in Nursing, 12*(3). Retrieved December 12, 2008, from www.medscape.com/viewarticle/569394.

Fonstand, N. O., McKersie, R. B., & Eaton, S. C. (2004). Case analysis: Interest-based negotiations in a transformed labor-management setting. *Negotiation Journal, 5–11.*

Hauck, A., Quinn Griffin, M., & Fitzpatrick, J. (2011). Structural empowerment and anticipated turnover among critical care nurses. *Journal of Nursing Management, 19*, 269–276.

Heckscher, D. (1996). *The new unionism: Employee involvement in the changing corporation*. Ithaca, New York: Cornell University Press.

Hunsberger, G. (October 1, 2001). Freightliner union approves reduced pay. *The Oregonian.*

Hunt, G. (1995). *Whistleblowing in the health service: Accountability, law and professional practice*. London: Edward Arnold.

Institute of Medicine (IOM). (2003). *Health professions education: A bridge to quality*. Washington, DC: The National Academies.

Institute of Medicine (IOM). (2011). *The future of nursing: Leading change, advancing health*. Washington, DC: The National Academies.

Kouzes, J. M., & Posner, B. Z. (2012). *The leadership challenge* (5th ed.). San Francisco, CA: Jossey-Bass.

Kramer, M., Schmalenberg, C., Maguire, P., Brewer, B. B., Burke, R., Chmielewski, L., et al. (2008). Structures and practices enabling staff nurses to control their practice. *Western Journal of Nursing Research, 30*(5), 539–559.

Kupperschmidt, B. R. (2004). Making a case for shared accountability. *Journal of Nursing Administration, 34*(3), 114–116.

Laschinger, H. K. S., Finegan, J., Shamian, J., & Wilk, P. (2004). A longitudinal analysis of the impact of workplace empowerment on work satisfaction. *Journal of Organizational Behavior, 25*(1), 527–545.

Leiter, M. P., & Laschinger, H. K. S. (2006). Relationships of work and practice environment to professional burnout. *Nursing Research, 55*(2), 137–146.

Levitan, S., & Johnson, C. (1983). Labor and management: The illusion of cooperation. *Harvard Business Review, 61*, 8–16.

Lewis, F., & Batey, M. (1982). Clarifying autonomy and accountability in nursing service, Part 2. *Journal of Nursing Administration, 12*(10), 10–15.

Manojlovich, M. (2005). The effect of nursing leadership on hospital nurses' professional practice behaviors. *Journal of Nursing Administration, 35*(7/8), 363–371.

McDowell, J. B., Williams, R. L., Kautz, D. D., Madden, P., Heilig, A., & Thompson, A. (2010). Shared governance: 10 years later. *Nursing Management, 41*(7), 32–37.

Minarik, P., & Catramabone, C. (1998). Collective participation in workforce decision-making. In D. Mason, D. Talbot, & J. Leavitt (Eds.), *Policy and politics for nurses: Action and change in the workplace, government, organizations and community*. (3rd ed.) Philadelphia: Saunders.

Moore, W. (1970). *The professions: Roles and rules*. New York: Russell Sage Foundation.

Mrayyan, M. T. (2004). Nurses' autonomy: Influence of nurse managers' actions. *Journal of Advanced Nursing, 45*(3), 326–336.

National Labor Relations Board v. Kentucky River Community Care, Inc., 121 S. Ct. 1861; No. 99–1815 (Argued February 21, 2001; decided May 29, 2001).

Nguyen, B. (1997). Long-awaited Providence ruling upholds right of charge nurses to bargain. *The American Nurse, 29*(1), 14.

Pittman, J. (2007). Registered nurse job satisfaction and collective bargaining unit membership status. *The Journal of Nursing Administration, 37*(10), 471–476.

Porter, C. A., Kolcaba, K., McNulty, R., & Fitzpatrick, J. J. (2010). The effect of a nursing labor management partnership on nurse turnover and satisfaction. *Journal of Nursing Administration, 40*(5), 205–210.

Porter-O'Grady, T. (2001). Collective bargaining: The union as partner. *Nursing Management, 32*, 30–32.

Porter-O'Grady, T. (2009). *Interdisciplinary shared governance: Integrating practice, transforming health care* (2nd ed.). Boston: Jones & Bartlett Publishers.

Porter-O'Grady, T. (2012). Reframing knowledge work: Shared governance in the postdigital age. *Creative Nursing, 18*(4), 152–159.

Porter-O'Grady, T. (2013). *Implementing shared governance: Creating a professional organization*. Retrieved September 15, 2013, from, www.tpogassociates.com/SharedGovernance.htm.

Porter-O'Grady, T., Hawkins, M., & Parker, M. (1997). *Whole systems shared governance: Architecture for integration*. Gaithersburg, MD: Aspen.

Porter-O'Grady, T., & Malloch, K. (2010). *Innovation leadership: Creating the landscape of healthcare*. Boston: Jones & Bartlett.

Regan, L., & Rodriguez, L. (2011). Nurse empowerment from a middle-management perspective: Nurse managers' and assistant nurse managers' workplace empowerment views. *The Permanente Journal, 15*(1), 101–107.

Roberts, S. J. (2000). Development of a positive professional identity: Liberating oneself from the oppressor within. *Advances in Nursing Science, 22*(4), 71–82.

Solomon, D. (October 4, 2004). Risk management: For financial whistle-blowers, new shield is an imperfect one. *The Wall Street Journal*.

Trus, M., Razbadauskas, A., Doran, D., & Suominen, T. (2012). Work-related empowerment of nurse managers: A systematic review. *Nursing and Health Sciences, 14*, 412–420.

U.S. Bureau of Labor Statistics. (2014). *Union members 2013* [Press release]. Retrieved May 13, 2014 from http://www.bls.gov/news.release/pdf/union2.pdf.

SUGGESTED READINGS

Budd, K. W., Warino, L. S., & Patton, M. E. (2004). Traditional and non-traditional collective bargaining: Strategies to improve the patient care environment. *Online Journal of Issues in Nursing, 9*(1). Retrieved October 1, 2009, from, www.nursingworld.org/MainMenuCategories/ANAMarketplace/ANAPeriodicals/OJIN/TableofContents/Volume92004/No1Jan04/CollectiveBargainingStrategies.aspx.

Collins, J. (2001). *Good to great: Why some companies make the leap … and others don't*. New York: Harper Business.

Fisher, R., Ury, W., & Patton, B. (1991). *Getting to yes: Negotiating agreement without giving in*. New York: Penguin Books.

Institute of Medicine (IOM). (2011). *The future of nursing: Leading change, advancing health*. Washington, DC: The National Academies.

Kouzes, J. M., & Posner, B. Z. (2007). *The leadership challenge* (4th ed.). San Francisco: Jossey-Bass.

Kramer, M., Schmalenberg, C., Maguire, P., Brewer, B. B., Burke, R., Chmielewski, L., et al. (2008). Structures and practices enabling staff nurses to control their practice. *Western Journal of Nursing Research, 30*(5), 539–559.

Perlow, L., & Williams, D. (2003). Is silence killing your organization? *Harvard Business Review, 81*, 52–58.

INTERNET RESOURCES

American Nurses Association (ANA). http://www.nursingworld.org.

National Nurses Organizing Committee (NNOC). *National RN movement*. http://www.nationalnursesunited.org/affiliates/entry/nnoc.

The future of nursing: Leading change advancing health. http://www.iom.edu/Reports/2010/The-Future-of-Nursing-Leading-Change-Advancing-Health.aspx.

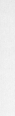

20

Managing Quality and Risk

Victoria N. Folse

This chapter explains key concepts and strategies related to quality and risk management. All healthcare professionals, including nurses, must be actively involved in the continuous improvement of patient care.

LEARNING OUTCOMES

- Apply quality management principles to clinical situations.
- Use the six steps of the quality improvement process.
- Practice using select quality improvement strategies to do the following:
  - Identify customer expectations.
  - Diagram clinical procedures.
  - Develop standards and outcomes.
  - Evaluate outcomes.
- Incorporate roles of leaders, managers, and followers to create a quality management culture of continuous readiness.
- Apply risk management strategies to an agency's quality management program.

KEY TERMS

accountability measure	never event	risk management
benchmarking	nursing-sensitive outcome	root-cause analysis
continuous quality improvement (CQI)	patient-care outcome	SBAR
failure mode and effects analysis (FMEA)	performance improvement (PI)	sentinel event
near miss	quality assurance (QA)	teach-back
	quality improvement (QI)	total quality management (TQM)
	quality management (QM)	

Kathleen M. Krawzak, RNC-NIC, BSN
Staff Nurse, Infant Special Care Unit, Evanston Hospital,
NorthShore University HealthSystem, Evanston, Illinois

Medical errors are one of the most common issues discussed among quality care and risk management healthcare professionals and are of great concern to me as a new nurse. The Institute of Medicine brought the issue of medical errors to the forefront of healthcare awareness with its landmark report *To Err is Human: Building a Safer Health System,* but the concern existed in hospitals long before that publication.

Unfortunately we have not made much progress. Many policies and procedures have been put into place to decrease the number of medical errors in hospitals. Some examples include electronic bar coding for medications, co-checking lab labels with a second RN, and performing time-outs before procedures. With increasing demands placed on nurses, it is critical that individual units address what they can do to foster quality care and prevent errors. We needed to do something.

What do you think you would do if you were this nurse?

INTRODUCTION

Healthcare agencies and health professionals strive to provide the highest quality, safest, most efficient, and cost-effective care possible. The philosophy of quality management and the process of quality improvement must shape the entire healthcare culture and provide specific skills for assessment, measurement, and evaluation of patient care. The goal of an organization committed to quality care is a comprehensive, systematic approach that prevents errors or identifies and corrects errors so that adverse events are decreased and safety and quality outcomes are maximized. Leadership must acknowledge safety challenges and allocate resources at the patient care and unit levels to identify and reduce risks. Managers must enhance work environments to support higher quality care, less patient risk, and more satisfied nurses. Quality management and risk management are focused on optimizing patient outcomes and emphasize the prevention of patient care problems and the mitigation of adverse events. Nursing must accept the primary leadership role for ensuring patient safety and achieving high quality in healthcare organizations.

QUALITY MANAGEMENT IN HEALTH CARE

Healthcare systems that demand quality recognize that survival and competitiveness are built on improved patient outcomes. Success depends on a philosophy that permeates the organization and values a continuous process of improvement. It is essential to integrate patient safety and risk management into broader quality initiatives. Nurses must be prepared to continuously improve the quality and safety of healthcare systems within which they work, and they must focus on the six competencies identified by Quality and Safety Education for Nurses (QSEN): patient-centered care, teamwork and collaboration, evidence-based practice, quality improvement, safety, and informatics (QSEN Institute, 2013). Quality necessitates maintaining safety in patient care, with a continual focus on clinical excellence from the entire interprofessional team. Patient safety is a key component of quality improvement and clinical governance. Moreover, the prevention of adverse events is paramount to improved patient outcomes.

The terms **quality management (QM)**, **quality improvement (QI)**, **performance improvement (PI)**, **total quality management (TQM)**, and **continuous quality improvement (CQI)** are often used interchangeably in health care. Quality-related terminology continues to evolve.

In this chapter, **quality management** refers to a philosophy that defines a healthcare culture emphasizing customer satisfaction, innovation, and employee involvement. Similarly, **quality improvement** refers to an ongoing process of innovation, prevention of error, and staff development that is used by institutions that adopt the quality management philosophy. Nurses maintain a unique role in quality management and quality improvement because of the amount of direct patient care provided at the bedside and because they have an understanding of the day-to-day issues and "real world" nursing involved in delivery of care. Active involvement of nurses in patient care improvement efforts (e.g., safe delivery of care during off peak hours and times of low staffing, high census, or high acuity, interprofessional communication problems associated with complex patients, improving medication safety, prevention of pressure ulcers) cannot only promote quality and safety of patient care but also positively impact job satisfaction and improve the work environment (Sving, Gunningberg, Hogman, & Mamhidir, 2012).

BENEFITS OF QUALITY MANAGEMENT

Healthcare systems that employ a comprehensive QM program experience many organizational benefits. First, greater efficiency and proactive planning may overcome some of the resource constraints, including limited reimbursement imposed by prospective payment plans and key staff shortages. Second, successful malpractice suits could be reduced with quality care because QM is based on the philosophy that actions should be right the first time and that improvement is always possible. Third, job satisfaction could be enhanced because QM involves everyone on the improvement team and encourages everyone to contribute. This style of participative management makes employees feel valued as team members who are empowered to make a difference.

PLANNING FOR QUALITY MANAGEMENT

Interprofessional planning is integral to the quest for quality. Issues are examined from various perspectives using a systematic process. Planning takes time and money; however, the price of poor planning can be very expensive. Costs of inadequate planning might involve correcting a patient care error, resulting in extended length of stay and added procedures. In turn, this increases the risk of liability for what was originally done, it risks a negative public image, and it magnifies employee frustration and promotes turnover. The costs of errors and ineffective nursing actions are avoidable costs.

EVOLUTION OF QUALITY MANAGEMENT

Nonhealthcare industries have excelled in focusing on process improvement as part of their core operating strategies. Numerous business management philosophies have been expanded and modified for use in healthcare organizations. For example, Six Sigma, a data-driven approach targeting a nearly error-free environment, empowers employees to improve processes and outcomes. As healthcare organizations "go lean," nurses are challenged to eliminate unnecessary steps and reduce wasted processes (saving time and money) to improve quality and the patient experience (Keller & Pyzdek, 2010). To achieve this, Six Sigma uses a five-step methodology known as *DMAIC*, which stands for **d**efine opportunities, **m**easure performance, **a**nalyze opportunity, **i**mprove performance, and **c**ontrol performance to improve existing processes. Parallels to the nursing process steps of assessment, diagnosis, planning, implementation, and evaluation can be seen in DMAIC and other QI processes.

In health care, emphasis is placed in the areas of patient safety and patient and employee satisfaction. The role of the leader or manager in this TQM method is to enable the team, remove barriers, and instill accountability. One of the most widely used evidence-based teamwork systems to improve communication and teamwork skills to improve patient safety within organizations is the Agency for Healthcare Research (AHRQ) Team Strategies and Tools to Enhance Performance and Patient Safety (TeamSTEPPS). Team training is modified for primary care office-based teams as well as for nursing homes and other long-term care settings. A customized TeamSTEPPS plan to train staff in teamwork skills to work with patients who have difficulty communicating in English (AHRQ, 2013).

Within healthcare systems, QI combines the assessment of *structure* (e.g., adequacy of staffing, effectiveness of computerized charting, availability of unit-based medication delivery systems), *process* (e.g., timeliness and thoroughness of documentation, adherence to critical pathways or care maps), and *outcome* (e.g., patient falls, hospital-acquired infection rates, patient and nurse satisfaction) standards. These three factors are usually considered interrelated, and comprehensive quality improvement initiatives actively involve direct care providers to improve quality and safety. The Literature Perspective on p. 364 presents an opportunity for nurses, including new graduates, to be involved in QI initiatives to reduce off-peak mortality.

LITERATURE PERSPECTIVE

Resources: De Cordova, P.B., Phibbs, C.S., & Stone, P.W. (2013). Perceptions and observations of off-shift nursing. *Journal of Nursing Management, 21,* 283-292; Eschiti, V., & Hamilton, P. (2011). Off-peak nurse staffing: Critical care nurses speak. *Dimensions in Critical Care Nursing, 30*(1), 62-69.

These two articles focused on concerns nurses have during off-peak shifts.

During off-peak weekday hours (7 PM to 7 AM) and on weekends and holidays, nurses often work in practice environments with limited ancillary services, fewer support staff, reduced supervision, and strained communication with on-call providers. An "off-peak effect" describing the increased risk for mortality among critically ill patients on nights and weekends is well documented, but the causes and solutions need further study. The global trend of increased patient mortality among critically ill patients admitted on weekends appear to be related to decreases in hospital staffing, access to diagnostic services, and intensivist coverage, as well as reluctance of patients to seek care on the weekends.

Implications for Practice

Because many new graduates work during off-peak hours on units where the patient population is extremely complex, it is critical to understand and mitigate the factors that impact quality and risk during these times. Nurse managers need to provide sufficient resources including ancillary personnel, to ensure a staffing balance based on experience, and to facilitate communication between shifts nurses. Involving nurses who work off-peak hours in the quality improvement initiatives will allow dialogue about improving interprofessional communication and collaboration and will provide an opportunity to verbalize the off-peak resources (e.g., experienced charge and resource nurses, clinical nurse specialists) needed to promote favorable patient outcomes.

Recognizing the relationship between quality patient care and nursing excellence, the American Academy of Nursing undertook a study that resulted in the distinction known as *Magnet*™. The American Nurses Credentialing Center (ANCC) created a process called the *Magnet Recognition Program*®. The term *Magnet*™ *hospital* was chosen to describe a hospital that attracts and retains nurses even in times of nursing shortages. Magnet™ hospital research has examined the characteristics of hospital systems that impede or facilitate professional practice in nursing and also promote quality patient outcomes. Common organizational characteristics of Magnet™ hospitals include structure factors (e.g., decentralized organizational structure, participative management style, and influential nurse executives) and process factors (e.g., professional autonomy and decision making,

ongoing professional development/education, active quality improvement initiatives). ANCC Magnet™ designated hospitals and other high reliability organizations in the United States and Europe generally have lower burnout rates, higher levels of job satisfaction, and provide higher levels of quality care resulting in greater levels of patient satisfaction (Aiken et al., 2012; Kelly, McHugh, & Aiken, 2012).

QUALITY MANAGEMENT PRINCIPLES

The combination of QI ideas from theory and research is sometimes referred to as total quality management (TQM) or, more simply, quality management (QM). The basic principles of QM are summarized in Box 20-1 and are developed further in the next section of this chapter.

Involvement

Leaders, managers, and followers must be committed to QI. Top-level leaders and managers retain the ultimate responsibility for QM but must involve the entire organization in the QI process. Although some healthcare organizations have achieved significant QI results without system-wide support, total organizational involvement is necessary for a culture transformation. If all members of the healthcare team are to be actively involved in QI, clear delineation of roles within a nonthreatening environment must be established (Table 20-1).

To work effectively in a democratic, quality-focused corporate environment, nurses and other healthcare workers must accept QI as an integral part of their role. Nurses have a direct impact on patient safety and healthcare outcomes and must follow evidence-based

BOX 20-1   PRINCIPLES OF QUALITY MANAGEMENT AND QUALITY IMPROVEMENT

1. Quality management operates most effectively within a flat, democratic, organization structure.
2. Managers and workers must be committed to quality improvement.
3. The goal of quality management is to improve systems and processes, not to assign blame.
4. Customers define quality.
5. Quality improvement focuses on outcomes.
6. Decisions must be based on data.

TABLE 20-1 ROLES/RESPONSIBILITIES IN QUALITY IMPROVEMENT PLAN

ROLE OF SENIOR LEADER	ROLE OF NURSE MANAGER	ROLE OF FOLLOWER
• Leads culture transformation • Sets priorities for house-wide activities, staffing effectiveness, and patient health outcomes • Builds infrastructure, provides resources, and removes barriers for improvement • Defines procedures for immediate response to errors involving care, treatment, or services and contains risk • Assesses management and staff knowledge of quality management process regularly, and provides education as needed • Implements and monitors systems for internal and external reporting of information • Defines and provides support system for staff who have been involved in a sentinel event	• Is accountable for quality and safety indicator performance within areas of responsibility • Communicates performance priorities and targets to staff • Meets regularly with staff to monitor progress and help with improvement work • Uses data to measure effectiveness of improvement • Works with staff to develop and implement action plans for improvement of measures that do not meet target • Provides time for unit staff to participate in quality improvement measures • Observes staff directly and coaches as needed • Consults quality management team (e.g., Six Sigma) or risk management team as appropriate • Writes and submits to senior leaders periodic action plan including performance measures and plans for improvement • Shares information and benchmarks with other units and departments to improve organization's performance	• Follows policies, procedures, and protocols to ensure quality and safe patient care • Remains current in the literature on quality and safety specific to nursing • Promotes evidence-based practice standards • Communicates with and educates peers immediately if they are observed not following quality and safety standards • Reports quality and safety issues to supervisor/manager • Invests in the process by continually asking self, "What makes this indicator important to measure?" "What has been done to improve it?" "What can I do to improve it?" • Participates actively in the quality improvement activities

guidelines to meet nursing-sensitive outcomes indicators. Nursing must be recognized and empowered to mobilize performance improvement knowledge and practice measures throughout the organization. When a separate department controls quality activities, healthcare managers and workers often relinquish responsibility and commitment for quality control to these quality specialists. Employees working in an organizational culture that values quality freely make suggestions for improvement and innovation in patient care. Exercise 20-1 may help nurses make QI suggestions.

Goal

The goal of QM is to improve the system, not to assign blame. Managers strive to provide a system in which workers can function effectively. To encourage commitment to QI, nurse managers must clearly articulate the organization's mission and goals. All levels of employees, from nursing assistants to hospital administrators, must be educated about QI strategies.

Communication should flow freely within the organization. When healthcare professionals understand each other's roles and can effectively communicate and work together, patients are more likely to receive safe, quality care. Because QM stresses improving the system, detection of employees' errors is not stressed; and if errors occur, re-education of staff is emphasized rather than imposition of punitive measures. When patient safety indicators are used to examine hospital performance, the focus of error analysis shifts from the individual provider to the level of the healthcare system. Human error is preventable through improved system design including the use of checklists, decreasing interruptions and distractions, preventing fatigue, and avoiding task saturation. (Riley, Davis, Miller, & McCullough, 2010).

Customers

Customers define quality. Successful organizations measure the factors that are most important to customers and focus their energies on enhancing quality in these areas. As patients become more sophisticated and view themselves as "consumers" who can take their business elsewhere, they want input into treatment decisions. Although typical patients may not be knowledgeable about a specific treatment, they know if they were satisfied with their experience with the healthcare provider.

Every nurse and healthcare agency has internal and external customers. Internal customers are people or units within an organization who receive products or services. A nurse working on a hospital unit could describe patients, nurses on the other shifts, and other hospital departments as internal customers. External customers are people or groups outside the organization who receive products or services. For nurses, these external customers may include patients' families, physicians, managed care organizations, and the community at large. Some customers (e.g., physicians, patient families) could be either internal or external customers depending on the actual care environment. Managers and direct care nurses can use Exercise 20-2 to identify their internal and external customers.

EXERCISE 20-2

For one week, list every person with whom you interact in your professional role. The internal customers are those people who work for or receive care in your organization. External customers come from outside the organization. What is the best method to obtain feedback from each of these customers?

Public reporting of quality and risk data is changing the way customers make decisions about health care and is intended to improve care through easily accessed information. Accredited hospitals are required to collect and report data on performance for core quality indicators, called accountability measures, that produce the greatest positive impact on

---

BOX 20-2   EXAMPLES OF ACCOUNTABILITY MEASURES

- Heart attack care
- Heart failure care
- Pneumonia care
- Surgical care
- Children's asthma care
- Inpatient psychiatric services
- VTE (venous thromboembolism) care
- Stroke care
- Perinatal care
- Immunization

Data from The Joint Commission. Retrieved February 20, 2014, from http://www.jointcommission.org/assets/1/6/2013_Accountability_measures_for_2014_TP.pdf.

---

patient outcomes (Box 20-2) and these data are made publicly available by The Joint Commission (TJC, 2013). In 2011, TJC launched a Top Performer on Key Quality Measures® program that recognizes accredited hospitals that attain excellence in accountability measure performance for certain conditions, including heart attack, heart failure, pneumonia, surgical care, children's asthma care, inpatient psychiatric services, venous thromboembolism, and stroke. Hospital Compare (Centers for Medicare & Medicaid Services [CMS], 2013a) allows customers to (1) find information on how well hospitals care for patients with certain medical conditions or surgical procedures, and (2) access patient survey results about the care received during a recent hospital stay. This information allows customers to compare the quality of care in over 4000 Medicare-certified hospitals. Patient satisfaction information on Hospital Compare is part of the Consumer Assessment of Healthcare Providers and Systems (CAHPS) Hospital Survey, known as HCAHPS. HCAHPS is a national, standardized, publicly reported survey of patient perspectives on care they experience during a hospital stay including communication with physicians, communication with nurses, responsiveness of hospital staff, pain management, communication about medicines, discharge information, cleanliness of the hospital environment, and quietness of the hospital environment (CMS, 2013b). In addition to Hospital Compare, Websites for Physician Compare, Nursing Home Compare, and Home Health Compare provide transparency for consumers. Consumer satisfaction of health care can be assessed through the use of questionnaires, interviews, focus group discussions, or observation. Patients' perspectives should be a key component of any quality improvement initiative. However, patients cannot always adequately assess the competence of clinical performance, and therefore patient feedback and patient satisfaction surveys must serve as only one data source for QI initiatives.

Focus

QI focuses on outcomes. Patient outcomes are statements that describe the results of health care. They are specific and measurable and describe patients' behavior. Outcome statements may be based on patients' needs, ethical and legal standards of practice, or other standardized data systems. Healthcare organizations that implement nursing-sensitive performance measures value nurses and have a strong commitment to patient care quality and workforce sustainability. This commitment is even more critical because the CMS no longer reimburses hospitals for the costs of additional care required due to hospital acquired injuries (CMS, 2013a). The Patient Protection and Affordable Care Act of 2010 also emphasizes pay-for-performance to reduce negative health outcomes.

Decisions

Decisions must be based on data. The use of statistical tools enables nurse managers to make objective decisions about QI activities. Collecting data without a preconceived idea is critical to making quality decisions. Quality information must be gathered and analyzed without bias before improvement suggestions and recommendations are made.

THE QUALITY IMPROVEMENT PROCESS

QI involves continual analysis and evaluation of products and services to prevent errors and to achieve customer satisfaction. As the term suggests, the work of continuous QI never stops because products and services can always be improved.

The QI process is a structured series of steps designed to plan, implement, and evaluate changes in healthcare activities. Many models of the QI process exist, including Six Sigma DMAIC, but most

---

BOX 20-3   STEPS IN THE QUALITY IMPROVEMENT PROCESS

1. Identify needs most important to the consumer of healthcare services.
2. Assemble an interprofessional team to review the identified consumer needs and services.
3. Collect data to measure the current status of these services.
4. Establish measurable outcomes and quality indicators.
5. Select and implement a plan to meet the outcomes.
6. Collect data to evaluate the implementation of the plan and the achievement of outcomes.

---

parallel the nursing process and all contain steps similar to those listed in Box 20-3. The six steps can easily be applied to clinical situations. In the following example, staff at a community clinic use the QI process to handle patient complaints about excessive wait times.

A community clinic receives a number of complaints from patients about waiting up to 2 hours for scheduled appointments to see a licensed practitioner. The clinic secretary and staff nurses suggest to the clinic manager that scheduling clinic appointments be investigated by the QI committee, which is composed of the clinic secretary, two clinic nurses, one physician, and one nurse practitioner. The clinic manager agrees to the staff's suggestion and assigns the problem to the QI committee. At their next meeting, the QI committee uses a flowchart to describe the scheduling process from the time a patient calls to make an appointment until the patient sees a physician or nurse practitioner in the examining room. Next, the committee members decide to gather and analyze data about the important parts of the process: the number of calls for appointments, the number of patients seen in a day, the number of cancelled or missed appointments, and the average time each patient spends in the waiting room. The committee discovers that too many appointments are scheduled because many patients miss appointments. This overbooking often results in long waiting times for the patients who do arrive on time. The QI committee also gathers information on clinic waiting times from the literature and through interviews with patients and colleagues. A measurable outcome is written: "Patients will wait no longer than 30 minutes to be seen by a licensed practitioner." After a discussion of options, the team recommends that appointments be scheduled at more reasonable intervals, that patients receive notification of appointments by mail and by phone, and that all clinic patients be educated about the importance of keeping scheduled appointments. The committee communicates its suggestions for throughput improvement to the manager and staff and monitors the results of the implementation of their improvement suggestions. Within 3 months, the average waiting room time per patient decreases to 90 minutes, and the number of missed patient appointments decreases by 20%. Because the desired outcome has not been met, the QI committee will continue the QI process.

Identify Consumers' Needs

The QI process begins with the selection of a clinical activity for review. Theoretically, any and all aspects of clinical care could be improved through the QI process. However, QI efforts should be concentrated on changes to patient care that will have the greatest effect. To determine which clinical activities are most important, nurse managers or direct care nurses may interview or survey patients about their healthcare experiences or may review unmet quality standards. The results of the research study in the Research Perspective below, give direction to reducing medication errors during transitions of care to nursing homes.

Assemble a Team

Once an activity is selected for possible improvement, an interprofessional team implements the QI process. QI team members should represent a cross section of workers who are involved with the problem. To maximize success, team members may need to be educated about their roles before starting the QI process.

To develop effective unit-based quality councils, the workplace environment must promote teamwork. Some departments within healthcare facilities are more open to teamwork than are others. Nursing leadership students as well as nurse leaders and managers can use Exercise 20-3 to decide whether their clinical unit is ready for a unit-based QI team.

EXERCISE 20-3

Ask yourself the following questions about the unit or department:
1. Is communication between nurses and other professionals promoted? If so, how?
2. Could the interprofessional communication process be improved in any way?
3. Does your system encourage nurses to act as a team?
4. Are other disciplines/departments included in team activities?
5. Can the team focus be improved in any way?

 RESEARCH PERSPECTIVE

Resources: Choi, J., Flynn, L., & Aiken, L.H. (2012). Nursing practice environments and registered nurses job satisfaction in nursing homes. *The Gerontologist, 52,* 484-492; Desai, R., Williams, C.E., Green, S.B., Pierson, S., & Hansen, R.A. (2011). Medication errors during patient transitions into nursing homes: Characteristics and association with patient harm. *The American Journal of Geriatric Pharmacotherapy, 9*(6), 413-422.

These two articles addressed concerns related to medical administration.

The risk of medication errors is highest during care transitions because of poor coordination of care across settings. Incidents that involve moving to a nursing home from home or other facility result in greater risk of patient harm compared with errors not involved in transition. Greater use of complex medications regimes and inability to direct their own care due to medical and cognitive impairment magnify the risk for nursing home residents. Errors in transition were most likely to be caused by transcription error, communication problems, unavailability of medicines, medication name confusion, and pharmacy dispensing, with more than half of errors beginning during the documentation phase of medication use. The quality of the practice environment in nursing homes has a tremendous impact on nurse job satisfaction.

Implications for Practice
Effective interprofessional communication and accurate transcription processes are critical during care transitions. Standardized communication for hand-off processes (e.g., SBAR) and a system for medication reconciliation are critical, particularly as patients transition across care settings. Reducing medication errors through improved hand-off communication and increased use of technology (e.g., electronic medical record, barcode scanning) is needed to address time pressures, work overload, and conflicting demands of nurses, including unlicensed assistive personnel in skilled care facilities. Nursing leaders and managers at nursing homes as well as skilled and extended care facilities need to infuse the QSEN competencies (QSEN Institute, 2013) of patient-centered care, teamwork and collaboration, evidence-based practice, quality improvement, safety, and informatics to reduce medication errors during transitions of care. Improving the practice environment will favorably impact quality and risk variables including registered nurse satisfaction.

Collect Data

After the interprofessional team forms, the group collects data to measure the current status of the activity, service, or procedure under review. Various data tools, including flowcharts, line graphs, histograms, Pareto charts, and fishbone diagrams, may be used to analyze and present this information. The use of empirical tools to organize QI data is an essential part of the QI process. Many newly licensed registered nurses lack formal training in the use of QI tools and lack sufficient knowledge, concepts, and tools required to fully participate in QI initiatives. QI skills of direct care providers are necessary to identify gaps between current care and best practice and to design, implement, test, and evaluate changes (Cline, Rosenberg, Kovner, & Brewer, 2011).

A detailed flowchart is used to describe complex tasks. The flowchart is a data tool that uses boxes and directional arrows to diagram all the steps of a process or procedure in the proper sequence. Sometimes, just diagramming a patient care process in detail reveals gaps and opportunities for improvement. The flowchart in Figure 20-1 depicts the process of a home health agency receiving a new patient referral.

Line graphs present data by showing the connection among variables. The dependent variable is usually plotted on the vertical scale, and the independent variable is usually plotted on the horizontal scale. In QI, this technique is often used to show the trend of a particular activity over time, and the result may be called a *trend chart*. The line graph in Figure 20-2 illustrates the number of referrals a home health agency receives during a year.

The histogram in Figure 20-3 illustrates the number of home health referrals that come from five different referral sources during a selected year. A histogram is a bar chart that shows the frequency of events.

A bar chart that identifies the major causes or components of a particular quality control problem is called a *Pareto chart*. It differs from a regular bar graph in that the highest frequencies of occurrence of a factor are designated in the bar at the left, with the other factors appearing in descending order. Used often in QI, the Pareto chart helps the QI team determine priorities, allowing the most significant problem to be addressed first. The Pareto chart in Figure 20-4 demonstrates that, on a medical-surgical unit over a 1-month period, omission of vital signs was the most common type of documentation error.

The fishbone diagram is an effective method of summarizing a brainstorming session. A specific problem or outcome is written on the horizontal line. All possible causes of the problem or strategies to meet the outcome are written in a fishbone pattern. Figure 20-5 uses a fishbone diagram to present possible causes of patients' complaints about extended waits for clinic appointments.

Although QI teams should be able to use these basic statistical tools, analysis that is more complex is sometimes necessary. In this situation, a statistical expert could be included on the QI team or the team may consult a statistician.

Establish Outcomes

After analyzing the data, the team next sets a goal for improvement. This goal can be established in a number of ways but always involves a standard of practice and a measurable patient-care outcome or nursing-sensitive outcome. Nursing-sensitive indicators reflect the structure, process, and outcomes of nursing care. The structure of nursing care is indicated by the supply of nursing staff, the skill level of the nursing staff, and the education/certification of nursing staff. Process indicators measure aspects of nursing care such as assessment, intervention, and RN job satisfaction. Patient outcomes that are determined to be nursing sensitive are those that improve if there is a greater quantity or quality of nursing care (e.g., pressure ulcers, falls, intravenous [IV] infiltrations). Some patient outcomes are more highly related to other aspects of institutional care, such as medical decisions and institutional policies (e.g., frequency of primary cesarean sections, cardiac failure) and are not considered nursing sensitive. The interprofessional team should use accepted standards of care and practice whenever possible. Clinical practice guidelines and standards should reflect evidence-based practice and should be updated as new research emerges. Sources that establish these standards include the following:

1. American Nurses Association (ANA) standards of nursing practice
2. State nurse practice acts
3. Accrediting bodies such as The Joint Commission (TJC) or recognition bodies such as the American Nurses Credentialing Center (ANCC)

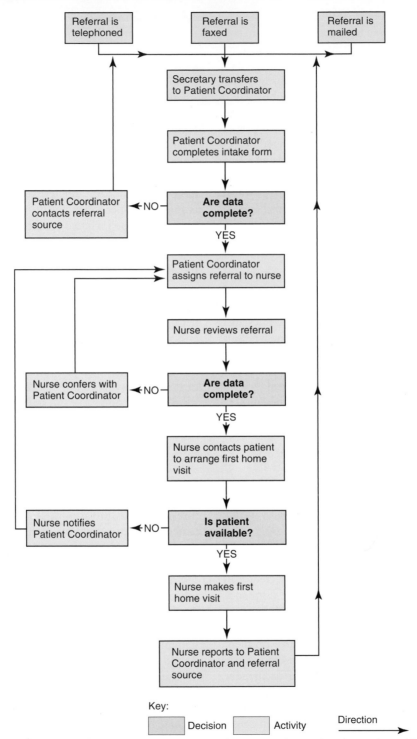

FIGURE 20-1 Steps in a flowchart diagramming process of a new patient referral, starting with the time a home health referral is made and ending with the first home visit.

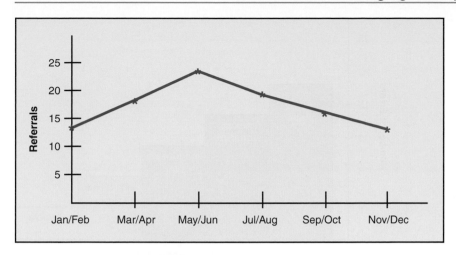

FIGURE 20-2 Line graph depicting the number of home health referrals received during 1 year.

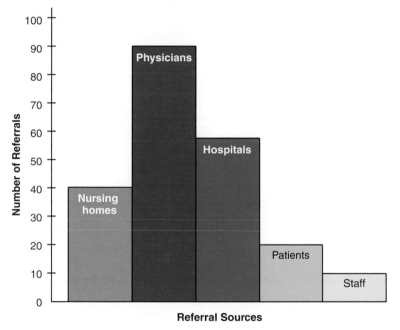

FIGURE 20-3 Histogram depicting the number of home health referrals received from five sources during 1 year.

4. Governmental bodies such as the Agency for Healthcare Research and Quality (AHRQ), the Centers for Medicare & Medicaid Services (CMS), the Centers for Disease Control and Prevention (CDC) Division of Healthcare Quality Promotion (DHQP), and the National Institute for Occupational Safety and Health (NIOSH)
5. Healthcare advisory groups such as the Institute of Medicine (IOM), the National Quality Forum (NQF), and the Quality & Safety Education of Nurses (QSEN)
6. Nationally recognized professional organizations
7. Nursing research/evidenced-based, best practice standards
8. Internal policies and procedures
9. Internal or external performance measurement data such as patient satisfaction surveys, employee opinion surveys, safety assessment surveys, and patient or employee rounding

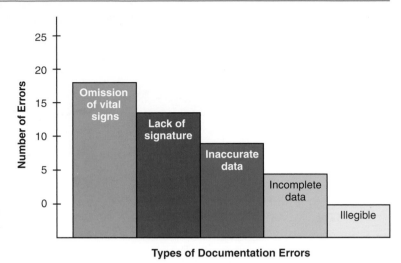

FIGURE 20-4 Pareto chart presenting major types of documentation errors that occurred on a medical/surgical unit over a 1-month period.

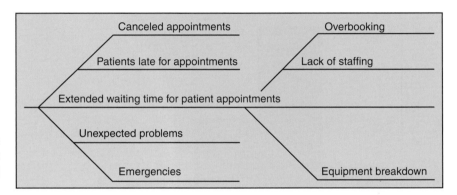

FIGURE   20-5 Fishbone diagram showing possible causes of extended waiting time for clinic patients.

Although individual healthcare organizations may have unique patient needs related to their specific population or environment, many targeted outcomes are similar. One way to evaluate the quality of outcomes is to compare one agency's performance with that of similar organizations. In a process called **benchmarking,** a widespread search is conducted to identify the best performance against which to measure others. Through this process of comparing the best practices with your practice and process, your organization learns to identify desired standards of quality performance. Available data include all reported hospital-acquired infection rates in other institutions as well as specific data, such as postoperative infection rates in adult surgical intensive care units of similar-size institutions.

However, recent mandates to publicly disclose outcomes, including nosocomial infection rates,

highlight potential issues with disclosure of data. Specifically, simply reporting hospital infection rates is not enough to promote hand-hygiene practices and may do little to improve outcomes and reduce hospital-acquired infections. Unfortunately, the usefulness of the information from other institutions continues to be hampered by differences in terminology and methodology, including use of present on admission data. Information technology plays a vital role in QI by increasing the efficiency of data entry and analysis. A consistent information system that trends high-risk procedures and systematic errors would provide a useful database regarding outcomes of care and resource allocation. The purpose of the NQF is designed to standardize measures so that true comparisons can be made.

The National Database of Nursing Quality Indicators (NDNQI) is a national nursing quality measurement program from the ANA that provides hospitals with unit-level performance reports with comparisons with regional, state, and national percentile rankings (ANA, 2013). All indicator data are collected and reported at the nursing unit level, which is valuable for unit-based patient safety and quality improvement initiatives. For example, a report could answer the question, "How is my hospital unit doing relative to the same unit type in peer hospitals?" NDNQI's nursing-sensitive indicators reflect the structure, process, and outcomes of nursing care. NDNQI's mission is to aid the nursing provider in patient safety and quality improvement efforts by providing research-based national comparative data on nursing care and the relationship to patient outcomes. Many of the NDNQI indicators are NQF-endorsed measures and are part of NQF's nursing-sensitive measure set (e.g., falls with injuries, nosocomial infections, restraint prevalence, nursing hours per patient day, staff mix). However, the NDNQI allows additional comparisons of indicators such as nurse job satisfaction, RN education and certification, and pressure ulcer, psychiatric patient assault, and pediatric IV infiltration rates.

Nursing has been a leader in the information system field by developing standardized nursing classification systems. The availability of standardized nursing data enables the study of health problems across populations, settings, and caregivers. Consistent use of standardized language enhances the process of QI and also demonstrates the contributions of nursing to lawmakers, healthcare policymakers, and the public. Three leading nursing classification systems have been identified: the North American Nursing Diagnosis Association International's (NANDA-I) nomenclature (Herdman, 2012); the Nursing Intervention Classification (NIC) system (Bulechek, Butcher, & Dochtermann, 2013); and the Nursing Outcomes Classification (NOC) system (Moorhead, Johnson, Maas, & Swanson, 2013). The use of standardized nursing terminologies like NANDA-I, NIC, and NOC provides a means of collecting and analyzing nursing data and evaluating nursing-sensitive outcomes.

Each classification system focuses on one component of the nursing process. Nursing diagnoses can be labeled using NANDA-I. These diagnosis labels represent clinical judgments about actual or potential health problems. Each diagnosis contains a definition, major and minor defining characteristics, and related factors. Accurate nursing diagnoses guide the selection of nursing interventions to achieve the desired treatment effects, determine nursing-sensitive outcomes, and ensure patient safety (Herdman, 2012).

The NIC system consists of interventions that represent both general and specialty nursing practice. Each intervention includes a label, a definition, and a set of activities that nurses perform to carry it out. For example, pain management is defined and specific activities are listed to alleviate pain or reduce the pain to a level that is acceptable to the patient (Bulechek et al., 2013).

The NOC system consists of outcomes that focus on the patient and include patient states, behavior, and perceptions that are sensitive to nursing interventions. Each outcome includes a definition, a five-point scale for rating outcome status over time, and a set of specific indicators to be used in rating the outcomes (Moorhead et al., 2013). Clinical testing for validation and refinement has occurred in various settings, and the standardization of terms continues to develop to reflect current knowledge and changes in nurses' roles and the structure of healthcare systems. The consistency of terms is essential in providing a large database across healthcare settings to predict resource requirements and establish outcomes of care.

Discuss Plans

The team discusses various strategies and plans to meet the new outcome. One plan is selected for implementation, and the process of change begins. Because QM stresses improving the system rather than assigning blame to employees, change strategies emphasize open communication and education of workers affected by the new standard and outcome. QI is impossible without continual education of all managers and followers.

Policies and procedures may need to be written or rewritten during the QI process. Policies should be reviewed frequently and updated so that they reflect best practice standards and do not become barriers to innovation. Communication about the change or improvement is essential.

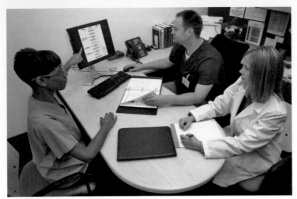

Diagramming a patient-care process in detail can reveal gaps and opportunities for improvement.

Evaluate

As the plan is implemented, the team continues to gather and evaluate data to document that the new outcomes are being met. If an outcome is not met, revisions in the implementation plan are needed. Sometimes improvement in one part of a system presents new problems. For example, nurses implemented screening for suicide risk in adolescents and adults presenting to the emergency department. A result of this improvement in care was a greatly increased number of referrals for counseling, which overwhelmed the existing hospital and community resources. The interprofessional team may need to reassemble periodically to handle the inevitable obstacles that develop with the implementation of any new process or procedure. Furthermore, individuals outside the medical center (external customers) may need to be included in the process. The example that follows also illustrates this idea.

A hospital is implementing a pneumatic tube system to dispense medications. An interprofessional team is assembled to discuss the process from various viewpoints: pharmacy, nursing, pneumatic tube operation managers, aides who take the medications from the pneumatic tube to the patient medication drawers, administrators, and physicians. The tube system is implemented. A nurse on one unit realizes that several patients do not have their morning medications in their medication drawers. The nurse borrows medications from another patient's drawer and orders the rest of the medications "stat" from pharmacy. Other nurses on that unit and other units have the same problem and are taking the

same or similar actions. Several problems are occurring— some of the medications are being given late, nurses waste precious time by searching other medication drawers, the pharmacy charges extra for the stat medications and is overwhelmed with stat requests, and the situation increases the nurses' frustration level. In some cases, patients suffer because of late administration of medications. QM principles would encourage the nurses to report the problems to the nurse manager or appropriate team member. The pneumatic tube team could compile data such as frequency of missing medications, timing of medication orders, and nursing units involved. The problems are analyzed with a system perspective to solve the late medication problem effectively.

In some organizations, when a change is implemented successfully, the QI team disbands. One of the crucial tasks of the nurse manager is to publicize and reward the success of each QI team. The nurse manager must also evaluate the work of the team and the ability of individual team members to work together effectively.

Some organizations that have used the QM philosophy for several years establish permanent QI teams or committees. These QI teams do not disband after implementing one project or idea but, rather, may meet regularly to focus on improvements in specific areas of patient care. The use of permanent QI teams or the adoption of a culture driven by QM can provide continuity and prevent duplication of efforts within the quality teams.

QM organizations stress system-level change and the evaluation of outcomes. However, in recent years, the need for process/performance improvement, including individual performance appraisal, has reemerged within healthcare organizations. Peer review and self-evaluation are performance-assessment methods that fit within the QM philosophy.

Any nurse can use the six steps of the QI process to self-evaluate and improve individual performance. For example, a nurse on a medical unit who wants to improve documentation skills might study past entries on patient records; review current institution policies, professional standards, and literature related to documentation; set specific performance-improvement goals after consultation with the nurse manager and expert colleagues; devise strategies and a timeline for achieving performance goals; and after implementing the strategies, review documentation entries to see whether self-improvement goals have been met.

QUALITY ASSURANCE

Although QI is a comprehensive process to prevent problems, it is naive to suggest the total abandonment of periodic inspection. One method used to monitor health care is quality assurance (QA) programs, which ensure conformity to a standard. QA focuses on clinical aspects of the provider's care, often in response to an identified problem. Many QA activities focus on process standards (e.g., documentation, adherence to practice standards). The focus may be asking questions such as "Did the nurse document the response to the pain medication within the required time period?" instead of "Did the patient receive adequate pain relief postoperatively?" In contrast, QI may examine process, structure, and outcome standards. The similarities and differences between QI and QA are summarized in Table 20-2.

One of the methods most often used in QA is chart review or chart auditing. Chart audits may be conducted using the records of active or discharged patients. Charts are selected randomly and reviewed by qualified healthcare professionals. In an internal audit, staff members from the same hospital or agency that generated the records examine the data. External auditors are qualified professionals from outside the organization who conduct the review. An audit tool containing specific criteria based on standards of care is applied to each chart under review. For example, auditors might compare documentation related to use of restraints for medical-surgical purposes with the criterion "Licensed independent practitioner evaluates patient in person within 4 hours of application." Auditors note compliance or lack of compliance with each audit criterion and report a summary of these findings to the appropriate manager or committee for corrective action.

Because the focus of the chart audit is on detecting errors and determining the person responsible for them, many staff members tend to view QA negatively. The nurse manager must reinforce that QA is not intended to be punitive but, instead, is an opportunity to improve patient care at the unit level. For example, to reinforce the importance of documentation, providing the standard of care for documentation and assisting the RN in reviewing several charts is an appropriate educational tool to reinforce policies and procedures or standards regarding documentation. The manager has the responsibility to communicate the importance of daily QA activities and how unit-based monitoring ties into the overall quality improvement program. Moreover, many institutions incorporate both the participation in and the results of QA into annual performance appraisals or clinical ladders.

RISK MANAGEMENT

QM and risk management are related concepts and emphasize the achievement of quality-outcome standards and the prevention of patient-care problems. Risk management also attempts to analyze problems and minimize losses after an adverse event occurs. These losses include incurring financial loss as a result of malpractice or absorbing the cost of an extended length of stay for the patient, negative public relations, and employee dissatisfaction. Moreover, the inclusion of safety standards in TJC guidelines further emphasizes the importance of risk management. As an example, Box 20-4 shows the 2014 National Patient

TABLE 20-2	COMPARISON OF TRADITIONAL QUALITY ASSURANCE AND QUALITY IMPROVEMENT PROCESSES	
	QUALITY ASSURANCE (QA) PROCESS	**QUALITY IMPROVEMENT (QI) PROCESS**
Goal	To improve quality	To improve quality
Focus	Discovery and correction of errors	Prevention of errors
Major tasks	Inspection of nursing activities	Review of nursing activities
	Chart audits	Innovation
		Staff development
Quality team	QA personnel or department personnel	Interprofessional team
Outcomes	Set by QA team with input from staff	Set by QI team with input from staff and patients

BOX 20-4   **2014 NATIONAL PATIENT SAFETY GOALS FOR HOSPITALS**

- Improve the accuracy of patient identification.
- Improve the effectiveness of communication among caregivers.
- Improve the safety of using medications.
- Reduce the harm associated with clinical alarm systems.
- Reduce the risk of healthcare-associated infections.
- The hospital identifies safety risks inherent in its patient population.
- The Universal Protocol for preventing wrong site, wrong procedure applies to all surgical and nonsurgical invasive procedures.

Safety Goals for hospitals (TJC, 2013). Additional goals of (1) reducing the risk of patient harm resulting from falls, and (2) preventing healthcare-associated pressure ulcers apply to long-term care facilities. The TJC Website carries the most up-to-date patient safety goals for all patient care settings.

The risk management department has several functions, which include the following:

- Defining situations that place the system at some financial risk, such as medication errors or patient falls
- Determining the frequency of occurrence of those situations
- Intervening and investigating identified events
- Identifying potential risks or opportunities to improve care

Each individual nurse is a risk manager and has the responsibility to identify and report unusual occurrences and potential risks. Active involvement in quality and risk management by direct caregivers, however, is a challenge complicated by staffing issues and increased demands on the nurse. Increased nursing staffing in hospitals is associated with better care outcomes. Consistent evidence shows that an increase in RN-to-patient ratios is associated with a reduction in hospital-related mortality, failure to rescue, and other nursing-sensitive outcomes, as well as reduced length of stay. Similarly, favorable patient care environments are associated with lower rates of serious complications or adverse events. Findings from seminal works by Aiken, Clarke, Sloane, Lake, and Cheney (2008) and Kane, Shamliyan, Mueller, Duval, and Wilt

(2007) are combined with more contemporary studies (e.g., Aiken et al., 2012; Kendall-Gallagher, Aiken, Sloane, & Cimiotti, 2011) in The Evidence section on p. 379 to reflect the current knowledge about nursing and the patient care environment.

Another barrier to improving patient safety is fear of punishment, which inhibits people from acknowledging, reporting, or discussing errors. One way to minimize errors is to monitor threats to patient safety continually and to recognize that individual errors often reflect organizational and system failures. For example, targeting nurse-to-patient load and work schedules, including 12-hour shifts and overtime, can reduce potential errors from human factors such as fatigue, stress, and distractions. Rotating shifts may have a negative effect on nurses' stress levels and job performance, and working longer hours may have a negative impact on patient outcomes (Witkoski Stimpfel, Sloane, & Aiken, 2012).

Both risk management and quality management deal with changing behavior, prevention, focus on the customer, and attention to outcomes. The following clinical examples illustrate how quality management and risk management complement each other. First, the implementation of lift teams reduces employee injuries associated with lifting heavy or fully dependent patients and simultaneously, for the patient, decreases adverse events associated with difficult transfers. The implementation of lift teams reflects managing both quality and risk. Second, adherence to the universal safety verification known as "time out" before the beginning of a surgical procedure ensures perioperative safety within a TQM framework. A third example, the use of teach-back, assures quality teaching and health literacy learning has occurred and that risks are minimized by asking patients to explain in their own words what they need to know or do. Asking a question like, "Please tell me, what will you do to take care of yourself when you get home? " provides the nurse with an opportunity to check understanding and reteach information if needed (Minnesota Health Literacy Partnership, 2011). Although nursing managers would prefer that all staff intrinsically embrace risk management practices aimed at patient and staff safety, accountability for safety can be one aspect of performance evaluations. Active involvement of staff in risk management activities is key to prevention of adverse events. Nurse managers should conduct safety rounds and praise employees for employing safe practice as part of best practice standards. This philosophy reinforces that risk management not only benefits the patient but also works to keep individual employees safe in the workplace.

Adverse-event reduction is a key strategy for reducing healthcare mortality and morbidity because patients who suffer adverse events are more likely to die or suffer permanent disability. Nurses have always played a pivotal role in the prevention of adverse events and can reduce negative outcomes with a focus on accurate assessment, early identification, and correction of potentially adverse situations. Also, adherence to best practice standards and ensuring quality standards for high-risk/high-volume practices (e.g., restraint use, medication reconciliation) can reduce adverse events. The NQF and CMS define never events as errors in medical care that are clearly identifiable, preventable, and serious in their consequences for patients and that indicate a real problem in the safety and credibility of a healthcare facility. Examples of never events include surgery on the wrong body part, foreign body left in a patient after surgery, mismatched blood transfusion, major medication error, severe pressure ulcer acquired in the hospital, and preventable postoperative deaths. Now that many third-party payers are following the CMS lead in withholding payment for preventable complications of care, no member of the healthcare team can fail to recognize the implications of quality care in their organization's overall success.

A comprehensive quality and risk program would proactively identify and reduce risks to patient safety through completion of a failure mode and effects analysis (FMEA) on select high-risk situations as advanced by TJC. If an adverse event occurs, nurses should also be able to recognize near misses and sentinel events and participate with an interprofessional team in the root-cause analysis. A sentinel event is a serious, unexpected occurrence involving death or physical or psychological harm, such as inpatient suicide, infant abduction, or wrong-site surgery. Similarly, a near miss may have resulted in no harm but highlights an imminent problem that must be corrected and can provide useful lessons in terms of risk analysis and reduction. TJC calls for voluntary self-reporting of sentinel events by both inpatient institutions and home health agencies. See Box 20-5

BOX 20-5 MOST COMMON HEALTHCARE SENTINEL EVENTS

- Unintended retention of foreign body
- Wrong patient, wrong site, wrong procedure
- Delay in treatment
- Suicide
- Operative/postoperative complications
- Fall
- Medication error
- Delay in treatment
- Criminal event
- Medication error
- Perinatal death/injury

Copyright © The Joint Commission, 2014. Reprinted with permission.

for the most common sentinel events reported in the healthcare arena. After a sentinel event is identified, a root-cause analysis is performed by a team that includes those directly involved in the event and those in leadership positions. A root-cause analysis is very similar to the QI process described in this chapter except that the root-cause analysis is a retrospective review of an incident to identify the sequence of events with the goal of identifying the root causes. The root-cause analysis leads to the development of specific risk-reduction strategies, and in certain situations, the plan must be reported to TJC.

Whereas reporting to TJC illustrates external reporting to regulatory or accrediting agencies, an internal method of communicating risks or adverse events is through electronic safety reporting systems or through incident reporting. Incident reports are kept separate from the patient's medical record and should serve as a means of communicating an incident that did cause or could have caused harm to patients, family members, visitors, or employees. Aggregated incident reports should be used to improve quality of care and decrease future risk. Trending data can illuminate systems issues that need to be modified to reduce risk and achieve quality patient care. Although an incident report may not be warranted for a unit-specific problem or an interdepartmental issue in which no adverse event occurred (e.g., delay in diagnosis or treatment), communication at the appropriate chain of command is essential to improve quality. Nurse managers are often responsible for investigating and remedying each identified hazard, which can result in safety being approached in a reactionary and overly narrow way. An effective approach to developing high reliability in healthcare quality and patient safety must also employ a systems perspective that allows the manager to look beyond the individual nurse and focus on the entire practice environment (Riley et al., 2010).

Evaluating Risks

In gathering data about unusual occurrences, the risk management team may involve perspectives from numerous disciplines to discover underlying problems that a single discipline might miss. Risk managers also use multiple data sources, data collection techniques, and perspectives to collect and interpret the data. Quantitative methods such as questionnaire or records of medication administration can be combined with qualitative methods such as open-ended question interviews. Actionable plans for reducing the incidence of common preventable adverse events such as medication administration errors (wrong patient, time, dose, drug, or mode of delivery) could result from assessment and analysis of both quantitative and qualitative data. Quality and risk strategies aimed at targeting high-volume and high-risk occurrences are essential. Moreover, accountability for quality efforts to third-party payers, including the federal government, on programs such as pay-for-performance, in which healthcare systems receive additional payment incentives if specific quality targets are achieved, and public reporting, in which quality data are made available for comparison, has significant implications for nurses. Opportunities include participation on quality improvement teams, data collection, and involvement in the implementation of quality initiatives.

However, recognizing errors does not always translate into reporting errors. The lack of agreement as to what constitutes error influences the willingness of healthcare professionals to report errors and subsequently affects whether they develop strategies that could reduce future risk. A lack of consensus exists regarding whether patients and families should be informed about healthcare errors.

Approaches to patient safety and risk management require healthcare providers to challenge their attitudes that errors are an unfortunate but inevitable part of patient care. Diminished resources and challenges in the work environment have the potential to compromise communication among providers and to contribute to an environment in which unsafe practices are overlooked or excused. For example, communication errors between nurses and other healthcare providers may result from hurried exchanges in crowded hallways or in the midst of a busy nursing station. Breakdown in communication among healthcare professionals is the most frequent cause of serious injuries and death in healthcare settings (Tschannen, Keenan, Aebersold, Kocan, Lundy, & Averhart, 2011). Not surprisingly, each of the National Patient Safety Goals (see Box 20-4) is directly or indirectly related to communication. Use of common language when communicating critical information helps prevent misunderstandings and creates a culture of quality and safety. **SBAR** (pronounced S-BAR) has become a best practice for standardizing communication between health care providers. SBAR stands for *s*ituation, *b*ackground, *a*ssessment, and *r*ecommendation (Institute for Healthcare Improvement, 2011). Because adverse patient outcomes commonly are a result of communication failures, The Joint Commission's National Patient Goals added standardization of handoff communication, the verbal and written exchange of pertinent information during transitions of care, in 2006. A team approach to quality and risk management is needed to promote optimal outcomes. Nurses have a responsibility to provide quality care and thus must serve in leadership roles to ensure a culture of integrated quality management and risk management.

CLINICAL MICROSYSTEMS

Developed by Dartmouth-Hitchcock Medical Center and the Institute for Healthcare Improvement, Clinical Microsystems (*www.clinicalmicrosystem.org*) serves as a resource to improve care. A microsystem is defined as a team providing care to a defined population of patients. It includes an information-rich environment and specified performance outcomes. A microsystem

---

EXERCISE 20-4

Describe an error that occurred in the agency where you practice that resulted in harm to the patient and one that did not. What would you suggest to avoid a reoccurrence? Decide under what circumstances you would inform the patient and family and under what circumstances you would withhold the information.

includes provision of care, a focus on quality and safety, and concern for satisfaction of both patients and staff. A microsystem might be a unit or a subelement of a unit or a specialized service that extends over more than one unit. At the core of a microsystem is the patient and the concern for improving the care patients in the population receive.

CONCLUSION

Quality management is critical to patient safety. As organizations addressed system errors having organized programs became even more important. Being able to address both clinical and system issues of risk contributes to improved quality.

THE SOLUTION

"Nursing M&Ms [morbidity and mortality]" is a program our unit has implemented to encourage nurses to feel comfortable discussing medical errors, near misses, and good catches. Nurses who have made medical errors are encouraged to share their experience at one of our quarterly meetings and address what steps they or the hospital could have taken to prevent the mistake from happening. Situations that occurred that were "good catches or near misses" are shared too, such as a laboratory order that was questioned by a nurse and found to be incorrect or a medication double-checked by another nurse who noted the dosage to be wrong. This meeting allows nurses to share with their co-workers strategies and techniques to improve the quality and safety of care. Minutes are recorded and provided to anyone unable to attend the meeting so that he or she, too, can learn from others' experiences. Because of these meetings, we have implemented new policies on our unit to provide more cautious care. For example, an incident occurred in which the wrong pumped breast milk was given to an infant. Because of this incident and our discussion in M&Ms, we worked with the hospital to create a label for pumped breast milk similar to the labels on medication. This way, we are able to scan the infant's wristband at the bedside, scan the barcode on the milk we are about to give, and then go on to verify our "5 *R*s." This change in practice allowed for better, safer care of the infants we care for. By using these M&Ms as a way to safely communicate, we can work together as a team to prevent future medical errors from occurring.

—*Kathleen M. Krawzek*

Would this be a suitable approach for you? Why?

■ THE EVIDENCE

A strong correlation has been established between nurse practice environments and patient and nurse outcomes. In a seminal study, Aiken et al. (2008) added to an established program of research and analyzed the effects of nurse practice environments on nurse and patient outcomes including nurse job satisfaction, burnout, intent to leave, and reports of quality of care including mortality and failure to rescue patients. This large multisite study reinforced findings from a systematic review examining the relationship of nurse staffing to patient outcomes in hospitals for the Agency of Healthcare Research and Quality (AHRQ). In an equally important early study supported by the (AHRQ), Kane et al. (2007) showed that increased nurse staffing was associated with reduced patient mortality, reduced failure to rescue, and decreased length of stay, whereas Aiken et al. (2008) advanced that nurses reported more positive job experiences and fewer concerns about quality care and that patients had a significantly lower risk of death and failure to rescue in hospitals with better care environments, the best nurse staffing levels, and the most highly educated nurses.

The evidence from these two seminal publications was expanded to examine additional factors that contribute to quality and risk. Kendall-Gallagher et al. (2011) found that nurse specialty certification was associated with better patient outcomes and that the effect on mortality and failure to rescue in general surgery patients was contingent upon baccalaureate education. Purdy, Laschinger, Finegan, Kerr, and Olivera (2010) found staffing levels were the largest predictors of nurse-assessed risks including the nursing-sensitive outcome indicator of falls. They also propose that empowering nurses and adequately resourcing practice environments to support patient care enhances job satisfaction and nursing retention. Similarly, Tzeng, Hu, and Yin (2011), examined the quality of the practice environment including the responsiveness of hospital staff and the cleanliness and quietness of the hospital environment and found that the quietness of the practice environment resulted in fewer injurious falls, whereas Aiken et al. (2012) provide additional support to the growing body of literature on the international hospital practice environment and safety and quality of care.

Nurse managers and leaders have several options for improving nurse retention and patient outcomes, including improving RN staffing, moving to a more educated nurse workforce, and facilitating a positive care environment. Hospitals whose practice environment includes investment in staff development, quality management, and good nurse-physician relations (e.g., Magnet™ designation) are associated with better nurse and patient outcomes. Nurse managers who promote an empowered workplace and facilitate teamwork support higher quality care, less patient risk, and more satisfied nurses. Investment in a baccalaureate-educated workforce and specialty certification has great potential to improve quality and reduce risk.

WHAT NEW GRADUATES SAY

- Completing a quality improvement project during leadership clinical prepared me to participate in my unit's safety committee immediately after orientation!
- QSEN competencies are really used on my unit!

- I asked to work 8-hour versus 12-hour shifts to avoid working over 10.5 hours so I am at less risk of committing an error.
- We are preparing for a visit by The Joint Commission and I feel prepared.

CHAPTER CHECKLIST

Many healthcare organizations are in the process of transforming their system to QM. Greater efficiency with improved quality is the goal of this approach. Effective QI includes identifying consumer expectations, planning, using an interprofessional approach, evaluating outcomes, and changing the system to provide an environment in which employees can perform their best.
- Quality management in health care
- Benefits of quality management
- Planning for quality management
- Evolution of quality management
- Quality management principles
  - Involvement
  - Goal

- Customers
- Focus
- Decisions
- The quality improvement process
  - Identify consumers' needs
  - Assemble a team
  - Collect data
  - Establish outcomes
  - Discuss plans
  - Evaluate
- Quality assurance
- Risk management
  - Evaluating risks
- Clinical microsystems

TIPS FOR QUALITY MANAGEMENT

- QM is based on data; anything measured and recorded can be improved.
- Concentrate QI energies on factors that are most important to patient quality and safety.

- Working together to prevent problems is more effective than fixing problems after they occur.

REFERENCES

Agency for Healthcare Research and Quality. (2013). *TeamSTEPPS*. Retrieved March 11, 2013, from, http://teamstepps.ahrq.gov.

Aiken, L., Clarke, S. P., Sloane, D. M., Lake, E. T., & Cheney, T. (2008). Effects of hospital care environment on patient mortality and nurse outcomes. *Journal of Nursing Administration*, *38*(5), 223–229.

Aiken, L. H., Sermeus, W., Van den Heede, K., Sloane, D. M., Busse, R., McKee, M., et al. (2012). Patient safety, satisfaction, and quality of hospital care: Cross-sectional surveys of nurses and patients in 12 countries in Europe and the United States. *British Medical Journal, 344*, e1717.

American Nurses Association. (2013). *National database of nursing quality indicators*. Retrieved March 14, 2013, from, www.nursingquality.org.

Bulechek, G. M., Butcher, H. K., & Dochtermann, J. M. (2013). *Nursing interventions classification (NIC)* (6th ed.). St. Louis, MO: Elsevier.

Centers for Medicare & Medicaid Services. (2013a). *Hospital compare*. Retrieved March 12, 2013 from, http://medicare.gov/hospitalcompare/.

Centers for Medicare & Medicaid Services. (2013b). *Hospital consumer assessment of healthcare providers and systems survey*. Retrieved May 28, 2013, from, www.hcahpsonline.org/home.aspx.

Choi, J., Flynn, L., & Aiken, L. H. (2012). Nursing practice environments and registered nurses job satisfaction in nursing homes. *The Gerontologist, 52*, 484–492.

Cline, D. D., Rosenberg, M. C., Kovner, C. T., & Brewer, C. (2011). Early career RNs' perceptions of quality care in the hospital setting. *Qualitative Health Research, 21*, 673–682.

Desai, R., Williams, C. E., Green, S. B., Pierson, S., & Hansen, R. A. (2011). Medication errors during patient transitions into nursing homes: Characteristics and association with patient harm. *The American Journal of Geriatric Pharmacotherapy, 9*(6), 413–422.

De Cordova, P. B., Phibbs, C. S., & Stone, P. W. (2013). Perceptions and observations of off-shift nursing. *Journal of Nursing Management, 21*, 283–292.

Eschiti, V., & Hamilton, P. (2011). Off-peak nurse staffing: Critical care nurses speak. *Dimensions in Critical Care Nursing, 30*(1), 62–69.

Herdman, T. H. (2012). *NANDA international: Nursing diagnoses: Definitions and classification 2012–2014*. Oxford: Wiley-Blackwell.

Institute for Healthcare Improvement. (2011). *SBAR technique for communication: A situational briefing model*. Retrieved March 14, 2013, from, http://www.ihi.org/resources/Pages/Tools/SBARTechniqueforCommunicationASituationalBriefingModel.aspx.

Kane, R. L., Shamliyan, T., Mueller, C., Duval, S., & Wilt, T. (2007). *Nursing staffing and quality of patient care*. Evidence report/technology assessment No. 151. (Prepared by the Minnesota Evidence-based Practice Center under Contract No. 290-02-0009.) AHRQ Publication No. 07-E005, Rockville, MD: Agency for Healthcare Research and Quality.

Keller, P., & Pyzdek, T. (2010). *The Six Sigma handbook: A complete guide for green belts, black belts, and managers at all levels* (3rd ed.). Columbus, OH: McGraw-Hill.

Kelly, L. A., McHugh, M. D., & Aiken, L. H. (2012). Nurse outcomes in Magnet and non-Magnet hospitals. *Journal of Nursing Administration, 42*(10 Suppl), S44–9.

Kendall-Gallagher, D., Aiken, L. H., Sloane, D. M., & Cimiotti, J. P. (2011). Nurse specialty certification, inpatient mortality, and failure to rescue. *Journal of Nursing Scholarship, 3*(2), 188–194.

Minnesota Health Literacy Partnership. (2011). *Training health care providers to use the teach-back method*. Retrieved on March 17, 2013, from www.healthliteracymn.org.

Moorhead, S., Johnson, M., Maas, M., & Swanson, E. (2013). *Nursing outcomes classification (NOC)* (5th ed.). St. Louis, MO: Elsevier.

Purdy, N., Laschinger, H., Finegan, J., Kerr, M., & Olivera, F. (2010). Effects of work environments on nurse and patient outcomes. *Journal of Nursing Management, 18*(8), 901–913.

QSEN Institute. (2013). *Competencies*. Retrieved on May 27, 2013, from www.qsen.org.

Riley, W., Davis, S. E., Miller, K. K., & McCullough, M. (2010). A model for developing high-reliability teams. *Journal of Nursing Management, 18*, 556–563.

Sving, E., Gunningberg, L., Hogman, M., & Mamhidir, A. (2012). Registered nurses' attention to and perceptions of pressure ulcer prevention in hospital settings. *Journal of Clinical Nursing, 21*(9), 1293–1303.

The Joint Commission. (2013). *Accountability measures for 2014*. Retrieved February 20, 2014, from, http://www.jointcommission.org/assets/1/6/2013_Accountability_measures_for_2014_TP.pdf, The Joint Commission. (2013). *2014 National patient safety goals*. Retrieved February 10, 2014, from http://www.jointcommission.org/assets/1/6/2014_HAP_NPSG_E.pdf.

Tschannen, D., Keenan, G., Aebersold, M., Kocan, M. J., Lundy, F., & Averhart, V. (2011). Implications of nurse-physician relations: Report of a successful intervention. *Nursing Economics, 29*(3), 127–135.

Tzeng, H., Hu, H., & Yin, C. (2011). The relationship of the hospital-acquired injurious fall rates with the quality profile of a hospital's care delivery and nursing staffing patterns. *Nursing Economic$, 29*(6), 299–316.

Witkoski Stimpfel, A., Sloane, D. M., & Aiken, L. H. (2012). The longer the shifts for hospital nurses, the higher the levels of burnout and patient dissatisfaction. *Health Affairs, 31*, 2501–2509.

SUGGESTED READINGS

Bisgaard, S. (2009). *Solutions to the healthcare quality crisis: Cases and examples of lean six sigma in healthcare*. Milwaukee, WI: American Society for Quality, Quality Press.

Cronenwett, L., Sherwood, G., Barnsteiner, J., Disch, J., Johnson, J., Mitchell, P., et al. (2007). Quality and safety education for nurses. *Nursing Outlook, 55*(3), 122–131.

Finkelman, A., & Kenner, C. (2007). *Teaching IOM: Implications of the Institute of Medicine reports for nursing education*. Silver Springs, MD: American Nurses Association.

Hughes, R. (2008). Tools and strategies for quality improvement and patient safety. In *Patient safety and quality: An evidence-based handbook for nurses*. Rockville, MD: Agency for Healthcare Research and Quality, AHRQ Publication No. 08-0043.

Institute of Medicine. (2000). *To err is human: Building a safer health system*. Washington, DC: National Academies Press.

Institute of Medicine. (2001). *Crossing the quality chasm: A new health system for the 21st century*. Washington, DC: National Academies Press.

Institute of Medicine. (2003). *Keeping patients safe: Transforming the work environment of nurses.* Washington, DC: National Academies Press.

Institute of Medicine. (2007). *Preventing medication errors.* Washington, DC: National Academies Press.

Sherwood, G. & Barnsteiner, J. (Eds.), (2012). *Quality and safety in nursing: A competency approach to improving outcomes.* Ames, IA: Wiley-Blackwell.

INTERNET RESOURCES

Agency for Healthcare Research and Quality. www.ahrq.gov/.

Agency for Healthcare Research and Quality. *TeamSTEPPS.* http://teamstepps.ahrq.gov/.

Centers for Disease Control and Prevention's Division of Healthcare Quality Promotion. http://www.cdc.gov/ncezid/dhqp/.

Centers for Medicare & Medicaid Services HCAHPS Survey. www.hcahpsonline.org/home.aspx.

Centers for Medicare & Medicaid Services Hospital Compare. http://medicare.gov/hospitalcompare/.

Centers for Medicare & Medicaid Services Physician Compare. www.medicare.gov/find-a-doctor/.

ECRI Institute. www.ecri.org/2013hazards.

Institute of Medicine. www.iom.edu/.

National Institute for Occupational Safety and Health. www.cdc.gov/NIOSH/.

National Quality Forum. www.qualityforum.org/.

The Joint Commission. www.jointcommission.org/.

The Joint Commission Accountability Measures. www.jointcommission.org/accountability_measures.aspx.

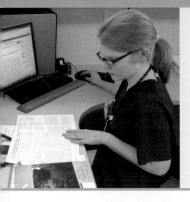

21

Translating Research into Practice

Margarete Lieb Zalon

The importance of research in the development of the scientific basis for nursing practice is described in this chapter. The role of the nurse as a follower, manager, and leader of a healthcare organization in applying research to practice is delineated in the context of twenty-first century demands for providing health care based on the best available scientific evidence. The practical aspects of evaluation and utilization of research, the development of evidence-based practice in nursing, and practice-based evidence are described. Strategies for translating research into practice that can be used by the individual nurse as a follower, leader, and manager in the context of the organization are outlined.

LEARNING OUTCOMES

- Value the individual nurse's obligation to use research in practice.
- Analyze the differences among evidence-based practice, practice-based evidence, comparative effectiveness, and outcomes research.
- Formulate a clinical question that can be searched in the literature.
- Evaluate resources for the best available evidence.
- Identify resources for critically appraising evidence.
- Assess organizational barriers to and facilitators of the implementation of research findings.
- Identify strategies for translating research into practice within the context of an organization.

KEY TERMS

clinical guidelines
comparative effectiveness
   research (CER)
diffusion of innovation
evidence-based practice (EBP)
meta-analysis
outcomes

participatory action research
   (PAR)
patient-centered outcomes
   research
practice-based evidence (PBE)
practice-based research network
   (PBRN)

randomized controlled trial
   (RCT)
research
translating research into practice
   (TRIP)
translation science

THE CHALLENGE

Holly Olsen, BSN, RN, CCRN
Staff Nurse, LifeFlight®, Miami Children's Hospital, Miami,
    Florida

I had been a staff nurse in neonatal intensive care units for 10 years, first in Miami and then Dallas, before returning to my hometown of Miami. I have been a member of the neonatal/pediatric transport team for LifeFlight®, which transports critically ill infants from the outlying community hospitals in Florida, as well as some international hospitals, back to our medical center. I was concerned about the care that we were able to provide to these fragile neonates. During the emergency of establishing an airway at the referral hospitals, using the correct endotracheal tube size and tube placement were not always done according to the Neonatal Resuscitation Program (NRP) guidelines. Sometimes we would need to reinsert a tube, wasting precious time. We knew that not selecting an appropriate-sized endotracheal tube for extremely-low-birth-weight (ELBW) infants could possibly lead to complications. We were not confident that everyone was familiar with best practices regarding neonatal resuscitation. I felt strongly that there had to be a way that we could improve on what we were doing.

What do you think you would do if you were this nurse?

INTRODUCTION

If you or a loved one required nursing care, you would want that care to be based on the best research evidence available. For example, if a family member needed to be on a ventilator, you would want to be sure that the nurses providing the care were using best practices to prevent ventilator-associated pneumonia. You would want to know that communication is good among nurses and physicians on the clinical unit where your family member has been placed, because you know that research demonstrates that teamwork and collaboration lead to lower mortality and fewer errors. If that family member also had a central venous catheter, you would want to be sure that the nurse who removes that catheter is using an established procedure that minimizes the risk for introducing an air embolism into the circulation. And, when that family member is discharged, you would want to know that the nurses are using well-tested strategies to help that person transition to home, recover from his or her illness, and manage that illness. As a follower, leader, and manager, you should be concerned about incorporating research evidence not only into clinical practices but also into the management of systems of care. The challenge is how to (1) find the best research evidence, (2) incorporate the best evidence into practice in a meaningful manner, and (3) motivate nurses, nursing leadership, and organizational leadership to care about using evidence in practice in the midst of all the other challenges faced in delivering high-quality nursing care.

Research is an integral part of professional practice. Research is the "diligent, systematic inquiry or investigation to validate and refine existing knowledge and generate new knowledge" (Burns & Grove, 2013, p. 1). Nurses, as professionals, have an obligation to society that involves rights and responsibilities as well as a mechanism for accountability. These obligations are outlined in *Nursing's Social Policy Statement: The Essence of the Profession* developed by the American Nurses Association (ANA, 2010) and includes: "To refine and expand nursing's knowledge base, nurses use theories that fit with professional nursing's values of health and health care that are relevant to professional nursing practice. Nurses apply research findings and implement the best evidence into their practice ... (p. 13).

The *Code of Ethics for Nurses* (ANA, 2001, p. 22) directs that the "nurse participates in advancement of the profession through contributions to practice, education, administration and knowledge development." Furthermore, the global importance of nursing research is illustrated by an International Council of Nurses' (ICN) position statement indicating support for "national nurses' associations in their efforts to enhance nursing research, particularly through improving access to education, which prepares nurses to conduct research, critically evaluate research outcomes and promote appropriate application of research findings to nursing practice" (2007, p. 3). Nursing research is designed to refine and expand the scientific foundation for nursing. Nursing practice draws upon nursing science and the physical, economic, biomedical, behavioral, and social sciences (ANA, 2010). Thus nurses need to apply findings of nursing research and research conducted by members of other disciplines that have relevance for their own practice.

Evidence-based practice (EBP) is derived from the definition of evidence-based medicine: the integration of the best research evidence with clinical expertise and the patient's unique values and circumstances in making decisions about the care of individual patients (Straus, Richardson, Glasziou, & Haynes, 2011). Use of the word "practice" denotes the use of evidence by all health care practitioners including nurses. In EBP, clinicians drive the search for solutions to clinical problems based on the best available evidence, which is then translated into practice. EBP is a broader, more encompassing view of using research in practice. It is focused on searching for, appraising, and synthesizing the best evidence to address a particular clinical practice problem.

The translation of evidence into practice involves all healthcare disciplines. The National Institutes of Health (NIH) (2011) created a roadmap to harness scientific discovery to improve the health of all people. The roadmap has three major themes: (1) new pathways to discovery, (2) research teams of the future, and (3) reengineering the clinical research enterprise. "New pathways to discovery" is focused on new strategies for diagnosing, treating, and preventing disease. It includes building blocks, biological pathways and networks, molecular libraries and imaging, structural biology, bioinformatics and computational biology, and nanomedicine. "Research teams of the future" focuses on high-risk research, interdisciplinary teams, and public-private partnerships. "Reengineering the clinical research enterprise" focuses on clinical research networks, policy analysis and coordination, dynamic assessment of patient-reported chronic disease outcomes, and translational research. The goal is to foster high-risk/high-reward research, develop transformative tools and methodologies, fill knowledge gaps, and foster collaboration in order to get research into the hands of practitioners so they can improve patient care.

The oft-quoted statistic of taking 17 years to apply research discoveries to clinical practice (Balas & Boren, 2000) is indicative of the need for healthcare professionals to accelerate research integration with practice. Even if that time has been reduced dramatically, the gap is still measured in years, not months. We might believe that once a research study is published in a journal, clinicians read it immediately and then nurses and/or policymakers use it to improve practice. Often, that is not the case. For example, Norma

Metheny has been researching techniques for testing nasogastric tube placement for many years. She and her colleagues demonstrated the unreliability of auscultating the epigastrium for air insufflated through the tube (Metheny & Titler, 2001). A variety of bedside methods are recommended to predict tube location during insertion and after feedings are started. Metheny's research has been incorporated into a practice alert of the American Association of Critical-Care Nurses (AACN) (2010) and enteral nutrition recommendations (Bankhead et al., 2009). EBP has the dual purpose of promoting the use of effective strategies to improve patient care and helping nurses to stop the use of ineffective strategies that might harm patients.

Research provides the foundation for nursing practice improvement. Examples include preoperative teaching, pain management, child development assessment, falls prevention, pressure-ulcer risk detection, incontinence care, transitional care, and family-centered care in critical care units. Research needs to be systematically evaluated to determine which interventions should be implemented to improve care outcomes. Practices that were once thought to be the standard of care may quickly become outdated. Some practices may have been carried out for many years without their scientific basis or effectiveness ever being examined. The latest research findings need to be incorporated into procedures using an evidence-based model when they are being updated by an organization.

> **EXERCISE 21-1**
> Identify a common activity that is part of your nursing practice, and determine whether any research supports that particular intervention or nursing care activity.

Nursing research designs can be categorized in several ways, such as basic versus applied, qualitative versus quantitative, cross-sectional versus longitudinal, experimental versus descriptive, and retrospective versus prospective. Regardless of the design, some research is ready for implementation and some research may not yet be ready to warrant a change in practice.

The quality of care and the quality of the outcomes of care can be dramatically improved with the implementation of practices derived from a systematic evaluation of research evidence. Patients, those entrusted to our care, are deserving of practices that are based on the best available evidence. Examining the evidence for a particular practice generally needs to go beyond examining the results of a single study. At times, a single, well-designed study might be adequate for recommending and implementing a practice change. However, developing an EBP requires the development of a clearly written clinical question and a more thorough search of the literature, the review of single studies, meta-analyses, meta-syntheses, critically appraised topics, systematic reviews, and clinical guidelines.

Evidence must be appraised and placed in the context of patient, family, and community values. Nurse managers/leaders may not necessarily be the ones actually conducting research, evaluating research evidence, or developing evidence-based guidelines, but they will be facilitating the application of research findings in practice. The outcomes of care are increasingly important to a public that wants to know what is best and what was improved. The classic definition of outcomes research is the "end results of health services that takes patients' experiences, preferences, and values into account" (Clancy and Eisenberg, 1998, p. 5).

This research has the intent of providing "scientific evidence relating to decisions made by all who participate in health care" (Clancy & Eisensberg, 1998, p. 245). Improving the outcomes of care involves different approaches such as identifying evidenced-based practices, comparative effectiveness research, participatory action research, practice-based evidence, and quality improvement. It also requires understanding how innovations are diffused into practice, and identifying appropriate strategies for translating research into practice and sustaining the practice improvement. Nurses and their leaders and managers will face many decisions along the way in order to effectively implement evidence derived from research into daily care practices.

FROM USING RESEARCH TO EVIDENCE-BASED PRACTICE

Individual nurses may apply research findings to their own practice. However, nurses' broader responsibility to society includes activating the change process in translating research into practice. Research use can be in a variety of forms: enlightenment, implementation of a research-based protocol, or the widespread adoption of standards based on research findings.

Ultimately, multiple factors influence how a particular research finding is adopted, translated into practice, and sustained.

Nurse researchers have a distinguished record of research utilization. In the 1970s, three major projects facilitated research utilization: the Western Interstate Commission on Higher Education in Nursing (WICHEN)(Krueger, 1977); Conduct and Utilization of Research in Nursing (CURN) (Horsley, Crane, Crabtree & Wood, 1983) and Nursing Child Assessment Satellite Training (NCAST), (King, Barnard & Hoehn, 1981) (NCAST Programs, 2014). These initiatives spawned the growth of many demonstration projects in an effort to use research, as well as research studies identifying factors that facilitate or create barriers to research utilization. The NCAST feeding and teaching scales, developed by Kathryn Barnard, partners nurses with low-income, first-time mothers to promote healthy pregnancies and improved child health. It is widely used by home health agencies and public health departments across the country and even internationally (NCAST Programs, 2014).

Stetler's model (2001) provides direction for individual nurses as well as for nurses in leadership roles responsible for patient care management in sustaining evidence-based practices. It consists of five phases: preparation, validation, comparative evaluation/decision making, translation/application, and evaluation (Figure 21-1). The preparatory phase involves searching, sorting, and selecting sources of evidence, defining external factors influencing the application of a research finding, and defining internal factors diminishing objectivity. The second phase, validation, focuses on utilization with an appraisal of study findings rather than the critique of a study's design. This phase includes completing review tables to facilitate understanding each study and to facilitate decision-making. The third phase, comparative evaluation and decision making, involves making a decision about the applicability of the studies by synthesizing cumulative findings; evaluating the degree and nature of other criteria, such as risk, feasibility, and readiness of the finding; and actually making a recommendation about using the research. The fourth phase, translation and application, involves practical aspects of implementing the plan for translating the research into practice at the individual, group, department, or organizational level. Multiple strategies are recommended

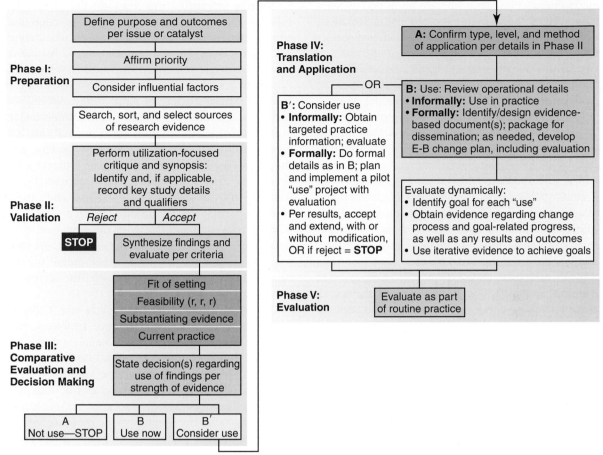

FIGURE 21-1 Stetler's model. *Feasibility (r,r,r),* evaluation of **r**isk factors, need for **r**esources, and **r**eadiness of others involved. *E-B,* Evidence-based.

for change implementation. Translating the research finding into practice should not exceed that warranted by the evidence. The last phase is evaluation, which can be informal or formal and may include a cost-benefit analysis. Evaluation can include whether the research innovation was implemented as intended and goal achievement. Stetler's model focuses heavily on the change process to facilitate successful translation of research into practice.

DEVELOPMENT OF EVIDENCE-BASED PRACTICE

EBP is derived from the work of Archie Cochrane, who described the lack of knowledge about healthcare treatment effects and advocated for using proven

treatments. Subsequently, the Cochrane Collaboration was established at Oxford University in 1993. About that time, Gordon Guyatt and his colleagues at McMaster University authored a series of articles in the *Journal of the American Medical Association* known as the *Users' Guides to the Medical Literature* that provided a foundation for teaching evidence-based medicine.

Thus, the focus in the 1990s changed to finding a research-based solution to clinical problems, not only in nursing, but also in medicine and other disciplines. Healthcare organizations began to be more systematic in using research and evaluating patient outcomes. The forerunner of the federal Agency for Healthcare Research and Quality (AHRQ) issued consensus-based clinical guidelines for common healthcare problems, such as acute pain, incontinence, pressure ulcers, depression, and human immunodeficiency virus (HIV) prevention. Professional associations and other groups also began to issue clinical guidelines. The *National Guideline Clearinghouse* was created on the Web by the AHRQ in partnership with the American Medical Association and the American Association of Health Plans. Professional associations, evidence-based practice work groups, private organizations, and other groups may submit clinical guidelines to the clearinghouse, which has a searchable database.

The EBP movement has grown exponentially with scientific publications, establishment of collaboration centers, resources on the Web, and grants focused specifically on translating research into practice. A number of evidence-based nursing centers have been established. The Joanna Briggs Institute, based in Australia, has a network of collaborating centers and evidence-based synthesis and utilization groups around the world. These centers have teams of researchers who critically appraise evidence and then disseminate protocols for the use of evidence in practice. Resources for evidence-based health care are listed in Box 21-1.

BOX 21-1   RESOURCES FOR EVIDENCE-BASED HEALTH CARE

Agency for Healthcare Research and Quality (AHRQ) evidence-based practice: www.ahrq.gov/
Centre for Evidence-Based Medicine (CEBM): www.cebm.net
The Cochrane Collaboration: www.cochrane.org
Cochrane Database of Systematic Reviews (CDSR): www.cochrane.org/cochrane-reviews/cochrane-database-systematic-reviews-numbers
Centre for Evidence-Based Medicine Toronto: www.cebm.utoronto.ca
Centre for Reviews and Dissemination (CRD): www.york.ac.uk/inst/crd
   Database of Abstracts of Reviews of Effects (DARE)
   Health Technology Assessment (HTA) Database
   NHS Economic Evaluation Database (EED)
Guidelines International Network: www.g-i-n.net/
International Council of Nurses: Closing the gap: From evidence to action: www.icn.ch/images/stories/documents/publications/ind/indkit2012.pdf
National Guideline Clearinghouse: www.guideline.gov
National Institute for Health and Clinical Excellence: www.nice.org.uk
National Institute of Clinical Studies: www.nhmrc.gov.au/nics/
Primary Care Practice-Based Research Networks: pbrn.ahrq.gov
Scottish Intercollegiate Guidelines Network (SIGN): www.sign.ac.uk/

Nursing specialty organizations that have developed evidence-based standards of practice and clinical guidelines, include the American Association of Neuroscience Nurses, Association of Women's Health, Obstetric and Neonatal Nurses (AWHONN), American Society of Perianesthesia Nurses, and the Infusion Nurses Society to name a few. AWHONN maintains a consumer Website *(www.health4women. org)* to provide information for women's and babies' health. The Oncology Nursing Society and the Registered Nurses' Association of Ontario have developed toolkits for EBP. The American Heart Association's Council on Cardiovascular and Stroke Nursing participates in interdisciplinary teams for guideline development. Many of the guidelines produced by evidence-based centers and other professional groups are available either online on the organization's Website or through the National Guideline Clearinghouse.

Today, researchers and clinicians are collaborating to solve particular practice problems and advance health care. Health maintenance organizations are monitoring provider practices for patients' adherence to screening guidelines. Voluntary organizations providing support services for individuals not covered by health insurance are expecting that the agencies they fund provide evidence for the outcomes of their projects to more effectively meet community needs.

Societal factors, such as the rising cost of health care, quality improvement initiatives, and the pressures to avoid errors, have resulted in an increased emphasis on research as a basis for practice decisions. Healthcare professionals are called upon to use evidence in practice in the midst of an exponentially expanding scientific knowledge base. The Institute of Medicine (IOM) (Greiner & Knebel, 2003) indicates that all healthcare professionals should be educated in EBP and be able to do the following:

- Know where and how to find the best possible sources of evidence
- Formulate clear clinical questions
- Search for relevant answers to those questions from the best possible sources, including those that evaluate or appraise evidence for its usefulness with respect to a particular patient or population
- Determine when and how to integrate those findings into practice

The IOM report along with many other initiatives, including healthcare reform legislation create the impetus for healthcare professionals to collaborate and work together as a team. These collaborative efforts need to be expanded to include evidence-based practice. The importance of an interdisciplinary approach to evidence-based practice is illustrated by Newhouse and Spring (2010) in the following Literature Perspective.

LITERATURE PERSPECTIVE

Resource: Newhouse, R.P. & Spring, B. (2010). Interdisciplinary evidence-based practice: Moving from silos to synergy. *Nursing Outlook, 58*(6), 309-317.

Despite calls for interprofessional education by leading policy organizations such as the Institute of Medicine, the health professions have not embraced the education of students in a collaborative approach to interdisciplinary evidence-based practice (EBP). The authors describe national initiatives fostering quality and healthcare reform that can be leveraged to foster interdisciplinary EBP. The work of two knowledge synthesis groups, the Cochrane Collaborative and the U.S. Preventive Services Task Force (USPSTF) are described. The Evidence-Based Behavioral Practice Model designed under the aegis of the NIH Office of Behavioral and Social Sciences Research to harmonize EBP approaches to behavioral health interventions includes a research synthesis by all team members. The five-step process is as follows: (1) ask, (2), acquire, (3) appraise, (4) apply, and (5) analyze and adjust.

Implications for Practice
Much of the work of EBP teams will be directed toward practice settings because that is where the evaluation and application of research evidence takes place. These efforts will require that the professions understand each other's language and coordinate their efforts as a team.

Nursing research exists on a continuum, and not all research is ready for, or of a quality that is appropriate for implementation; or it may not be ready for implementation in a particular setting. However, the quality of care and the quality of the outcomes of care can be dramatically improved with the implementation of evidence-based nursing practices. Nurses are heeding the call to develop evidenced-based practices. Nurse leaders and managers have a critical responsibility in promoting the use of the best evidence for practice. Resources for evidence-based nursing are listed in Box 21-2.

BOX 21-2   RESOURCES FOR EVIDENCE-BASED NURSING

American Nurses Association Research Toolkit: www.nursingworld.org/Research-Toolkit

Arizona State University College of Nursing Center for the Advancement of Evidence-Based Practice (CAEP): https://nursingandhealth.asu.edu/evidence-based-practice/

University of Iowa College of Nursing Evidence-Based Practice Guidelines: www.nursing.uiowa.edu/excellence/evidence-based-practice-guidelines

The Joanna Briggs Institute: www.joannabriggs.edu.au

The Sarah Cole Hirsch Institute for Best Nursing Practices Based on Evidence: http://fpb.case.edu/Centers/Hirsh/

ONS PEP ® Putting Evidence into Practice. www.ons.org/Research/PEP

The Ohio State University Center for Transdisciplinary Evidence-based Practice (CTEP): http://nursing.osu.edu/sections/ctep/

The Registered Nurses Association of Ontario Nursing Best Practice Guidelines: www.rnao.org/bestpractices/

University of Texas Health Science Center at San Antonio's Academic Center for Evidence-Based Practice (ACE): www.acestar.uthscsa.edu/

EXERCISE 21-2
Select a clinical guideline appropriate for implementation in your clinical setting (see National Guideline Clearinghouse [www.guideline.gov]). Identify as many strategies as possible for disseminating the guideline's key points to direct care nurses at a clinical agency. Compare your list of strategies with that of a colleague.

COMPARATIVE EFFECTIVENESS RESEARCH

Though clinicians are concerned with identifying the best evidence for a practice, very often the benefits of a particular practice are not particularly clear. Comparing the effectiveness of interventions can help to address the needs of clinicians in determining best practices for their patients. Comparative effectiveness research (CER) is the "generation and synthesis of evidence that compares the benefits and harms of alternative methods to prevent, diagnose, treat, and monitor a clinical condition or to improve the delivery of care" (Institute of Medicine, 2009, p. 29). In 2009, the American Recovery and Reinvestment Act of 2009 set aside $1.1 billion for comparative effectiveness research. To understand CER, one needs to understand the difference between efficacy and effectiveness. Efficacy is testing an intervention or treatment in a traditional randomized clinical trial under carefully controlled conditions and is used to determine whether an intervention or treatment works. Whereas effectiveness is testing whether the intervention or treatment works in the real world of practice (Morton & Ellenburg, 2012). CER is focused on addressing the decision needs of clinicians and their patients in daily practice (IOM, 2009, p. 33). An example of CER in nursing is a study comparing two protocols for nursing home residents with advanced dementia (Kovach et al., 2012), A five-step decision support tool was compared with a nine-step decision support tool to address the undertreatment of pain and other unmet needs. The nine-step tool was more helpful to nurses in changing their practice and improving patient outcomes.

PRACTICE-BASED EVIDENCE

With the growth of large databases, the use of electronic health records, and sophisticated statistical techniques, examining practices in real-world situations and comparing the effectiveness of interventions is enhanced. Practice-based evidence (PBE) is a research methodology that helps inform practice decisions by examining outcomes in the real world. In clinical practice, patients may not be similar and the application of an intervention may have multiple variations, which provides an important approach for studying comparative effectiveness. A PBE study uses an observational cohort study design that compares clinically relevant interventions, includes diverse study participants, uses heterogeneous practice settings, collects data on a broad range of health outcomes, and includes frontline clinicians in study development (Horn, DeJong, & Deutscher, 2012). This methodology was used to determine factors associated with nursing home implementation of the components of a pressure ulcer prevention program that integrated health information technology (Sharkey et al., 2013). High level administrators, nurse managers, quality improvement personnel, nurse educators, an internal champion, and an in-house dietician were related to a high level of program implementation.

PARTICIPATORY ACTION RESEARCH

The inclusion of stakeholders, for example, frontline clinicians in the study by Horn et al. (2012), is an example of participatory action research (PAR), sometimes also called community-based participatory research. In PAR, the members of the community being studied are integral members of the research team and are involved in identifying the questions and addressing the issues involved in the implementation of the research project (Chevalier & Buckles, 2013). The importance of community stakeholders and the need to make research relevant to the community of interest was recognized with key provisions of the Affordable Care Act (ACA) of 2010. The Patient-Centered Outcomes Research Institute (PCORI), under the auspices of the Centers for Medicare & Medicaid (CMS), was created by Congress to conduct research to provide information about the best available evidence to help patients and their health providers make more informed decisions (PCORI, 2012). The focus is on CER, improving healthcare systems, communication, and dissemination; addressing disparities; and accelerating patient-centered outcomes research (PCORI, 2012). Strong stakeholder input is considered critical to the success of this type of research. PAR is particularly strong in public health and community settings, but increasingly is being used in other healthcare settings such as hospitals. An example of PAR is a study designed to implement evidence-based oncology nursing practices on a nursing unit (Abad-Corpa et al., 2013). The researcher and clinicians agreed together on 7 practice changes and 11 implementation strategies.

QUALITY IMPROVEMENT

Quality improvement activities are focused on using data to improve the processes and outcomes of care, whereas evidence-based practice is focused on the incorporation of the best scientific evidence into specific care processes (Shirey et al., 2011). Many times these activities overlap. The National Database of Nursing Quality Indicators (NDNQI®) established by the ANA (n.d.) collects data on nursing structures, processes and outcomes, which provide a comprehensive overview of quality. It includes data on nursing-sensitive outcomes. These outcomes, such as falls, nosocomial infections, and pressure ulcers, are directly related to the quality of nursing care in contrast to those outcomes that are dependent on a multidisciplinary team effort. Hospitals receive benchmark comparisons with state, regional, and national data. The staff can then design practice improvement projects with outcomes measured using a standard methodology. These projects often use evidence-based practices as a foundation for their quality improvement activities. For example, researchers at one hospital used NDNQI® data related to nurse satisfaction to assess the effectiveness of a team building intervention (Barrett, Piatek, Korber, & Padula, 2009).

Similarly, a number of physician specialty organizations collect quality indicators for specific procedures such as coronary artery bypass graft surgery and joint replacement providing their members with benchmark data. The U.S. Department of Veterans Affairs launched its Quality Enhancement Research Initiative in 1998 to use research evidence to improve practice. A variety of strategies, very often incorporating different types of research activities, is used to make practice improvements to enhance patient care.

DIFFUSION OF INNOVATIONS

The now classic theory of diffusion of innovations (Rogers, 2003) describes how innovations spread through society, occurring in stages: knowledge, persuasion, decision, implementation, and confirmation. This theory, highlighted in the following Theory Box, provides a useful model in planning for the integration of evidence into practice over time.

An innovation might be continued because of the positive reinforcement received when outcomes are favorable. An innovation also might be discontinued, for example, when a better idea is adopted or when disenchantment occurs because of dissatisfaction with the process or outcome.

An intervention's characteristics can influence its adoption. These include the relative advantage (whether it is better than what it replaces), compatibility (consistency with values, experiences, needs), complexity (difficulty in understanding its use), trialability (the degree to which it can be easily tested), and observability (the ease of seeing the results) (Rogers, 2003).

Widespread media attention to a particular finding can be instrumental in the adoption of a practice change. Extensive publicity accompanied the publication of a study about family presence during emergency procedures and resuscitation (Meyers et al., 2000). Publication of the study was accompanied by press releases, television news stories and a

THEORY BOX

Rogers' Diffusion of Innovations

STAGE	KEY IDEA	ACTIVITIES
Knowledge	Exposure to an innovation and how it functions	The process includes seeking and analyzing information. Literature reviews are focused on addressing practice problems. Information can be disseminated through journals, conferences, educational programs, audiovisual or electronic media, journal clubs, and/or other outlets.
Persuasion	Development of attitudes about an innovation through psychological involvement and selective perception	Informal communication networks are used to facilitate change. Positive or negative attitudes can develop. An event or activity can be used to spark interest in moving from a favorable attitude to behavior change.
Decision	Commitment to adoption	The innovation can be adopted, adopted and then discontinued, rejected outright, or not even considered by the organization at this stage.
Implementation	Putting the innovation into practice	Change agents provide support for the implementation process. Behavior changes as the innovation is adopted. Key features of an innovation are identified to evaluate its effectiveness. Problems with implementing the innovation are addressed. Change and modification (reinvention) occur to use the innovation in a particular practice environment. Reinvention facilitates the sustainability of the innovation.
Confirmation	Evaluating the innovation	A decision is made about continuing or discontinuing the innovation. The innovation, if adopted, is integrated into the organization's practices.

Theory data from Rogers, E. (2003). *Diffusion of innovations* (5th ed., pp. 171-195). New York: Free Press.

video. Since then, family presence research has been replicated, and expanded to other settings (Pankop, Chang, Thorlton, & Spitzer, 2013). This strengthens the scientific basis for the innovation and facilitates the practice of allowing families to be present during resuscitation, but it is not without challenges and barriers to widespread implementation. McHugh and Ma (2013) found that hospitals with a good work environment for nurses had fewer 30-day readmissions for Medicare patients over age 65 years with heart failure, myocardial infarction, and pneumonia than those with poor work environments. The results suggest that improving environments for nursing practice and reducing nursing workloads could result in fewer readmissions for Medicare patients. This research was reported in *The Philadelphia Inquirer* and *U.S. News & World Report* providing consumers with information about the importance of nurse staffing and working conditions in hospitals, noting that readmissions cost Medicare more than $15 billion per year. This is particularly significant with increased hospital accountability for preventable readmissions under the ACA.

Nurse researchers write clinical articles in addition to research articles. Many journals that are directed toward clinicians provide nurses with easy-to-understand summaries of studies from the general healthcare and nursing research literature. Nursing schools develop press releases when researchers publish studies, which are then used by the media for their news articles. For example, Rachel Jones (Jones & Lacroix, 2012) conducts research on the use of urban soap opera videos delivered on a handheld device to convey messages about HIV risk reduction in young adult urban women. Publicity in various media outlets in the community, her receipt of an award from *The New York Times,* and a Website increase visibility of this important public health problem.

EXERCISE 21-3

Locate a research column in a clinical nursing journal. Identify one study that has implications for your practice. Retrieve the original article to learn more about the patient population, details of the study design, and results.

The translation of research into practice requires that nurse leaders and managers understand group dynamics, individual responses to innovation and change, and the culture of their healthcare organization.

BOX 21-3   CHARACTERISTICS OF INNOVATION ADOPTERS

TYPE	CHARACTERISTICS
Innovators	Active in seeking new information. Organization's visionaries.
Early adopters	Organization's opinion leaders who learn about an innovation and apply it to their practice. Can be effective in communicating the value of an innovation.
Early majority	Will not bring forth an innovation but will readily adopt it when brought forth by others.
Late majority	Skeptics who do not adopt something unless there is pressure. Feel safe when there is limited uncertainty.
Laggards	Most secure in holding on to the past. Most comfortable when an idea cannot fail.

From Rogers, E. (2003). *Diffusion of innovations* (5th ed.). New York: Free Press.

Rogers (2003) categorizes people according to how quickly they are willing to adopt an innovation. Box 21-3 describes these categories. Understanding the characteristics of innovation adopters is critical when planning to introduce new practices based on research evidence.

Nursing as a profession has an obligation to the public to shorten the typical 17-year gap between discovery in a research finding to adoption in clinical practice. Those committed to the EBP movement in nursing have attempted to speed the adoption of innovations. Rogers' (2003) theory of diffusion of innovations is useful in helping us understand how research can be disseminated to the larger community. It also provides guidance on how to take advantage of organizational dynamics to accelerate the process.

The diffusion of an innovation does not necessarily follow a linear path. External factors may sometimes contribute to the adoption of an innovation. These may include the development of standards regarding the practice that are widely disseminated, cost-effectiveness studies, changes in the products or technology, the publication of clear and compelling evidence, and changes in staff members and leadership at an institution. For example, the Needlestick

Safety and Prevention Act of 2000 required employers to identify, evaluate, and implement safety-engineered medical devices, keep injury logs, and involve users of sharps in the decision making regarding the use of such devices. Percutaneous injury surveillance data from 1993 to 2006 indicate that after the legislation, injury rates in nonsurgical settings dropped by 31.6%, but they increased by 6.5% in surgical settings, with three quarters of the injuries occurring when devices were passed among team members (Jagger, Berguer, Phillips, Parker, & Gomaa, 2011). In a comparison of direct care nurses' needlestick injuries in four countries, researchers found injuries to direct care nurses working on medical-surgical units in the United States decreased, but they increased for nurses working in the operating room/perioperative care settings (Clarke, Schubert, & Körner, 2007). However, the sharps injuries were higher in Germany and Canada where there is less use and adoption of safer technologies. These studies indicate that additional efforts are needed to change practices in order to decrease injury rates.

A meta-analysis of the use of saline and the elimination of a low-dose heparin flush solution for capped angiocatheters is a well-known example of compelling evidence for innovation diffusion (Goode et al., 1991). A meta-analysis used statistics to combine results of similar studies to determine whether aggregated findings are significant. Although some institutions continued to use heparin flushes for a number of years, their use became less common and all but disappeared in the late 1990s. This was considerably later than one would expect, given the compelling nature of the evidence. The innovation needed to be communicated to nurses, physicians, and key leaders in the institutional hierarchy that using heparin was no longer appropriate. For some institutions, it was not until the costs were analyzed and concerns were raised about complications from small doses of heparin that transition to saline flushes was finally accomplished. This research has been extended to central venous catheters in adults and capped peripheral and central venous catheters in children and neonates. A systematic review of heparin use in peripheral intravenous catheters in neonates indicated that because of variations in the neonates' clinical conditions and treatments, a recommendation to

use heparin could not be made (Shah, Ng, & Sinha, 2005). Unfortunately, serious and deadly errors were made when heparin doses suitable for adults were mistakenly administered instead of low-dose flush solutions. Research in this area has continued with the demonstration that catheters flushed with normal saline lasted significantly longer than heparin-flushed catheters (Cook, Bellini, & Cusson, 2011). Careful analysis of research results, the timely implementation of important findings, and ongoing clinical research are critical to the nurse's role in promoting patient safety. The best evidence needs to be incorporated into practice and practices that have potential for harm need to be eliminated.

Another example of innovation diffusion is a review of the evidence for intramuscular (IM) injection technique conducted by Malkin (2008). The practice of administering IM injections for pain management to adults in acute care settings has virtually disappeared with the use of the intravenous and epidural routes. Nurses learn the technique in their initial nursing program but may never subsequently alter their practices (Malkin, 2008). IM injections are used in many settings throughout the world to deliver long-acting antibiotics; biologics such as immunoglobulins, vaccines, and toxoids; and hormonal agents. Use of the dorsogluteal site is no longer recommended, yet we do not know whether nurses are still using this technique.

Madsen et al. (2005) questioned the practice of listening to the bowel sounds of abdominal surgery patients to assess the return of gastrointestinal motility, concluding that the presence or absence of bowel sounds was not associated with any interventions. The authors recommend problems experienced by patients after abdominal surgery indicating absent bowel motility (e.g., nausea, abdominal distention) be treated with interventions such as antiemetic administration or nasogastric tube insertion. The research team developed and evaluated a practice guideline outlining steps for gastrointestinal assessment. Massey (2012) found that time to first flatus and time to first bowel sounds in patients recovering from gastrointestinal (GI) surgery were not significantly different. Auscultation of bowel sounds to indicate return of GI motility is a practice tradition that could possibly be replaced with other more reliable indicators (Massey, 2012). Astute practitioners should observe for the adoption of these recommendations and whether textbooks continue to recommend bowel sound assessment for patients after abdominal surgery.

TRANSLATING RESEARCH INTO PRACTICE

The science of how research is adopted is known as translation science, the science of translating research into practice (TRIP). Translation research is the "scientific investigation of methods and variables that affect adoption of evidence-based healthcare practices by individual practitioners and healthcare systems to improve clinical and operational decision-making. This includes testing the effects of strategies to promote and sustain evidence-based practices" (Titler, 2004, p. 38).

Research takes a long time to be translated into practice as illustrated by the classic example of scurvy. Lancaster demonstrated that lemon juice supplements eliminated scurvy in sailors in 1601, and Lind replicated that finding in 1747, but it was not until 1795 that the British navy added a citrus-juice supplement to the diet of its sailors (Brown, 2005). To accelerate the diffusion of research into practice, AHRQ (2012a) created a model (ACTION II) designed to promote innovation in health care delivery by conducting practice-based implementation research in a wide variety of settings. Three critical gaps in knowledge translation have been identified: (1) from need for knowledge to discovery of new knowledge, (2) from discovery to clinical application of knowledge and (3) from clinical application to development of routine clinical actions or policy (Pearson, Jordan, & Munn, 2012).

When planning to translate a research finding into practice, nurses need to know what types of strategies have been most successful. It is also helpful to know how much time was involved, how often the strategy was used, how long the treatment lasted, and whether the results were sustainable. Nurses are now testing the effectiveness of specific interventions within an organizational context and evaluating adherence to the EBP. For example, although results may be good from a particular protocol used in a randomized controlled trial to decrease ventilator-associated pneumonia, those same results may not be as dramatic when the protocol is implemented at institutions with varying resources and degrees of commitment to implementing the protocol. Nurses need to pay careful attention to the development of a clinical protocol or an evidence-based guideline and also address the implementation process. For example, implementation of EBPs with regard to pain management continues to be challenging. The implementation of an EBP pain management protocol for older adults with hip fractures not only improves the quality of pain management for these patients but also reduces hospital costs (Brooks, Titler, Ardery, & Herr, 2009; Titler et al., 2009). This EBP protocol used multifaceted strategies including practitioners' review and "reinvention" of the EBP guideline, quick reference guides, and clinical reminders. In addition, the use of opinion leaders and change champions, a three-day train-the-trainer educational program, and educational outreach for physicians and nurses was incorporated into the protocol. The intervention had a strong effect on nurse practice but had less effect on physician practices (Titler et al., 2009).

Dobbins, Ciliska, Estabrooks, and Hayward (2005) evaluated the strength of the research evidence for various strategies that promote behavioral change among health professionals. Consistently effective strategies included academic detailing or educational outreach visits (providing healthcare providers with accurate information in face-to-face visits), reminders, multifaceted interventions, and interactive education meetings and workshops. Strategies having mixed effects included audit and feedback, local opinion leaders, local consensus processes, and patient-mediated interventions. Strategies having little or no effect included the distribution of educational materials and didactic educational programs. The key point here is that active involvement leads to greater success. In a systematic review of interventions to increase nurses' research use, only four studies met inclusion criteria (Thompson, Estabrooks, Scott-Findlay, Moore, & Wallin, 2007). Educational meetings led by an opinion leader and formation of multidisciplinary committees were effective at increasing research use. Clearly, such limited evidence illustrates the need for additional research to examine best practices in increasing nurses' use of research.

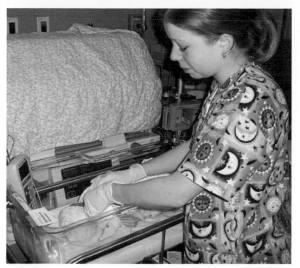

The purpose of gathering and analyzing evidence is to improve patient care.

The translation of research into practice operates at four levels: the individual healthcare professional, healthcare groups or teams, organizations, and the larger healthcare system or environment (Ferlie & Shortell, 2001). Each level has strategies that are the most appropriate, such as protocol and guideline development at the individual and team level, knowledge management at the organizational level, and the establishment of EBP centers at the systems level. This implies a multifaceted approach to disseminating EBPs and the responsibility to the larger healthcare community in fostering EBP. Various funding agencies support TRIP projects designed to evaluate the effectiveness of strategies to implement research findings because of the societal need for the timely implementation of scientific findings. TRIP science has the potential to speed up the adoption of innovations and sustain their use over time.

EBP is a proactive approach to improving patient care. Rather than relying on nurses, be they clinicians, managers, or administrators, to read the research and apply it to practice, they are now called upon to analyze practice problems and identify the research that will help them answer questions about how they should go about delivering care. Translation science takes EBP a step further in accountability for using evidence-based strategies to implement scientifically based practices.

For research to be translated into practice, it needs to reach the nurse, nurse leaders, nurse managers, and administrators in an institution, as well as policymakers who can provide the infrastructure and support necessary for the implementation of research results. Nurses today, in contrast to previous research findings, are ready for and value evidence-based practice (Melnyk, Fineout-Overholt, Gallagher-Ford, & Kaplan, 2012; Pravikoff, Tanner, & Pierce, 2005). However, Melnyk et al. (2012) also found that the organizational barriers identified over the last 20 years continue to exist today. Nurses' readiness for EBP can be harnessed for implementing and sustaining necessary practice changes. When changes in practice are demonstrated to improve outcomes and also save costs, the public and government agencies will provide additional impetus for their implementation.

EVALUATING EVIDENCE

Evidence is best evaluated with a systematic process. The EBP steps are illustrated in Box 21-4. The first steps in the implementation of EBP are creating a spirit of inquiry and identifying the problem so that the relevant information can be obtained. The clinical question should be put into the widely used PICOT format of *patient, intervention, comparison intervention or group, outcome,* and *time* to facilitate searching for

---

BOX 21-4 STEPS OF EVIDENCE-BASED PRACTICE

0. Cultivate a spirit of inquiry.
1. Ask the burning clinical question in PICOT (patient, intervention, comparison, outcome, and time frame) format.
2. Search for and collect the most relevant best evidence.
3. Critically appraise the evidence (i.e., rapid critical appraisal, evaluation, and synthesis).
4. Integrate the best evidence with one's clinical expertise and patient preferences and values in making a practice decision or change.
5. Evaluate outcomes of the practice design or change based on evidence
6. Disseminate the outcomes of the EBP (evidence-based practice) decision or change.

From Melnyk, B.M., Fineout-Overholt, E. (2011). Making the case for evidence-based practice and cultivating a spirit of inquiry. In Melnyk, B.M., & Fineout-Overholt, E. (Eds.), *Evidence-based practice in nursing and healthcare: A guide to best practice* (pp. 3-24). Philadelphia: Lippincott, Williams & Wilkins.

BOX 21-5   ASKING THE RIGHT QUESTION: THE PICOT FORMAT

Patient population	What is the patient population or the setting? This could be adults, children, or neonates with a certain health problem; or home care versus an acute care setting.
Intervention/ **I**nterest Area	What is the intervention? This can be an intervention or a specific area of interest (e.g., postoperative complications, the experience of postoperative pain).
Comparison	What is a comparison intervention? This is what the intervention might be compared with, such as a treatment, or the absence of a risk factor.
Outcome	What are the results? There might be multiple strategies to measure the results, such as complication rate, satisfaction, a nursing diagnosis, or a nursing quality indicator.
Time	What is the time frame for this intervention? Is time a relevant factor for this particular evaluation? For example, are you interested in short-term or long-term outcomes?

Adapted from Thabane, L., Thomas, T., Ye, C., & Paul, J. (2009). Posing the research question: Not so simple. *Canadian Journal of Anaesthesia, 56*(1), 71-79.

the appropriate evidence (Melnyk, Fineout-Overholt, Stillwell, & Williamson, 2010; Thabane, Thomas, Ye, & Paul, 2009). These steps are illustrated in Box 21-5.

Identifying the question may be the most challenging part of the process. Different strategies can be used to identify practice problems. For example, one might conduct a survey of staff members or use a focus group methodology. Conducting a staff survey would necessitate that staff members have sufficient knowledge of research and EBP to understand what is desired. The data from surveys or focus groups, or even informal interviews with staff, can be examined along with patient outcome data for a particular setting to address relevant practice problems. Collaborating with nurses and extending that to collaboration with members of other disciplines to

identify desired outcomes will enhance the ultimate success of an evidence-based project. This is because the staff members who will eventually be involved in implementing the practice are involved in its design and conception. Once the clinical question has been identified, writing it down will help in moving on to the next step of gathering evidence.

EXERCISE 21-4
Develop a clinical question using the PICOT (patient, intervention [interest], comparison, outcome, and time) format. Do a search in PubMed *(www.ncbi.nlm.nih.gov/pubmed)* with the key PICOT terms.

The third step of the process is searching for evidence. A number of databases are available to search for evidence. Some databases contain preprocessed evidence, such as abstracts of studies and systematic reviews of evidence. Others contain citations for original single studies. Commonly used databases are listed in Box 21-6. Obtaining a librarian's assistance to navigate the databases is helpful because the databases are constantly being upgraded with new features. Several of the suggested readings include more detailed information on locating research evidence. Preprocessed evidence can also be located in the evidence-based resources listed in Boxes 21-1 and 21-2.

The evidence for a particular practice problem can come from a single research study, an integrative review of the literature, a meta-analysis, a meta-synthesis, a clinically appraised topic, a clinical guideline, or a systematic review. Sometimes a single research study might be appropriate for application to a particular problem. For other clinical questions, multiple guidelines from different organizations on essentially the same clinical problem with slightly different recommendations might need to be studied.

A hierarchy of preprocessed evidence that ranges from evidence from a single research study to systems that integrate and regularly update EBP is illustrated in Figure 21-2. Researchers examining evidence and developing guidelines use a variety of different rating systems that include a hierarchy and key quality domains. Rating evidence is a rapidly growing field. No single established method of rating evidence is best for all situations. Using an evidence hierarchy might be most useful in rating the strength of research when comparing the quality between two or more best practice interventions (Jackson, Fazal, & Giesbrecht, n.d.).

BOX 21-6   COMMONLY USED DATABASES AND SEARCH PLATFORMS FOR NURSING

CANCERLIT www.cancer.gov/search/cancer_literature/	Bibliographic database with over a million citations and abstracts related to cancer. Includes proceedings of meetings, government reports, selected monographs, and theses.
CINAHL Cumulative Index to Nursing and Allied Health Literature www.ebscohost.com/cinahl/	A comprehensive nursing and allied health abstract database that includes some full-text material such as state nursing journals, nurse practice acts, research instruments, government publications, and patient education material from 1982 to the present.
EMBASE www.embase.com	Biomedical and pharmaceutical studies. By institutional subscription.
EBSCO www.ebscohost.com	A search platform for a variety of databases including CINAHL and MEDLINE. By institutional subscription.
MEDLINE http://www.nlm.nih.gov/databases	The largest component within PubMed, indexing over 5200 journals according to medical subject headings, MeSH. Free through PubMed.
OVID www.ovid.com	A search platform for a variety of databases including CINAHL and MEDLINE. By institutional subscription and individual pay-per-view.
PsyclNFO www.apa.org/pubs/databases/psychinfo	Abstract database of the behavioral sciences and mental health literature from the 1800s to the present. By institutional subscription or individual article purchase.
PubMed www.ncbi.nlm.nih.gov/entrez	The abstract database of the National Library of Medicine, providing access to over 15 million citations from the 1950s to the present. Links to publishers' websites for many articles. Free.

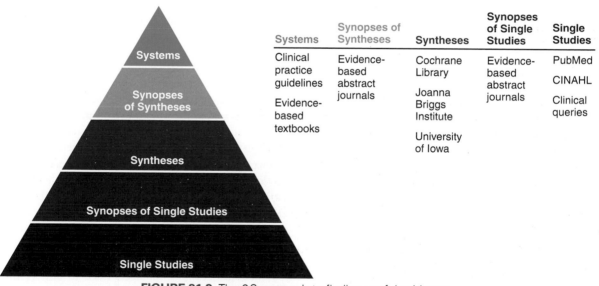

Systems	Synopses of Syntheses	Syntheses	Synopses of Single Studies	Single Studies
Clinical practice guidelines	Evidence-based abstract journals	Cochrane Library	Evidence-based abstract journals	PubMed
Evidence-based textbooks		Joanna Briggs Institute		CINAHL
		University of Iowa		Clinical queries

FIGURE 21-2 The 6 S approach to finding useful evidence.

Ultimately, whoever conducts the analysis will have to make some decisions about the strength of the evidence and whether it can be applied to a particular patient population. What is important is that once the evidence has been located, an appropriate and systematic method for rating or appraising the evidence is used. This rating system should include an analysis of whether the evidence can be applied to a particular clinical situation.

Appraisal tools exist for evaluating different types of evidence from a single qualitative study, qualitative meta-syntheses, descriptive studies, randomized clinical trials, and clinical guidelines to systematic reviews. The suggested readings provide examples of such tools. These appraisal tools generally include a series of steps for evaluating the quality of the research that is specific to the study design, type of review or guideline, or strategy for determining the applicability of the evidence to one's practice. Key elements of guideline appraisal tools include an assessment of the reliability and validity of the evidence. The *Appraisal of Guidelines for Research and Evaluation (AGREE)* tool was developed to address variability in the quality of clinical guidelines (AGREE Research Trust, 2010). The quality domains of AGREE II are predictors associated with guideline adoption (Brouwers et al., 2010).

Much of the EBP literature has been devoted to evaluating **randomized controlled trials (RCT)**. These include at least two groups and the random assignment of study participants to one group or another, either by a coin toss or by some other strategy, to test a treatment's effectiveness. Generally, it is preferable that such studies are double-blinded, meaning that the participants and those who are evaluating the outcomes do not know who has received the treatment. Although this design is generally considered the gold standard in terms of ranking individual studies, one needs to consider the quality of the study rather than merely the design. The number of RCTs conducted in nursing has been limited. Also, in certain clinical trials, blinding recipients to the interventions may be difficult to accomplish. An example is an intervention that involves clinician interaction with the study participant. An RCT is not always an appropriate design for answering a particular research question. Hence it is important that the appraisal method examine the rigor or the quality of the research in accordance with standards for that type of study.

Once the evidence has been appraised, this information needs to be integrated with clinical expertise and the preferences and values of patients, families, and communities in making the change. For example, in evaluating a research-based protocol for teaching oncology patients about preparing for a bone marrow transplant, the amount and type of information that would be desired by the patient need to be considered. In this instance, a qualitative research study might provide guidance for decision making. For certain types of interventions, the inclusion of patient preferences might not be appropriate,

as in the example of implementing a protocol for the reduction of ventilator-associated pneumonia. However, direct care nurses need to be involved in planning the details. Determining patient preferences depends on the nature of the intervention or change that is proposed.

The sheer quantity and complexity of information available indicate that nurses in direct practice need to collaborate with researchers. Nurses bring their clinical expertise, their assessment of clinically relevant questions, and their understanding of the patient population. Researchers bring their capacity to appraise evidence to facilitate its application to the clinical setting. Together, practitioners and researchers can forge a partnership in the development of an evidence-based solution to a clinical practice problem, which can then be systematically evaluated and disseminated to the wider community.

ORGANIZATIONAL STRATEGIES

The partnership between nurses and researchers needs to be extended to top leaders and stakeholders within an organization. To implement EBPs, an organization needs to be committed to the process. Staff and management need to partner with researchers to identify the appropriate evidence. Key decision makers within the organization then need to receive the evidence in a usable format. For example, in deciding whether it is best for nurses to administer preprocedure sedation or for parents to administer sedatives to children before their arrival in a department for a procedure, one needs to consider the evidence, the safety of the procedure, and the risks of unmonitored or parent-administered sedation, particularly if the child is being transported to the procedure in the back seat of a car. Providing key organizational decision makers with evidence regarding the safety of such a practice would be critical for decision-making.

Nurse leaders and managers need to understand the organizational context for using research evidence and the complex interactions between clinicians and their practice settings. The **P**romoting **A**ction on **R**esearch **I**mplementation in **H**ealth **S**ervices (PARIHS) framework illustrates this complexity (Kitson et al., 2008). Successful implementation in the PARIHS framework depends on the evidence that is being implemented, the context for implementation

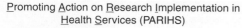

Promoting Action on Research Implementation in Health Services (PARIHS)

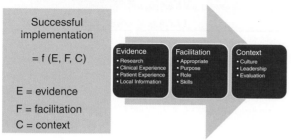

FIGURE 21-3 Promoting Action on Research Implementation in Health Services. CLAHRC for Greater Manchester in collaboration with NHS Manchester.

and the facilitation process (Figure 21-3). The following are key features of this framework:

- Evidence includes a variety of knowledge sources including research, clinical experience, patient preferences, and local information.
- Implementing evidence involves negotiation, a shared understanding of the knowledge, and a team effort
- Some contexts are more conducive to successful implementation (e.g., transformational leaders, learning organization, monitoring, feedback and evaluation).
- Appropriate facilitation improves the likelihood of success.

The PARIHS framework was used to evaluate implementation of preoperative fasting guidelines in a large implementation randomized controlled trial involving 19 hospitals in the United Kingdom. The interventions did not impact fasting times but were mediated by a complex interplay of individuals' behaviors, attitudes, emotional responses, communication, interprofessional functioning, surgical systems, and processes (Rycroft-Malone et al., 2013). The study authors indicate potentially successful strategies are working within existing structures and initiatives all ready in place, alignment with organizational goals, working with pivotal leaders, and raising awareness.

Things to consider in sustaining the practice change include (1) the strength of the evidence behind the change; (2) external and internal factors driving the change; (3) additional contextual factors such as history of practice change efforts, working relationships, and competing initiatives; and (4) method of change facilitation (education, feedback) (Rutledge, 2011). A comprehensive toolkit is available to assist nurses in the implementation of evidence-based guidelines (Registered Nurses Association of Ontario, 2012). Strategies for working with key stakeholders are described and their early involvement is emphasized because of their understanding of the extent of the problem, unmet needs, and motivation required to address the problem. An environmental assessment for readiness for EBP appears in Box 21-7. Instruments to assess beliefs about EBP and implementation are also available (Melnyk et al., 2008). A microsystem assessment can be used to understand interactions among patients, professionals, purpose, processes, and patterns in the smallest functional unit possible to gain insights regarding how a particular clinical problem or change to an EBP can be best addressed (Nelson, Batalden, & Godfrey, 2011). To sustain EBP in an organization, the leadership needs to support a research culture, the organization needs capacity to engage in EBP, and an infrastructure needs to be created to facilitate EBP (Stetler, 2003). The latter includes integrating research into key documents, creating expectations and roles, and providing recognition and technical support.

> **EXERCISE 21-5**
> Use the environmental readiness assessment in Box 21-7 to assess the capacity of your agency to implement an evidence-based guideline. Identify one strategy to address a specific barrier to implementation.

The Magnet Recognition Program® was developed by the American Nurses Credentialing Center (ANCC) to recognize excellence in nursing services. As more hospitals seek Magnet™ designation, greater emphasis will be placed on the integration of research with the delivery of nursing care. Research in the Magnet™ model includes a focus on new knowledge, innovations, and improvements with evidence of nurses taking the lead in research efforts. The model also reflects nurses' ethical and professional contributions of new findings, evidence and quality improvement to the nursing profession, and empirical outcomes with a focus on the differences that nurses have made (American Nurses Credentialing Center, n.d.).

BOX 21-7   IMPLEMENTATION OF CLINICAL PRACTICE GUIDELINES (CPG): ENVIRONMENTAL READINESS ASSESSMENT WORKSHEET

ELEMENT	QUESTION	FACILITATORS	BARRIERS
Structure	To what extent does decision-making occur in a decentralized manner? Is there enough staff to support the change process?		
Workplace culture	To what extent is the CPG consistent with the values, attitudes and beliefs of the practice environment? To what degree does the culture support change and value evidence?		
Communication	Are there adequate (formal and informal) communication systems to support information exchange relative to the CPG and the CPG implementation processes?		
Leadership	To what extent do the leaders within the practice environment support (both visibly and behind the scenes) the implementation of the CPG?		
Knowledge, skills, and attitudes of target group	Does the staff have the necessary knowledge and skills? Which potential target group is open to change and new ideas? To what extent are they motivated to implement the CPG?		
Commitment to quality management	Do quality improvement processes and systems exist to measure results of implementation?		
Availability of resources	Are the necessary human, physical, and financial resources available to support implementation?		
Interdisciplinary relationships	Are there positive relationships and trust between and among the disciplines that will be involved or affected by the CPG?		

Reprinted with permission from Registered Nurses Association of Ontario. (2002). *Toolkit: Implementation of clinical practice guidelines.* Toronto, Canada: Author. Available online at www.rnao.org/bestpractices.

The adoption of EBPs ultimately depends on a complex interaction of individual and organizational factors. Factors associated with the adoption of innovation include larger organizational size, presence of a research champion, less traditionalism, and uncommitted organizational resources. Organizational determinants positively influencing research utilization by nurses include staff development, opportunity for nurse-to-nurse collaboration, and staffing and support services. Less research utilization was associated with increased emotional exhaustion, higher nursing workloads, and higher rates of patient and nurse adverse events (Estabrooks et al., 2008; Cummings, Estabrooks, Midodzi, Wallin, & Hayduk, 2007). Nurse managers and administrators are increasingly called upon to support individual nurses, implement strategies to enhance individuals' use of evidence, and create an organizational infrastructure that promotes EBP.

ISSUES FOR NURSE LEADERS AND MANAGERS

Some of the issues faced by nurse leaders and managers include a lack of resources, limited expertise of staff members with respect to EBP, lack of knowledge about nursing research, and limited time for planning. Not all organizations can hire a full-time nurse researcher. Some organizations may not employ clinical nurse specialists. This is shortsighted in view of the potential benefits of improved patient outcomes and cost savings because of a reduction in adverse outcomes. However, this resource limitation is a reality faced in many organizations. Regardless, it is important to remember that using the best available evidence can be most successful in a partnership model. Therefore working with nurse researchers at a local college or university could be valuable. An example of a partnership between second-degree nursing students and

BOX 21-8 COLLABORATION IN DEVELOPING AN EVIDENCE-BASED PROTOCOL FOR KANGAROO CARE

Clinician Perspective

We discovered there was interest in, but not common practice of, kangaroo care for premature babies. Many of the staff members in our facilities have a wealth of clinical experience. But, they really did not have the chance to learn about evidence-based practice in school. The students came to us to talk about our needs. When they finished their work, they presented their findings about the evidence for kangaroo care and thermoregulation at our regional perinatal center nursing leadership retreat. Initially, they were intimidated about presenting to a group of such experienced nurses. However, it was rewarding to see them become more confident about their work.

Since the student presentation, we have had an upsurge of interest in providing kangaroo care. It has helped us in overcoming resistance to its use. We are now working on how to most effectively implement kangaroo care because it takes concerted work and staff time to teach and prepare the parents. One of our hospitals is using the poster developed by the students as a training tool. I enjoyed working with the students in a way that produced a tangible outcome for everyone involved. Learning how to conduct research for evidence-based practice gave the students a skill that they will have as new nurses and can offer as a complement to their more experienced nursing colleagues as they begin their professional careers.

Sally Girvin, MPH, BS, RN, NP
Coordinator, New York Presbyterian Regional Perinatal Centers, New York

Student Perspective

The eight of us who worked on this project were in the middle of our accelerated nursing program when it was assigned to us. We had to come up with an answerable clinical question, but due to our lack of clinical experience, we had only a vague idea of what to ask. We were able to develop our question after we talked with Sally and listened to her needs. We had spent some time in the neonatal intensive care unit and realized how hard it would be for the already busy nurses to take on this project. As students, we had the time.

When we went to the retreat to present our project, we thought no one would be interested in what we had done, that it might not be applicable, or that we had discovered something they already knew. The response was incredible. Our presentation created open debate. Some hospitals had kangaroo-care policies, some did not, some had them and did not follow them, and some people were unsure what they had in place. It really prompted people to look at their practices. It was a great experience to work with Sally and her colleagues and to see that what we did had an influence on policy. It was an experience that we can take with us wherever we go.

Elizabeth K. Kelly, BS, RN
Student at Columbia University School of Nursing, New York, when this project was developed

clinicians facilitated by Patricia Stone at Columbia University is illustrated in Box 21-8. New graduates who have recently completed research courses can use this model to partner with experienced nurses, thus demonstrating leadership skills and strengthening mentorship bonds. Faculty can partner with staff in a facility to provide consultation for a specific patient care problem, and agencies can partner together to address a specific practice problem.

Collaboration is critical in ensuring that evidence-based practices are incorporated into nursing care. Collaboration within organizations should involve the interdisciplinary healthcare team. For example, the adoption of suctioning guidelines should include all members of the healthcare team involved in suctioning, including nurses, pulmonologists, hospitalists, and respiratory therapists. Ideally, documentation is integrated and focused on patient outcomes in order to improve practice.

Collaboration also can take place through a **practice-based research network (PBRN).** Originally

formed to address research issues in primary care, PBRNs are being used in large healthcare organizations because they can integrate systems across multiple practice sites. AHRQ (2012b) has registered 136 primary care PBRNs, covering 11,500 primary care practices with 48 million patients. Advanced practice nurses, school nurses, and community nursing centers have established PBRNs (Deshefy-Longhi, Swartz, & Grey, 2008; Vessey et al., 2007; Anderko, Lundeen, & Bartz, 2006). Five large health systems, the Mayo Clinic, Geisinger, Kaiser Permanente, Intermountain Healthcare, and GroupHealth Cooperative (all pioneers in using electronic records), created the Care Connectivity Consortium (Poorsina, 2012). Not only do these networks provide health information exchange for the benefit of individual patients who travel to different regions of the country, but they also facilitate answering research questions that require larger samples and can draw upon the depth of the group's practice and research expertise. PBRNs are ideally suited to advance CER and PBE and have the potential for expansion into other settings such as home care, hospice, rehabilitation, and long-term care.

Examples of collaborative research include the U.S. Department of Veterans Affairs (VA) *Quality Enhancement Research Initiative (QUERI)*; the Guthrie/Geisinger health system partnership; and the Setting Universal Cessation Counseling Education and Screening Standards (SUCCESS) program of the Association of Women's Health, Obstetrical and Neonatal Nurses (AWHONN). The QUERI program is focused on heart failure, diabetes, HIV/hepatitis, heart disease, mental health, polytrauma, stroke, and substance use disorders (VA, n.d.). A partnership among three health systems in Pennsylvania and New York (Geisinger/Guthrie/Susquehanna Health) addresses a regional public health problem with a health surveillance network designed to investigate the health effects of Marcellus Shale gas drilling (Geisinger, 2014).

The SUCCESS program for smoking cessation for pregnant women was developed to reduce the adverse birth outcomes associated with smoking during pregnancy (Albrecht, Kelly-Thomas, Osborne, & Ogbagaber, 2011). AWHONN created a science team, which evaluated the evidence and concluded that smoking cessation education had the best chance of reducing low birth weight rates. Using a train-the-trainer approach to implement the program in nine states and two Canadian provinces, AWHONN was able to increase the number of practitioners providing smoking cessation interventions. In addition, numerous formal and informal groups have been established to address specialized needs and common concerns (e.g., researchers at Magnet™-designated facilities, researchers within specialty organizations).

The preparedness of nurses for evidence-based practice is an organizational issue. Many nurses might not have had research and/or statistics courses in their basic nursing education. Nurses may have had research courses many years ago and have not since used their research knowledge. Even if nurses had research courses, they might not be familiar with the critical appraisal of evidence and evidence-based practice. Nurses on a clinical unit might not be familiar with reading research or with using advanced search strategies for locating evidence for a particular practice problem. This might be especially true for nurses who

have been out of school for a long time and have not had the opportunity to develop computer literacy skills. Information on evidence-based nursing as an approach has only recently been incorporated into nursing research textbooks. A first step in developing the capacity to evaluate evidence for practice can be accomplished by starting a monthly journal club. This involves reading a relevant research article and discussing how it might be applied to the practice situation. Although nursing has a number of general and specialty nursing research journals, *Evidence-Based Nursing* and *Worldviews on Evidence-Based Nursing* are specifically devoted to evidence-based nursing practice. *Implementation Science* is a journal devoted specifically to the examination of strategies to promote the incorporation of research findings into routine health care. Journal club discussions can be used as a springboard for the identification of clinical practice problems. Even small hospitals have libraries and perhaps a part-time librarian who can assist with gathering information and identifying useful articles for the journal club's agenda. Nurses returning to school have access to university libraries, as do nurses who are employed as adjunct faculty in nursing programs.

When translating research into practice, outcomes need to be evaluated. Collecting outcomes data before implementing a protocol is preferable in order to have a basis for comparison. This is especially important when it is not possible to carry out an experimental design in which the intervention is implemented in one setting but not another. This may be the case because of sample size considerations or staff of different units casually talking with one another about the intervention. It is also important to consider whether the implementation of an evidence-based practice will turn into a research project. Sometimes quality improvement and evidence-practice activities are categorized as research. On the other hand, quality improvement activities and the adoption of evidence-based practices might not meet the standards for a research project, and the results might not be generalizable to other settings (Newhouse, 2007). Regardless, nurses preparing to engage in a project that might be considered research should consult with the organization's institutional review board early in the planning phase regardless of whether data are collected directly from patients, medical records, or staff members.

This ensures that the necessary human subjects protections are in place before the project is started.

Nurses, other healthcare professionals, and the public might not be familiar with nursing research or evidence-based nursing. Therefore it is important to publicize key nursing research findings. When nursing research is publicized in the media or through news alerts, it should also be communicated to organizational key decision makers. Sending e-mails, posting articles, and providing people with the resources helps people to learn for themselves. Joining a professional association and signing up for alerts from key agencies provide nurses with access to the latest news, research, and standards. Research has a much better chance of being implemented if key stakeholders have the opportunity to understand its relevance. It may be necessary to introduce concepts related to translating research into practice in small increments. For example, a first step might be incorporating research into the revision of procedures and agency guidelines as they come up for review. Subsequently, nurses and key stakeholders can be asked to identify clinical practice problems that create challenges in providing care in order to develop an evidence-based solution. Multiple strategies are needed to implement research findings. Multiple strategies are also needed to change a culture to one that is driven by research and evidence-based standards for practice. Finally, if one should have the opportunity to implement an EBP, as much consideration needs to be given to planning for implementation as protocol development (see Chapter 17). Advance planning should include a thorough and frank discussion of the barriers and facilitators, as well as how to minimize the barriers and maximize the facilitators. Also, strategies to sustain the adoption of the practice over time need to be considered. Although the implementation of EBP is a very complex process, the increased emphasis on the use of scientifically based evidence creates an exciting opportunity for nurses to demonstrate the value of nursing in improving patient care and healthcare outcomes.

CONCLUSION

Nurses are accountable to their patients to provide the best care possible. This means that nurses must translate research into practice. Numerous approaches to do so are possible. The challenge lies in more rapidly incorporating solid evidence into practice so that patients may benefit from that translation sooner than the current translation time.

THE SOLUTION

I began by working with a team that included a fellow staff nurse, a nurse researcher, and a nurse practitioner. We reviewed the literature and found that guidelines for selecting an appropriate-sized endotracheal tube for ELBW infants were unclear. We also decided to do a retrospective chart audit to determine what, if any, were the effects of size variations of the endotracheal tube and the depth of endotracheal tube placement on oxygen saturation and carbon dioxide levels upon intubation. We used guidelines from the NRP.

Conducting research is not without its challenges. I have not had much experience with data collection. It was also difficult to get the time to do the study. However, we really wanted to carry out this project. Sometimes, we would take our laptop on transport with us and do data entry during the "dead leg" (on the way to get the patient), as well as during our down times between transports. We shared the results with the staff at our hospital and with our community partners. Subsequently, we made large charts to be used by everyone who would be involved in neonatal resuscitation. We had a very positive response. I believe that the work we did was really important in improving the quality of care provided by the staff of our transport team and our outlying community hospitals for these tiny, fragile babies.

—Holly Olsen

Would this be a suitable approach for you? Why?

THE EVIDENCE

Holtzclaw (2013) described evidence-based approaches for the management of fever and febrile symptoms for persons living with HIV (PLWH). The author, a nurse who has focused her research on examining the nature of fever and control of febrile shivering, conducted a comprehensive review of the literature using several databases in addition to examining retrieved articles for additional sources. The search strategy and decision making for the selection of articles were clearly delineated. The evolution of scientific thinking about the nature of fever and particularly as a symptom in HIV was described along with the physiological threats and benefits of febrile responses. The evidence for antipyretic/analgesic drugs to treat fever, malaise, and lassitude, and the assessment and replacement of febrile fluid loss from sweat were also described. The article concluded with clinical considerations: (1) phases of febrile episodes, (2) the counterproductive effects of attempts to cool a fever, (3) insulating extremities to reduce shivering and perceptions of chill, (4) impact of higher body temperature on infectious organisms, and (5) specific measures for patients with HIV infection. Holtzclaw notes the lack of recent evidence on febrile symptom management in HIV care and in nursing in general and the need to test current fever management practices in HIV care.

WHAT NEW GRADUATES SAY

- Being a new nurse is an advantage because of the ability to apply what was learned about evidence-based practice in school.
- It is helpful when research is made visible by providing poster boards of the use and implications of evidence-based practices such as catheter-associated urinary tract infection (CAUTI), hand hygiene, falls prevention, and pressure ulcer prevention.
- It feels good to teach a preceptor about the latest research evidence.
- Taking part in a residency program provides additional opportunities not only to discuss developing research, but how to introduce it and apply it on the unit.

CHAPTER CHECKLIST

Society increasingly demands that health care be based on the best available evidence. Nurses have a societal obligation to use practices that are based on sound scientific evidence. The time from scientific discovery or publication of research to implementation in practice is lengthy and needs to be shortened. Nurses can speed this process by using scientifically based strategies to facilitate the translation of research into practice. The nurse manager needs to understand the organizational context for the implementation of evidence-based protocols. Multiple strategies need to be developed to enhance the use of evidence as the foundation for nursing care delivery.

- From using research to evidence-based practice
- Development of evidence-based practice
- Comparative effectiveness research
- Practice-based evidence
- Participatory action research
- Quality improvement
- Diffusion of innovations
- Translating research into practice
- Evaluating evidence
- Organizational strategies
- Issues for nurse leaders and managers

TIPS FOR DEVELOPING SKILL IN USING EVIDENCE

- Make a personal commitment to read research articles.
- Complete an online tutorial in EBP.
- Use your clinical experiences to develop relevant clinical questions.
- Obtain assistance from researchers, advanced practice registered nurses, and nurse leaders.
- Use the Patient, Intervention, Comparison, Outcome, and Time (PICOT) format to search for evidence on a clinical practice problem.
- Use a journal club to encourage your colleagues to join you in learning about EBP and evaluating research evidence.

REFERENCES

Abad-Corpa, E., Delgado-Hito, P., Cabrero-García, J., Meseguer-Liza, C., Zárate-Riscal, C. L., Carrillo-Alcaraz, A., et al. (2013). Implementing evidence in an oncohaematology nursing unit: A process of change using participatory action research. *International Journal of Evidence-Based Healthcare*, *11*(1), 46–55.

Agency on Healthcare Research Quality. (2012a). *Accelerating change and transformation in organizations and networks II*. Retrieved February 7, 2014 from, www.ahrq.gov/research/findings/factsheets/translating/action2/index.html.

Agency on Healthcare Research Quality (AHRQ). (2012b). 2012 AHRQ-registered PBRNs and the annual "PBRN slides". *PBRNews*, 7, 8.

Albrecht, S. A., Kelly-Thomas, K., Osborne, J. W., & Ogbagaber, S. (2011). The SUCCESS program for smoking cessation for pregnant women. *Journal of Obstetrical Gynecological Neonatal Nursing*, *40*(5), 520–531.

American Association of Critical-Care Nurses (AACN). (2010). *AACN clinical practice alert: Verification of feeding tube placement*. Aliso Viejo, CA: Author. Retrieved February 7, 2014 from, http://www.aacn.org/wd/practice/content/practicealerts.pcms?menu=practice.

American Nurses Association (ANA). (2001). *Code of ethics for nurses with interpretive statements*. Washington, DC: Author.

American Nurses Association (ANA). (2010). *Nursing's social policy statement: The essence of the profession*. Silver Spring, MD: Author.

American Nurses Association (ANA). (n.d.). *National Database of Nursing Quality Indicators*. Silver Spring, MD: Author.

American Nurses Credentialing Center. (n.d.). *Frequently asked questions about ANCC's Magnet Recognition Program®*. Retrieved March 15, 2013 from www.nursecredentialing.org.

Anderko, L., Lundeen, S., & Bartz, C. (2006). The Midwest Nursing Centers Consortium Research Network: translating research into practice. *Policy, Politics & Nursing Practice*, 7, 101–109.

Balas, E., & Boren, S. (2000). Managing clinical knowledge for health care improvement. In J. vanBemmel & A. McCray (Eds.), *Yearbook of medical informatics 2000: Patient-centered systems* (pp. 65–70). Stuttgart, Germany: Schattauer.

Bankhead, R., Boullata, J., Brantley, S., Corkins, M., Guenter, P., Krenitsky, J. & A.S.P.E.N. Board of Directors (2009). Enteral nutrition practice recommendations. *JPEN Journal of Parenteral and Enteral Nutrition*, *33*(2), 122–167.

Barrett, A., Piatek, C., Korber, S., & Padula, C. (2009). Lessons learned from a lateral violence and team-building intervention. *Nursing Administration Quarterly*, *33*(4), 342–351.

Brooks, J. M., Titler, M., Ardery, G., & Herr, K. (2009). Effect of evidence-based acute pain management practices on inpatient costs. *Health Services Research*, 44, 245–263.

Brouwers, M. C., Kho, M. E., Browman, G. P., Burgers, J. S., Cluzeau, F., Feder, G., et al. for the AGREE Next Steps Consortium (2010). Development of the AGREE II, part 1: Performance, usefulness and areas for improvement. *CMAJ*, *182*(1), 1045–1052.

Brown, S. R. (2005). *Scurvy: How a surgeon, a mariner, and a gentlemen solved the greatest medical mystery of the age of sail*. New York: St. Martin's Press.

Burns, N., & Grove, S. K. (2013). *The practice of nursing research: Conduct, critique, and utilization* (7th ed.). St. Louis: Saunders.

Chevalier, J. M., & Buckles, D. J. (2013). *Participatory action research: Theory and methods for engaged inquiry*. London: Routledge.

Clancy, C., & Eisenberg, J. M. (1998). Outcomes research: Measuring the end results of health care. *Science*, *282*(5387), 245–246.

Clarke, S. P., Schubert, M., & Körner, T. (2007). Sharp-device injuries to hospital staff nurses in 4 countries. *Infection Control and Hospital Epidemiology*, *28*(4), 473–478.

Cook, L., Bellini, S., & Cusson, R. M. (2011). Heparinized saline vs. normal saline for maintenance of intravenous access in neonates: An evidence-based practice change. *Advances in Neonatal Care*, *11*(3), 208–215.

Cummings, G. G., Estabrooks, C. A., Midodzi, W. K., Wallin, L., & Hayduk, L. (2007). Influence of organizational characteristics and context on research utilization. *Nursing Research*, *56*(Suppl. 4), S24–S39.

Deshefy-Longhi, T., Swartz, M. K., & Grey, M. (2008). Characterizing nurse practitioner practice by sampling patient encounters: An APRNet study. *Journal of the American Academy of Nurse Practitioners*, *20*, 281–287.

DiCenso, A., Bayley, L., & Haynes, R. B. (2009). ACP Journal Club. Accessing pre-appraised evidence: fine-tuning the 5S model into a 6S model. [Editorial]. *Annals of Internal Medicine*, *151*(6) JC3-2, JC3-3.

Dobbins, M., Ciliska, D., Estabrooks, C., & Hayward, S. (2005). Changing nursing practice in an organization. In A. DiCenso, G. Guyatt, & D. Ciliska (Eds.), *Evidence-based nursing: A guide to clinical practice* (pp. 172–200). St. Louis: Mosby.

Estabrooks, C. A., Scott, S., Squires, J. E., Stevens, B., O'Brien-Pallas, L., Watt-Watson, J., et al. (2008). Patterns of research utilization on patient care units. *Implementation Science*, *3*, 31.

Ferlie, E. B., & Shortell, S. M. (2001). Improving the quality of health care in the United Kingdom and the United States: A framework for change. *Milbank Quarterly*, *79*, 281–315.

Geisinger Health System. (2014). *Marcellus shale and health outcomes*. Retrieved May 4, 2014 from, http://www.geisinger.org/research/centers_departments/environmental/marcellus_shale.

Goode, C. J., Titler, M., Rakel, B., Ones, D. S., Kleiber, C., Small, S., et al. (1991). A meta-analysis of effects of heparin flush and saline flush: Quality and cost implications. *Nursing Research*, *40*, 324–330.

Greiner, A. C., & Knebel, E. (Eds.), Board on Health Care Services, Committee on the Health Professions Summit, Institute of Medicine. (2003). *Health professions education: A bridge to quality*. Washington, DC: National Academies Press.

Holtzclaw, B. (2013). Managing fever and febrile symptoms in HIV: Evidence-based approaches. *Journal of the Association of Nurses in AIDS Care*, *24*(1 Suppl.), S86–S102.

Horn, S. D., DeJong, G., & Deutscher, D. (2012). Practice-based evidence research in rehabilitation: An alternative to randomized controlled trials and traditional observational studies. *Archives of Physical Medicine and Rehabilitation*, *93*(Suppl. 2), S127–S137.

Horsley, J. A., Crane, J., Crabtree, M. K., & Wood, D. J. (1983). *Using research to improve nursing practice: A guide*. San Francisco: Grune & Stratton.

Institute of Medicine. (2009). *Initial national priorities for comparative effectiveness research*. Washington, DC: The National Academies Press.

International Council of Nurses (ICN). (2007). *Nursing research (position statement)*. Retrieved March 1, 2013 from, www.icn.ch/images/stories/documents/publications/position_statements/B05_Nsg_Research.pdf.

Jackson, S. F., Fazal, N. & Giesbrecht, N. (n.d.). A hierarchy of evidence: Which intervention has the strongest evidence of effectiveness? *Public Health Agency of Canada*. Retrieved March 16, 2013 from http://66.240.150.14/intervention/evidence-eng.html.

Jagger, J., Berguer, R., Phillips, E. K., Parker, G., & Gomaa, A. E. (2011). Increase in sharps injuries in surgical settings versus nonsurgical settings after passing needlestick legislation. *AORN Journal*, 93(3), 322–330.

Jones, R., & Lacroix, L. J. (2012). Streaming weekly soap opera video episodes to smartphones in a randomized controlled trial to reduce HIV risk in young urban African American/black women. *AIDS Behavior*, 16(5), 1341–1358.

King, D., Barnard, K. E., & Hoehn, R. (1981). Disseminating the results of nursing research. *Nursing Outlook*, 29(3), 164–169.

Kitson, A., Rycroft-Malone, J., Harvey, G., McCormack, B., Seers, K., & Titchen, A. (2008). Evaluating successful implementation of evidence into practice using the PARiHS framework: Theoretical and conceptual challenges. *Implementation Science*, 3, 1.

Kovach, C. R., Simpson, M. R., Joosse, L., Logan, B. R., Noonan, P. E., Reynolds, S. A., et al. (2012). Comparison of the effectiveness of two protocols for treating nursing home residents with advanced dementia. *Research in Gerontological Nursing*, 5(4), 251–263.

Krueger, J. C. (1977). Utilizing clinical nursing research findings in practice: A structured approach. *Communicating Nursing Research*, 9, 381–394.

Madsen, D., Sebolt, T., Cullen, L., Folkedahl, B., Mueller, T., Richardson, C., et al. (2005). Listening to bowel sounds: An evidence-based practice project. *American Journal of Nursing*, 105(12), 40–49.

Malkin, B. (2008). Are techniques used for intramuscular injection based on research evidence? *Nursing Times*, 104(50/51), 48–51.

Massey, R. L. (2012). Bowel sounds indicating an end of postoperative ileus: Is it time to cease this long-standing practice. *Medsurg Nursing*, 21(3), 146–150.

McHugh, M. D., & Ma, C. (2013). Hospital nursing and 30-day readmissions among Medicare patients with heart failure, acute myocardial infarction, and pneumonia. *Medical Care*, 51(1), 52–59.

Melnyk, B. B., Fineout-Overholt, E., Gallagher-Ford, L., & Kaplan, L. (2012). The state of evidence-based practice in US nurses: Critical implications for nurse leaders and educators. *Journal of Nursing Administration*, 42(9), 410–417.

Melnyk, B. B., Fineout-Overholt, E., & Mays, M. Z. (2008). The evidence-based practice beliefs and implementation scales: Psychometric properties of two new instruments. *Worldview on Evidence-Based Nursing*, 5(4), 208–216.

Melnyk, B. B., Fineout-Overholt, E., Stillwell, S. B., & Williamson, K. M. (2010). Evidence-based practice: Step-by-step: The seven steps of evidence-based practice. *American Journal of Nursing*, 110(1), 51–53.

Metheny, N. A., & Titler, M. G. (2001). Assessing placement of feeding tubes. *American Journal of Nursing*, 101(5), 36–46.

Meyers, T. A., Eichhorn, D. J., Guzzetta, C. E., Clark, A. P., Klein, J., Taliaferro, E., et al. (2000). Family presence during invasive procedures and resuscitation: The experience of family members, nurses, and physicians. *American Journal of Nursing*, 100(2), 32–43.

Morton, S. C., & Ellenberg, J. H. (2012). Infusion of statistical science in comparative effectiveness research. *Clinical Trials*, 9, 6–12.

National Institute for Health Research. (n.d.). *CLAHRC for Greater Manchester in collaboration with NHS Manchester*. Retrieved from http://clahrc-gm.nihr.ac.uk/heartfailure/about/#Implementation%20and%20Research%20 Themes.

National Institutes of Health (NIH). (2011). *About the NIH roadmap*. Retrieved March 1, 2013 from, http://commonfund.nih.gov/aboutroadmap.aspx.

NCAST Programs. (2014). *History*. Seattle, WA: Author. Retrieved February 16, 2014 from, http://www.ncast.org/index.cfm?fuseaction=page.display&page_id=29.

Nelson, E., Batalden, P., & Godfrey, M. M. (2011). *Value by design: Developing clinical microsystems to achieve organizational excellence*. Hoboken, NJ: Jossey-Bass.

Newhouse, R. (2007). Diffusing confusion among evidence-based practice, quality improvement, and research. *Journal of Nursing Administration*, 37, 432–435.

Newhouse, R. P., & Spring, B. (2010). Interdisciplinary evidence-based practice: Moving from silos to synergy. *Nursing Outlook*, 58(6), 309–317.

Pankop, R., Chang, K., Thorlton, J., & Spitzer, T. (2013). Implemented family presence protocols: An integrative review. *Journal of Nursing Care Quality*, 28(3), 281–288.

Patient-Centered Outcomes Research Institute. (2012). *National priorities for research and research agenda*. Retrieved February 14, 2014 from, www.pcori.org/research-we-support/priorities-agenda/.

Pearson, A., Jordan, Z., & Munn, Z. (2012). Translational science and evidence-based healthcare: A clarification and reconceptualization of how knowledge is generated and used in health care. *Nursing Research and Practice*, Retrieved February 14, 2014 from http://www.ncbi.nlm.nih.gov/pmc/articles/PMC3306933/.

Poorsina, R. (2012). *Care Connectivity Consortium takes care coordination to new levels for patients and providers*. Kaiser Permanente. [Press Release]. Retrieved February 14, 2014 from, http://xnet.kp.org/newscenter/pressreleases/nat/2012/091112_care_connectivity_consortium.html.

Pravikoff, D. S., Tanner, A. B., & Pierce, S. T. (2005). Readiness of U.S. nurses for evidence-based practice. *American Journal of Nursing*, 105(9), 40–51, quiz 52.

Registered Nurses' Association of Ontario. (2002). *Toolkit: Implementation of clinical practice guidelines*. Toronto, ON: Author.

Registered Nurses' Association of Ontario. (2012). *Toolkit: Implementation of clinical practice guidelines* (2nd ed.). Toronto, ON: Author.

Rogers, E. (2003). *Diffusion of innovations* (5th ed.). New York: Free Press.

Rutledge, D. (2011). From our readers…Sustaining evidence-based practice initiatives. *American Nurse Today, 6*(2), 2p.

Rycroft-Malone, J., Seers, K., Chandler, J., Hawkes, C. A., Crichton, N., Allen, C., et al. (2013). The role of evidence-context and facilitation in an implementation trial: Implications for the PARIHS framework. *Implementation Science, 8,* 28.

Shah, P. S., Ng, E., & Sinha, A. K. (2005). Heparin for prolonging peripheral intravenous catheter use in neonates. *Cochrane Database of Systematic Reviews,* CD002774.

Sharkey, S., Hudak, S., Horn, S. D., Barrett, R., Spector, W., & Limcangco, R. (2013). Exploratory study of nursing home factors associated with successful implementation of clinical decision support tools for pressure ulcer prevention. *Advances in Skin and Wound Care, 26*(2), 83–92, quiz pp. 93–94.

Shirey, M. R., Hauck, S. L., Embree, J. L., Kinner, T. J., Schaar, G. L., Phillips, L. A., et al. (2011). Showcasing differences between quality improvement, evidence-based practice, and research. *Journal of Continuing Education in Nursing, 42*(2), 57–68, quiz 69–70.

Stetler, C. B. (2001). Updating the Stetler model of research utilization to facilitate evidence-based practice. *Nursing Outlook, 49*(6), 272–279.

Stetler, C. B. (2003). Role of the organization in translating research into evidence-based practice. *Outcomes Management, 7*(3), 97–103.

Straus, S. E., Richardson, W. S., Glasziou, P., & Haynes, R. B. (2011). *Evidence-based medicine: How to practice and teach EBM* (4th ed.). Edinburgh: Churchill Livingstone.

Thabane, L., Thomas, T., Ye, C., & Paul, J. (2009). Posing the research question: Not so simple. *Canadian Journal of Anaesthesia, 56*(1), 71–79.

The AGREE Research Trust. (2010). *Introduction to AGREE II.* Retrieved February 7, 2014 from, http://www.agreetrust.org/about-the-agree-enterprise/introduction-to-agree-ii/.

Thompson, D. S., Estabrooks, C. A., Scott-Findlay, S., Moore, K., & Wallin, L. (2007). Interventions aimed at increasing research use in nursing: A systematic review. *Implementation Science, 2,* 15.

Titler, M. G. (2004). Methods in translation science. *Worldviews on Evidence-Based Nursing, 1,* 38–48.

Titler, M. G., Herr, K., Brooks, J. M., Xie, X. J., Ardery, G., Schilling, M. L., et al. (2009). Translating research into practice intervention improves management of acute pain in older hip fracture patients. *Health Services Research, 44,* 265–287.

U.S. Department of Veterans Affairs. (n.d.). *QUERI-Quality Enhancement Research Initiative.* Retrieved February 14, 2014 from www.queri.research.va.gov/.

Vessey, J. A. Founding Oversight Board Members of MASNRN (2007). Development of the Massachusetts School Nurse Research Network (MASNRN): A practice-based research network to improve the quality of school nursing practice. *Journal of School Nursing, 23,* 65–72.

SUGGESTED READINGS

Ackley, B. J., Ladwig, G. B., Swan, B. A., & Tucker, S. J. (2008). *Evidence-based nursing care guidelines: Medical-surgical interventions.* St. Louis: Mosby.

Brown, S. J. (2010). *Evidence-based nursing: The research practice connection* (2nd ed.). Boston: Jones & Bartlett.

Duncan, J., Montalvo, I., & Dunton, N. (2011). *NDNQI case studies in nursing quality improvement.* Silver Spring, MD: American Nurses Association.

Dunton, N. & Montalvo, I. (Eds.), (2009). *Sustaining improvement in nursing quality: Hospital performance on NDNQI indicators, 2007–2008.* Silver Spring, MD: American Nurses Association.

Fawcett, J., & Garrity, J. (2009). *Evaluating research for evidence-based nursing.* Philadelphia: F.A. Davis.

Houser, J., & Bokovy, J. (2006). *Clinical research in practice: A guide for the bedside scientist.* Boston: Jones & Bartlett.

International Council of Nurses. (2012). *Closing the gap: From evidence to action.* Geneva: Author. Retrieved February 14, 2014 from, http://nursingworld.org/MainMenuCategories/ThePracticeofProfessionalNursing/Improving-Your-Practice/Research-Toolkit/ICN-Evidence-Based-Practice-Resource/Closing-the-Gap-from-Evidence-to-Action.pdf.

Kleinpell, R. (2013). *Outcome assessment in advanced practice nursing* (3rd ed.). New York: Springer.

Melnyk, B. & Fineout-Overholt, E. (Eds.), (2010). *Evidence-based practice in nursing and healthcare: A guide to best practice.* Philadelphia: Lippincott, pp. 3–24.

Schmidt, N. A., & Brown, J. M. (2011). *Evidence-based practice for nurses.* Boston: Jones & Bartlett.

PART 4

Interpersonal and Personal Skills

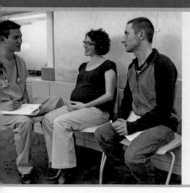

Consumer Relationships

Margarete Lieb Zalon

This chapter explores the changes that have altered consumer relationships with healthcare providers and looks specifically at nurses' responsibilities to the consumer. Nurses set the tone for effective staff-patient interaction. Because nurses are the healthcare providers who spend the most time with the consumer, this chapter provides concepts and strategies to assist in developing effective nurse-consumer relationships.

LEARNING OUTCOMES

- Categorize health consumers' interactions into three relationship structures.
- Interpret the results of selected changes that influence consumer relationships in health care.
- Evaluate the impact of a service-oriented philosophy on the quality of the nurse-consumer relationship.
- Appraise the four major responsibilities of nursing—service, advocacy, teaching, and leadership—in relation to the promotion of successful nurse-consumer relationships.

KEY TERMS

advocate	healthcare consumer	patient satisfaction
care coordination	healthcare provider	quality indicator
consumer focus	high tech	service
cultural competence	high touch	service recovery
gatekeeper	medical home	
health literacy	patient activation	

THE CHALLENGE

Suzanne Freeman, RN, MBA
President of Carolinas Medical Center, Charlotte, North
Carolina

Customer satisfaction is the number one goal in our healthcare facilities. The hospital board officially acknowledged this goal, and systems were set in place to measure, monitor, and improve customer satisfaction. The staff ultimately defined principles to illustrate their commitment to this goal: teamwork, integrity, caring, commitment, and communication. Each individual would be treated with dignity and as a valued member of a "family."

The husband of a patient seen in the emergency department (ED) some time ago called the nurse manager a few days after his wife's visit. When she arrived at the ED, her chief complaint was intermittent chest pain for 2 days. She had indicated that she did not have pain upon arrival to the ED and was ultimately admitted to the hospital with the diagnosis statement "Chest pain, rule out MI [myocardial infarction]."

The husband complained that his wife had been required to "sign herself in," even though he had asked the nurse to have his wife seen immediately. He thought that the nurse had not taken his wife's complaints seriously and that the resulting delay had caused her condition to worsen. He attributed this issue to the fact that his wife required coronary artery bypass surgery the following day.

The nurse manager immediately met with the triage nurse involved. They talked through the encounter and examined the documentation. The triage nurse thought that her assessment of "nonemergent" was valid. She noted that the patient was registered by the patient registration personnel and that the physician saw her within 30 minutes of her arrival. The triage nurse's assessment indicated "Vital signs stable, no history of heart disease, right-sided chest pain × 2 days." The pain scale records indicated "No pain now." The assessment made by the triage nurse appeared valid to the nurse manager. The nurse manager also noted that the nurse's competency in assessing patients for triage was historically reliable. The triage nurse did not recall the husband asking for his wife to be seen immediately.

The nurse manager visited the patient and her spouse in the coronary care unit. She apologized for their expectations not being met during the triage process. She assured the couple that their concerns were taken seriously and offered her sincerest apologies. Her words seemed to be well received by the couple. Each thanked her for her concern and visit.

Apparently, the couple was not satisfied, however, because the husband called the vice president for patient services that same day. He related the story, including the nurse manager's visit. He added that he had recently viewed a news report about how women were undertreated and misdiagnosed with regard to chest pain. The vice president listened carefully and promised to follow up quickly with a response.

What do you think you would do if you were this nurse?

INTRODUCTION

Consumer relationships in healthcare delivery refers to the multitude of encounters between the consumer (client, patient, or customer) and healthcare system representatives. Who are the consumers of health care, and what do they expect from providers? What are their likes and dislikes, and how do they evaluate their health care?

Today, hospitals and other healthcare organizations are concerned with protecting consumer rights and are actively engaged in assessing patient/consumer satisfaction as a strategy to improve quality, enhance market share, and meet regulatory and/or accreditation requirements. The role of nurses as trusted professionals in the development of consumer relationships in healthcare organizations is increasingly recognized for its importance. The Patient Protection and Affordable Care Act (ACA) of 2010 provides the opportunity for more Americans to have control over their health care while providing access to affordable insurance for millions of Americans.

Consumers hold nurses in high regard. They view nurses as knowledgeable, worthy of respect, concerned for others, honest, caring, confidential, friendly, hardworking, and especially trustworthy. Nurses consistently top the list in Gallup polls of the public's ratings of honesty and ethical standards of various professions, with a great majority of Americans believing nurses' honesty and ethical standards are "high" or "very high" (Gallup® Politics, 2013). Nurses have been at the top of the list in every year since they were added to the annual survey in 1999, except in 2001 when firefighters ranked higher. Nurses, by virtue of this favorable status with the public, occupy positions of influence and can foster and promote successful consumer relationships across healthcare settings.

We are all consumers of health care—friends, neighbors, families, people like us, and people very different from us. Consumers are diverse culturally, ethnically, socially, physically, and psychologically. Consumers are indeed becoming better connoisseurs of health care than they were in the past. Consumers are increasingly making use of online health care information. Consumers can access their own test results, schedule appointments, and communicate with their health care provider, but these services are only available to a small number of patients and are not used by all those who have such access. Chronic health conditions require that consumers take an active role in managing their health. Chronic illnesses account for 63% of global mortality and one third of the world's disease burden, with 80% of cardiovascular and diabetes deaths, and almost 90% of chronic obstructive pulmonary disease deaths occurring in low-income and middle-income countries (World Health Organization, 2011).

Employers view consumerism as a vehicle for reducing healthcare costs and for improving quality by empowering employees to make more appropriate choices about healthcare services while improving health care. Employers make wellness programs available to their employees to promote healthy lifestyles. These programs can reduce illness, improve productivity, and reduce health insurance premium costs. Under the ACA, employers are allowed to make adjustments in contributions and premiums for wellness program participation. Employers may provide incentives and/or penalties for such participation. The Leapfrog Group, a consortium of employers and organizations that buys health care, works to prevent mistakes in health care and improve the quality and affordability of health care. It supports informed healthcare decisions by those using and paying for health care and promoting high-value health care through incentives and rewards (The Leapfrog Group, n.d.). Hospitals and other healthcare organizations will increasingly be called upon to provide value for their services.

Under ACA, health insurance coverage is expected to extend to an additional 27 million people with coverage including certain essential benefits. The system is built on a requirement for purchasing minimum essential health coverage or paying a penalty. Insurers are prohibited from excluding people based upon pre-existing conditions; basic preventive services such as screening mammography are included. Insurers are not allowed to cancel policies when people get sick, and lifetime limits are banned. Consumers can shop for health insurance in online marketplaces known as "exchanges," which make it easy to compare costs. These changes will place increased demands on the resources of healthcare systems.

Access to health insurance, does not necessarily mean that people will take advantage of available services. Parents in a young family may ensure that their children receive needed care and immunizations but forgo obtaining preventive health care for themselves. We still have significant healthcare disparities in our country that are manifest in numerous ways. For example, blacks and Hispanics are less likely to have employer-sponsored health insurance, and people with Medicaid insurance may use facilities that are underresourced. Interventions that can be used to reduce disparities include team care, patient navigation, cultural tailoring, collaboration with families and community members, and interactive skills-based training. These interventions are all focused on improving the nature of healthcare delivery, particularly relationships with consumers.

Equitable access to health information and improved communication are key strategies identified in *Healthy People 2020* to improve population health outcomes and healthcare quality, and to achieve health equity (U.S. Department of Health & Human Services, 2010). Further, as an example, the American Recovery and Reinvestment Act of 2009 authorized nearly $38 billion in spending to support the deployment of health information technology. In the United States, 69% of adults track a health indicator for themselves or a loved one, with 49% keeping track of their progress "in their heads" and 21% using some form of technology (Fox & Duggan, 2013).

Disparities still exist in access to the Internet and technology, which are primarily related to age, household income, educational attainment, and disability (Zickuhr & Smith, 2012). However, mobile technology is changing the digital divide with young adults, minorities, those with no college experience, and those with lower household income being more likely to indicate that phones are their main source of Internet access (Zickuhr & Smith). These data have implications for access to healthcare information. These changes also affect the nature of the relationship between consumers and nurses, consumers and other healthcare providers, and consumers and healthcare organizations.

Consumers can access unlimited information about health; and such access may vary by ethnicity and socioeconomic status. Although some information available from the Internet and other resources might not be reliable, healthcare consumers tend to be better informed now more than they ever have been. Numerous government agencies and voluntary organizations provide consumers with guidance in managing chronic conditions, making decisions about health, and preventing harm from lapses in patient safety. Publicity about medical errors, the shortage of healthcare professionals (including nurses), and information campaigns directed toward consumers to promote safety have heightened consumer awareness of the importance of being involved in all aspects of one's health care. Consumers question providers regarding the care they receive or do not receive, and they ask, "Why are you doing that?" "Where can I get the best care?" "Why did my nurse do that differently yesterday?" and "How do I know what is the best decision for me?"

RELATIONSHIPS

The Consumer Focus

Consumer relationships are constantly changing and thus affect the providers of health services: primary care and public health services, managed care organizations, hospitals, home health agencies, and long-term care facilities, as well as individual providers such as nurses and physicians. As inpatient services have become more complex and outpatient services have grown, competition for patients becomes fiercer. This has resulted in a shift in focus from healthcare providers to **healthcare consumers**. As noted in The Challenge at the beginning of the chapter, consumers drive what happens in our healthcare settings. Healthcare processes are being redefined with the consumer as the center. How consumers view and value their care is important data. Consumers enter into distinct relationships to meet their healthcare needs, including relationships with healthcare agencies, insurers or payers, nurses, physicians, and allied health providers. Changes in access, insurance coverage, nurses' roles and responsibilities, physician services, communication technology, pay-for-performance, and globalization are just a few factors influencing these relationships.

Health Literacy

Consumers rely on information from a variety of sources to make healthcare decisions. The relationships that consumers develop with their healthcare providers, including nurses, are important in helping them navigate the healthcare system. However, nearly half of America's adults—that is, 90 million people—have difficulty understanding and using health information (Nielson-Bohlman, Panzer, & Kindig, 2004). The definition of **health literacy** used by the federal government is "the degree to which individuals have the capacity to obtain, process, and understand basic health information and services needed to make appropriate health decisions" (U.S. Department of Health & Human Services, 2010).

Understanding consumers' health-literacy needs goes beyond assessment of reading ability. The first component of the health literacy definition is the *capacity to obtain*. Global aging, climate change, war, terrorism, and life-extending medical and technologic advances also influence this capacity (Perlow, 2010). Decades of research demonstrate that people with low health literacy do not understand health information very well and tend to get less preventive health care, which in turn affects their health (Nielson-Bohlman et al., 2004). Promoting health literacy involves education, consideration of the context, and sociocultural factors. Using a Health Literate Care Model involves weaving health literacy strategies into care by assuming that patients do not understand their health conditions or what to do about them, and then, subsequently assessing patients' understanding (Koh, Brach, Harris, & Parchman, 2013). For example, a nurse who is an expert clinician in a specialty practice area, when diagnosed with a serious chronic illness, may not have the appropriate background to make informed healthcare decisions. Promoting health literacy is an important component of health care because individuals with limited literacy are vulnerable. They are more likely to be sicker when they enter into the healthcare system and are likely to use more healthcare services.

Healthcare Provider–Consumer Relationships

Healthcare provider–consumer relationships have changed as physicians' typical mode of practice moved from a single, private enterprise to multigroup practices that also include nurse practitioners, certified nurse-midwives, certified registered nurse anesthetists, clinical nurse specialists, registered nurse first assistants, physician assistants, and other healthcare professionals. Some group practices are incorporated into integrated service models that include health maintenance organizations (HMOs), managed care programs, physician-hospital organizations, accountable care organizations, and patient-centered medical homes. When consumers visit a group practice, they might not have the option of selecting a specific healthcare provider. Rural healthcare consumers have seen local hospitals closed or purchased by large healthcare systems resulting in the need to develop relationships with new healthcare providers. They may become more critical and less accepting of their care. They may feel alienated and insecure in unfamiliar circumstances, even if they are receiving the best care. Patients no longer know their healthcare providers as they did in the past, and providers may be less familiar with their patients, resulting in decreased opportunity for the development of mutual respect and trust. Many hospitals now use hospitalists, which makes care coordination following discharge more challenging. Almost half of all hospitalized patients experience a medical error after discharge, and these errors can be traced back to communication breakdowns and lack of follow-up systems (McLeod, 2013).

Registered nurses (RNs) and advanced practice registered nurses (APRNs) are in an ideal position to provide oversight and facilitate communication through care coordination. According to the National Quality Forum (2010), care coordination is an information-rich, patient-centric endeavor that seeks to deliver the right care to the right patient at the right time. Models of care coordination include case management, transitional care, disease management, health information technology, and other strategies to manage the delivery of health services while providing support to patients and providers (National Quality Forum, 2010). Increasingly nurses will be expected to work within teams of healthcare providers and provide care coordination in systems that reward quality, safety, and efficiency (Buerhaus et al., 2012).

Trust is an important component of consumer relationships. Trust is influenced by the healthcare provider's competence and interpersonal skills. Perceptions of service quality positively influence trust, and perceptions of trust positively influence patient satisfaction (Chang, Chen, & Lan, 2013). Patients want and expect attentiveness to their concerns and respectful treatment. Healthcare practitioners must be sensitive to the needs of patients in order to establish trusting relationships.

Agency-Consumer Relationships

Healthcare consumers may have been accustomed to receiving extended acute care in an inpatient setting. This option is no longer available for many. Patients may be angry and frightened at the thought of being on their own or receiving very limited services from home health agencies. The type of insurance coverage and the insurance carrier may dictate the specific hospital or healthcare agency used. Managed care options require that the consumer use particular and specific healthcare facilities or be responsible for all or a larger portion of the bill.

Patients discharged from emergency departments are often poorly prepared to manage their care at home because they do not understand discharge instructions (Engel et al., 2012). Nurses in acute care settings have limited time to provide complex discharge instructions. Home health nurses may not be able to make a sufficient number of visits to enable patients to successfully manage a chronic illness.

One solution to containing costs is a consumer-directed healthcare plan, which generally has high deductibles with the goal of reducing healthcare costs by providing consumers with information about choices, risks, benefits, and costs. The goal is greater emphasis on case management, disease management, and patient education. These plans use report cards, risk assessments, nurse-help telephone lines, Websites, and an array of other consumer education materials. As the ACA is fully implemented, consumers will be comparison shopping for healthcare services through health insurance exchanges just as they might comparison shop for prescription drugs. Despite growth in consumer awareness, the impact of consumer-directed healthcare plans on patient satisfaction and healthcare costs is unknown. Less than 20% of people who had consumer-directed health plans understand that their plan exempted preventive services, medical tests, and screenings from their deductible (Reed, Graetz, Fung, Newhouse, & Hsu, 2012). More consumer education will be needed to ensure that people take advantage of the services available through these types of plans.

The days of healthcare organizations operating under an outmoded paradigm with only the needs of physicians and third-party payers driving the agencies' priorities are limited. In increasingly competitive healthcare markets, greater application of data sharing and access to electronic health records result in the use of advanced analytical tools to mine data for trends and provide decision-making support. New services include self-monitoring with technology in the home, videoconferencing, text messaging, and instant messaging with healthcare providers, and clinics staffed by nurse practitioners in grocery and drug stores. These changes will require that healthcare organization leaders focus efforts on relationships with patients who are more knowledgeable and demanding.

Nurse-Consumer Relationships

Nurses spend a lot of time with the consumer, and these encounters are generally personal and intensely meaningful. Nurses are in a distinct position to influence and promote positive consumer relationships. The nurse manager sets the tone for effective staff-patient interactions centered on the patient.

Changes from hospital or nursing home care to outpatient and in-home care have particularly altered the nurse-consumer relationship. Nurses are taking leadership roles as primary care providers (e.g., nurse practitioners, midwives), teachers and educators, and home healthcare managers and advocates, particularly in compensation and insurance areas. Nurses are emerging as the gatekeepers of the healthcare system, the liaisons between the consumer and a complex healthcare market.

The National Priorities Partnership (NPP) has recognized that ensuring that patients receive well-coordinated care across all providers, settings, and levels of care is integral to the quality of care. The NPP is a coalition of 52 major healthcare organizations including the American Nurses Association (ANA) with the shared vision of achieving better health and a safe, equitable, and value-driven health system (NPP, 2011). The nurse manager is a key position to facilitate care coordination by working with case managers and members of the interdisciplinary healthcare team. The nurse in the gatekeeper or care coordinator role can be an influential advocate for consumers who could receive less-than-desired care in a complicated healthcare system. This group typically has included those who receive no care and need it most, such as those who are homeless, uninsured, or underinsured; persons who abuse drugs or alcohol; children of poverty; migrant workers; and people with acquired immunodeficiency syndrome (AIDS). Some institutions and private corporations capitalize on the case-management skills of nurses by developing "nurse navigator" or "patient navigator" roles, which are designed to assist patients through a complex healthcare system or with healthcare decisions.

Policymakers are examining the role of "medical homes" in facilitating the integration of care across systems. The patient-centered medical home (PCMH) is a delivery model that focuses on improved access, care coordination, quality, satisfaction, and comprehensive patient-centered care in primary care settings (Schram, 2012). PCMH demonstration projects have proliferated across the country. Although discussions have focused on physician-directed care, nurse practitioners are well suited to lead teams transforming to PCMH models. However, this idea has met with resistance from physician-led groups. Advanced practice nurses provide an integral safety net for patients who are uninsured or underinsured or who have chronic health conditions. Research has demonstrated the effectiveness of care delivered by advanced practice nurses (Newhouse et al., 2011). Advanced practice nurses need to be included in policy decisions about PCMHs and their implementation.

Nursing has long recognized the value of the integral nature of the nurse-patient relationship and the value of caring as an element of that relationship. The *Code of Ethics for Nurses* holds that the "nurse's primary commitment is to the patient" with an expectation that the nurse involves patients in planning for care (ANA, 2001, pp. 9-10). Patient-centered care includes alleviating vulnerabilities, both physiologic and interpersonal; it also includes therapeutic engagement and developing a relationship in a manner that is reinforced by the information practices of a particular setting (Hobbs, 2009). Healthcare reform initiatives under the ACA focus on the involvement of patients in their care.

Involving patients in their own care is a cornerstone of healthcare reform and important for improving health outcomes, reducing costs, and improving patient experiences (Hibbard & Greene, 2013). **Patient activation** refers to patients' willingness and ability to take independent actions to manage their health care and includes understanding their role in the process and having the confidence to do so. Whereas patient engagement includes activation, interventions designed to increase activation, and the resulting behavior (Hibbard & Greene, 2013). Nurses are well-prepared to implement strategies that activate patient engagement because they take the time to establish productive relationships with consumers.

Nurses have four major responsibilities in promoting successful consumer relationships, as follows:
Service
Advocacy
Teaching
Leadership

EXERCISE 22-1
List as many clinical situations as you can think of in which the nurse might carry out the four aforementioned responsibilities. Compare your list with those of your peers.

SERVICE

A **service** orientation responds to the needs of the customer. In The Challenge at the beginning of the chapter, activities are centered on the patient and family, including how nursing care and all other services are delivered so that patient care is holistic. The NPP's goals (2011), in addition to the previously mentioned care coordination, include engaging patients and their families in managing their health and making decisions about their care, improving the health of the population, improving the safety and reliability of America's healthcare system, guaranteeing appropriate and compassionate care for patients with life-limiting illnesses, and eliminating overuse.

The patient must be at the center of care to achieve these goals. Healthcare professionals, including nurses, want to deliver patient-centered care. However, assessing how well that is accomplished in an organization is challenging. The Picker Institute, a nonprofit organization, conducted an extensive evaluation of care from the patient's perspective. Its patient-centered care model is illustrated in Box 22-1. Each dimension is an important part of

BOX 22-1   EIGHT PRIMARY DIMENSIONS OF PATIENT-CENTERED CARE

- Respect for patient's values, preferences, and expressed needs: includes attention to quality of life, involvement in decision making, preservation of patient's dignity, and recognition of patient's needs and autonomy
- Coordination and integration of care: involves clinical care, ancillary and support services, and "front-line" patient care
- Information, communication, and education: includes information on clinical status, progress, and prognosis; information on processes of care; and information and education to facilitate autonomy, self-care, and health promotion
- Physical comfort: considers pain management, help with activities of daily living, and hospital environment
- Emotional support and alleviation of fear and anxiety: demands attention to anxiety over clinical status, treatment, and prognosis; anxiety over the effect of the illness on self and family; and anxiety over the financial impact of the illness
- Involvement of family and friends: recognizes the need to accommodate family and friends and involve family in decision making; to support the family as caregiver; and to recognize family needs
- Transition and continuity: addresses patient anxieties and concerns about information on medication, treatment regimens, follow-up, danger signals after leaving the hospital, recovery, health promotion, and prevention of recurrence; coordination and planning for continuing care and treatment; and access to continuity of care and assistance
- Access to care: addresses timeliness of admission to a patient room in an in-patient setting and appointment waiting times in the outpatient setting.

Data from Shaller, D. (2007, October). *Patient-centered care: What does it take?* New York: The Commonwealth Fund.

the consumer's interaction with the healthcare system and provides guidance in promoting consumer relationships.

Even with an increasing emphasis on customer service, most healthcare facilities are not as "customer-friendly" as they might be; that is, they are built and organized in a manner that best serves the organization, not the consumer. They are compartmentalized, with each department having specialized functions. Patients are transported to departments to receive services. They risk loss of privacy, excessive exposure, and increased discomfort and fatigue during the transfer and waiting episodes. On an average day, a seriously ill hospitalized patient may have encounters with 50 or more personnel in the course of receiving care and treatment. This approach is not "service-oriented." A service orientation means delivering services in a manner that is least disruptive. When possible, services should come to the patient and should be as easy, comfortable, pleasant, and effective as possible. Meeting the emotional, psychosocial, and spiritual needs of the patient is important. Consumers may view problems with care services such as delays in administering medication or lack of information as a safety problem rather than a service quality problem (Rathert, Brandt, & Williams, 2012). Care needs to be technologically advanced and compassionate, and address what matters to patients.

EXERCISE 22-2

List five examples of what you think are not consumer-friendly practices or situations in your nursing setting. (Example: Patients asked to repeat information several times to different healthcare team members; not faxing discharge prescriptions to a pharmacy.) Identify at least two strategies to help address each problem.

Providing satisfying and meaningful service is not easy. Every consumer is different, and every situation is different. How things are done and how needs are met vary. Service is not a prescribed set of rules and regulations. Service is a multidimensional concept and means placing a premium on the design, development, and delivery of care. For example, a home care patient needs intravenous (IV) antibiotic therapy. Inserting the IV catheter is the task-oriented, production part of the care. The service aspect involves considering the patient's specialized needs, such as placing the needle in the left arm so that he can continue to use a cane with his right arm or using a local anesthetic before inserting the needle to reduce discomfort.

Quality nursing care must be both clinically correct and satisfying to the customer. "Clinically correct" is the product aspect, and "satisfying to the consumer" is the service orientation. Each individual nurse is responsible for being competent and providing quality patient care that is clinically correct and satisfying. The nurse manager is accountable for the overall quality of care delivered to patients.

Healthcare agencies must be sensitive to whether the agency milieu is indeed a healing environment that supports and reinforces the actual quality of clinical care. The challenge in the busy, unpredictable, cost-constrained healthcare environment is to provide care that has a **consumer focus** by meeting or exceeding customer expectations. Nurses, as leaders, need to recognize the economic value of their services as well as the economic value of improving the quality of the patient experience. Patient-centeredness means that care should be focused around "patient's needs, preferences, circumstances, and well-being" (Cosgrove et al., 2013). Positive patient experiences are dependent on identifying and acting on patient preferences. Engaged and empowered patients are integral to improving our healthcare system (Smith et al., 2012). The following Literature Perspective describes strategies for reducing costs and waste while improving outcomes within a framework of patient engagement.

 LITERATURE PERSPECTIVE

Resource: Cosgrove, D. M., Fisher, M., Gabow, P., Gottlieb, G., Halvorson, G. C., James, B. C., Kaplan, G. S, Perlin, J. B., Petzel, R., Steele, G. D. & Toussaint, J. S. (2013). Ten strategies to lower costs, improve quality and engage patients: The view from leading health system CEOs. *Health Affairs, 32*(2), 321-327.

Health system CEOs outlined 10 key strategies that improve outcomes with a focus on patient-centered care. Patient engagement is a theme that is present in many of the strategies. The checklist includes (1) visible leadership, (2) culture of continuous improvement and learning, (3) information technology focused at the point of care, (4) use of evidence-based protocols, (5) optimal use of resources, (6) integrated care with right care in the right setting with the right providers and right teamwork, (7) patient clinician collaboration on care, (8) tailored services for patients needing intensive resources, (9) embedded safeguards, and (10) internal transparency with visible progress in performance, outcomes, and costs. An example of success is an evidence-based approach to labor and delivery at Intermountain Healthcare resulting in a drop of inappropriate elective inductions of labor, with women spending 750 fewer hours in delivery each year. The CEOs call for research on patient engagement and its relationship to continuous improvement.

Implications for Practice

Nurse managers are critical to the successful patient-engagement. Team approaches with an organizational commitment can lead to improved patient satisfaction and significantly better outcomes. Patients want an environment that meets their needs for safety and security, support, and psychological and physical comfort. Focusing on strategies to enhance patient engagement can meet these patient needs.

Hospital leaders value the role of the Magnet Recognition Program® in improving outcomes and patient satisfaction. The Magnet™ designation demonstrates excellence of nursing care through transformational leadership; structured empowerment; exemplary professional nursing practice; and new knowledge, innovations, and improvement, which lead to empirical quality outcomes (Gokenbach & Drenkard, 2011). To achieve Magnet™ status, the organization needs to demonstrate excellence in patient satisfaction, nurse satisfaction, and nurse-sensitive clinical outcome data. These attributes cannot be achieved without excellence in a consumer service orientation. This culture of excellence must be exemplified in every aspect of the organization, from the chief executive officer, to the chief nursing officer, to the nurse manager for nurses at the front lines of care to feel empowered to promote excellence in consumer service.

A service orientation is consumer-driven and consumer-focused and emphasizes the quality of the nurse-patient relationship. Caring has been described as critical to nursing and is important in establishing nurse-patient relationships. However, caring is not enough, nor is caring the unique purview of nurses. Thinking critically and taking appropriate, timely action is a part of the therapeutic process. The nurse must do the right thing right at the right time.

Caring in nursing is manifest "high tech–high touch." High tech denotes a mechanistic perspective, whereas high touch denotes a caring, humanistic perspective. Caring for patients is challenging in today's fast-paced healthcare environment. The more high technology is used in health care, the more the patient wants and needs high touch—someone who is trusted and respected. The quality of human contacts becomes the measure by which the consumer forms perceptions and judgments about nursing and the health agency. Consumers may not be able to evaluate the quality of interventions, but they always can evaluate the quality of the relationship with the person delivering the service.

Patient satisfaction ratings, along with measurable healthcare outcomes, are important data used by healthcare organizations to provide quality care and to maintain a competitive edge. Nurses, because of their 24-hour accountability for patient care, are integral to high patient-satisfaction ratings. Healthcare organizations want high ratings, and advertise their ratings in the community. Standard-setting organizations,

such as The Joint Commission, the National Quality Forum, and the Magnet Recognition Program®, include patient satisfaction as a quality indicator. Patient satisfaction and perception of the quality of care are affected by the quality of the nurse-patient relationship (The Quality Patient Experience, 2012).

One needs also to consider the range and the depth of patient satisfaction data collected. Some hospitals only collect data required by government or regulatory organizations. Others collect more specific data on satisfaction with nursing care, including such elements as how promptly the call light was answered and whether patients were satisfied with a specific aspect of nursing care. Pain management and the discharge process are two specific areas where nurses can make significant improvement in patient satisfaction. Post-discharge patient call backs used to verify discharge instructions and address concerns have been shown to improve patient satisfaction (Cochran, Blair, Wissinger, & Nuss, 2012).

A standardized survey of patients' perceptions of the quality of hospital care known as the Hospital Consumer Assessment of Healthcare Providers and Systems (HCAHPS) was developed by the Centers for Medicare & Medicaid Services (CMS) and the Agency for Healthcare Research and Quality (AHRQ) (CMS, 2012). Hospitals are now required to collect and publicly report HCAHPS results in order to receive their full CMS payment. The HCAHPS reports appear on the Hospital Compare Website, allowing consumers to make meaningful comparisons and creating incentives for hospitals to improve quality. Valid measurement of patient satisfaction is an evolving science; nurses do not always accurately gauge what factors are most important to patients. Satisfaction measures are often skewed in a positive direction with scores clustered at the top of the scale. This makes it difficult to interpret results and make improvements.

The National Database of Nursing Quality Indicators (NDNQI®) is a national repository for unit-based quality data that can be used by organizations to benchmark the outcomes of care against those of other institutions (ANA, n.d.). Unit-based quality indicators, including satisfaction with nursing care, are a key feature of the NDNQI®. In addition to hospitals being provided with their own and comparison data, researchers are able to access de-identified data in order to answer important questions about nursing care quality. For example, the relationships between hospital Magnet™ status, nursing unit staffing, and patient falls were examined, indicating falls are lower in Magnet™ hospitals, and additional registered nurse (RN) hours per patient day was associated with a 3% lower fall rate (Lake, Shang, Klaus, & Dunton, 2010).

Nurses have a responsibility to exercise critical thinking and decision making with respect to patient satisfaction with nursing care. For example, postoperative patients may not want to cough and deep breathe, yet we know that failure to do so can result in pneumonia. Patients may have severe postoperative pain, yet report moderate satisfaction levels (Tocher, Rodgers, Smith, Watt, & Dickson, 2012). This paradox illustrates nurses' responsibilities for (1) advocating for their patients, (2) ensuring pain relief, (3) correcting patient misconceptions, and (4) implementing pain-management strategies consistent with established standards. Reviewing and analyzing patient satisfaction survey results are invaluable tools. Managers need to share the results of such surveys with their staff, examine what they are doing right so that they continue doing it, and determine how improvements could be made.

Understanding the process by which patients determine their satisfaction can only enhance the abilities of leaders and followers in their efforts to improve the patient experience. The theory of navigating care can be used to describe the process of patient satisfaction with nurse-led chronic disease management. Key elements and their application are described in the Theory Box below.

Healthcare organizations are increasingly concerned about patient satisfaction not only as a barometer of excellence in service, but also as an impact to their bottom line. Some organizations use scripting to provide standardized responses to certain situations in order to improve patient satisfaction. An example is the use of a standardized script related to patient rounding. Some nurses have indicated that they dislike such standardization, that it limits their critical decision making and professional judgment, making them the "Stepford Nurses," and treating them as incompetent. Others indicate that it provides consistency and assurance to patients by providing nurses with the tools to handle difficult situations, such as delayed procedures and how to de-escalate situations with angry patients and family members (Hendren, 2011). The truth is probably somewhere in the middle. Useful strategies in using responses that are consistent with nursing's values rather than a market assembly-line approach are described in Table 22-1 (Leebov, 2008).

In addition to addressing patient satisfaction, organizations need a **service recovery** program to be responsive to its customers. Service recovery is a strategy for identifying complaints and rectifying service failures to retain or "recover" dissatisfied customers. Axioms for service recovery are described in Box 22-2. Effective service recovery

---

THEORY BOX

Navigating Care

CONCEPT	KEY POINTS	APPLICATION
Determining care needs	Self-monitoring Monitoring by health professionals	Patients assess their chronic conditions and decide on care needs based upon their own assessment of their health.
Forming relationships	Building a rapport Working together	Sufficient time and private space are needed for practice consultations. Nurses need to adjust their communication style to individual needs of patients.
Having confidence	Trusting the model of care Trusting the nurse role Trusting the physician Evaluating the practice nurse	Patients understand the parameters of the care model, understand when referrals are made back to primary care provider, and understand the collaboration among healthcare team members.

From Mahomed, R., St. John, W., & Patterson, E. (2012). Understanding the process of patient satisfaction with nurse-led chronic disease management in general practice. *Journal of Advanced Nursing, 68*(11), 2538-2549.

TABLE 22-1 SIX WAYS TO MAKE CARING VISIBLE

COMMUNICATION SKILL	EXPLANATION	EXAMPLES
1. Listening actively	Acknowledge and reflect back the person's feeling in a nonjudgmental way.	"I can image this might feel scary to you." "You seem upset this morning."
2. Showing caring nonverbally	Use facial expression, intonation, posture, eye contact, and other body language to mirror the patient's feelings.	Showing a sense of urgency nonverbally as you respond to a call light Screwing up your forehead to show concern when patient appears upset
3. Making explicit your positive intent	Explain your purpose. How is what you're doing in the patient's best interest?	"I want to make you comfortable. Here's a blanket." "I want to help you with your pain."
4. Using the words "for you"	Make it clear that the patient is your focus.	"I will call your daughter for you." "Let me check on the test results for you."
5. Using the blameless apology	Express genuine regret for the negative experience without taking blame or blaming someone.	"I am so sorry it's been a frustrating morning for you." "I'm really sorry about the delay."
6. Expressing appreciation	Give the personal gift of positive regard.	"I really admire your courage." "Thank you so much for speaking up."

From Leebow W (2008). *Beyond customer service: the challenge to care givers.*
Copyright © 2008 HealthCom Media. All rights reserved. *American Nurse Today,* January 2008, www.americannursetoday.com.

BOX 22-2 APPLICATION OF SERVICE RECOVERY AXIOMS TO THE CLINICAL SETTING

AXIOM	CLINICAL APPLICATION
1. All customers have basic expectations related to reliability, assurance, tangibles (e.g., cleanliness of a unit), empathy, and responsiveness.	Return to the patient when expected. Provide consistency between words and actions. Indicate that you understand that the patient has concerns. Keep patients informed about what is going to happen.
2. Successful recovery is psychological as well as physical.	Listen to the patient. Allow patients to describe how the mistake or adverse action affected them.
3. Working with customers in a spirit of partnership in problem solving and based on needs improves health care experiences.	Involve patients in addressing the problem. Ask patients what they need to have happen. Acknowledge patient concerns.
4. Customers react more strongly to "fairness mistakes" than "honest mistakes."	Communicate about what went wrong, the plan for problem resolution, and prevention of recurrence.
5. Effective recovery is a planned process.	Practice responses to common problems such as delayed medications or tests.

Adapted from Agency for Healthcare Research and Quality (AHRQ). (2012, June 27). *The CAHPS improvement guide: Practical strategies for improving the patient care experience.* Adapted from Zemke, R., & Bell, C. (2000). *Knock your socks off service recovery.* New York: American Management Association. Retrieved February 16, 2013, from www.cahps.ahrq.gov.

includes encouraging healthcare providers, rather than just hospital administrators, to talk with patients about a serious error. In the past, healthcare organizations were concerned with potential liability when the person making an error talks with the patient or family about it. However, research suggests that the content of the message has a significant effect on how the person feels about an error. Patients should be treated with fairness and respect, be provided with an explanation and information on how such an error will be prevented in the future. Consideration must be given to which person is the most appropriate to offer an apology as well as planning its content. A nurse making a medication error that did not harm a patient is the best person to make the disclosure and apology. However, if a patient's discharge is delayed by a day because of an omission or error in preparation for a diagnostic test, then it might be more appropriate for the nurse manager and/or nurse administrator to initiate the discussion. Some organizations use scripts for situations when care has not gone as planned. For example, when there is an excessive delay in the emergency department, staff training on when and how to use a script for this situation can help a patient or family member feel less distressed.

EXERCISE 22-3

Make a "what-if" list of actions that would enhance services to the consumers of health care. (Example: What if every single nurse would ask each patient at the beginning of the shift about the patient's most important concern that day.)

ADVOCACY

Nurses practice in healthcare environments dominated by unrest and insecurity. Some of these forces are shown in Box 22-3. Such forces bring about ethical and moral questions: Who gets care? Where do they get care? How much care? Who has the right to die? Who has the right to live? Who makes the decisions? Differing values and beliefs, along with economic constraints and limited resources, affect decisions that are made.

Consumers have basic rights that need to be protected—the right to individualized care; the right

---

BOX 22-3 FORCES OF UNREST AND INSECURITY IN THE HEALTHCARE ENVIRONMENT

1. Increased costs
2. Shift to outpatient services
3. Complex social problems (AIDS, violence, poverty, global climate change)
4. Decreased access to health care
5. Aging population (increasing life span)
6. Technologic and genetic advances
7. Shortage of nurses and other healthcare professionals
8. Culturally and ethnically diverse work/consumer groups
9. Underrepresentation of women and ethnic groups in health-related research
10. Economic instability
11. Increase in regulatory and reporting requirements
12. Uncertainty and divisiveness about implementation of healthcare reforms.

---

to their own values, beliefs, and cultural ways; and the right to be informed and participate in care decisions. Unresolved within the healthcare system is the issue of two levels of care that are based on economics but tend to result in racial-cultural discrimination. Not only has care been on a two-tiered basis, but also minorities and women have been significantly underrepresented in health-related research; this results in additional healthcare disparities because less information is available for decision making.

Who in the healthcare system is in a position to be the guardian of consumer rights? The nurse is! The nurse acts as the primary person to be alert to circumstances that may prevent a successful outcome for the patient and to intervene on the patient's behalf. The nurse is in the position to address the issues of cultural, ethnic, and racial sensitivity. The nurse is concerned with addressing the individualized needs and wants of the patient.

The definition of *nursing* includes advocacy in the care of individuals, families, communities, and populations (ANA, 2010b). Nurses, in accordance with the ANA *Code of Ethics for Nurses,* have the responsibility to promote, advocate, and strive to protect the health, safety, and rights of the patient (2001). Patient advocacy includes (1) safeguarding patients' autonomy, (2), acting on behalf of patients, and (3) championing social justice in the provision of health care (Bu & Jezewski, 2007). An advocate is one who does the following:

- Defends or promotes the rights of others
- Changes systems to meet the needs of others
- Empowers and promotes self-determination in others
- Promotes autonomy of diverse cultural and social groups
- Ensures respect, equality, and dignity for others
- Cares for the humaneness of all

Nursing practice involves interacting with consumers who are culturally, economically, and socially diverse. Diversity encompasses more than differences in nationality or ethnicity and may include a variety of ways that patients are different from their healthcare providers. Nurses are responsible for assisting consumers in accessing and participating in the healthcare system. Some patients enter the healthcare system much like immigrants entering a foreign country. Patients who enter a system with a set of values, beliefs, behaviors, and language unlike their own may experience culture shock. Patients who speak little or no English and those who may have low health literacy are vulnerable for poor health outcomes. Nurses need to recognize the culture of their work setting, realizing that it may differ markedly from the culture of the consumer, and move beyond ethnocentrism to provide culturally competent care. Cultural and linguistic competence brings together congruent attitudes, behaviors, and policies within an organization in such a way that allows people to work effectively in cross-cultural situations (Office of Minority Health, 2005). This competence includes cultural knowledge, actively learning about a community; cultural sensitivity—valuing and respecting beliefs, norms, and practices of the people being served—and collaboration within a community (Flaskerud, 2007). Cultural competence is critical to reducing the potential impact of healthcare disparities and providing consumer service.

The advocate role requires the nurse to perceive and be comfortable with conflict and then mediate, negotiate, clarify, explain, and intervene. The nurse can advocate by being a liaison between the consumer and the system. The nurse's role is to interpret the rules and customs of the agency to the consumer. The role is also to negotiate changes when the consumer and agency differ in values and beliefs.

To provide culturally appropriate care, the nurse must possess knowledge about various culturally diverse groups (see Chapter 9). It takes time to develop cultural sensitivity and awareness. Some guidelines that are useful in learning to appreciate and value diversity are the following:

- Avoid stereotyping.
- Avoid making assumptions.
- Learn by observing interactions of minority group members.
- Adjust expectations to be culturally sensitive.
- Create a more level playing field—modify your behavior to accommodate diversity.

Powerlessness or an imbalance in power between the consumer and the system can result in value systems being forced on the recipient of care. Consumers who lack economic means by being uninsured, underinsured, or undocumented often become powerless in the healthcare delivery system. They are at the mercy or will of those who control the power and the money. These consumers (described earlier) may be denied access to care, or if they achieve access, they may not receive equal care. As implementation of the ACA unfolds, researchers will be examining its impact on reducing health care disparities.

Consumers interacting with our healthcare systems, regardless of their status, have a right to know about their eligibility for services and care. The nurse must be willing to ensure that economic constraints do not prevent consumers from receiving what they need. Some advocacy for the recipients of inequality in our healthcare system is done on the here-and-now level—initiating a referral to a social agency when a patient does not have transportation to his home or appealing to the ethics committee when a patient's wishes for end-of-life decisions are not being followed. On a broader scale, advocacy means becoming involved professionally and politically to change the systems and policies to provide healthcare access and equality.

> **EXERCISE 22-4**
> A patient does not speak English and is a member of an immigrant group that is not well represented in your community. Using the Culturally and Linguistically Appropriate Services (CLAS) standards, identify four strategies that the culturally competent nurse can use to ensure that the patient receives high quality care.

Race and ethnicity as factors in health and health care have been the subject of concern; however, people very often may erroneously assume that members of a particular group have the same beliefs, attitudes, and values about health when in fact there is extraordinary diversity.

The U.S. Census Bureau predicts that by the year 2040, more than half the U.S. population will be ethnic minorities. Among residents aged 5 years and older in the United States, 20% speak a language other than English at home (Shin & Kominski, 2010). Diversity refers to not just race or ethnicity, but also age, gender, socioeconomic status, religion, sexual orientation, physical characteristics, and disability. Cultural competence will play an increasingly important role in nurse-consumer relationships. An organization that creates a culture of mutual respect, recognizing the contributions of all its employees, will be much more effective in providing culturally competent health care.

The following are some of the keys to becoming a successful nurse advocate:

- Developing networking systems within work agencies
- Being involved in professional associations to enhance awareness of issues affecting practice and, thus, consumers
- Acquiring the knowledge needed to access systems
- Learning about community resources and support networks
- Developing skill in referring and engaging patients

A patient advocate's ultimate aim is to empower patients (i.e., the consumers of health care) to help them use their own abilities to promote health. Patient empowerment is a critical component of health care and is integral to error reduction. Patient participation occurs when nurses treat the patient as a valuable partner achieving a trusting relationship where the patient and nurse share in control and responsibility; participation is inhibited when patients feel neglected or like the helpless object of a nurse's actions (Larsson, Sahlsten, Segesten, & Plos, 2011). Nurses must be sensitive to patient preferences and expectations as illustrated in the Research Perspective below.

The nurse manager should keep in mind the most basic element of empowerment—helping people assert control. Support for patients and their families is critical when a hospitalized patient suffers an illness requiring major transition in roles and responsibilities. Families have different management styles: thriving, accommodating, enduring, struggling, and floundering (Knafl et al., 2011). Understanding a family's management style can be useful in tailoring interventions according to the changing needs of patients and their families.

Nurses can evaluate the consumer's quality of care by comparing it with quality indicators or critical pathways in the quality review process. For example, if standards indicate patients with a particular bronchial condition need a chest radiograph examination on day 2 and another on day 5, all patients should receive this same level of care. Pressure ulcers and nosocomial infections, such as hospital-acquired pneumonia are indicators of the quality of nursing care. The NDNQI® data can be used to track nurse-sensitive quality indicators on each clinical unit of a hospital. Nurse managers are in a distinct position to ensure that all patients receive appropriate care by setting the tone for staff reporting discrepancies, omissions, and challenges in delivering care.

 RESEARCH PERSPECTIVE

Nurse managers must acknowledge and respect legal, ethical, and moral responsibilities of the staff to advocate for patients. If a patient receives the wrong medication just before being discharged, the patient needs to be informed and this information needs to be included in the patient's record. If the patient has an adverse reaction and needs to return to the emergency department, the record aids diagnosis and facilitates the institution of prompt treatment. Some states require written notification of consumers for serious errors. Although efforts have been made to increase error reporting to facilitate the institution of system changes to decrease errors, the use of blame hinders the staff in disclosing medication errors to the leadership of an organization (Wagner, Harkness, Hébert, & Gallagher, 2013). This is a major challenge in identifying problematic practices in order to reduce error and promote patient safety. Nurses in leadership positions are also obligated legally and ethically to report unacceptable or questionable clinician and organizational practices. As Yoder-Wise (2010) points out, having the courage to advocate for patients can sometimes impose personal risks, as it did in the case known nationally as the "Winkler County Nurses." Nurses Vickilyn Galle and Anne Mitchell reported their concerns about a physician's practices to the medical board; they became their patients' heroes—and ours as well.

The savvy manager knows that the way in which consumers define quality may not always match the way "experts" define it. Quality health care and quality nursing care do not depend on the ability to pay or social acceptance. Good care occurs irrespective of the economic circumstance of the consumer. Nurses are the guardians of that right for consumers. Nurses have historically been the champions for the poor and the underserved. It is no different today.

TEACHING

Consumers of health care have a right and a need to know how to care for their own health needs. Nurses have an obligation to teach the consumer. Patient teaching is included in nursing practice standards (ANA, 2010a) and is often included in professional nursing definitions of state nurse practice acts. As indicated earlier, the Magnet Recognition Program® model includes exemplary professional practice,

which in turn includes the role of nurses as teachers. Consumers are demanding information about their health status and plan of care. They are entitled to (1) receive information regarding health concerns, (2) participate in caring for their health needs, and (3) contribute to finding solutions to their health problems. Education empowers consumers to exercise self-determination with greater control over what happens, to make informed decisions, and to choose options wisely. Knowledge is power. Sharing knowledge means sharing power. Nurses providing patient care also need to consider patient preferences for information and decision-making as well as the unique needs of the community served by their organization. For example, in a study of patients and their partners after myocardial infarction, more active roles in decision making were desired by females, younger patients and partners, and patients and partners with higher educational levels (Nilsson, Ivarsson, Alm-Roijer, Svedberg, & the SAMMI-study group, 2013).

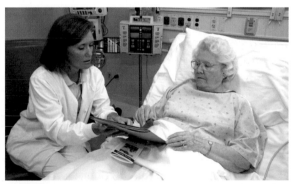

Education empowers consumers to exercise self-determination.

Healthcare delivery systems affect the ways nurses teach consumers. Short hospital stays and care provided in outpatient and transitional settings require effective use of time and resources. Patients need to be able to manage their own health care earlier and more independently. Hands-on, technical training is needed in many instances. Nurses' perceptions of their patients' understanding of post-discharge treatment plans differ from the perceptions of patients themselves. They may perceive patients to be much more knowledgeable than patients themselves report. Three P's for successful consumer education are shown in Box 22-4.

BOX 22-4   **THREE *P*'S FOR A SUCCESSFUL CONSUMER EDUCATION FOCUS**

Philosophy—Patient education is an investment with a significant positive return. Money invested in teaching is money well spent. Time and energy invested are time and energy well spent.

Priority—Education is important. Quality nursing care always has an educational component. Informed consumers want to participate and look to nurses to teach them.

Performance—Clinical teaching excellence is a required nurse competency. Nurses must be skilled in using a variety of techniques and methods to meet the needs of the diverse consumers served.

Nurses need to be sensitive to the teaching needs of those at risk for disparities in health care: persons of a different race or ethnic group, women, children, older adults, rural residents, and those with limited or no health insurance, low health literacy, and/or low socioeconomic status. It is important that lower expectations are not unintentionally communicated to persons who are disadvantaged, have a low literacy level, or have limited English proficiency.

Patients often hesitate asking for help with language skills. Some healthcare agencies include an assessment of a patient's ability to learn, but the lack of assessment criteria may hinder nurses' efforts to institute appropriate teaching. The U.S. Census Bureau's language screening questions can be used. The person is asked if a language other than English is spoken at home, and if the answer is "yes," the person is asked to rate how well he or she speaks English: very well, well, not well, or not at all (Shin & Kominski, 2010). The National Standards for Culturally and Linguistically Appropriate Services (CLAS) include standards for cultural competence, language access, and organizational support (Office of Minority Health, 2001). Hospital length of stay is significantly longer for patients with limited English proficiency when professional interpreters are not used at admission, or at both admission and discharge (Lindholm, Hargraves, Ferguson, & Reed, 2012). Nurse managers can make a commitment to culturally and linguistically appropriate care highly visible to their staff by advocating for ongoing training to meet the unique needs of their patient population and access language services for patients with limited English proficiency.

Teaching can be simple or complex. In teaching elemental, task-oriented behaviors, the nurse uses basic materials, simple relationships, guides, sequencing of steps, and cause-and-effect relationships. Chronic disease self-management education programs can have a significant impact on health behavior and health focusing on a partnership between the patient and the healthcare provider. Nurses are involved in innovative program models that include Internet support, health coaching, patient navigation, and telemonitoring. Patients with chronic illnesses and their families may require extensive teaching for illness management. Factors that might impede learning need to be considered. The nurse manager can ensure that staff have the resources for patient teaching, that it is done effectively and then appropriately documented, and that it is consistent with the patient's care plan.

In addition to being easy to read, written teaching materials need to reflect relevance, accuracy, and thoroughness, and they need to be updated regularly. They need to be appropriate for the patient's literacy level. Geriatric populations have the highest rates of low health literacy compared to other age groups (Cutilli & Schaefer, 2011). Education needs to be provided at a level that can be understood by patients and reflects mutually agreed upon goals. "Teach-backs," directly asking patients to repeat key points of care management instructions, can be employed to assess understanding, correct misinformation, and reinforce teaching. Having content knowledge, understanding consumer preferences, and being able to individualize information to meet consumers' learning abilities are critical to quality teaching. Families should be included as appropriate when providing information. Teaching is one of the most positive experiences nurses can have. Teaching can be fun and rewarding, but it is hard work.

As a step-by-step method, the nursing process can be applied to teaching (Figure 22-1).

LEADERSHIP

Nurses are critically positioned to provide leadership for the twenty-first–century changes in health care. Understanding paradigm shifts in health care and the need to be responsive to change will prepare nurse

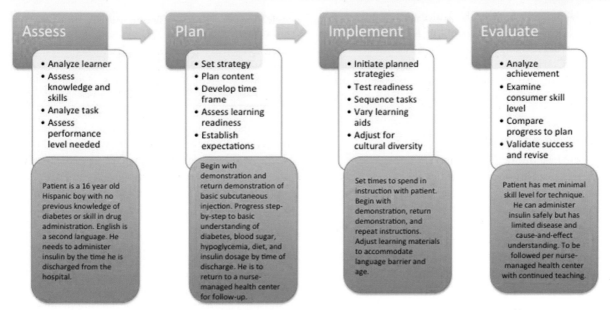

FIGURE 22-1 Application of the nursing process to teaching.

managers to participate fully in shaping healthcare organizations of the future.

Nurse managers influence the quality of care delivered by the staff setting the tone for the unit's vision and mission and focus. They must believe in and model a consumer-based service philosophy. Each consumer is different. What will satisfy one person will not satisfy another. Nurse managers, because they receive referrals when patients are dissatisfied with some aspect of their care, are in a unique position not only to find a solution but also to understand the types of problems being experienced by the patients and suggest strategies for solving them. Being successful as leaders requires openness and flexibility; leaders are expected not only to do things right but also to do the right things and be effective role models for their followers. Leadership also requires the ability to relinquish control and a tolerance for ambiguity and change.

Change is the modus operandi of the nursing environment in any healthcare setting. What works today may not work 6 months from now. Given the rapidly changing environment, the pressure to control costs, and advances in technology, science, and information, nurse managers need a whole new set of beliefs, behaviors, and skills.

Patient outcomes, standards of care, and evidence-based practice are attracting greater attention and receiving much more public scrutiny. Healthcare reform focuses on the provision of quality care along with controlling costs. Nursing, as a profession, needs to be much stronger in making the case for value of services provided by nurses.

Managers must be willing to give up direct control of every process. Staff must be supported in their use of power to be in control and to make decisions at the consumer-staff level of interaction. Giving up control involves being willing to take a risk and having a belief in the other person's ability to perform.

Leadership behaviors contributing to individual and personal excellence include the following:
- Allowing professionals more influence over their practice
- Giving staff opportunities to learn new and varied skills
- Giving recognition and reward for success and support and consolation for lack of success
- Fostering motivation and belief in the importance of each individual and the value of his or her contribution

The leader's role is to create within the worker a passion to do and contribute to the work effort successfully. This is supported by the seminal work of Aiken, Clarke, and Sloane (2002), who indicated that nurse staffing and organizational/managerial support for nursing are key to improving the quality of patient care.

Focusing on Consumers

We do best those things that we know how to do skillfully and those things about which we feel passionately. Fitting the right person to the right job is important. Maximum contribution is required from each staff member in today's healthcare agencies. Because the leader is the one who sets the standard for the success or failure of the staff's contributions, it is important to assess each staff member carefully—what is his or her skill level and commitment level, and what can be done to assist in making a maximum contribution? Figure 22-2 is an example of a completed staff assessment tool. Nurse managers can compile similar information for their staff members.

Subsequently, the information can be used to form staff development plans.

> **EXERCISE 22-7**
> Form small groups and assess each member of the group using the headings shown in the staff assessment tool (see Figure 22-2)

When staff members know the leader is sincerely concerned about their welfare, they are better able to use their time, energy, and talents to serve the needs of the consumer. Staff members who are nurtured and cared for will be better able to nurture and care for the consumer.

CONCLUSION

Consumers are the core of our care. They create the need for the profession. Our ability to form solid relationships allows us to enhance the care people need and deserve. Being sensitive to how consumers view quality helps nurse leaders and managers address services that meet needs.

Staff Member	Skill Level	Commitment Level	Suggested Action
(1) S. Baker, RN	High technical competence Able to teach others Learns quickly Needs improved people skills	Appears bored Does only what is assigned No enthusiasm Critical of any change	Assign challenges to use technical strengths Provide situations in which teaching others occurs Plan: Team assign with D. Carroll
(2) D. Carroll, RN	6-month postbasic program Learns quickly Slow with technical skills Needs technical supervision Excellent people skills	Excited about work Asks for new experiences Accepting of new ideas Volunteers to help others	Improve technical skills Provide safe and successful learning experiences Plan: Team assign with S. Baker
(3) J. Ratke, RN	Moderate technical competence Works best alone Not interested in teaching co-workers Good people skills	Restless, distracted Looking for a change Accepts new ideas Self-commitment—not group-oriented	Set up an independent project of her choosing (e.g., unit research idea) Provide some special technical training to increase skills
(4) C. Thomas, RN	High-level technical skills Enjoys helping others Excellent people skills Looks for challenges	Team player Interested in welfare of group Critical of poor performers Acts as cheerleader for change	Utilize willingness and group skills to plan and present a unit activity (e.g., in-service education production, unit open house)

FIGURE 22-2 Staff assessment tool.

THE SOLUTION

The vice president immediately met with the triage nurse and nurse manager. The nurse manager was surprised that her visit had not resolved the complaint. The vice president asked the triage nurse if she would have assessed a man with the same profile differently. Her immediate answer was "no." She stated that the staff was aware of the research evidence related to gender bias but that the protocol for assessing chest pain was well-designed and very objective, without bias to gender. With the approval of the nurse manager and triage nurse, the vice president invited the husband into the meeting. The husband and the nurse talked through the scenario of events and conversation that occurred during triage, especially the husband's perception that the triage nurse dismissed his request for immediate attention. They agreed that the husband might have said, "Does she really have to register herself?" The triage nurse had not interpreted his statement as a request for immediate action. Each realized that a miscommunication had occurred. Furthermore, the nurse responded to the husband's concern about gender bias. She explained that there had been information in the medical literature but that cardiologists, ethicists, and other healthcare experts had reviewed and approved the chest pain assessment protocol, ensuring no bias of gender. This situation was brought to resolution by an open line of communication. The result can often be "service recovery."

Several important points may be learned from this incident:

- Effective communication is critical for success. Clarification is always appropriate in situations of intense emotion. Active listening is an essential component of effective communication.
- Imagine yourself in the patient's situation and environment.
- Engage the involved persons in the evaluation and solution related to a miscommunication.
- Healthcare practices, policies, and procedures should be updated to reflect new knowledge.
- Consumers are increasingly knowledgeable about health care; therefore expectations are more sophisticated and maintaining public trust is of great concern.
- Leadership must exude missionary zeal in educating personnel to the expectations for behavior in terms of consumer satisfaction.

—*Suzanne Freeman*

Would this be a suitable approach for you? Why?

THE EVIDENCE

Nurses are often the "face" of an organization and they are perceived as having great prestige. They are seen as members of the most trusted profession. Additionally, trust in healthcare providers is linked to their interpersonal skills. This important skill contributes to patient engagement, which leads to improved outcomes of care.

Patients want to be treated fairly, with respect and attentiveness. Their perceptions of care are affected by care focusing on individual needs and preferences.

Additionally, patients may be satisfied with care that is not of high quality. Patient satisfaction is a key indicator of the quality of care; and sicker patients are less satisfied with the quality of their care.

Nearly half of the adults in the United States have difficulty using and understanding health information. Further, many patients discharged from the emergency department or hospital are not prepared to manage their care at home. This occurs despite deliberate discharge planning.

WHAT NEW GRADUATES SAY

- Sometimes the standard communication approach is really useful. It is especially so when a patient is upset because I can become upset and forget to focus on the patient rather than myself.

- My unit has a computer for use by family so that we can help them find reliable Internet resources. I just have to remember to coach them in finding good sites rather than doing it myself.

CHAPTER CHECKLIST

Times have changed, as has the role of the nurse manager. Healthcare's movement into the community, home, clinic, and outpatient setting has placed a whole new perspective on how to provide quality, cost-effective nursing care. Patients must participate in their care and need service-oriented nurses to be teachers, advocates, and leaders on their behalf. Managing care delivery in these diverse settings requires the use of flexible and creative skills. The implementation of health care reform will result in an increased emphasis on patient-centered care and care coordination, areas where nurses can make important contributions. The key is to keep the patient as the center of focus and provide culturally competent nursing care.

- Relationships
  - The consumer focus
    - Health literacy
- Healthcare provider–consumer relationships
- Agency-consumer relationships
- Nurse-consumer relationships
- Service
- Advocacy
- Teaching
- Leadership
  - Focusing on consumers

TIPS FOR PROMOTING A CONSUMER FOCUS

- Introduce yourself to patients using your full name and title.
- Ask patients about their most important concerns.
- Explain the purpose of your care.
- Provide explanations of what will be happening next.
- Tell patients when you expect to return.
- Ask patients if they have additional questions.
- Acknowledge patient concerns or negative experiences in a respectful manner.
- Ask yourself: Is your response one that you would like for yourself or a family member?

REFERENCES

Agency for Healthcare Research and Quality (AHRQ). (2012, June 27). *The CAHPS improvement guide: Practical strategies for improving the patient care experience*. Retrieved February 16, 2014, from, www.cahps.ahrq.gov.

Aiken, L. H., Clarke, S. P., & Sloane, D. M. (2002). Hospital staffing, organization, and quality of care: Cross-national findings. *Nursing Outlook, 50*, 187–194.

American Nurses Association (ANA). (2001). *Code of ethics for nurses with interpretive statements*. Washington, DC: Author.

American Nurses Association (ANA). 2010a. *Nursing: Scope and standards of practice* (2nd ed.). Silver Spring, MD: Nursesbooks.

American Nurses Association (ANA). 2010b. *Nursing's social policy statement: The essence of the profession* (3rd ed.). Silver Spring, MD: Nursesbooks.

American Nurses Association (ANA). (n.d.). *NDNQI: Transforming data into quality care*. Silver Spring, MD: Author. Retrieved February 17, 2014 from http://www.nursingworld.org/ndnqi2.

Bu, X., & Jezewski, M. A. (2007). Developing a mid-range theory of patient advocacy through concept analysis. *Journal of Advanced Nursing, 57*, 101–110.

Buerhaus, P. I., DesRoches, C., Applebaum, S., Hess, R., Norman, L. D., & Donelan, K. (2012). Are nurses ready for healthcare reform? A decade of survey research. *Nursing Economic$, 30*(6), 318–329.

Centers for Medicare and Medicaid Services. (2012). *HCAPHS: Fact sheet*. Retrieved February 16, 2014 from, www.hcahpsonline.org/Facts.aspx.

Chang, C. S., Chen, S. Y., & Lan, Y. T. (2013). Service quality, trust and patient satisfaction in interpersonal-based medical service encounters. *BMC Health Services Research, 13*, 22. http://dx.doi.org/10.1186/1472-6963-13-22.

Cochran, V. Y., Blair, B., Wissinger, L., & Nuss, T. D. (2012). Lessons learned from implementation of postdischarge telephone calls at Baylor Health Care System. *Journal of Nursing Administration, 42*(1), 40–46.

Cosgrove, D. M., Fisher, M., Gabow, P., Gottlieb, G., Halvorson, G. C., et al. (2013). Ten strategies to lower costs, improve quality and engage patients: The view from leading health system CEOs. *Health Affairs, 32*(2), 321–327.

Cutilli, C. C., & Schaefer, C. T. (2011). Case studies in geriatric health literacy. *Orthopedic Nursing, 30*(4), 281–285.

Engel, K. G., Buckley, B. A., Forth, V. E., McCarthy, D. M., Ellison, E. P., Schmidt, M. J., et al. (2012). Understanding emergency department discharge instructions: Where are knowledge deficits greatest? *Academic Emergency Medicine, 19*(9), E1035–E1044.

Flaskerud, J. (2007). Cultural competence: What is it? *Issues in Mental Health Nursing, 28*, 121–123.

Fox, S., & Duggan, M. (2013, January 28). *Tracking for health*. Washington, DC: Pew Research Center's Internet & American Life Project. Retrieved February 17, 2014 from, http://pewinternet.org/Reports/2013/Tracking-for-Health.aspx.

Gallup® Politics. (2013, December 16). *Honesty and ethics rating of clergy slides to new low: Nurses again top list; lobbyists are worst*. Retrieved February 18, 2014 from, www.gallup.com/poll/166298/honesty-ethics-rating-clergy-slides-new-low.aspx.

Gokenbach, V., & Drenkard, K. (2011). The outcomes of Magnet environments and nursing staff engagement: A case study. *Nursing Clinics of North America, 46*(1), 89–105.

Hendren, R. L. (2011, September 6, 2011). *10 ways to help nurse improve patient satisfaction*. HealthLeaders Media. Retrieved February 19, 2014 from, www.healthleadersmedia.com/page-3/NRS-270551/10-Ways-to-Help-Nurses-Improve-Patient-Satisfaction##.

Hibbard, J. H., & Greene, J. (2013). What the evidence shows about patient activation: Better health outcomes and care experiences; fewer data on costs. *Health Affairs, 32*(2), 207–214.

Hobbs, J. L. (2009). A dimensional analysis of patient-centered care. *Nursing Research, 58*, 52–62.

Knafl, K., Deatrick, J. A., Gallo, A., Dixon, J., Grey, M., Knafl, G., et al. (2011). Assessment of the psychometric properties of the family management measure. *Journal of Pediatric Psychology, 36*, 494–505.

Koh, H. K., Brach, C., Harris, L. M., & Parchman, M. L. (2013). A proposed 'Health Literate Care Model' would constitute a systems approach to improving patients' engagement in care. *Health Affairs, 32*(2), 357–367.

Lake, E. T., Shang, J., Klaus, S., & Dunton, N. E. (2010). Patient falls: Association with hospital Magnet status and nursing unit staffing. *Research in Nursing and Health, 33*(5), 413–425.

Larsson, I. E., Shalsten, M. J. M., Segesten, K., & Plos, K. A. E. (2011). Patients' perceptions of nurses' behavior that influence patient participation in nursing care: A critical incident study. *Nursing Research and Practice*, Article ID 534060.

Leebov, W. (2008). Beyond customer service: Use these 5 message points to adapt principles of customer service to patient care. *The American Nurse Today, 3*(1), 21–23.

Lindholm, M., Hargraves, J. L., Ferguson, W. J., & Reed, G. (2012). Professional language interpretation and inpatient length of stay and readmission rates. *Journal of General Internal Medicine, 27*(10), 1294–1299.

McLeod, L. A. (2013). Patient transitions to outpatient: Where are the risks? Can we address them? *Journal of Healthcare Risk Management, 32*(3), 13–19.

National Priorities Partnership. (2011). *Input to the Secretary of Health and Human Services on priorities for the national quality strategy*. National Priorities Partnership. Retrieved February 12, 2013 from, www.qualityforum.org/Setting_Priorities/NPP/Input_into_the_National_Quality_Strategy.aspx.

National Quality Forum. (2010, October). *Care coordination. Quality connections*. Retrieved February 11, 2013 from, www.qualityforum.org/Publications/2010/10/Quality_Connections__Care_Coordination.aspx.

Newhouse, R. P., Stanik-Hutt, J., White, K. M., Johantgen, M., Bass, E. B., Zangaro, G., et al. (2011). Advanced practice nurse outcomes 1990–2008: A systematic review. *Nursing Economic$, 29*(5), 230–250 quiz 251. Review.

Nielson-Bohlman, L., Panzer, A. M., & Kindig, D. A. (Eds.). Committee on Health Literacy, Board on Neuroscience and Behavioral Health, Institute of Medicine. (2004). *Health literacy: A prescription to end confusion*. Washington, DC: National Academies Press.

Nilsson, U. G., Ivarsson, B., Alm-Roijer, C., Svedberg, P., & the SAMMI-study group (2013). The desire for involvement in healthcare, anxiety and coping in patients and their partners after a myocardial infarction. *European Journal of Cardiovascular Nursing, 12*(5), 461–467.

Office of Minority Health. (2001). *National standards for culturally and linguistically appropriate services in health care (CLAS)*. Washington, DC: U.S. Department of Health and Human Services. Retrieved February 18, 2014 from, www.thinkculturalhealth.hhs.gov.

Office of Minority Health. (2005). *What is cultural competency?* Retrieved February 19, 2013 from, http://minorityhealth.hhs.gov/templates/browse.aspx?lvl=2&lvlID=11.

Perlow, E. (2010). Accessibility: Global gateway to health literacy. *Health Promotion Practice, 11*, 123–131.

Rathert, C., Brandt, J., & Williams, E. S. (2012). Putting the 'patient' in patient safety: A qualitative study of consumer experiences. *Health Expectations, 15*(3), 327–336.

Reed, M. E., Graetz, I., Fung, V., Newhouse, J. P., & Hsu, J. (2012). In consumer-directed health plans, a majority of patients were unaware of free or low-cost preventive care. *Health Affairs, 31*(12), 2641–2648.

Schram, A. P. (2012). The patient-centered medical home: Transforming primary care. *Nurse Practitioner, 37*(4), 33–39.

Shaller, D. (2007, October). *Patient-centered care: What does it take?* New York: The Commonwealth Fund.

Shin, H. B., & Kominski, R. A. (2010). *Language use in the United States; 2007, American Community Survey reports, ACS-12*. Washington, DC: U.S. Census Bureau.

Smith, M., Saunders, R., Stuckhardt, L, McGinnis, J. M. (Eds.), Committee on the Learning Health Care System in America. (2012). *Best care at lower cost: The path to continuously learning health care in American*. Washington, DC: National Academies Press.

The Leapfrog Group. (n.d.). *The Leapfrog Group: Fact sheet*. Retrieved February 17, 2014 from http://www.leapfroggroup.org/about_leapfrog/leapfrog-factsheet

The Quality Patient Experience. (2012). *Nurse patient relationship is central to patient satisfaction*. Retrieved February 15, 2013 from, www.quality-patient-experience.com.

Tocher, J., Rodgers, S., Smith, M. A., Watt, D., & Dickson, L. (2012). Pain management and satisfaction in postsurgical patients. *Journal of Clinical Nursing, 21*(23–24), 3361–3371.

U.S. Department of Health & Human Services. (2010). *Healthy People 2020: Health communication and health information technology*. Retrieved February 11, 2013 from, www.healthypeople.gov/2020/topicsobjectives2020/overview.aspx?topicid=18.

U.S. Department of Health & Human Services, Office of Disease Prevention and Health Promotion. (2010). *National action plan to improve health literacy*. Washington, DC: Author.

Wagner, L. M., Harkness, K., Hébert, P. C., & Gallagher, T. H. (2013). Nurses' disclosure of error scenarios in nursing homes. *Nursing Outlook, 61*(1), 43–50.

World Health Organization. (2011). *Global status report on noncommunicable disease 2010*. Geneva: WHO Press.

Yoder-Wise, P. S. (2010). More serendipity: The Winkler County trial. *The Journal of Continuing Education in Nursing, 41*, 147.

Zickuhr, K., & Smith, A. (2012, April 13). *Digital differences*. Washington, DC: Pew Research Center's Internet & American Life Project. Retrieved February 11, 2013 from, http://pewinternet.org/Reports/2012/Digital-differences.aspx.

SUGGESTED READINGS

Clark, P. A. (2006). *Patient satisfaction and the discharge process: Evidence-based best practices.* Marblehead, MA: Opus Communications.

Curley, M. A. (2007). *Synergy: The unique relationship between nurses and patients.* Indianapolis: Sigma Theta Tau International, Center for Nursing Press.

Duncan, J., Montalvo, I., & Dunton, N. (2011). *NDNQI case studies in nursing quality improvement.* Silver Spring: Nursesbooks.org.

Hark, L., & DeLisser, H. (2009). *Achieving cultural competency: A case-based approach to training health professionals.* New York: Wiley.

Laviest, T. (2005). *Minority populations and health: An introduction to health disparities in the United States.* Hoboken, NJ: Jossey-Bass.

Leebov, W. (2008). *Wendy Leebov's essentials for great patient experiences: No-nonsense solutions with gratifying results.* Chicago: American Hospital Association.

Mackoff, B. L. (2010). *Nurse manager engagement: Strategies for excellence and commitment.* Boston: Jones & Bartlett.

Press, I. (2005). *Patient satisfaction: Understanding and managing the experience of care* (2nd ed.). Baltimore, MD: Health Administration Press.

Studer, Q., Robinson, B. C., & Cook, K. (2010). *The HCAHPS handbook: Hardwire your hospital for pay-for performance success.* Gulf Breeze, FL: Fire Starter Publishing.

INTERNET RESOURCES

Agency on Healthcare Research and Quality Information for Consumers and Patients. www.ahrq.gov/consumer/.

Cultural Diversity in Health Care. www.ggalanti.org.

Cultural Diversity in Nursing. www.culturediversity.org/.

Department of Health and Human Services. www.healthfinder.gov.

Health Canada. www.hc-sc.gc.ca/index_e.html.

Health on the Net Foundation. www.hon.ch.

Hospital Compare. www.medicare.gov/hospitalcompare.

Institute of Medicine. www.iom.edu.

Medline Plus: Trusted health information for you. www.nlm.nih.gov/medlineplus/.

National Database of Nursing Quality Indicators. www.nursingquality.org/.

National Health Information Center, U.S. Department of Health and Human Services. http://healthfinder.gov/.

National Institutes of Health, Health Information. http://health.nih.gov/.

Office of Minority Health. www.omhrc.gov.

The Quality Patient Experience. www.quality-patient-experienc

Think Cultural Health. www.thinkculturalhealth.hhs.gov/.

World Health Organization. www.who.int.

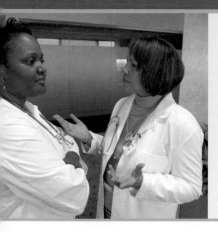

Conflict: The Cutting Edge of Change

Victoria N. Folse

Appropriate conflict-handling strategies are essential in professional nursing practice because conflict cannot be eliminated from the workplace. To resolve conflicts, nurse leaders must be able to determine the nature of a particular issue, choose an appropriate approach for each situation, and implement a course of action. This chapter focuses on maximizing the nurse leader's ability to deal with conflict by providing effective strategies for conflict resolution.

LEARNING OUTCOMES

- Use a model of the conflict process to determine the nature and sources of perceived and actual conflict.
- Assess preferred approaches to conflict, and commit to be more effective in resolving future conflict.
- Determine which of the five approaches to conflict is the most appropriate in potential and actual situations.
- Identify conflict management techniques that will prevent lateral violence and bullying from occurring.

KEY TERMS

accommodating	compromising	lateral violence
avoiding	conflict	mediation
bullying	horizontal violence	negotiating
collaborating	interpersonal conflict	organizational conflict
competing	intrapersonal conflict	

THE CHALLENGE

Miranda J. Kennedy, BSN, RN, CCRN
Staff Nurse, Medical Surgical Intensive Care Unit, Presence
Saint Joseph's Medical Center, Joliet, Illinois

Fresh out of orientation, I was walking down the hall and I heard the wife of one of my patients holler, "Miranda!! In here quick! It's happening again!" I raced into the room to find my patient diaphoretic and hypotensive, but still coherent. I quickly called my charge nurse and then called a rapid response. It was another busy day on the unit; I had just finished giving two stat meds to two different patients and recognized that another one of my patients required

a sitter. Because the charge nurse was busy, the assistant nurse manager came in the room to assist. The MD happened to be nearby so he was also present for the rapid response along with two critical care nurses. While we were reviewing what had occurred, the MD asked what medications that patient had received that AM, his 0800 vitals, and symptoms at the time of the episode. As I was looking vitals up, the assistant nurse manager said to me, "Yeah, did you even check your blood pressure before you gave all of his meds?!?"

What do you think you would do if you were this nurse?

INTRODUCTION

Conflict is a disagreement in values or beliefs within oneself or between people that causes harm or has the potential to cause harm. Folger, Poole, and Stutman (2012) add that conflict results from the interaction of interdependent people who perceive incompatibility and the potential for interference. Conflict is a catalyst for change and has the ability to stimulate either detrimental or beneficial effects. If properly understood and managed, conflict can lead to positive outcomes and practice environments, but if it is left unattended, it can have a negative impact on both the individual and the organization (Scott & Gerardi, 2011a, 2011b; Wright, 2011). In professional practice environments, unresolved conflict among nurses is a significant issue resulting in job dissatisfaction, absenteeism, and turnover. Patient dissatisfaction is lower in hospitals in which nurses are frustrated and burned out, which signals a problem with quality of care (McHugh, Kutney-Lee, Cimiotti, Sloane, & Aiken, 2011; Wright, 2011). Successful organizations are proactive in anticipating the need for conflict resolution and innovative in developing integrated conflict resolution strategies that apply to all members (Brinkert, 2010).

Conflict can be desirable at times and can be a strategic tool when addressed appropriately. Some of the first authors on organizational conflict (e.g., Blake & Mouton, 1964; Deutsch, 1973) claimed that a complete resolution of conflict might, in fact, be undesirable because conflict also stimulates growth, creativity, and change. Seminal work on the concept of organizational conflict management suggested conflict was necessary to achieve organizational goals

and cohesiveness of employees, facilitate organizational change, and contribute to creative problem solving and mutual understanding. Moderate levels of conflict contribute to the quality of ideas generated and foster cohesiveness among team members, contributing to an organization's success (Almost, 2006). An organization without conflict is characterized by no change; and in contrast, an optimal level of conflict will generate creativity, a problem-solving atmosphere, a strong team spirit, and motivation of its workers. Conflict on an interdisciplinary team can result in better patient care when collaborative treatment decisions are based on carefully examined and combined expertise (Tschannen, Keenan, Aebersold, Kocan, Lundy, & Averhart, 2011).

The complexity of the healthcare environment compounds the impact that caregiver stress and unresolved conflict has on patient safety. Conflict is inherent in clinical environments in which nursing responsibilities are driven by patient needs that are complex and frequently changing and in practice settings in which nurses have multiple professional roles (Brinkert, 2010). Healthcare providers are exposed to high stress levels from increased demands on a limited and aging workforce, a decrease in available resources, a more acutely ill and underinsured patient population, and a profound period of change in the practice environment. Conflict among healthcare providers is inevitable and is compounded by employee diversity, high nurse-to-patient ratios, pressure to make timely decisions, and status differences (Wright, 2011). Nurses employed in better care environments report more positive job experiences and fewer concerns about quality care. Interprofessional collaboration has been characterized by effective communication and is a key factor in reducing error and improving patient outcomes (Tschannen et al., 2011). Moreover, hospitals with good nurse-physician relations are associated with better nurse and patient outcomes, making collaboration and conflict resolution among nurses and physicians crucial in promoting quality of care outcomes (Aiken et al., 2012).

An important factor in the successful management of stress and conflict is a better understanding of its context within the practice environment. The diversity of people involved in health care may stimulate conflict, yet the shared goal of meeting patient care needs provides a solid foundation for conflict resolution. Because nursing remains a predominately female profession, this may contribute to the use of avoidance and accommodation as primary conflict handling strategies. An international study, however, found that both physicians and nurses were likely to use avoidance as the main strategy to handle conflict (Kaitelidou et al., 2012). The stereotypical self-sacrificing behavior seen in avoidance and accommodation is strongly supported by the altruistic nature of nursing. Avoidance may be appropriate during times of high stress, but when overused, it threatens the well-being of nurses and retention within the discipline.

TYPES OF CONFLICT

The recognition that conflict is a part of everyday life suggests that mastering conflict-management strategies is essential for overall well-being and personal and professional growth. A need exists to determine the type of conflict present in a specific situation, because the more accurately conflict is defined, the more likely it will be resolved. Conflict occurs in three broad categories and can be intrapersonal, interpersonal, or organizational in nature; a combination of types can also be present in any given conflict.

Intrapersonal conflict occurs within a person when confronted with the need to think or act in a way that seems at odds with one's sense of self. Questions often arise that create a conflict over priorities, ethical standards, and values. When a nurse decides what to do about the future (e.g., "Do I want to pursue an advanced degree or start a family now?"), conflicts arise between personal and professional priorities. Some issues present a conflict over comfortably maintaining

the status quo (e.g., "I know my newest charge nurse likes the autonomy of working nights. Do I really want to ask him to move to days to become a preceptor?"). Taking risks to confront people when needed (e.g., "Would recommending a change in practice that I learned about at a recent conference jeopardize unit governance?") can produce intrapersonal conflict and, because it involves other people, may lead to interpersonal conflict.

Interpersonal conflict is the most common type of conflict and transpires between and among patients, family members, nurses, physicians, and members of other departments. Conflicts occur that focus on a difference of opinion, priority, or approach with others. A manager may be called upon to assist two nurses in resolving a scheduling conflict or issues surrounding patient assignments. Members of healthcare teams often have disputes over the best way to treat particular cases or disagreements over how much information is necessary for patients and families to have about their illness. Yet, interpersonal conflict can serve as the impetus for needed change and can accelerate innovation in approach.

Organizational conflict arises when discord exists about policies and procedures, personnel codes of conduct, or accepted norms of behavior and patterns of communication. Some organizational conflict is related to hierarchical structure and role differentiation among employees. Nurse managers, as well as their staff, often become embattled in institution-wide conflict concerning staffing patterns and how they affect the quality of care. Complex ethical and moral dilemmas often arise when profitable services are increased and unprofitable ones are downsized or even eliminated.

A major source of organizational conflict stems from strategies that promote more participation and autonomy of direct care nurses. Increasingly, nurses are charged with balancing direct patient care with active involvement in the institutional initiatives surrounding quality patient care. A growing number of standards set by The Joint Commission (TJC) target improving communication and conflict management (Scott & Gerardi, 2011a, 2011b). Specifically, TJC requires that healthcare organizations have a code of conduct that defines acceptable and inappropriate behaviors and that leaders create and implement a process for managing intimidating and disruptive behaviors that undermine a culture of safety. Standards pertaining to medical staff also include interpersonal skills and professionalism (TJC, 2012). The Magnet Recognition Program® of the American Nurses Credentialing Center (ANCC) identifies interdisciplinary relationships as one of the Forces of Magnetism necessary for Magnet™ designation (2012). Specifically, collaborative working relationships within and among the disciplines are valued, demonstrated through mutual respect, and result in meaningful contributions in the achievement of clinical outcomes. Magnet™ hospitals must have conflict management strategies in place and use them effectively, when indicated. The following are other "forces" that are particularly germane to conflict in the practice environment:

- Organizational structure (nurses' involvement in shared decision making)
- Management style (nursing leaders create an environment supporting participation, encourage and value feedback, and demonstrate effective communication with staff)
- Personnel policies and programs (efforts to promote nurse work/life balance)
- Image of nursing (nurses effectively influencing system-wide processes)
- Autonomy (nurses' inclusion in governance leading to job satisfaction, personal fulfillment, and organization success)

> **EXERCISE 23-1**
>
> Recall a situation in which conflict between or among two or more people was apparent. Describe verbal and nonverbal communication and how each person responded. What was the outcome? Was the conflict resolved? Was anything left unresolved?

STAGES OF CONFLICT

Conflict proceeds through four stages: frustration, conceptualization, action, and outcomes (Thomas, 1992). The ability to resolve conflicts productively depends on understanding this process (Figure 23-1) and successfully addressing thoughts, feelings, and

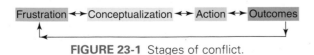

FIGURE 23-1 Stages of conflict.

behaviors that form barriers to resolution. As one navigates through the stages of conflict, moving into a subsequent stage may lead to a return to and change in a previous stage. To illustrate, the evening shift of a cardiac step-down unit has been asked to pilot a new hand-off protocol for the next 6 weeks, which stimulates intense emotions because the unit is already inadequately staffed (frustration). Two nurses on the unit interpret this conflict as a battle for control with the nurse educator, and a third nurse thinks it is all about professional standards (conceptualization). A nurse leader/manager facilitates a discussion with the three nurses (action); she listens to the concerns and presents evidence about the potential effectiveness of the new hand-off protocol. All agree that the real conflict comes from a difference in goals or priorities (new conceptualization), which leads to less negative emotion and ends with a much clearer understanding of all the issues (diminished frustration). The nurses agree to pilot the hand-off protocol after their ideas have been incorporated into the plan (outcome).

Frustration

When people or groups perceive that their goals may be blocked, frustration results. This frustration may escalate into stronger emotions, such as anger and deep resignation. For example, a nurse may perceive that a postoperative patient is noncompliant or uncooperative, when in reality the patient is afraid or has a different set of priorities at the start from those of the nurse. At the same time, the patient may view the nurse as controlling and uncaring, because the nurse repeatedly asks if the patient has used his incentive spirometer as instructed. When such frustrations occur, it is a cue to stop and clarify the nature and cause of the differences.

Conceptualization

Conflict arises when different interpretations of a situation occur, including a different emphasis on what is important and what is not, and different thoughts about what should occur next. Everyone involved develops an idea of what the conflict is about, and this view may or may not be accurate. This may be an instant conclusion, or it may develop over time. Everyone involved has an individual interpretation of what the conflict is and why it is occurring. Most often, these interpretations are dissimilar and involve the person's own perspective, which is based on personal values, beliefs, and culture.

Regardless of its accuracy, conceptualization forms the basis for everyone's reactions to the frustration. The way the individuals perceive and define the conflict has a great deal of influence on the approach to resolution and subsequent outcomes. For example, within the same conflict situation, some individuals may see a conflict between a nurse manager and a direct care nurse as insubordination and become angry at the threat to the leader's role. Others may view it as trivial complaining, voice criticism (e.g., "We've been over this new protocol already; why can't you just adopt the change?"), and withdraw from the situation. Such differences in conceptualizing the issue block its resolution. Thus it is important for each person to clarify "the conflict as I see it" and "how it makes me respond" before all the people involved can define the conflict, develop a shared conceptualization, and resolve their differences. The following are question to consider:

- What is the nature of our differences?
- What are the reasons for those differences?
- Does our leader endorse ideas or behaviors that add to or diminish the conflict?
- Do I need to be mentored by someone, even if that individual is outside my own department or work area, to successfully resolve this conflict?

Action

A behavioral response to a conflict follows the conceptualization. This may include seeking clarification about how another person views the conflict, collecting additional information that informs the issue, or engaging in dialog about the issue. As actions are taken to resolve the conflict, the way that some or all parties conceptualize the conflict may change. Successful resolution frequently stems from identifying a common goal that unites (e.g., quality patient care, good working relations). It is important to understand that people are always taking some action regarding the conflict, even if that action is avoiding dealing with it, deliberately delaying action, or choosing to do nothing. The longer ineffective actions continue, though, the more likely people will experience frustration, resistance, or even hostility. The more the actions appropriately match the nature of the conflict,

the more likely the conflict will be resolved with desirable results.

Outcomes

Tangible and intangible consequences result from the actions taken and have significant implications for the work setting. Consequences include (1) the conflict being resolved with a revised approach, (2) stagnation of any current movement, or (3) no future movement.

Constructive conflict results in successful resolution, leading to the following outcomes:

- Growth occurs.
- Problems are resolved.
- Groups are unified.
- Productivity is increased.
- Commitment is increased.

Unsatisfactory resolution is typically destructive and results in the following:

- Negativity, resistance, and increased frustration inhibit movement.
- Resolutions diminish or are absent.
- Groups divide, and relationships weaken.
- Productivity decreases.
- Satisfaction decreases.

Assessing the degree of conflict resolution is useful for improving individual and group skills in resolutions. Two general outcomes are considered when assessing the degree to which a conflict has been resolved: (1) the degree to which important goals were achieved and (2) the nature of the subsequent relationships among those involved (Box 23-1).

BOX 23-1   ASSESSING THE DEGREE OF CONFLICT RESOLUTION

I. Quality of decisions
   A. How creative are resulting plans?
   B. How practical and realistic are they?
   C. How well were intended goals achieved?
   D. What surprising results were achieved?
II. Quality of relationships
   A. How much understanding has been created?
   B. How willing are people to work together?
   C. How much mutual respect, empathy, concern, and cooperation have been generated?

Modified from Hurst, J., & Kinney, M. (1989). *Empowering self and others.* Toledo, OH: University of Toledo.

CATEGORIES OF CONFLICT

Categorizing a conflict can further define an appropriate course of action for resolution. Conflicts arise from discrepancies in four areas: facts, goals, approaches, and values. Sources of fact-based conflicts are external written sources and include job descriptions, hospital policies, standard of nursing practice, and TJC mandates. Objective data can be provided to resolve a disagreement generated by discrepancies in information. Goal conflicts often arise from competing priorities (e.g., desire to empower employees vs. control through micromanagement); frequently, a common goal (e.g., quality patient care) can be identified and used to frame conflict resolution. Even when all agree on a common goal, different ideas about the best approach to achieve that goal may produce conflict. For example, if the unit goal is to reduce costs by 10%, one leader may target overtime hours and another may eliminate the budget for continuing education. Values, opinions, and beliefs are much more personal, thus generating disagreements that can be threatening and adversarial. Because values are subjective, value-based conflicts often remain unresolved. Therefore a need to find a way for competing values to coexist is necessary for conflict management.

MODES OF CONFLICT RESOLUTION

Understanding the way healthcare providers respond to conflict is an essential first step in identifying effective strategies to help nurses constructively handle conflicts in the practice environment. Five distinct approaches can be used in conflict resolution: avoiding, accommodating, competing, compromising, and collaborating (Thomas & Kilmann, 1974, 2002). These approaches can be viewed within two dimensions: assertiveness (satisfying one's own concerns) and cooperativeness (satisfying the concerns of others). Most people tend to employ a combined set of actions that are appropriately assertive and cooperative, depending on the nature of the conflict situation (Thomas, 1992). See the conflict self-assessment in Box 23-2.

As you read the rest of this section, use this pattern of scores and your reflections to examine the appropriate uses of each approach, assess your use of each

---

EXERCISE 23-2

Self-assessment of preferred conflict-handling modes is important. As you read and answer the 30-item conflict survey in Box 23-2, think of how you respond to conflict in professional situations. After completing the survey, tally, total, and reflect on your scores for each of the five approaches. Consider the following questions:

- Which approach do you prefer? Which do you use least?
- What determines if you respond in a particular manner?
- Considering the reoccurring types of conflicts you have, what are the strengths and weaknesses of your preferred conflict-handling styles?
- Have others offered you feedback about your approach to conflict?

---

approach more extensively, and commit to new behaviors to increase your future effectiveness.

Avoiding

Avoiding, or withdrawing, is very unassertive and uncooperative because people who avoid neither pursue their own needs, goals, or concerns immediately nor assist others to pursue theirs. Avoidance as a conflict-management style only ensures that conflict is postponed, and conflict has a tendency to escalate in intensity when ignored. That is not to say that all conflict must be addressed immediately; some issues require considerable reflection, and action should be delayed. The positive side of withdrawing may be postponing an issue until a better time or simply walking away from a "no-win" situation (Box 23-3). The self-assessment in Box 23-4 will help you recognize your own avoidance behaviors and use them more effectively.

Accommodating

When accommodating, people neglect their own needs, goals, and concerns (unassertive) while trying to satisfy those of others (cooperative). This approach has an element of being self-sacrificing and simply obeying orders or serving other people. For example, a co-worker requests you cover her weekends during her children's holiday break. You had hoped to visit friends from college, but you know how important it is for her to have more time with her family, so you agree. Box 23-5 lists some appropriate uses of accommodation.

Individuals who frequently use accommodating may feel disappointment and resentment because they "get nothing in return." This is a built-in by-product

BOX 23-2 CONFLICT SELF-ASSESSMENT

Directions: Read each of the following statements. Assess yourself in terms of how often you tend to act similarly during conflict at work. Place the number of the most appropriate response in the blank in front of each statement. Put *1* if the behavior is never typical of how you act during a conflict, *2* if it is seldom typical, *3* if it is occasionally typical, *4* if it is frequently typical, or *5* if it is very typical of how you act during conflict.

_____ 1. Create new possibilities to address all important concerns.
_____ 2. Persuade others to see it and/or do it my way.
_____ 3. Work out some sort of give-and-take agreement.
_____ 4. Let other people have their way.
_____ 5. Wait and let the conflict take care of itself.
_____ 6. Find ways that everyone can win.
_____ 7. Use whatever power I have to get what I want.
_____ 8. Find an agreeable compromise among people involved.
_____ 9. Give in so others get what they think is important.
_____ 10. Withdraw from the situation.
_____ 11. Cooperate assertively until everyone's needs are met.
_____ 12. Compete until I either win or lose.
_____ 13. Engage in "give a little and get a little" bargaining.
_____ 14. Let others' needs be met more than my own needs.
_____ 15. Avoid taking any action for as long as I can.
_____ 16. Partner with others to find the most inclusive solution.
_____ 17. Put my foot down assertively for a quick solution.
_____ 18. Negotiate for what all sides value and can live without.
_____ 19. Agree to what others want to create harmony.
_____ 20. Keep as far away from others involved as possible.
_____ 21. Stick with it to get everyone's highest priorities.
_____ 22. Argue and debate over the best way.
_____ 23. Create some middle position everyone agrees to.
_____ 24. Put my priorities below those of other people.
_____ 25. Hope the issue does not come up.
_____ 26. Collaborate with others to achieve our goals together.
_____ 27. Compete with others for scarce resources.
_____ 28. Emphasize compromise and trade-offs.
_____ 29. Cool things down by letting others do it their way.
_____ 30. Change the subject to avoid the fighting.

Conflict Self-Assessment Scoring

Look at the numbers you placed in the blanks on the conflict assessment. Write the number you placed in each blank on the appropriate line below. Add up your total for each column, and enter that total on the appropriate line. The greater your total is for each approach, the more often you tend to use that approach when conflict occurs at work. The lower the score is, the less often you tend to use that approach when conflict occurs at work.

COLLABORATING	COMPETING	COMPROMISING	ACCOMMODATING	AVOIDING
1. _____	2. _____	3. _____	4. _____	5. _____
6. _____	7. _____	8. _____	9. _____	10. _____
11. _____	12. _____	13. _____	14. _____	15. _____
16. _____	17. _____	18. _____	19. _____	20. _____
21. _____	22. _____	23. _____	24. _____	25. _____
26. _____	27. _____	28. _____	29. _____	30. _____
Total _____	Total _____	Total _____	Total _____	Total _____

Throughout the rest of this section, there are descriptions of each approach and related self-assessment and commitment-to-action activities. Use these totals to stimulate your thinking about how you do and could handle conflict at work. Most important, consider if your pattern of frequency tends to be consistent, or inconsistent, with the types of conflicts you face. That is, does your way of dealing with conflict tend to match the situations in which that approach is most useful?

From Hurst, J.B. (1993). *Conflict self-assessment*. Toledo, OH: Human Resource Development Center, University of Toledo.

BOX 23-3 APPROPRIATE USES FOR THE AVOIDING APPROACH

1. When facing trivial and/or temporary issues, or when other far more important issues are pressing
2. When there is no chance to obtain what one wants or needs, or when others could resolve the conflict more efficiently and effectively
3. When the potential negative results of initiating and acting on a conflict are much greater than the benefits of its resolution
4. When people need to "cool down," distance themselves, or gather more information

BOX 23-4 AVOIDANCE: SELF-ASSESSMENT AND COMMITMENT TO ACTION

If You Tend to Use Avoidance Often, Ask Yourself the Following Questions:

1. Do people have difficulty getting my input into and understanding my view?
2. Do I block cooperative efforts to resolve issues?
3. Am I distancing myself from significant others?
4. Are important issues being left unidentified and unresolved?

If You Seldom Use Avoidance, Ask Yourself the Following Questions:

1. Do I find myself overwhelmed by a large number of conflicts and a need to say "no"?
2. Do I assert myself even when things do not matter that much? Do others view me as an aggressor?
3. Do I lack a clear view of what my priorities are?
4. Do I stir up conflicts and fights?

Commitment to Action

What two new behaviors would increase your effective use of avoidance?
1.
2.

BOX 23-5 APPROPRIATE USES OF ACCOMMODATION

1. When other people's ideas and solutions appear to be better, or when you have made a mistake
2. When the issue is far more important to the other(s) person than it is to you
3. When you see that accommodating now "builds up some important credits" for later issues
4. When you are outmatched and/or losing anyway; when continued competition would only damage the relationships and productivity of the group and jeopardize accomplishing major purpose(s)
5. When preserving harmonious relationships and avoiding defensiveness and hostility are very important
6. When letting others learn from their mistakes and/or increased responsibility is possible without severe damage

BOX 23-6 ACCOMMODATION: SELF-ASSESSMENT AND COMMITMENT TO ACTION

If You Use Accommodation Often, Ask Yourself the Following Questions:

1. Do I feel that my needs, goals, concerns, and ideas are not being attended to by others?
2. Am I depriving myself of influence, recognition, and respect?
3. When I am in charge, is "discipline" lax?
4. Do I think people are using me?

If You Seldom Use Accommodation, Ask Yourself the Following Questions:

1. Am I building goodwill with others during conflict?
2. Do I admit when I have made a mistake?
3. Do I know when to give in, or do I assert myself at all costs?
4. Am I viewed as unreasonable or insensitive?

Commitment to Action

What two new behaviors would increase your effective use of accommodation?
1.
2.

of the overuse of this approach. The self-assessment in Box 23-6 asks you to examine your current use of accommodation and challenges you to think of new ways to use it more effectively.

Competing

When competing, people pursue their own needs and goals at the expense of others. Sometimes people use whatever power, creativeness, or strategies that are available to "win." Competing may also take the form of standing up for your rights or defending important principles, as when opposition to mandatory overtime is voiced (Box 23-7).

People whose primary mode of addressing conflict is through competition often react by feeling threatened, acting defensively or aggressively, or even resorting to cruelty in the form of cutting remarks, deliberate gossip, or hurtful innuendo. Competition within work groups can generate ill will, favor a

BOX 23-7 APPROPRIATE USES OF COMPETING

1. When quick, decisive action is necessary
2. When important, unpopular action needs to be taken, or when trade-offs may result in long-range, continued conflict
3. When an individual or group is right about issues that are vital to group welfare
4. When others have taken advantage of an individual's or group's noncompetitive behavior and now are mobilized to compete about an important topic

BOX 23-8 COMPETING: SELF-ASSESSMENT AND COMMITMENT TO ACTION

If You Use Competing Often, Ask Yourself the Following Questions:

1. Am I surrounded by people who agree with me all the time and who avoid confronting me?
2. Are others afraid to share themselves and their needs for growth with me?
3. Am I out to win at all costs? If so, what are the costs and benefits of competing?
4. What are people saying about me when I am not around?

If You Seldom Compete, Ask Yourself the Following Questions:

1. How often do I avoid taking a strong stand and then feel a sense of powerlessness?
2. Do I avoid taking a stand so that I can escape risk?
3. Am I fearful and unassertive to the point that important decisions are delayed and people suffer?

Commitment to Action

What two new behaviors would increase your effective use of competition?

1.
2.

win-lose stance, and commit people to a stalemate. Such behaviors force people into a corner from which there is no easy or graceful exit. Use Box 23-8 to help you learn to use competing more effectively.

Compromising

Compromising involves both assertiveness and cooperation on the part of everyone and requires maturity and confidence. Negotiating is a learned skill that is developed over time. A give-and-take relationship results in conflict resolution, with the result that each person can meet his or her most important priorities as much of the time as possible. Compromise is very often the exchange of concessions as it creates a middle ground. This is the preferred means of conflict resolution during union negotiations, in which each side is appeased to some degree. In this mode, nobody gets everything he or she thinks he or she needs, but a sense of energy exists that is necessary to build important relationships and teams.

Negotiation and compromise are valued approaches. They are chosen when less accommodating or avoiding is appropriate (Box 23-9). Compromising is a blend of both assertive and cooperative behaviors, although it calls for less finely honed skills for each behavior than does collaborating. Negotiating is more like trading (e.g., "You can have this if I can have that," as in "I will chair the unit council taskforce on improving morale if you send me to the hospital's leadership training classes next week so I can have the skills I need to be effective."). Compromise is one of the most effective behaviors used by nurse leaders because it supports a balance of power between themselves and others in the work setting. The self-assessment in Box 23-10 will help you become more aware of your own use of negotiation and compromise and improve it.

Collaborating

Collaborating, although the most time-consuming approach is the most creative stance. It is both assertive and cooperative because people work creatively and openly to find the solution that most fully satisfies all important concerns and goals to be achieved. Collaboration involves analyzing situations and defining the conflict at a higher level where shared goals are identified and commitment to working together is generated (Box 23-11). When

BOX 23-9 APPROPRIATE USES OF COMPROMISE

1. When two powerful sides are committed strongly to perceived mutually exclusive goals
2. When temporary solutions to complex issues need to be implemented
3. When conflicting goals are "moderately important" and not worth a major confrontation
4. When time pressures people to expedite a workable solution
5. When collaborating and competing fail

BOX 23-10   NEGOTIATION/ COMPROMISE SELF-ASSESSMENT AND COMMITMENT TO ACTION

If You Tend to Use Negotiation Often, Ask Yourself the Following Questions:
1. Do I ignore large, important issues while trying to work out creative, practical compromises?
2. Is there a "gamesmanship" in my negotiations?
3. Am I sincerely committed to compromise or negotiated solutions?

If You Seldom Use Negotiation, Ask Yourself the Following Questions:
1. Do I find it difficult to make concessions?
2. Am I often engaged in strong disagreements, or do I withdraw when I see no way to get out?
3. Do I feel embarrassed, sensitive, self-conscious, or pressured to negotiate, compromise, and bargain?

Commitment to Action
What two new behaviors would increase your compromising effectiveness?
1.
2.

BOX 23-11   APPROPRIATE USES FOR COLLABORATION

1. When seeking creative, integrative solutions in which both sides' goals and needs are important, thus developing group commitment and a consensual decision
2. When learning and growing through cooperative problem solving, resulting in greater understanding and empathy
3. When identifying, sharing, and merging vastly different viewpoints
4. When being honest about and working through difficult emotional issues that interfere with morale, productivity, and growth

---

nurses use cooperative conflict-management approaches, decision making becomes a collective process in which action plans are mutually understood and implemented. An organizational culture that supports collaborative behavior among nurses and physicians is needed to merge the unique strengths of both professions into opportunities to improve patient outcomes (Nair, Fitzpatrick, McNulty, Click, & Glembocki, 2012). For example, when nurses and

physicians work together, they can collaborate by asking, "What is the best thing we can do for the patient and family right now?" and "How does each of us fit into the plan of care to meet their needs?" This requires discussion about the plan, how it will be accomplished, and who will make what contributions toward its achievement and proposed outcomes. Use the self-assessment in Box 23-12 to determine your own use of collaboration.

At the onset of conflict, involved collaborating individuals can carefully analyze situations to identify the nature and reasons for conflict and choose an appropriate approach. For example, a conflict arises when a direct care nurse and a charge nurse on a psychiatric unit disagree about how to handle a patient's complaints about the direct care nurse's delay in responding to the patient's requests. At the point that they reach agreement that it is the direct care nurse's responsibility and decision to make, collaboration has occurred. The charge nurse might say, "I didn't realize your plan of care was to respond

---

BOX 23-12   COLLABORATION SELF-ASSESSMENT AND COMMITMENT TO ACTION

If You Tend to Collaborate Often, Ask Yourself the Following Questions:
1. Do I spend valuable group time and energy on issues that do not warrant or deserve it?
2. Do I postpone needed action to get consensus and avoid making key decisions?
3. When I initiate collaboration, do others respond in a genuine way, or are there hidden agendas, unspoken hostility, and/or manipulation in the group?

If You Seldom Collaborate, Ask Yourself the Following Questions:
1. Do I ignore opportunities to cooperate, take risks, and creatively confront conflict?
2. Do I tend to be pessimistic, distrusting, withdrawing, and/or competitive?
3. Am I involving others in important decisions, eliciting commitment, and empowering them?

Commitment to Action
What two new behaviors would increase your collaboration effectiveness?
1.
2.

to the patient at predetermined intervals or that you told the patient that you would check on her every 30 minutes. I can now inform the patient that I know about and support your approach." Or the direct care nurse and the charge nurse might talk and subsequently agree that the direct care nurse is too emotionally involved with the patient's problems and that it may be time for her to withdraw from providing the care and enlist the support of another nurse, even temporarily. Discussion can result in collaboration aimed at allowing the direct care nurse to withdraw appropriately. Another, less desirable choice could be to compete and let the winner's position stand (e.g., "I'm in charge; I'm going to assign another nurse to this patient to preserve our patient satisfaction scores" or "I know what is best for this patient; I took care of her during her past two admissions").

DIFFERENCES OF CONFLICT-HANDLING STYLES AMONG NURSES

The way in which conflict-management styles are used in health care has changed very little in the past 20 years. Previous studies suggest that avoidance and accommodation remain the predominant choices for direct care nurses and that the prevalent style for nurse managers is compromise, despite the emphasis placed on collaboration as an effective strategy for conflict management (Mahon & Nicotera, 2011). Nursing students and new graduates may be unprepared to handle conflict in the practice environment; Hasson, McKenna, and Keeney (2013) reported a number of barriers novice nurses faced when delegating tasks such as fear of causing conflict. This highlights the need to develop delegation strategies including conflict-handling skills to adapt to the evolving professional role. The prevalent conflict-management style for nursing students is avoidance and accommodation (Pines et al., 2011). Nurses who successfully managed disruptive workplace conflict reported a deliberate approach that included delaying confrontation, approaching the colleague calmly, and acknowledging the colleague's point of view (Lux, Hutcheson, & Peden, 2012). Nurses working in specialty areas may adapt communication and conflict management strategies to respond to diverse patient populations and the unique mix of interprofessional colleagues. For example, in primary care settings, conflicts regarding scope of practice issues, role confusion, and disagreements over accountability for care are amplified (Brown, Lewis, Ellis, Stewart, Freeman, & Kasperski, 2011). See the Research Perspective, which describes conflicts and communication gaps common in intensive care units and in palliative care situations.

 RESEARCH PERSPECTIVE

Resource: Aslakson, R.A., Wyskiel, R., Thornton, I., Copley, C., Shaffer, D., Zyra, M., Nelson, J., & Pronovost, P.J. (2012). Nurse-perceived barriers to effective communication regarding prognosis and optimal end-of-life care for surgical ICU patients: A qualitative exploration. *Journal of Palliative Medicine, 15*(8), 910-915.

Two sources of conflict that arise in critical care environments are end-of-life decisions and communication issues, both of which are most evident in interprofessional conflict and tension between team members and patients' families. Intensive care nurses identified barriers to optimal communication regarding palliative care including discomfort with discussing prognosis, inadequate skill and training, and fear of conflict. The ICU is particularly vulnerable because of the stressful work environment, complex network of interprofessional relationships, and a need for making life and death decisions under considerable time pressure and familial burden. Additionally, critical care resources

(e.g., bed shortages, costs, and length of stay), values (e.g., ethical disputes over goals of treatment), and task conflicts (e.g., timing of ventilator withdrawal, pain management) can exaggerate conflicts.

Implications for Practice
Conflicts in intensive care units most negatively affect the Quality and Safety Education for Nurses (QSEN) competencies of patient-centered care, teamwork and collaboration, and safety (QSEN Institute, 2013). Reduced conflict in the ICU could be achieved with regular interprofessional unit and team meetings and when end-of-life decisions are made collaboratively with physicians, nurses, the family, and a healthcare ethicist as needed. Leaders and manager must model and coach bedside nurses in effective conflict handling strategies in order to favorably impact the practice environment.

Nurses and physicians do not routinely collaborate with each other in conflict situations conducive to collaboration. Conflicts between nurses and physicians may be intensified because of the overlapping nature of their domains and lack of clarification between roles. Also, when asked to describe relationships with physicians, nurses frequently reported power as a dominant theme. The compromising mode is a common conflict-handling mode used in nurse/physician interactions. Compromise supports a balance of power in the workplace. A need exists to strengthen a healthy professional alliance that relies on collaborative practice to ensure favorable patient outcomes. Effective communication with other members of the health care team positively influences teamwork, staff satisfaction, and improves quality of patient care and safety (Institute of Healthcare Improvement, 2011; TJC, 2012).

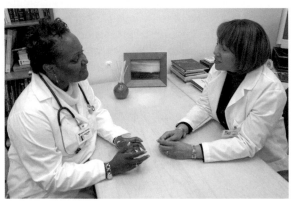

Compromise supports a balance of power between self and others in the workplace.

THE ROLE OF THE LEADER

Encouraging positive working relations among healthcare providers requires effective conflict management as part of a healthy working environment. The role of the nurse leader is to create a practice environment that fosters open communication and collaborative practices for achieving mutual goals that enable nurses to employ constructive approaches to conflict management. Specifically, leaders must adopt a strategic proactive approach that aligns conflict management approaches with the overall mission of the organization (Scott & Gerardi, 2011a, 2011b). TJC adopted new accreditation standards requiring that hospitals manage conflict between leadership groups to promote a culture of safety (TJC, 2012). The training of nurse managers as conflict coaches shows promise in creating a positive practice environment when integrated with other conflict intervention processes (Brinkert, 2011). This innovative model can increase the nurse manager's conflict competencies and skill set in effectively impacting conflicts concerning diverse issues (e.g., scheduling; adherence to policies and procedures; difficult interdepartmental and interprofessional behaviors) with a multitude of stakeholders, including patients and their families, direct care nurses, other departments, physicians, and insurance companies (Brinkert, 2011). By providing an environment of open communication and acknowledgement of each team member's viewpoint, the nurse manager can model and coach staff to independently and effectively resolve future conflicts themselves (Johansen, 2012).

With the aging workforce and current nursing shortage, it is essential to create practice environments that will retain nurses and prevent premature departure from the discipline. Moreover, managers need to help challenge the stereotypical gender behavioral expectations and self-esteem issues frequently associated with a female-oriented profession and model effective management and leadership styles. One way to promote a positive work setting is to promote conflict prevention and ensure conflict resolution (Almost, 2006). The Literature Perspective on page 443 highlights the most recent and comprehensive concept analysis on conflict. Nurse leaders must provide the best example of advocacy and empowerment to their staff by coaching newer nurses to think strategically about a mode of conflict handling that is appropriate for the situation. Poor communication often creates conflict that jeopardizes patient safety, whereas inadequate leadership appears to be a contributing factor to most sentinel events (Scott & Gerardi, 2011a, 2011b). Nursing managers need to support their staff's use of effective conflict-management strategies by modeling open and honest communication, including staffing decision making, and securing resources that meet the staff's need in delivering quality care. Providing education on conflict management could empower nurses and physicians to use these newly acquired skills in negotiation and creative problem-solving techniques (Kaitelidou et al., 2012). Research confirms that healthcare providers do not always voice concerns about patients and actively avoid conflict in clinical settings (Lyndon, Zlatnik, & Wachter, 2011). Healthcare leaders and managers who promote effective conflict resolution skills and who discourage the use of avoidance as a strategy have the potential to reduce employee stress and burnout as well as promote higher job satisfaction (Wright, 2011).

For example, a manager's need to give clear direction to a team automatically places less emphasis on the team deciding on the direction themselves. However, for the team to be successful, eventually that manager must recognize the need for the team to work on its own even though the manager may at times need to intervene. Imagine a nurse manager was confronted by an angry team whose members felt like they were being treated like children, always being told what to do. Working together, they initiated team meetings and decision-making procedures (actions emphasizing participatory management, as in self-scheduling practices) that resulted in more ideas, a sense of ownership, and a noticeable self-direction from the team and its individual members. However, after a few months of continually emphasizing participation, the team began to lose its focus and cohesiveness and once again came to the manager for more direction. The manager listened and provided clarification, and the team regained its focus and efficiency.

The nature of the differences, underlying reasons, importance of the issue, strength of feelings, and commitment to shared goals all have to be considered when selecting an approach to resolving conflict. Preferred and previously effective approaches can be considered, but they need to match the situation. Sometimes, a third party may be introduced into a conflict so that mediation can occur. Mediation is a learned skill for which advanced training and/or certification is available. Principled negotiation can produce mutually acceptable agreements in every type of conflict. The method involves separating the people from the problem; focusing on interests, not positions; inventing options for mutual gain; and insisting on using objective criteria. The mediator is usually an impartial person who assists each party in the conflict to better hear and understand the other. In society, for example, much focus is on who can control whom and on who is the "winner." The successful individual involved in conflict resolution and negotiation often

---

 LITERATURE PERSPECTIVE

Resource: Almost, J. (2006). Conflict within nursing environments: Concept analysis. *Journal of Advanced Nursing*, 53(4), 444-453.

A concept analysis, including the development of a conceptual diagram of antecedents and consequences of conflict (Figure 23-2), in nursing work environments was performed following an exhaustive review of the literature published from 1980 to 2004. Sources of conflict originate from individual characteristics, interpersonal factors, and organizational dynamics. Individual differences, typically generated by differing opinions and values, create potential conflict. Demographic dissimilarity (e.g., gender, educational levels, age, race, ethnicity) can stimulate conflict as well. Interpersonal factors such as distrust, perceptions of injustice or disrespect, and inadequate or poor communication style can lead to conflict. Organizational factors including the interdependence among team members and the changes that result from restructuring can set the stage for conflict within the practice environment. Similarly, the effects of unresolved conflict are visible in individual characteristics, interpersonal factors, and organizational dynamics. Individual effects include job stress and dissatisfaction, absenteeism, and intent to leave, whereas interpersonal factors such as hostility and avoidance are dominant. The organizational impact of negative conflict management includes reduced productivity and ineffective teamwork.

Implications for Practice

Sources of conflict within the practice environment must be anticipated and addressed to enhance organizational effectiveness. Healthcare leaders must engage in conflict-management strategies to prevent or resolve conflict within nursing environments to ensure quality and safety. Nurses in managerial positions spend inadequate time on conflict resolution. Many lack the educational preparation to manage conflict or do not feel qualified or sufficiently experienced to effectively deal with conflict. Moreover, some staff can be difficult, so managers must remain focused on the problem and not the personalities of the team members. Nurse managers must also remain cognizant of other pitfalls of effective conflict resolution. For example, a common way for managers to avoid conflict in the workplace is to delay responding to colleagues' concerns voiced in staff meetings, to not reply to voice mails or e-mail messages, or to cancel or postpone important meetings. If this behavior is known and continues, the avoiding behavior is said to be endorsed or approved, leading to an unhealthy practice environment. Fostering collaboration requires a commitment of time and interpersonal energy to be effective, which many nurse leaders report as a barrier.

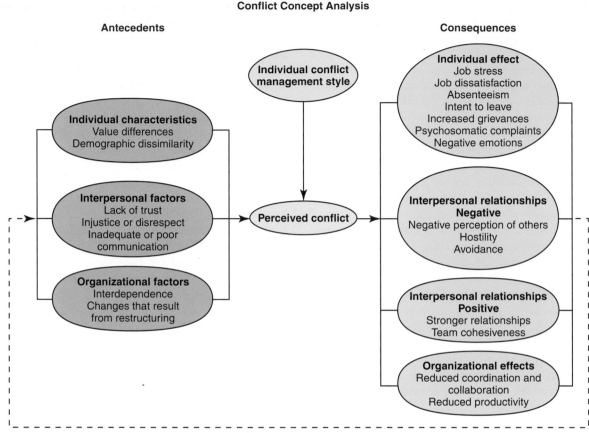

FIGURE 23-2 Diagram of antecedents and consequences of conflict

moves beyond avoidance, accommodation, and compromise. In the nursing practice arena, added difficulty occurs in negotiating conflicts when at least one of the parties is on an unequal or uneven playing field. This disadvantage is made even worse when the other party to the conflict does not even acknowledge the disparities involved.

Interest-based bargaining, a negotiation strategy that produces agreements that satisfy common interests and balance opposing positions, has been effectively used in complex organizational conflicts such as in collective bargaining situations. This approach has been implemented by the healthcare giant Kaiser Permanente whose national agreements with its labor unions cover not only wages and benefits but also performance goals related to service, care quality, and affordability. They also address workforce

and community health and workforce development (Kaiser Permanente, 2012).

MANAGING LATERAL VIOLENCE AND BULLYING

A significant source of interpersonal conflict in the workplace stems from lateral violence—aggressive and destructive behavior or psychological harassment of nurses against each other. Nurses are particularly vulnerable because lateral or horizontal violence involves conflictual behaviors among individuals who consider themselves peers with equal power—but with little power within the system. Bullying is closely related to lateral or horizontal violence, but a real or perceived power differential between the instigator and recipient must be present in bullying. Bullying is associated with psychological and physical stress, underperformance, professional disengagement, increased job turnover, and the potential for diminished quality of care (Dzurec & Bromley, 2012).

Understanding the sources of intraprofessional conflict in the practice environment is essential (see also Chapter 25). Nurses are in positions to identify and intervene on the part of their colleagues when they see or experience horizontal violence or bullying. With increased awareness and sensitivity, nurses may be better able to monitor themselves, as well as assist their peers to recognize when they are participating in negative behaviors. Identifying and understanding particular incidences when nurses are most vulnerable and apt to engage in negative behavior (e.g., heavy workload, short staffing) and establishing performance expectations has the potential to reduce lateral violence in the workplace (Walrafen, Brewer, & Mulvenon, 2012). Incorporating workplace civility in nursing orientation programs and modeling professional behaviors provides a foundation to promote a healthy work culture. Nursing students and new graduates often lack the confidence and skill set to prevent interpersonal conflict and must rely on experienced nurse managers and leaders to reduce the likelihood of horizontal violence or bullying (Weaver, 2013). Nurse educators have a similar responsibility to develop nursing curricula that educate and encourage dialogue about horizontal violence to increase awareness and provide nursing students the skills to combat horizontal violence (Walrafen et al., 2012).

In hostile work environments, the ability to provide quality patient care is compromised. TJC (2012) acknowledges that unresolved conflict and disruptive behavior adversely affect safety and quality of care. The vulnerability of newly licensed nurses as they are socialized within the nursing workforce and deal with interpersonal conflicts is a significant challenge. Longo and Smith (2011) reported it is common for nursing students to report being put down by a direct care nurse and, in turn, for direct care nurses to experience horizontal violence at work. Lateral violence affects newly licensed nurses' job satisfaction and stress, as well as their perception of whether to remain in their current position and in the profession. Similarly, nursing students are particularly vulnerable to lateral

violence and bullying in the transition to becoming a nurse and may begin to question their long-held belief that nurses are caring and supportive professionals. See The Challenge and The Solution, which present the experiences of a new graduate nurse in a situation related to this chapter.

Lateral violence may be a response to the practice environment, in which ineffective leadership may exacerbate the problem. TJC (2012) acknowledges that incivility and disruptive behavior that intimidates others and affects morale or staff turnover can be harmful to patient care. It mandates that organizations have a code of conduct that defines acceptable, disruptive, and inappropriate behaviors and that leaders create and implement a process for managing these conflictual situations. One-on-one conflict resolution must be encouraged, but a mechanism for confidential reporting is also necessary. Training on conflict management that includes how to recognize and defend against lateral violence is necessary to ensure a positive professional practice environment. Senior level leaders and nurse managers are responsible for ensuring appropriate policies are in place to confront negative workplace behaviors, including lateral violence and bullying.

EXERCISE 23-3

Consider a conflict you would describe as "ongoing" in a clinical setting. Talk to some people who have been around for a while to get their historical perspective on this issue. Then consider the following questions:

- What are their positions and years of experience?
- How are resources, time, and personnel wasted on mismanaging this issue?
- What blocks the effective management of this issue?
- What currently aids in its management?
- What new things and actions would add to its management in the future?

CONCLUSION

Conflict occurs in all walks of life. The major issue of conflict in nursing is that patients could suffer. Knowing how to respond appropriately in conflict situations helps leaders, managers, and followers focus on quality and safety rather than disagreements and disruptions.

THE SOLUTION

I replied that his pressure was in the 130s that morning, which meant every medication I had given him was appropriate, based on the parameters in the MAR. The physician probably responded better to her than I did, he said, "I'm not looking to assign any blame to anyone, I am just trying to get a picture of what we are working with here." Her comment stung though and left a lasting impression. I thought in nursing and healthcare we are supposed to be a TEAM. During times of stress, if we spend our time trying to assign blame instead of recruiting each other onto the team, we can shut other people down in a way that is detrimental to the patient. That day was also very reaffirming for me personally that I was going to be leaving that job, as that is not the foundation to grow as a new nurse. Overall, that experience really impacted my attitude as a nurse and made me consider what type of leader, colleague, and person I wanted to be perceived as at work. The positive attitude that the physician took towards my level of abilities as a professional was much more empowering than my own assistant manager. I try to empower and value my colleague's inputs and their skills each day I work, realizing how much power our words and attitudes affect those around us, and overall affect the care delivered to the patient.

—Miranda J. Kennedy

Would this be a suitable approach for you? Why?

THE EVIDENCE

Conflict in the professional practice environment results in negative outcomes for nurses and other healthcare professionals, organizations, and patients. Lateral violence is toxic to the profession through its negative impact on the retention of staff and on detrimental outcomes for patients. It is essential for registered nurses to work in an effective and collaborative manner with other members of the healthcare team to enhance retention and eliminate lateral violence and bullying from the workplace (Wright, 2011). The need for a culture change to abolish lateral violence has been endorsed by a number of professional organizations (e.g., American Nurses' Association, The Joint Commission, International Council of Nurses, National Student Nurses Association). Bullying, lateral violence, and all forms of disruptive behaviors have a negative impact on the retention of nursing staff and the quality and safety of patient care. Nurses must enhance their knowledge and skills in managing conflict and promote workplace policies to eliminate bullying and lateral violence. Nurse leaders and followers must eliminate hostile work environments, workplace intimidation, reality shock for new graduates, and the acceptance of inappropriate professional interactions.

WHAT NEW GRADUATES SAY

- Interprofessional communication simulations were helpful, but I'm still afraid to call a physician in the middle of the night. I have to remember we share a commitment to quality patient care.
- I could have used more practice communicating with older nurses. I am working on disagreeing without coming across as disrespectful.

- It was good to complete the Thomas-Kilmann Conflict Mode Instrument as a student because I am aware of my need to reduce my use of avoidance when a conflict arises on my unit.

CHAPTER CHECKLIST

A more thorough understanding of conflict within the professional practice environment will enable the nurse to prevent or successfully manage nonproductive conflict. Navigating desirable conflict within the work environment will promote change resulting in organizational growth and personal and professional enrichment of nurses.

- Types of conflict
- Stages of conflict
  - Frustration

- Conceptualization
- Action
- Outcomes
- Categories of conflict
- Modes of conflict resolution
  - Avoiding
  - Accommodating
- Competing
- Compromising
- Collaborating
- Differences of conflict-handling styles among nurses
- The role of the leader
- Managing lateral violence and bullying

TIPS FOR ADDRESSING CONFLICT

- Recognize that conflict is a necessary and beneficial process typically marked by frustration, different conceptualizations, a variety of approaches to resolving it, and ongoing outcomes.
- Assess the work environment to see what behaviors are endorsed and fostered by the leaders. Determine if these behaviors are worthy of imitation.
- Determine any similarities and differences in facts, goals, methods, and values in sorting out the different conceptualizations of a conflict situation.
- Assess the degree of conflict resolution by asking questions about the quality of the decisions (e.g., creativity, practicality, achievement of goals,

breakthrough results) and the quality of the relationships (e.g., understanding, willingness to work together, mutual respect, cooperation).
- Remind yourself of your preferences for resolving conflict (e.g., which of the five approaches do you not use often enough and which do you overuse?) and assess each situation to match the best approach for that type of conflict regardless of which is your favorite approach.
- Assist others around you in assessing conflict situations and determining how they can best approach them.

REFERENCES

Aiken, L. H., Sermeus, W., Van den Heede, K., Sloane, D. M., Busse, R., McKee, M., et al. (2012). Patient safety, satisfaction, and quality of hospital care: Cross-sectional surveys of nurses and patients in 12 countries in Europe and the United States. *British Medical Journal, 344,* e1717.

Almost, J. (2006). Conflict within nursing environments: Concept analysis. *Journal of Advanced Nursing, 53*(4), 444–453.

American Nurses Credentialing Center (ANCC). (2012). *Forces of magnetism.* Retrieved October 17, 2013, from. www.nursecredentialing.org/Magnet/ForcesofMagnetism.

Aslakson, R. A., Wyskiel, R., Thornton, I., Copley, C., Shaffer, D., Zyra, M., et al. (2012). Nurse-perceived barriers to effective communication regarding prognosis and optimal end-of-life care for surgical ICU patients: A qualitative exploration. *Journal of Palliative Medicine, 15*(8), 910–915.

Blake, R. R., & Mouton, J. S. (1964). *Solving costly organization conflict.* San Francisco: Jossey-Bass.

Brinkert, R. (2010). A literature review of conflict communication causes, costs, benefits and interventions in nursing. *Journal of Nursing Management, 18,* 145–156.

Brinkert, R. (2011). Conflict coaching training for nurse managers: A case study of a two-hospital health system. *Journal of Nursing Management, 19,* 80–91.

Brown, J., Lewis, L., Ellis, K., Stewart, M., Freeman, T. R., & Kasperski, M. J. (2011). Conflict on interprofessional primary health care

teams—Can it be resolved? *Journal of Interprofessional Care, 25,* 4–10.

Deutsch, M. (1973). *The resolution of conflict: Constructive and destructive processes.* New Haven, CT: Yale University Press.

Dzurec, L. C., & Bromley, G. E. (2012). Speaking of workplace bullying. *Journal of Professional Nursing, 28*(4), 247–254.

Folger, J. P., Poole, M. S., & Stutman, R. K. (2012). *Working through conflict: Strategies for relationships, groups, and organizations* (7th ed.). Boston, MA: Allyn and Bacon.

Hasson, F., McKenna, H. P., & Keeney, S. (2013). Delegating and supervising unregistered professionals: The nursing student experience. *Nurse Education Today, 33*(3), 229–235.

Institute of Healthcare Improvement. (2011). *SBAR technique for communication: A situational briefing model.* Retrieved on June 8, 2013, at. www.ihi.org/knowledge/Pages/Tools/SBARTechniqueforCommunicationASituationalBriefingModel.aspx.

Johansen, M. L. (2012). Keeping the peace: Conflict management strategies for nurse managers. *Nursing Management, 43*(2), 50–54.

Kaiser Permanente & The Coalition of Kaiser Permanente Unions. (2012). *Labor management partnership bargaining 2012.* Retrieved June 8, 2013, from. http://bargaining2012.org/.

Kaitelidou, D., Kontogianni, A., Galanis, P., Siskou, O., Mallidou, A., Pavlakis, A., et al. (2012). Conflict management and job satisfaction in paediatric hospitals in Greece. *Journal of Nursing Management, 20,* 571–576.

Longo, J., & Smith, M. C. (2011). A prescription for disruptions in care: Community building among nurses to address horizontal violence. *Advances in Nursing Science, 34*(4), 345–356.

Lux, K. M., Hutcheson, J. B., & Peden, A. R. (2012). Successful management of disruptive behavior: A descriptive study. *Issues in Mental Health Nursing, 33*(4), 236–243.

Lyndon, A., Zlatnik, M. G., & Wachter, R. M. (2011). Effective physician-nurse communication: A patient safety essential for labor and delivery. *American Journal of Obstetrics and Gynecology, 205*(2), 91–96.

Mahon, M. M., & Nicotera, A. M. (2011). Nursing and conflict communication: Avoidance as preferred strategy. *Nursing Administration Quarterly, 35*(2), 152–163.

McHugh, M. D., Kutney-Lee, A., Cimiotti, J. P., Sloane, D. M., & Aiken, L. H. (2011). Nurses' widespread job dissatisfaction, burnout, and frustration with health benefits signal problems for patient care. *Health Affairs, 30*(2), 202–210.

Nair, D. M., Fitzpatrick, J. J., McNulty, R., Click, E. R., & Glembocki, M. M. (2012). Frequency of nurse-physician collaborative behaviors in an acute care hospital. *Journal of Interprofessional Care, 26*(2), 115–120.

Pines, E. U., Rauschhuber, M. L., Norgan, G. H., Cook, J. D., Canchola, L., Richardson, C., et al. (2011). Stress resiliency, psychological empowerment and conflict management styles among baccalaureate nursing students. *Journal of Advanced Nursing, 68*(7), 1482–1493.

QSEN Institute. (2013). *Competencies.* Retrieved on May 27, 2013, from, www.qsen.org.

Scott, C., & Gerardi, D. 2011a. A strategic approach for managing conflict in hospitals: Responding to joint commission

leadership standard, part 1. *The Joint Commission Journal on Quality and Patient Safety, 37*(2), 59–69.

Scott, C., & Gerardi, D. 2011b. A strategic approach for managing conflict in hospitals: Responding to joint commission leadership standard, part 2. *The Joint Commission Journal on Quality and Patient Safety, 37*(2), 70–80.

The Joint Commission. (2012). *Comprehensive accreditation manual for hospitals (CAMH).* Retrieved June 8, 2013, from, www.jcrinc.com/Joint-Commission-Requirements/Hospitals/.

Thomas, K. W. (1992). Conflict and conflict management: Reflections and update. *Journal of Organizational Behavior, 13*(3), 265–274.

Thomas, K. W., & Kilmann, R. H. (1974). *Thomas-Kilmann conflict mode instrument.* Tuxedo, NY: Xicom.

Thomas, K. W., & Kilmann, R. H. (2002). *Thomas-Kilmann conflict mode instrument.* (revised edition). Mountain View, CA: CPP, Inc.

Tschannen, D., Keenan, G., Aebersold, M., Kocan, M. J., Lundy, F., & Averhart, V. (2011). Implications of nurse-physician relations: Report of a successful intervention. *Nursing Economics, 29*(3), 127–135.

Walrafen, N., Brewer, M. K., & Mulvenon, C. (2012). Sadly caught up in the moment: An exploration of horizontal violence. *Nursing Economic$, 30*(1), 6–12.

Weaver, K. B. (2013). The effects of horizontal violence and bullying on new nurse retention. *Journal of Nurses Professional Development, 29*(3), 138–142.

Wright, K. B. (2011). A communication competence approach to healthcare worker conflict, job stress, job burnout, and job satisfaction. *Journal for Healthcare Quality, 33*(2), 7–14.

SUGGESTED READINGS

Apker, J., Propp, K. M., & Ford, W. S. (2009). Investigating the effect of nurse-team communication on nurse turnover: Relationships among communication processes, identification, and intent to leave. *Health Communications, 24*(2), 106–114.

Arnold, E. C., & Boggs, K. U. (2011). *Interpersonal relationships: Professional communication skills for nurses* (6th ed.). St. Louis: Elsevier.

Beckett, C. D., & Kipnis, G. (2009). Collaborative communication: Integrating SBAR to improve quality/patient safety outcomes. *Journal for Healthcare Quality, 31*(5), 19–28.

Center for American Nurses. (2008). *Lateral violence and bullying in the workplace.* Silver Spring, MD: Author.

Cronenwett, L., Sherwood, G., Barnsteiner, J., Disch, J., Johnson, J., Mitchell, P., et al. (2007). Quality and safety education for nurses. *Nursing Outlook, 55*(3), 122–131.

Fassier, T., & Azoulay, E. (2010). Conflicts and communication gaps in the intensive care unit. *Current Opinion in Critical Care, 16,* 654–665.

Laschinger, H., Finegan, J., & Wilk, P. (2009). New graduate burnout: The impact of professional practice environment, workplace, and empowerment. *Nursing Economic$, 27*(6), 377–383.

Leever, A. M., Hulst, M. V. D., Berendsen, A. J., Boendemaker, P. M., Roodenburg, J. L. N., & Pols, J. (2010). Conflicts and conflict

management in the collaboration between nurses and physicians: A qualitative study. *Journal of Interprofessional Care, 24*(6), 612–624.

Lindy, C., & Schaefer, F. (2010). Negative workplace behaviours: An ethical dilemma for nurse managers. *Journal of Nursing Management, 18,* 285–292.

Runde, C. E., & Flanagan, T. A. (2008). *Building conflict competent teams.* San Francisco, CA: Jossey-Bass.

The Joint Commission. (2008). *Behaviors that undermine a culture of safety.* Retrieved March 17, 2013, from, www.jointcommission.org/assets/1/18/SEA_40.PDF.

The Joint Commission. (2009). *Leadership committed to safety.* Retrieved March 17, 2013, from, www.jointcommission.org/sentinel_event_alert_issue_43_leadership_committed_to_safety/.

Thomas, S., & Burk, R. (2009). Junior nursing students' experiences of vertical violence during clinical rotations. *Nursing Outlook, 57*(4), 226–231.

Vessey, J. A., DeMarco, R. F., Gaffney, D. A., & Budin, W. C. (2009). Bullying of staff registered nurses in the workplace: A preliminary study for developing strategies for the transformation of hostile to healthy workplace environments. *Journal of Professional Nursing, 25*(5), 299–306.

INTERNET RESOURCES

American Nurses Association. www.nursingworld.org/Mobile/ Nursing-Factsheets/lateral-violence-and-bullying-in-nursing. html.

Association for Conflict Resolution. http://acrnet.org.

Center for Conflict Resolution. www.conflict-resolution.org/.

Healthcare Conflict Management. *Solutions to help you manage conflict to protect the quality and safety of care.* www.healthcare-conflict-management.com/.

Managing Personal/Personnel Problems

Karren Kowalski

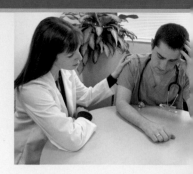

The purpose of this chapter is to discuss various personal and personnel problems that a leader must face in all nursing settings. Some specific tips and tools are provided as ways to intervene, coach, correct, and document problem behaviors. Emphasis is placed on effective communication, both written and verbal.

LEARNING OUTCOMES

- Differentiate common personal/personnel problems.
- Relate role concepts to clarification of personnel problems.
- Examine strategies useful for approaching specific personnel problems.
- Prepare specific guidelines for documenting performance problems.
- Value the leadership aspects of the role of the novice nurse.

KEY TERMS

absenteeism	nonpunitive discipline	role strain
chemically dependent	progressive discipline	role stress

THE CHALLENGE

Kathleen Bradley, RN, MSN, NE-BC
Director of Professional Resources, Porter Adventist Hospital,
Denver, Colorado

I work in a hospital that uses a float pool of well-prepared staff who are ready to be assigned to various areas so that the appropriate level of care can be provided. As you might expect, these nurses, especially when new to the hospital, are not always familiar with all of

the aspects of every unit. One of the nurses employed at the hospital in the resource float pool was floated one day to the surgical unit. During her shift, she cared for a patient, who, while unattended, fell out of bed. The nurse manager of the float pool was asked to determine what happened.

What do you think you would do if you were this nurse?

INTRODUCTION

As a novice nurse, the question may be one of perception. "As a new direct care nurse, I don't think of myself as a leader, so how is this information applicable?" In reality, even nurses with limited experiences (referred to here as *novice*) are responsible for and thus lead assistive and support personnel. They often lead a team consisting of licensed practical/vocational nurses (LPNs/LVNs) and nursing assistants who are responsible for a group of patients. They are responsible for including other team members such as housekeeping personnel and allied health professionals (e.g., respiratory therapists, pharmacists, dietitians, and physical therapists) in providing excellent quality care for patients. The novice nurse must know how to handle difficult situations, including the decision to involve the unit leadership. It can be quite satisfying to work effectively with people. On the other hand, working with people presents some of the greatest challenges in the workplace. Problems such as absenteeism, uncooperative or unproductive employees, clinical incompetence, employees with emotional problems, and chemically dependent employees are only a few. If a nurse or a new leader wants to be successful, these problems must be dealt with in ways to minimize their effects on patient care and on staff morale. Just as documentation of patient care is critical, documentation of performance problems is critical. Overall goals are to assist the employee in the improvement of performance, to maintain the highest standards for the delivery of patient care, and to provide a supportive environment in which all staff members deliver the best care and attain work satisfaction. From this perspective, in this chapter we examine several specific employee prob-

lems and address the leader's role and options as well as the responsibilities of the novice nurse.

PERSONAL/PERSONNEL PROBLEMS

Absenteeism

One of the most vexing personnel problems is that of absenteeism (Black, 2012; Dellve, Hadzibajramovic, & Ahlborg, 2011; Gorman, Yu, & Alamgir, 2010). Inadequate staffing adversely affects patient care both directly and indirectly. When an absent caregiver is replaced by another who is unfamiliar with the routines, employee morale suffers and care may not meet established standards. Working with inadequate staffing or working overtime to cover for absent workers creates physical and mental stress. Replacement personnel usually need more supervision, which not only is costly but also may decrease productivity and the quality of patient care. Indirectly, co-workers may become resentful about being forced to assume heavier workloads and/or may be pressured to work extra hours. Chronic absenteeism may lead to increased staff conflicts, to decreased morale, and eventually to increased absenteeism among the entire staff. Given that nurses prefer to avoid conflict and negative behavior and to accommodate or make excuses for these situations (Sportsman, 2005), one way to confront persistent absenteeism is to discuss the situation directly with the employee (also see Chapter 18) by verbalizing:

- "I feel concerned when I see that you have been absent 3 days this month."
- "Can you see how excessive absences affect the smooth functioning of the unit, the workload of other team members, and the safety of patients?"
- "This rate of absences cannot continue. What is your plan for addressing this situation?"

Absenteeism also has a deleterious effect on the financial management of a nursing unit. Replacement of absent personnel by temporary personnel or overtime paid to other employees is very costly, and the cost of fringe benefits used by absent workers is very high. When employee costs are excessive, they compromise the ability to support other creative efforts of the unit such as staff education and new equipment and may affect staff-patient ratios. Also, as care delivery systems become more complex and technically oriented, successful nurse leaders realize that technology is not a replacement for human caregivers. Absent caregivers cannot be replaced with machines.

Absenteeism cannot be totally eliminated. Unplanned illnesses, accidents, bad weather, sick family members, a death in the family, and even jury duty, which are legitimate reasons for missing work and beyond the control of management, will always occur. However, some portion of absenteeism is voluntary and preventable; thus the cause must be identified so that it may be addressed. Issues leading to absenteeism including personal situations such as sick dependent family members, poor health, job stress, or high work demands such as long hours, excessive workload, lack of control over work, and poor support from managers have been identified (Hilton, Scuffham, Vecchio, & Whiteford, 2010; Wallace, 2009). These stressors lead to a poor work environment and lower the morale of fully engaged nurses.

Absenteeism may also indicate poor work satisfaction. Dissatisfied staff may in fact be completely disengaged, which can lead to increased absences. If the leader believes that the issue is attributable to work dissatisfaction, unit-based discussions may lead to insight about the sources. Such discussions provide an excellent opportunity for the novice nurse to listen, to learn, and to speak to issues. If the underlying cause can be identified, it may be possible to prevent the loss of the dissatisfied employee if retention is the goal. Some employees who convey that they are never happy with their jobs may continually disrupt the overall unit with their absenteeism and should be terminated. The Evidence section on p. 461 illustrates some of those factors to consider.

With role theory as a framework, absenteeism has been linked to role stress and role strain. Absence from work is a way of withdrawing from an undesirable situation short of actually leaving, and many employees increase their absenteeism just before submitting their resignation. If the healthcare worker is experiencing some form of role stress, it might be manifested through absenteeism. Role strain may be reflected by (1) withdrawal from interaction, (2) reduced involvement with colleagues and the organization, (3) decreased commitment to the mission and the team, and (4) job dissatisfaction. All of these could be manifested through absenteeism. With this framework, management of absenteeism is based on the belief that competent role performance requires interpersonal competence. Role competence is demonstrated through the ability of a person to act in a way that honors both the tasks and the interpersonal relationships. Role behavior occurs in a social context rather than in isolation. Therefore the nurse leader needs to understand the existing situation, when the situation changed to its current status, when it needs to change further, and how to accomplish such change. Because people who are more satisfied in their work usually commit to "be there" for their team, enhancing job satisfaction may be an effective strategy toward reducing absenteeism.

One model for nonpunitive discipline can be found in Figure 24-1. This model demonstrates how undesirable behaviors, such as absenteeism, can be successfully altered. Box 24-1 identifies specific steps that are involved in nonpunitive discipline.

This model of nonpunitive discipline allows employees to free themselves from some role stress by clarification of role expectations and assumptions (SESCO Management Consultants, 2013). Employees can receive satisfaction from the realization that a problem may not be inadequate performance caused by personal faults but, rather, a lack of clarification of role expectations within the organization. Novice nurses may be called on to implement the process described in Box 24-1. For example, the novice nurse may be involved with the nurse manager or a support staff member or, in extenuating circumstances, the new nurse may be directly involved in the process. Remember, the focus is on the clear understanding of the situation, the growth of the individual, and the smooth and effective functioning of the team.

EXERCISE 24-1

Review the policy manual at a local healthcare organization. Determine what constitutes excessive absenteeism. What are the identified consequences?

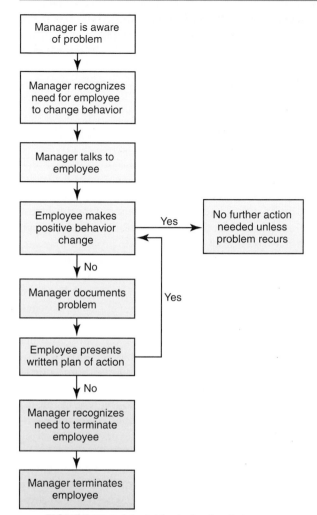

FIGURE 24-1 Model for behavioral change.

BOX 24-1 STEPS TO CLARIFY ROLE EXPECTATIONS

Step 1: Remind the employee of the employment policies and procedures of the agency. Sometimes an employee does not know or has forgotten the existing standards, and a reminder with no threats or discipline is all that is needed. The employee must remain ultimately accountable to the organization's policies and procedures.

Step 2: When the oral reminder does not result in a behavior change, put the reminder in writing for the employee. These oral and written reminders are simply statements of the problem and the goals to which both the manager and the employee agree. The employee must voluntarily agree with the manager that the behavior in question is not acceptable and must agree to change.

Step 3: If the written reminder fails, only then grant the employee a day of decision, which is a day off with pay to arrive at a decision about future action. Pay is given for this day so that it is not interpreted as punishment. The employee must return to work with a written decision as to whether or not to accept the standards for work attendance. Remember that this is a voluntary decision on the employee's part. Emphasize to the employee that it is the employee's decision to adhere to the standards.

Step 4: If the employee decides not to adhere to standards, termination results. However, if the employee agrees to adhere to the standards and in the future does not, he or she, in essence, has terminated employment. Keep a copy of the written agreements, and give the employee a copy. The manager should be clearly aware of the organization's policy for termination and request assistance from the human resources department as deemed necessary.

Uncooperative or Unproductive Employees

The problem of uncooperative or unproductive employees is another area of frustration for the nurse leader. Hersey, Blanchard, and Johnson (2008) identified two major dimensions of job performance that relate to this problem: motivation and ability. The type and intensity of motivation vary among employees because of differing needs and goals that employees express. The leader can best handle employees with motivation problems by attempting to determine the cause of the problem and by working to provide an environment that is conducive to increased motivation for the employee. If the employee is uncooperative or unproductive because of a lack of ability, education and training are appropriate interventions.

The manager can determine lack of ability on the part of an employee in various ways. Frequent errors in judgment or techniques are often an indication of lack of knowledge, skill, or critical thinking. This illustrates the need for the nurse leader to document all variances or untoward events carefully after discussing them with the employee. When the nurse manager has thorough documentation, trends may be discovered that, in turn, suggest that a specific employee is having problems. The nurse manager can cite problem behaviors and perhaps even trends to the employee. Corrective action is easier to pursue and resolution is more effective with this strategy. When the problem is determined to result from a need for more education or training, the manager can work with the education department or the clinical specialist for the involved unit to help the employee improve his or her skills. Most employees are extremely cooperative in situations such as this because they want to do a good job but sometimes do not know how. Employees may deny they need help or may be too embarrassed to ask for help. When the manager can show an employee concrete evidence of a problem area, cooperation is enhanced.

Immature Employees

Sometimes an unproductive employee simply lacks maturity. This lack of maturity may be described as *emotional intelligence underdevelopment* that results in such problems as being socially inept or unable to control one's impulses (Goleman, 2011). These employees are frequently defensive and emotional or tearful. They lack self-insight into their behavior. Sometimes immaturity in an employee may not be readily apparent to the leader but may be manifested in any of the following actions: defiance, testing of workplace guidelines, passivity or hostility, or little appreciation for any management decisions. The challenge for the nurse leader is not to react in kind but, rather, to relate to this employee in a positive and mature manner. A sense of humor and the ability to ease the employee into a more receptive mood are sometimes helpful. However, the leader needs to determine whether the undesirable behaviors are reflecting a state of being uncomfortable or incompetent. For example, if an employee states, "Administration is always making decisions to make our jobs harder," rather than making a hostile or defensive comment in reply, the manager could take the employee aside and say, "I notice that you seem to be angry about this new policy. Let's talk about it some more." Immature employees either act immaturely all of the time or regress to an immature level when stressed. The nurse leader must recognize immaturity in an employee and react calmly and without anger. The leader must keep in mind that this employee may be displaying dynamics rooted in unresolved personal areas and that the behavior is not a personal attack on the leader. The best way to deal with this behavior is to confront the employee with the specific problem and define realistic limits of acceptable behavior with consequences for nonadherence. Generally, employees comply with specific limits but will test management in other areas. As this testing occurs, the leader must continue the same limit-setting technique. Remember that the immature employee usually has problems because of a lack of self-worth, power, and self-control. Praise

and affirmation are valuable tools that the leader can use to help these employees feel better about themselves. Chapter 3 addresses generational issues if they are factors to consider.

EXERCISE 24-2

A nurse comes to you, the nurse leader, and states that one of the other nurses is tying a knot in the air vent (pigtail) of nasogastric tubes. This nurse does not know how to approach the employee to discuss the problem. What would you do?

Clinical Incompetence

Clinical incompetence is possibly one of the most frustrating problems that the nurse leader faces, although it may be entirely correctable. The problem may surface immediately in a new employee. It is possible that despite an effective interview process, a lack of fit exists between the new nurse's strengths or skill set and the needs of the unit. Such a nurse can be coached and supported to find a different position, one that fully utilizes his or her strengths and skills. At other times, clinical incompetence comes as a surprise if coworkers "cover" for another employee. Some nurses are unwilling to report instances of clinical incompetence because they do not want to feel responsible for getting one of their peers in trouble. When other employees are engaged in enabling behavior by covering for the mistakes of one of their peers, the nurse leader may be surprised to discover that the employee does not know or cannot do what is expected of him or her. Sadly, the employee in question has been able to cover incompetence by hiding behind the performance of another employee. The nurse leader must remind employees that part of professional responsibility is to maintain quality care and thus they are obligated to report instances of clinical incompetence, even when it means reporting a co-worker. Ignoring violations of a safety rule or poor practice is unprofessional and cannot be tolerated.

Most healthcare agencies use skills checklists or a competency evaluation program to ascertain that their employees have and maintain essential skills for the job they are expected to do. A skills checklist is one way to determine basic clinical competency (Table 24-1). This checklist typically contains a number of basic skills along with ones that are essential for safe functioning in the specific area of employment (Hamstrom, Kankkunen, Suominen, & Ritta, 2012).

TABLE 24-1 EXAMPLE OF A SKILLS CHECKLIST

Purpose

1. The clinical skills inventory is a three-phase tool to enable the newly hired RN and the nurse manager to determine individual learning needs, verify competency, and plan performance goals.
2. The RN will complete the self-assessment of clinical skills during the first week of employment. The RN will use the appropriate scale to document current knowledge of clinical skills.
3. The nurse manager will document observed competency of the orientee or delegate this to a peer. All columns must be completed on the inventory level.
4. At the end of orientation, the new RN and the manager will use the inventory to identify performance goals on the plan sheet. The skills inventory will be in a specified place on the

nursing unit so that it is available to the manager and other RNs. It should be updated at appropriate intervals as specified by the manager.

Scale for Self-Assessment

1 = Unfamiliar/never done
2 = Able to perform with assistance
3 = Can perform with minimal supervision
4 = Independent performance/proficient

Score for Validation of Competency

1 = Unable to perform at present
2 = Able to perform with assistance
3 = Progressing/repeat performance necessary
4 = Able to perform independently

CLINICAL SKILLS (EXAMPLES)	SELF-ASSESSMENT		COMMENT	VALIDATION			COMMENT
	SCALE	DATE		SCORE	DATE	INITIALS	
Epidural catheter care							
NG/Dobbhoff							
Insertion							
Management							
Preoperative care/ teaching							
Postoperative care/ teaching							

Plan Sheet for Skills Inventory

Name _____
Date _____

Goals	Date to Be Completed

_____
_____
_____
_____
_____
_____
_____

Orientee's signature _____
Manager's signature _____
Date _____

Any type of skills review should be directly linked to quality-improvement indicators. The employee may be asked to do a self-assessment of the listed skills or competencies and then have performance of the skills validated by a peer or co-worker. This is a very effective method for the leader to assess the skill level of employees and to determine where additional education and training may be necessary. In addition, if the leader discovers that an employee cannot perform a skill adequately, the skills list can easily be checked and directly observed behaviors can be assessed to determine at what level the employee is functioning. At the completion of the assessment, a specific plan for remediation can be developed. Sometimes, an employee may be able to perform all of the tasks on a skills checklist but still cannot manage overall patient care effectively. If, in questioning the employee or in evaluating the employee's performance, the manager/leader determines a lack of knowledge or problems with time management, formal education may be the proper course of action. In either event, the leader must establish a written contract containing a plan of action that sets time limits within which certain expectations must be achieved. This ensures compliance on the part of the employee. A more comprehensive program for competency evaluation might include not only the skills checklist but also unit-specific objectives, an overall framework for evaluation, and critical-thinking exercises that are interactive in nature (Johnson, Opfer, VanCura, & Williams, 2000). The role of the novice nurse leader, particularly with ancillary personnel, is to support the nurse manager as well as be helpful and supportive of the team members who are striving to improve.

Emotional Problems

Emotional problems among nursing personnel may affect not only the involved individual but also co-workers and ultimately the delivery of patient care. The nurse leader must be aware that certain behaviors, such as poor judgment, increased errors, increased absenteeism, decreased productivity, and a negative attitude, may be manifestations of emotional problems in employees.

A nurse manager began hearing complaints from patients about a nurse named Nancy. Patients were saying that Nancy was abrupt and uncaring with them. The manager had not received any complaints about Nancy before this time, so she questioned Nancy about why this was occurring. Nancy reported that her mother was very ill and she was so worried about her and so upset that she could not sleep and was tired all of the time. She went on to say that she was having trouble being sympathetic with complaining patients when they did not seem to be as sick as her mother.

When an employee's behavior changes significantly, personal problems with which the person cannot cope may be the cause. The nurse leader is not and should not be a therapist but must intercede, not only to help the individual with the problems but also to maintain proper functioning of the unit. In dealing with the employee who exhibits behaviors that indicate emotional problems, the manager assists the individual to obtain professional help to cope with the problem. The individual's work setting and schedule may need to be adjusted. This may require support from other staff members so no negative patient care results. The manager acknowledges that an employee is experiencing emotional difficulties and yet the standards of patient care cannot be compromised. Staff are reassured to witness the care and concern shown a fellow staff member who is in great difficulty. They can interpret that similar support would be given to them if they were in a difficult situation.

The most important approach that the manager can take with an emotionally troubled employee is to provide support and encouragement and to assist the individual to obtain appropriate help (Hilton et al., 2010). Many agencies have some kind of employee assistance program (EAP) to which the manager should refer any troubled employee. (The Literature Perspective on p. 457 describes a counseling service and how it helps retain nurses.) During this process, the manager must remember to check with the human resources department about any implications that may occur because of the Americans with Disabilities Act (ADA). If an employee has a documented mental illness, the employing agency may be under certain legal constraints as specified in the ADA. The nurse manager should always remember that many resources are available to assist with personnel problems. The manager should never feel required to know all of the legal implications regarding employment policies. Rather, the manager must know that help is available and how to access it.

LITERATURE PERSPECTIVE

Resource: Luquette, J.S. (2005). The role of on-site counseling in nurse retention. *Oncology Nursing Forum, 32,* 234-236.

This article describes various aspects of an on-site counseling service and how it demonstrates value to nurses. The key cornerstone beliefs of the service are confidentiality, minimal financial cost, professionalism of the provider, and convenient appointment times and office locations. Services can be both group and individually based. To be effective, the services must be available when nurses work and also be available by phone. The offices need to be in less trafficked areas to help maintain confidentiality. Numerous professional and personal issues are cited. In addition, the service should include crisis intervention and services devoted to team-building.

Implications for Practice

The availability of on-site counseling during any work schedule helps charge nurses and nurse managers refer individuals for help and allows individual nurses to seek the support they may need during challenging times.

EXERCISE 24-3

As a nurse manager in a community health agency, you have just had a meeting that was called by several of your direct care nurses. They expressed concern regarding another nurse colleague who has come to work tearful several times during the past week. They state she often goes into the break room when she is in the agency and appears as if she has been crying when she comes out. She has refused to discuss her distress with her colleagues. These nurses express concern and want you to help her. What is your response? What would you do?

Chemical Dependency

Chemical dependency among nursing personnel places patients and the organization at risk. Such an employee adversely affects staff morale by increasing stress on other staff members when they have to assume heavier workloads to cover for the chemically dependent employee who is not performing at full capacity or who is often absent. As a result, patient care may be jeopardized because staff is focusing more on the problems of a co-worker than on those of the patients. For the novice nurse, it is critical to be aware of the professional responsibilities of reporting incidents in which peers or team members exhibit signs of chemical dependency.

The manager is responsible for early recognition of chemical dependency and referral for treatment when appropriate (National Council of State Boards of Nursing, 2011). State laws vary as to the reportability of chemical dependency. As is true of all nurses, a nurse manager is responsible for upholding the nurse practice act and should be familiar with the legal aspects of chemical dependency in the state in which he or she is employed. As with the employee with emotional problems, the nurse manager should be aware of ADA issues and check with the human resource department for help with how to handle the employment of a chemically dependent employee. Most states and agencies have reporting requirements regarding substance abuse. The state board of nursing is a key place to determine specific details required by a given state. All nurse managers should familiarize themselves with the nurse practice act in the state in which they are employed and with the personnel policies relating to substance abuse in their employing agency. Furthermore, nurse managers should ensure that staff are familiar with legal requirements.

In the present social climate, more interest exists in helping affected individuals than in punishing them; showing empathy and understanding also facilitates their work. Identification of an employee with a chemical dependency is usually difficult, especially because one of the primary symptoms is denial. The primary clue to which a manager should be alert when chemical dependency is suspected is any behavioral change in an employee. This change could be any deviation from the behaviors the employee normally exhibits. Some specific behaviors to note might be mood swings, a change from a tidy appearance to an untidy one, an unusual interest in patients' pain control, frequent changes in jobs and shifts, or an increase in absenteeism and tardiness.

When a manager suspects that an employee may be chemically dependent, the manager must intervene because patient care may be jeopardized. A manager facing a problem with an impaired nurse must be compassionate yet therapeutic. Knowing that denial may be one of the primary signs of substance abuse, the manager must focus on performance problems that the nurse is exhibiting and urge the nurse to seek counseling or treatment voluntarily. EAPs always protect the employee's privacy and are usually available free or at a minimal charge to the employee. The manager should strive to refer any troubled employee to the EAP. This removes the manager from the counseling role and helps employees get the professional help they need without fear of a breach in confidentiality. If a nurse refuses to seek help voluntarily for a substance abuse problem, the manager is responsible for following the established policy for such employees. The manager must remember that if the substance-abusing employee is terminated and not reported to the State Board of Nursing, the manager not only may be violating a law but also may be enabling this employee to obtain employment in another agency and potentially be in a position to harm patients and co-workers.

Many states have rehabilitation programs for chemically impaired nurses so that they may return to nursing if rehabilitated. Nurse managers are sometimes asked to assist with monitoring the progress of a chemically impaired nurse. Specific guidelines are established through the rehabilitation program with the cooperation of the employee, the agency, and the manager. The manager is typically asked to provide feedback about the employee's progress to the employee and to the state or rehabilitation program involved. These programs vary, but, for example, a nurse who has been an admitted abuser of meperidine may be allowed to work in a setting in which this drug is never used, or the nurse may not be permitted to administer any controlled substances to patients. This, of course, puts an added burden on other staff members, but it can be a positive experience for all because nurses face some of their professional responsibility by helping another nurse while upholding patient care. Often, as a part of their therapy, these nurses are required to share openly with other staff members what their problem is and what they are doing to control it. When handled in a positive, professional way, the nurse manager can turn a potentially destructive situation into a positive, constructive one.

Regardless of the type of personnel issue, the manager needs to have a plan in place for ongoing monitoring and follow-up of issues/problems.

EXERCISE 24-4

Review your state's nurse practice act and rules and regulations. What are you required to do if you believe a nurse has a problem with chemical dependency?

Incivility

Incivility or lateral violence in the workplace is disruptive behavior or communication that creates a negative work environment, thus interfering with quality patient care and safety (Chipps & McRury, 2012). Such behavior is often nurse to nurse or provider to provider. These behaviors include nonverbal innuendo such as eye-rolling or eyebrow raising, verbal affronts, undermining activities, withholding information, sabotage, infighting, scapegoating, backstabbing, failure to respect privacy, and broken confidences (Hickson, 2013; Lewis & Malecha, 2011) (see the Literature Perspective below). Uncivil behavior must be addressed. The first step by the manager when he or she has observed the unwanted behavior may be a discussion with the nurse; the next step is written documentation in the personnel file if the behaviors do not abate. This is followed by a stepwise disciplinary action in association with the human resources department (Clark, Farnsworth, & Springer, 2008). It is important for the new nurse to be cognizant and aware of behaviors of incivility and to understand the guidelines/rules relevant to such behavior in the facility. Also, it is important for the new nurse to support increased teamwork by behaving in a positive, upbeat manner and to not become enmeshed in negative behavior on the unit.

 LITERATURE PERSPECTIVE

Resource: Hickson, J. (2013). New nurses' perceptions of hostility and job satisfaction. *The Journal of Nursing Administration, 43*(5), 293-301.

This article investigated the perceptions of new graduate nurses regarding nurse-to-nurse hostility and job satisfaction for both Magnet™ and non-Magnet™ settings. The new RNs completed an online survey, which indicated that nurses in the Magnet™ and non-Magnet™ facilities all experienced hostility and similar job satisfaction results. Nurse hostility affected job satisfaction as related to autonomy; interpersonal communication and collaboration; status and recognition; task requirements, including professional practice; opportunity for advancement; and the environment, such as pay and fairness.

Implications for Practice

Based on these findings, nursing leadership needs to focus on orientation and residency programs for transition into practice, adequately prepared preceptors, and zero tolerance for uncivil behavior within the nursing culture.

DOCUMENTATION

Documentation of personnel problems is unquestionably one of the most important but also one of the most onerous aspects of the nurse manager's job. As much as some managers may wish they would, personnel problems probably will not "disappear" and therefore will eventually have to be resolved. Through careful, ongoing documentation of problems, the manager makes the task of identifying and correcting problems much less burdensome.

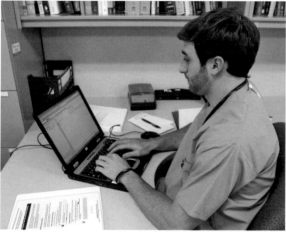

Documentation of personnel problems is an important aspect of the nurse manager's job.

Documentation cannot be left to memory! At the time that an employee is involved in a problem situation or receives a compliment or does something extremely well, a brief notation to this effect must be placed in the personnel file. This entry includes the date, time, and a brief description of the incident. Adding a small notation as to what was done about a problem when it occurred is also helpful. Along with this, the nurse manager should keep a log or summary sheet of all reported errors, unusual incidents, and accidents. These extremely important data should include the date, time, and names of involved individuals and should be tallied monthly for analysis by the manager. The few extra minutes each day that the manager spends tracking these data provide invaluable information to him or her about organizational and individual functioning. This tracking can then be used to pinpoint an individual's problem areas, areas of excellence in individual performance, and overall organizational problem areas. The manager who keeps careful records about organizational functioning has greater control in the management of personal and personnel problems. Box 24-2 describes content and format for such documentation and provides an example as an illustration.

BOX 24-2   DOCUMENTATION OF PROBLEMS

- Description of incident—an objective statement of the facts related to the incident
- Actions—statements describing the plan to correct and/or prevent future problems
- Follow-up—dates and times that the plan is to be carried out, including required meeting with the employee

Example

Several patients reported that Becky, one of the night-shift registered nurses, was "curt" and "gruff" and seemed uncaring with them. I called Becky into my office and reiterated the complaints that I had received, including the specifics of times and incidents. I reminded Becky about what my expectations were relating to patient care, emphasizing the importance of a caring attitude with all patients. We discussed what the possible cause of Becky's behavior might be, such as problems at home or lack of sleep. Becky denied being curt or gruff but agreed that some of her mannerisms might be misinterpreted. I suggested to Becky that perhaps she needed to be particularly aware of her body language and to soften her tone of voice. After discussing this incident and reminding Becky of the importance of caring in nursing, I cited the policy regarding behavior and told Becky that this behavior would not be tolerated. I told Becky we needed to meet every Friday morning at the end of Becky's shift to discuss how the week had gone and to determine how she was interacting with the patients assigned to her. I also told Becky I would be checking with patients to see what they had thought of Becky, pointing out that I do this routinely.

These weekly meetings are to be conducted for 6 weeks, followed by monthly meetings for a 3-month period. If problems do not recur, the meetings will be discontinued after this time.

Joseph P. Riley, RN, MSN
Nurse Manager, Hanson Way Hospital

PROGRESSIVE DISCIPLINE

When an employee's performance falls below the acceptable standard despite corrective measures that have been taken, some form of discipline must be enacted. Most organizations use some form of **progressive discipline** to correct problem behaviors.

BOX 24-3   STEPS IN PROGRESSIVE DISCIPLINE

1. Counsel the employee regarding the problem.
2. Reprimand the employee. A verbal reprimand usually precedes a written one, but some organizations issue both a verbal and a written reprimand simultaneously. When the documentation is written, the employee must sign to verify that the problem was discussed. This does not mean that the employee agrees with the reprimand. It means only that he or she is aware of a written reprimand that is to be placed in the employee's personnel file. The employee always receives a copy of a written reprimand.
3. Suspend the employee if the problem persists. He or she will be suspended without pay for a specified period, usually several days or longer according to the agency policy. During this time, the employee may realize the seriousness of the problem based on the resulting discipline.
4. Allow the employee to return to work with written stipulations regarding problem behavior.
5. Terminate the employee if the problem recurs.

When the nurse leader suspects that specific behaviors may lead to progressive discipline, it is critical that all interactions be documented and that the human resources department is involved in the process to ensure accurate adherence to all policies. Progressive discipline consists of evaluating performance and providing feedback within a specified structure of increasing sanctions. These sanctions, progressing from least severe to most severe, are described in Box 24-3. Examples of the kind of workplace behavior that usually involves progressive discipline and could even result in immediate termination are harassment and chemical abuse.

TERMINATION

At times, even though the manager has done everything possible to gain the cooperation of a problem employee, the problems may persist. In such cases, termination is the only choice. Because termination is one of the most difficult things a manager does, the following guidelines should be followed:

1. The manager must be confident that everything possible has been done to help the employee correct the problem behaviors.
2. The manager must recognize that if employment continues, this employee will have a deleterious

effect on overall organizational functioning and, more important, on nursing care.
3. The employee must have been made fully aware of the problem performance and of the fact that all of the correct disciplinary steps have been followed.
4. The nurse manager should check with the human resources and legal departments before proceeding to ensure that termination is justifiable legally and that proper steps have been followed.

The nurse manager needs to be confident in the knowledge that all policies regarding termination have been followed before having an actual termination meeting with the employee. It is always preferable to err on the side of caution when proceeding with termination of an employee. Remember that termination is something that the employee has caused as a result of persistent problem behaviors or certain behaviors for which the organization has zero tolerance. Termination is not done at the whim of management; it results from failure on the part of the employee to change a problem behavior.

Situations that may warrant immediate dismissal include theft, violence in the workplace, and willful abuse of the patient, to name a few. Again, the manager should use the assistance of the human resource department to ensure that all of the organization's policies are being upheld correctly. The following example illustrates that a manager needs to anticipate a termination to ensure ongoing standards:

Linda has gone through all of the steps in the progressive discipline process as a result of her abusive behavior toward her co-workers. She returned to work and seemed to be doing well until about 6 weeks later, when she slammed down her clipboard during report and angrily accused the charge nurse of always giving her the worst assignments. The nurse manager was present and asked Linda to come into her office. At this point, she told Linda she was relieving her of her assignment that day and asked her to go home to cool off. The manager told her that she would call her the following day about what would be done. Linda went home, and the manager reviewed the incident with her nurse administrator. They both agreed that Linda's behavior not only was intolerable but also violated the terms of her probation and therefore she should be terminated. The manager called Linda the following day as she had agreed to do and asked her to come and meet with her.

The manager and administrator met with Linda and reviewed the incidents and the disciplinary measures leading up to this incident. The nurse manager asked the administrator to be present at the scheduled meeting because it is a good practice to have a witness in a confrontational situation such as termination. The manager stated to Linda that she regretted it had come to this but pointed out to her that her behavior had violated all of the agreed-upon stipulations and, as a result, she would be terminated immediately. Linda was tearful and had numerous excuses, but the manager remained firm and merely repeated that Linda, in not fulfilling the agreement, had chosen to end her employment.

> **EXERCISE 24-5**
> Review a healthcare organization's policies regarding termination. What are the conditions, such as stealing or violence, that are described as cause for immediate dismissal? Is abusing substances at work one of those conditions?

CONCLUSION

All employees share a role with managers to prevent and control personal/personnel problems in their work setting. Everyone must be willing to refuse to allow unethical behavior from co-workers and to speak out and act appropriately when problems occur.

THE SOLUTION

The nurse manager in charge of the resource float pool wanted to assess the float pool nurses' critical-thinking skills and did this through weekly rounding. The charge nurses of each unit also completed a peer assessment form whenever a nurse floated to the unit so that the nurse who floated there could receive feedback. In this manner, if a pattern emerged from either the rounding assessment or the peer reviews, the float nurse could receive immediate coaching. Finally, the nurse manager decided to have the staff review published information about hourly rounding and review the patient fall protocols from the various units where the float nurse worked.

—*Kathleen Bradley*

Would this be a suitable approach for you? Why?

THE EVIDENCE

Davey, Cummings, Newburn-Cook, and Lo (2009) sought to identify predictors of short-term absenteeism in direct care nurses. Such absenteeism contributes to lack of continuity in patient care and decreases staff morale, which is costly to the facility. A systematic review of studies conducted between 1986 and 2006 led to the inclusion of 16 peer-reviewed research studies. Findings were that the individual "nurse's history of prior absences," "work attitudes" (e.g., job satisfaction, organizational commitment, and work involvement), and other "retention factors" such as shared governance reduced absenteeism, whereas poor leadership, "burnout," and "job stress" increased absenteeism. It became clear that the reasons underlying absenteeism are still poorly understood and that a robust theory for nurse absenteeism is lacking. Further theory development and research are needed.

Major, Abderrahman, and Sweeney (2013) have constructed guidelines for new graduates to assist them in having difficult conversations in conflict situations. These new nurses are encouraged to "start with heart," which translates into encouraging a free flow of conversation. "Learn to look" means to be conscious of when a conversation needs to occur, whereas "make it safe" means to be respectful and to value the other person's perspective. "Master your story" translates as being clear about your feelings and why they were evoked. "State your path" indicates that while sharing your perspective, ask the other nurses how they reached their perspectives. "Explore other's paths" requires asking questions to better understand the other nurses. "Move to action" means the nurses together will decide how the issue being discussed will be resolved.

It is most helpful if the new nurse can address issues before the situation becomes a confrontational issue that can escalate into aggressive, undesirable behavior.

WHAT NEW GRADUATES SAY

- I really thought "real" people (not students) would not have so many personal problems. I was shocked!
- My nurse manager terminated one of the staff within the first month I worked on my unit. This nurse called in or was late at least five times that month. I might not have noticed but I was paired with her. Every absence made the charge nurse change many assignments. It was so stressful.

CHAPTER CHECKLIST

To obtain satisfaction from working with people, a nurse manager must be knowledgeable about personal and personnel issues that are likely to occur in the work setting. The nurse manager must be able to detect, prevent, and correct problems that affect nursing care and staff morale in a nursing agency. Proper documentation and follow-up are key elements in the successful management of all personnel issues.

- Personal/personnel problems
  - Absenteeism
- Uncooperative or unproductive employees
- Immature employees
- Clinical incompetence
- Emotional problems
- Chemical dependency
- Incivility
- Documentation
- Progressive discipline
- Termination

TIPS IN THE DOCUMENTATION OF PROBLEMS

- Identify the incident and related facts.
- Describe actions taken by the manager when the problem was identified.
- Develop an action plan for everyone involved.
- Schedule a follow-up meeting to evaluate progress of the action plan.
- Remember to document everything objectively and completely!

REFERENCES

Black, C. (October 2012). Why healthcare organisations must look after their staff. *Nursing Management, 19*(6), 27–30.

Chipps, E. M., & McRury, M. (2012). The development of an educational intervention to address workplace bullying. *Journal for Nurses in Staff Development, 28*(3), 94–98.

Clark, C. M., Farnsworth, F., & Springer, P. J. (2008). Policy development for disruptive student behaviors. *Nurse Educator, 33*(6), 259–262.

Davey, M. M., Cummings, G., Newburn-Cook, C. V., & Lo, E. A. (2009). Predictors of nurse absenteeism in hospitals: A systematic review. *Journal of Nursing Management, 17*(3), 312–330.

Dellve, L., Hadzibajramovic, E., Ahlborg, G., Jr. (2011). Work attendance among healthcare workers: Prevalence, incentives, and long-term consequences for health and performance. *Journal of Advanced Nursing, 67*(9), 1918–1929.

Goleman, D. (2011). *The brain and emotional intelligence: New insights.* Northampton, MA: More than Sound, LLC.

Gorman, E., Yu, S., & Alamgir, H. (2010). When healthcare workers get sick: Exploring sickness absenteeism in British Columbia, Canada. Occupational Health and Safety Agency for Healthcare (OHSAH). *Work, 35*, 117–123, 2010.

Hamstrom, N., Kankkunen, P., Suominen, T., & Ritta, M. (2012). Short hospital stays and new demands for nurse competencies. *International Journal of Nursing Practice, 18*(5), 501–508.

Hersey, P., Blanchard, K., & Johnson, D. E. (2008). *Management of organizational behavior: Utilizing human resources* (9th ed.). Englewood Cliffs, NJ: Prentice Hall.

Hickson, J. (2013). New nurses' perceptions of hostility and job satisfaction. *The Journal of Nursing Administration, 43*(5), 293–301.

Hilton, M., Scuffham, P., Vecchio, N., & Whiteford, H. (2010). Using the interaction of mental health symptoms and treatment status to estimate lost employee productivity. *Australian and New Zealand Journal of Psychiatry, 44*, 151–161.

Johnson, T., Opfer, K., VanCura, B., & Williams, L. (2000). A comprehensive interactive competency program. Part I: Development and framework. *Medsurg Nursing, 9*(5), 265–268.

Lewis, P., & Malecha, A. (2011). The impact of workplace incivility on the work environment, manager skill and productivity. *The Journal of Nursing Administration, 41*(1), 41–47.

Major, K., Abderrahman, E. A., & Sweeney, J. I. (2013). Greening the 'Proclamation for Change': Healing Through Sustainable Health Care Environments – *The American Journal of Nursing, 113*(4), 66–70.

National Council of State Boards of Nursing. (2011). Clues to chemical dependency. *ASBN Update*, *15*(1), 9–11.

SESCO Management Consultants. (2013). *A positive approach to employee discipline*. (Retrieved on July 19, 2013) https://sescomgt.com/printarticle.php?id=98&action=print.

Sportsman, S. (2005). Build a framework for conflict assessment. *Nursing Management*, *36*(4), 32–40.

Wallace, M. (2009). Occupational health nurses: The solution to absence management. *AAOHN Journal*, *57*(3), 122–127.

SUGGESTED READINGS

DeCampti, P., Kirby, K. K., & Baldwin, C. (2010). Beyond the classroom to coaching: Preparing new nurse managers. *Critical Care Nursing Quarterly*, *33*(2), 132–137.

Hojat, M. (2009). Ten approaches for enhancing empathy in health and human services cultures. *Journal of Health and Human Services Administration*, *31*(4), 412–450.

Huseman, R. C. (2009). The importance of positive culture in hospitals. *Journal of Nursing Administration*, *39*(2), 60–63.

Lewis, R., Yarker, J., Donaldson-Feilder, E., Flaxman, P., & Munic, F. (2010). Using a competency-based approach to identify the management behaviours required to manage workplace stress in nursing: An incident study. *International Journal of Nursing Studies*, *47*(3), 307–313.

Simpson, K. R. (2008). Horizontal hostility. MCN. *The American Journal of Maternal Child Nursing*, *33*(5), 328.

Wildman, S., & Hewison, A. (2009). Rediscovering a history of nursing management: From Nightingale to the modern matron. *International Journal of Nursing Studies*, *46*(12), 1650–1661.

Wilson, S. (2009). Developing interpersonal skills. *Nursing New Zealand*, *15*(11), 3–4.

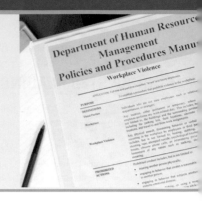

Workplace Violence and Incivility

Crystal J. Wilkinson

Nurses working in hospitals and other healthcare facilities have a disproportionately higher risk of experiencing physical violence because of the very nature of their jobs. To maintain personal safety and an environment free from the potential of physical violence, nurses must be alert to signs of trouble. Not all healthcare workplace violence is of a physical nature initiated by patients or their families; like any other business, the workplace is subject to horizontal violence or interdisciplinary incivility. Any type of violence in health care interferes with optimal job performance and has negative effects on the delivery of high-quality patient care. No organization can completely prevent or eliminate workplace violence, but with proper planning and effective programs, the chances of such violent occurrences can be dramatically reduced.

LEARNING OUTCOMES

- Describe the types of violence/incivility that may occur in the workplace and its effects on productivity and morale.
- Analyze risk factors for potential violence or disruption.
- Assess an organization's plan for preventing workplace violence and incivility.
- Summarize interventions that help prevent horizontal violence and incivility.

KEY TERMS

bullying	interpersonal conflict
horizontal violence	lateral aggression
incivility	toxic workplace

THE CHALLENGE

The Emergency Department Staff and Safety Manager*
University Medical Center at Brackenridge, Austin, Texas

University Medical Center Brackenridge (UMCB), a member of the Seton Healthcare Family, is a Level 1 trauma center located in a large urban area. We are near the heart of the downtown district and serve a broad cross section of the population. Our emergency department is busy all the time, and we never know what will come through the door. A nurse was assaulted by a patient with mental

illness. After exhibiting threatening behavior, he was apprehended by the police and brought to our emergency department. He had been calm and compliant up until about 6 hours after admission. At that point he became aggressive and seriously injured the nurse. We needed to develop a safety policy.

What do you think you would do if you were a nurse on this team?

*Kevin Craven, MBA, BSN, RN, Director, Emergency Services; Kristina Walker, CSP, OHST Site Safety Officer

INTRODUCTION

Workplace violence and incivility in health care have emerged as an important safety issue over the past decade. They are seen on a continuum from threats or intimidation to the most extreme form, homicide. Violence, whether from persons external or internal to an organization, has been shown to have negative effects, including increased job stress, reduced productive work time, decreased morale, increased staff turnover, and loss of trust in the organization and its management. By increasing personal awareness of workplace violence and incivility and by acquiring tactics for decreasing or preventing violence and incivility, nurses can contribute to better, safer healthcare organizations.

DEFINING WORKPLACE VIOLENCE AND INCIVILITY

The Occupational Safety & Health Administration (OSHA) enforces safety standards and provides training and outreach to employers to ensure safe and healthful working conditions. OSHA (2013) defined workplace violence as any act or threat of physical violence, harassment, intimidation, or other threatening disruptive behavior that occurs at the worksite. The definition includes overt and covert behaviors ranging from offensive or threatening language to homicide. In recent years, additional descriptions of other forms of workplace violence have been added. Horizontal violence or lateral aggression has been used to describe aggressive and destructive behavior of co-workers against each other. Other terms associated with this type of violence include bullying and

interpersonal conflict. These behaviors exist in what has been termed toxic workplaces. Incivility includes a wide range of behaviors from ignoring others, to rolling one's eyes, to yelling, and eventually to personal attacks, both physical and psychological. Both types of workplace violence are unacceptable.

SCOPE OF THE PROBLEM

The true scope of workplace violence in health care is difficult to determine. The main source of data for workplace violence and injuries is the Bureau of Labor Statistics (BLS). A BLS report (2012b) indicated healthcare workers, especially nurses, experience high rates of violence compared to workers in most other industries. In 2011, 203 workplace homicides occurred in the category of healthcare and social assistance workers (BLS, 2012a). Although this number is a concern, the incidence of fatal injuries is low when compared with the combined number of fatalities or for those in other types of industries. Underreporting, varying data collection methodologies, and source data give a wide range of estimates for violence against and among healthcare workers (Gacki-Smith, Juarez, & Boyett, 2009; Gates, Gillespie, & Succop, 2011; Hartley & Ridenour, 2011; Stokowski, 2010). Underreporting violence in health care is thought to be related to a perception within nursing that assaults with or without injuries are "part of the job." Some nurses may be fearful to report violence thinking they could have prevented it or they are pessimistic about the response they will receive from supervisors or managers. Similar perceptions exist related to lateral violence or incivility. Nurses tend to feel that this animosity is the predictable consequence of people working together and something they must get used to if they wish to remain in the profession (Dellasega, 2011). Workplace bullying is often reported to result in enough psychological distress to nurses to cause them to leave the profession (Dellasega, 2009). Bullying also interferes with teamwork and communication and can impact patient safety. These concerns underscore the urgent need for prevention of both patient-to-nurse and nurse-to-nurse violence.

THE COST OF WORKPLACE VIOLENCE

Our knowledge of the scale of workplace violence remains incomplete because no consistent system of data collection exists. Data regarding the less severe forms of workplace violence are particularly sparse. Even less clear is the financial toll workplace aggression exacts on businesses. Lewis and Malecha (2011) calculated lost productivity due to workplace violence at $11,581 per nurse per year. In a survey by Rosenstein (2010), participants indicated that 80% had witnessed disruptive behaviors and more than one third knew a nurse who left employment because of it. The direct cost of recruiting and hiring a new nurse is estimated at between $60,000 and $100,000. Pearson and Porath (2009) suggested that estimates of the cost of workplace violence should also consider how many times people report they are sick when they are really avoiding bad behavior. This absenteeism, and the decreases in productivity because employees no longer feel comfortable in the environment, are difficult to quantify but need to be considered. When added together, these costs mount rapidly.

Incivility and its associated disruptive behaviors have also been determined to have a negative effect on the delivery of high-quality patient care. The Joint Commission (TJC) in its root cause analysis of sentinel events found that nearly 70% of the events impacting patient care quality could be traced back to a communication problem (TJC, 2008). The cost of poor communication among healthcare providers has been estimated at $12 billion annually (Agarwal, Sands, & Diaz-Schneider, 2008). Although not all communication problems are related to incivility, many nurses have reported uncivil communication as a problem. Studies have yet to capture the full cost of

RESEARCH PERSPECTIVE

Resource: Purpora, C. & Blegen, M.A. (2012). Horizontal violence and the quality and safety of patient care: A conceptual model. *Nursing Research and Practice,* 2012:306948.

For many years nurses have voiced concern about horizontal violence in the clinical setting and its impact on care, but researchers had no framework for linking workplace violence with quality outcomes. Additionally, no direct empirical links between horizontal violence, disruptive behavior, dysfunctional communication, and patient care had been identified. The researchers proposed a conceptual model for horizontal violence and the quality and safety of patient care that was based on four theories:

1. Freire's oppression model (Freire, 2003)
2. Maslow's theory of human motivation (Maslow, 1943)
3. DeVito's theory of essential human communication (DeVito, 2008)
4. Reason's Swiss cheese model of systems accidents (Reason, 2000)

These four theories, linked for the first time in this conceptual model, illustrate how horizontal violence can impact quality and safety in the healthcare setting.

Implications for Practice

This framework provides a foundation to guide research in the area of workplace violence, patient safety, and quality. The model's propositions generate other questions based on empirical links that are meant to stimulate new research to bridge the gap in our understanding of the consequences of workplace violence.

workplace violence in its many forms, and more data are needed to assess the economic impact of violence in health care and the effectiveness of intervention strategies (see the Research Perspective).

ENSURING A SAFE WORKPLACE

Although no national legislation or federal regulations specifically address the prevention of workplace violence, OSHA has published voluntary guidelines for workers in healthcare and several other high-risk professions. Although employers are not legally obligated to follow these guidelines, the Occupational Safety and Health Act (OSH Act, 1970) mandates that, in addition to complying with hazard-specific standards, all employers have a general duty to provide their employees with a workplace free from recognized hazards likely to cause death or serious physical harm. An organization can be cited if its leaders fail to address such hazards.

Because healthcare workers are at increased risk, OSHA (2004) developed *Guidelines for Preventing Workplace Violence for Health Care and Social Service Workers* to assist healthcare organizations in developing violence prevention plans. Several states are also enacting or developing laws, standards, or recommendations that address healthcare workplace security and safety. Many of these laws have been created with strong support from state-based nursing organizations with support from the American Nurses Association (ANA) and other professional healthcare organizations. A few states have passed laws that enhance criminal penalties for crimes committed against licensed or certified health professionals (ANA, 2012) (Figure 25-1). Many other states have or are working on legislation requiring healthcare organizations to have a workplace violence prevention plan. In 2010, TJC issued a sentinel event alert that identifies the issue of preventing violence in the health care setting should be a priority for leaders. It notes that problems in the area of policy and procedure, inadequate assessment of the environment, and lack of education and training contribute to the majority of issues related to violence. TJC's Environment of Care standard requires healthcare facilities to have a plan describing how the institution provides for security of patients, visitors, and staff.

MAKING A DIFFERENCE

So what is the nurse in a leader, manager, or follower role to do given the serious and complex issue of violence in the workplace? Making a difference includes promotion of an organizational culture of safety and civility, development and implementation of a safety strategy, and personal strategies to prevent being victimized by violence in any setting are critical.

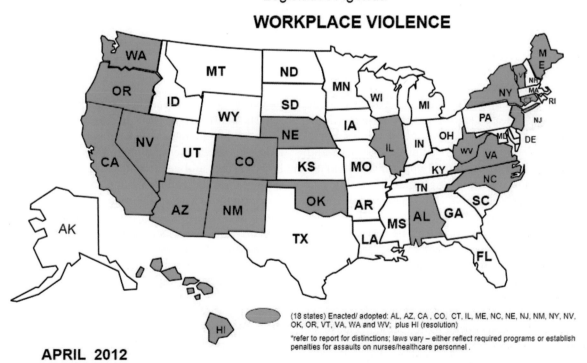

The American Nurses Association's Nationwide State Legislative Agenda

WORKPLACE VIOLENCE

(18 states) Enacted/ adopted: AL, AZ, CA , CO, CT, IL, ME, NC, NE, NJ, NM, NY, NV, OK, OR, VT, VA, WA and WV; plus HI (resolution)

*refer to report for distinctions; laws vary – either reflect required programs or establish penalties for assaults on nurses/healthcare personnel.

APRIL 2012

FIGURE 25-1 The American Nurse Association's Nationwide State Legislative Agenda for workplace violence, April 2012.

PREVENTION STRATEGIES

The old adage "an ounce of prevention is worth a pound of cure" is particularly relevant when dealing with workplace violence. Preventing even one act of violence can save money and time and diminish the possible negative psychological impact of such an event. The costs from lost work time and wages, reduced productivity, medical costs, workers' compensation payments, and legal and security expenses may be difficult to estimate but are clearly excessive when compared with the cost of prevention. Other future costs of workplace violence include increased staff turnover rates. Loss of the organizational investment required to train qualified staff and departure of experienced existing staff can increase operating expenses and reduce the quality of care. By taking a proactive approach that includes preventing violence, organizations can also prevent being victimized. To address the issue of violence, it is necessary to have a broad understanding of types of violence that may be encountered and the signs that portend a potentially violent situation. In short, prevention is the right thing to do.

Types of Violence

Since 1990, the University of Iowa Injury Prevention Research Center (IPRC) has been one of 11 injury "Centers of Excellence" funded by the National Center for Injury Prevention and Control, a branch of the Centers for Disease Control and Prevention (CDC). Workplace violence has been one of their research focus areas (IPRC, 2001). The university collects and uses epidemiologic data on groups at high risk in order to develop prevention strategies and training to control and prevent injuries. In their investigations, they categorize workplace violence into four types (Box 25-1). These categories can be very helpful in the design of strategies to prevent workplace violence, because each type of violence requires a different approach for prevention and acknowledges the fact that some workplaces may be at higher risk for certain types of violence. Understanding the types of violence allows leaders to conduct a more focused risk assessment based on what types of crimes may occur.

Risk Assessment

Although anyone working in health care is at risk for becoming a victim of violence, those with direct

---

BOX 25-1   CATEGORIES OF WORKPLACE VIOLENCE

Criminal Intent (Type I): The perpetrator has no legitimate relationship to the business or its employees and is usually committing a crime in conjunction with the violence. These crimes can include robbery, shoplifting, and trespassing. The vast majority of workplace homicides (85%) fall into this category.

Customer/Client (Type II): The perpetrator has a legitimate relationship with the business and becomes violent while being served by the business. This category includes customers, clients, patients, students, inmates, and any other group for which the business provides services. A large proportion of customer/client incidents are believed to occur in the healthcare industry, in settings such as nursing homes or psychiatric facilities; the victims are often patient caregivers. Police officers, prison staff, flight attendants, and teachers are some other examples of workers who may be exposed to this kind of workplace violence.

Worker-on-Worker (Type III): The perpetrator is an employee or past employee of the business who attacks or threatens another employee(s) or past employee(s) in the workplace. Worker-on-worker fatalities account for approximately 7% of all workplace violence homicides.

Personal Relationship (Type IV): The perpetrator usually does not have a relationship with the business but has a personal relationship with the intended victim. This category includes victims of domestic violence assaulted or threatened while at work.

From Iowa Injury Prevention Research Center. (February 2001). *Workplace violence: A report to the nation.* University of Iowa—Iowa City. Retrieved February 15, 2013, from *www.public-health.uiowa.edu/iprc/resources/workplace-violence-report.pdf.*

---

patient contact are at higher risk. The BLS (2012b) reports healthcare workers in hospitals, specifically those in the emergency department, are at particularly high risk. Violence is also a frequent occurrence in psychiatric and geriatric settings. Unlike in other settings, hospital violence differs in that it is usually the result of patients or their family members feeling frustration or anger. This is usually related to feelings of vulnerability, stress, and loss of control that accompany illness. Many factors have been identified that can increase the risk for violence erupting in healthcare facilities. Risk factors identified in OSHA's guidelines (2004) are listed in Box 25-2. Other risk factors for violence include the location of the facility, its size, and the type of care provided. Facilities in inner-city areas that serve a wide variety of the disadvantaged, especially those with mental illness or a history of violent behavior or those who are under the influence of drugs or alcohol, are at increased risk for violence to occur. Reviewing reports of violent

BOX 25-2   **RISK FACTORS FOR VIOLENCE IN HEALTHCARE FACILITIES**

- Work in understaffed situations, especially during visiting hours and meal times
- Transportation of patients between areas in a facility
- Long waits for patient care
- Overcrowded, uncomfortable waiting areas
- Solo work or in isolation from other staff
- Solo work with patients in areas with no back-up or way to get assistance, such as communication devices or alarm systems
- Poor environmental design
- Inadequate security
- Lack of staff training in handling potentially violent situations
- Lack of policies for preventing and managing crises with potentially violent individuals
- Unrestricted movement of patients or visitors
- Poorly lit corridors, rooms, parking lots, or other areas
- Prevalence of handguns or other weapons among patients, their families, or friends
- Increased presence of gang members, drug or alcohol abusers, trauma patients, or distraught family members
- Use of hospitals or healthcare facilities for holding criminals, violent individuals, and the acutely mentally disturbed
- Chronically mentally ill patients being released without adequate resources for follow-up care
- Availability of money or drugs within the facility

Adapted from Occupational Safety & Health Administration (OSHA). (2004). *Guidelines for preventing workplace violence for health care and social service workers.* Retrieved February 15, 2013, from *www.osha.gov/Publications/osha3148.pdf.*

BOX 25-3   **WORKPLACE VIOLENCE PROGRAM CHECKLISTS**

OSHA and ANA have provided comprehensive checklist documents that can assist leaders and managers in conducting an organizational workplace violence assessment. The checklist titles are provided here. The checklists provide detailed step-by-step instructions to conduct an in-depth assessment and establish a monitoring program. To see the complete document, go to *www.osha.gov* (OSHA Publication No. 3148-01R 2004).

Checklist 1: Organizational Assessment Questions Regarding Management Commitment and Employee Involvement
Checklist 2: Analyze Workplace Violence Records
Checklist 3: Identifying Environmental Risk Factors for Violence
Checklist 4: Assessing the Influence of Day-to-Day Work Practices on Occurrences of Violence
Checklist 5: Post-Incident Response
Checklist 6: Assessing Employee and Supervisor Training
Checklist 7: Record-keeping and Evaluation

Adapted from American Nurses Association: *Promoting Safe Work Environments for Nurses, 2002.* From Occupational Safety and Health Administration (OSHA). (2004). *Guidelines for preventing workplace violence for health care and social service workers* (OSHA Publication No. 3148-01R). Washington, DC: U.S. Department of Labor *(www.osha.gov).*

incidents reveals they often take place during times of high activity and interaction with patients, such as at mealtimes and during visiting hours and patient transportation. Assaults may occur when service is denied, when a patient is involuntarily admitted, or when a healthcare worker attempts to set limits on eating, drinking, or use of tobacco or alcohol.

Similar to the nursing process, prevention of workplace violence begins with a systematic assessment. Assessing risk and planning for prevention of workplace violence call for input and expertise from a variety of staff. A risk assessment based on an interdisciplinary team approach to workplace violence prevention is often the most effective. A team with representation from administration, staff, security, facilities engineering, human resources, legal counsel, and risk management is needed to address risks from all perspectives. A worksite assessment involves a step-by-step, common sense look at the facility

and the surrounding areas for existing problems and potential hazards. OSHA's guidelines (2004) provide a comprehensive assessment with checklists and forms developed by the ANA to assist with the process. These are helpful to managers and leaders who are not familiar with this type of assessment (Box 25-3). The ECRI Institute *(www.ecri.org)*, a federally designated Patient Safety Organization, and the International Association for Healthcare Security & Safety (IAHSS) *(www.iahss.org)* also have numerous resources and tools to assist healthcare organizations in creating security management plans to reduce the potential for violence.

When looking at possible threats or hazards, those from within an organization also must be considered. Determining if current employees pose a danger in the workplace is a critical factor that is often overlooked. In addition to personal and psychological factors, behaviors can be observed in employees that may be related to violence or aggression in the workplace (Paludi, Nydegger, & Paludi, 2006). The most obvious of these is a previous history of aggression and substance abuse. Screening potential employees through drug testing, background checks, and references can help reduce these risks.

Firing Right

Organizational conditions or outcomes may magnify the potential for violence to erupt. This includes prolonged high levels of stress or factors that create what is known as a *toxic workplace environment*. Rapid change, layoffs, changes in schedules and workloads, or wage freezes could have this effect. The employment situation with the highest potential to create this kind of stress is the firing or layoff process. Most organizations have specific protocols that deal with the process of terminating employees, because firing is cause for strong emotions that can increase the potential for violence. Managers may be responsible for staff terminations in some organizations; others require this process to occur in the human resources department. Either approach requires close collaboration between nursing and human resources. The goal always is to conduct the process in the most professional manner possible, although organizational rules may specify a detailed procedure. A few tips on how to prepare for this potentially problematic situation are provided in Box 25-4.

Unfortunately no profile or litmus test exists to identify whether a current employee might become violent. Employers and employees alike must remain alert to problematic behavior that, in combination, could point to possible violence. Because no single behavior suggests a greater potential for violence, behaviors must be looked at in totality. Problem situations, circumstances that may heighten the risk of violence, can involve a particular event or employee or the workplace as a whole.

EXERCISE 25-1

Assess several clinical settings for workplace violence risks. Can you identify any based on what you have read? What security measures are currently in place? Can any of them be improved? How safe would you feel in the different geographical areas?

Once the risk assessment is completed, the next step is to analyze the data and prioritize the problems that need to be addressed. Priorities can be established by asking a few basic questions: What are the risks? Who might be harmed and how? What is the level of risk? What measures need to be taken to reduce or eliminate risk? Do we need to implement changes now or later? Once the priorities are set, the business of designing or improving prevention programs can begin. (See the "Developing a Safety Plan" section on p. 475.)

HORIZONTAL VIOLENCE: THE THREAT FROM WITHIN

In 2008, TJC strengthened requirements in their leadership standards for dealing with disruptive behavior. Citing studies that suggest intimidating and disruptive behaviors contribute to poor patient satisfaction and preventable adverse outcomes, the standards call for codes of conduct and processes for managing such behaviors. Horizontal or lateral violence describes a wide variety of behaviors, from verbal abuse to physical aggression between co-workers. This term, though commonly used, may be limiting because it suggests the violence is perpetrated between those at the same level of authority. It may be better termed *relational aggression* (Dellasega, 2009, Dellasega, 2011), which can occur between people at different levels. This includes bullying behavior and intimidation. *Horizontal violence* or *bullying* is used in this section because these are terms common in the literature. Horizontal violence and its effects have been reported in the nursing literature for more than 20 years. In a review of five research studies on horizontal violence, researchers (Woelfle & McCaffrey, 2007) found that horizontal violence is experienced by not only nursing students but also the novice and veteran nurses. Many of the research reports found infighting and a

---

BOX 25-4   FIRING RIGHT

Firings should be planned with forethought for any potential problems. Steps should be taken to avoid potential violence during employee separation. A key step is protecting the employee's dignity and avoiding humiliation. The reasons for termination should be clear and leave no room for debate. All details should be arranged, including timing, the room used, and who is present. The room should provide privacy but not contain any objects that could be used as a weapon. The person being terminated should not be blocked from accessing the exit door. Termination notices and severance checks along with any other documentation should be on hand. Arrangements should be made to clean out the person's desk or locker. No option should be available for the person to return to the worksite. This saves everyone from embarrassment and any potential scenes. It is important to try to determine how the person will react to make appropriate arrangements. If a perceived need exists, a security officer or off-duty police officer can be called to stand by.

Adapted from Winfeld, L. (2001). *Training tough topics*. New York: American Management Association.

general lack of support of nurses for each other to be common occurrences. The studies also indicated that new graduates were likely to experience horizontal violence, which resulted in high absentee rates and thoughts of leaving nursing after their first year. This caused the researchers to ask this question: How can nurses treat patients kindly and give them the respect they need when they treat each other so poorly? In light of the looming nursing shortage, these consistent findings among nurses were cause for concern.

Many theories exist as to why horizontal violence is prevalent in nursing, ranging from nursing's traditional hierarchical structure, to oppression of nursing as a profession (Roberts, Demarco & Griffin, 2009), to feminism (Farrell, 2001). However, workplace aggression is common in other professions and is most likely the result of complex individual, social, and organizational characteristics (Papa & Venella, 2013). Regardless of the reasons why it happens, the concerns are that impaired personal relationships between nurses at work can cause errors, accidents, and poor work performance and may play a significant role in attrition (Johnson, 2009; Lewis & Malecha, 2011; Porto & Lauve, 2006; Purpora & Blegen, 2012; Roberts, Demarco, & Griffin, 2009; Shields & Wilkins, 2009; TJC, 2008). There is no place in a professional practice environment for lateral violence and bullying among nurses or between healthcare professionals. These disruptive behaviors are toxic to the nursing profession and have a negative impact on retention of quality staff. Horizontal violence and bullying should never be considered normally related to socialization in nursing nor be accepted in professional relationships. All healthcare organizations should implement a zero tolerance policy related to disruptive behavior, including a professional code of conduct and educational and behavioral interventions to assist nurses in addressing disruptive behavior (Papa & Venella, 2013). A number of other state and national nursing organizations also have issued statements regarding the detrimental effect of disruptive behavior on both patients and nurses and have called for solutions to address the problem. TJC (2008) revised its standards for disruptive behavior calling for identification of manifestations of abuse and violence in healthcare organizations. Holloway and Kusy (2010) provided practical organizational strategies to address toxic behaviors to change the culture of incivility (see the Literature Perspective). With professional groups

LITERATURE PERSPECTIVE

Resource: Holloway, L.E. & Kusy, M.E. (2010). Disruptive and toxic behaviors in healthcare: Zero tolerance, the bottom line, and what to do about it. *Medical Practice Management, 25*(6), 335-340.

This article provides the results of a survey of over 400 healthcare leaders representing 39% of healthcare organizations. The authors found that 94% of those surveyed had to deal with some form of incivility or toxic behavior at work. Citing the literature that indicates toxic environments and disruptive behavior impact patient safety and quality of care, the authors provide a whole system approach that is tailored to complex healthcare environments. The Toxic Organization Change System (TOCS) addresses incivility at the level of the organization, the team, and the individual. It describes specific strategies that can be used preventively or remedially. At the organization level, the main strategies include establishing a set of values that call for professionalism, courtesy, and respect for all. Defining these values from the ground up is an important activity to bring together stakeholders from across the organization. Once the values are established they are incorporated into the performance appraisal process. Managers are trained how to evaluate and reinforce these behaviors and values in both formative and summative stages. The team's strategy consists of identifying individuals or processes that perpetuate toxic cultures and working to rebuild positive norms and functional teams in those environments. This includes use of a 360-degree team assessment and facilitation to improve communication and address toxic behavior. Individual strategies involve managers providing regular feedback, establishing goals and working on professional growth and development with their staff. This includes instituting clear consequences for toxic behaviors and being willing to terminate staff members who perpetuate toxic culture.

Implications for Practice

Addressing a toxic culture requires training in conflict management, leadership, communication, and team building. To move an organization from a culture of incivility to one of respect is no easy task but in this era of healthcare reform, tight budgets, and need for better healthcare outcomes, it is work that organizations must do to meet their bottom line and to ensure nurses feel valued, respected, and safe.

calling for change from within nursing and accreditation groups calling on administration to fix problems, we must examine how to implement a change. See stopbullyingnurses.com for resources.

Increasing Awareness of Horizontal Violence

The causes of horizontal violence within nursing are pervasive and long-standing. No definitive actions have been shown to significantly decrease the occurrence of violence. One thing is certain—recognizing the tendency toward bullying, harassment, or intimidation in the workplace is a prerequisite to preventing it. The true depth of the problem is difficult to determine. Commonly, horizontal violence is significantly underreported for any number of reasons, and organizational leaders often are not aware of its extent. To get an accurate picture of employee satisfaction and concerns about bullying and other forms of violence, anonymous surveys should be conducted. Surveying staff can help identify problems and provide a basis for developing appropriate interventions. To understand if violence or intimidation is a reason for leaving, organizations should conduct exit interviews with the assurance that the information will remain confidential if an employee fears retaliation. This is an important step in gauging if the problem is bullying or intimidation by managers. Johnson (2009) found that 50% of respondents indicated that they were bullied by their manager or director. The researcher suggested that when management is part of the problem, victims have a harder time feeling they have adequate support to end the negative cycle of violence. This may serve to perpetuate the existence of a toxic environment within an organization.

Nursing leaders can set the stage for addressing workplace bullying by examining and addressing their own behaviors and by fostering an environment that encourages open communication and collaboration. With personal insight in hand, they can lead their nurses to examine their own behavior and work together to create a work environment in which bullying is not tolerated. An atmosphere of openness can encourage dialog and brainstorming to find solutions. Lack of support leads many victims of bullying to decide that the best alternative is to leave the organization and to give this advice to others who find themselves in similar situations (Johnson, 2009). Employees who are supported in reporting workplace aggression may feel they have options other than leaving. The worst outcome would be for the nurse to feel that using formal and informal organizational channels to bring about an end to bullying was emotionally draining, time-consuming, and futile.

Organizational culture and working conditions also can contribute to bullying and horizontal violence. High stress levels, inadequate staffing, organizational change, and unrealistic expectations can contribute to a toxic environment and foster increased incivility among staff. A culture of zero tolerance for horizontal violence is an effective leadership strategy to prevent its occurrence. For organizations that have tolerated horizontal violence, developing a new shared set of values and goals that promote empowerment, communication, and collaboration is a positive step (Longo, 2007). Leaders need to set the tone for establishing a civil workplace in which all members are treated with respect and in which conflicts are dealt with in a healthy and open manner (Holloway & Kusy, 2010). TJC (2010) suggests 11 actions that can be used as a blueprint for developing a program to address disruptive behavior within organizations (Box 25-5). No violence prevention program will work if management does not endorse it.

Encouragement to report violence in all its forms is crucial to understanding the root of the problem and implementing plans to eradicate it. Acts of good faith by organizational management in supporting staff include a policy of nonretaliation for reporting. Making sure that reporting is easier and doing an impartial investigation is critical. Ensuring appropriate discipline for identified problems that is proportional to the seriousness of the event goes a long way in building employee trust. People are the greatest resource in an organization, and wise management invests time and effort in addressing culture, safety, and satisfaction of nursing staff. Finally, organizations that implement interventions aimed at addressing workplace bullying need to collect data to determine whether these interventions are successful.

Nurses themselves must work to actively develop a culture in which violence is not tolerated. This involves a critical self-assessment of personal behaviors and looking for patterns or situations that could trigger subtle types of lateral aggression. Awareness and understanding of the types of horizontal violence can help them to actively not participate in the behaviors. This is a powerful tool in eradicating a toxic environment. Many subtle forms of horizontal violence that may not be readily recognized as violent behavior but are psychologically and emotionally harmful are listed in Box 25-6. Recognizing these behaviors and efforts to eliminate them can create a healthier working environment

BOX 25-5   THE JOINT COMMISSION SUGGESTED ACTIONS

1. Educate all team members—both physicians and nonphysician staff—on appropriate professional behavior defined by the organization's code of conduct.
2. Hold all team members accountable for modeling desirable behaviors, and enforce the code consistently and equitably among all staff, regardless of seniority or clinical discipline, in a positive fashion through reinforcement as well as punishment.
3. Develop and implement policies and procedures/processes appropriate for the organization that address the following:
   - "Zero tolerance" for intimidating and/or disruptive behaviors
   - Medical staff policies regarding intimidating and/or disruptive behaviors
   - Reducing fear of intimidation or retribution and protecting those who report or cooperate in the investigation of intimidating, disruptive, and other unprofessional behavior
   - Responding to patients and/or their families who are involved in or witness intimidating and/or disruptive behaviors
   - How and when to begin disciplinary actions (e.g., suspension, termination, loss of clinical privileges, reports to professional licensure bodies)
4. Develop an organizational process for addressing intimidating and disruptive behaviors that solicits and integrates substantial input from an interdisciplinary team including representation of medical and nursing staff, administrators, and other employees.
5. Provide skills-based training and coaching for all leaders and managers in relationship-building and collaborative practice, including skills for giving feedback on unprofessional behavior, and conflict resolution.
6. Develop and implement a system for assessing staff perceptions of the seriousness and extent of instances of unprofessional behaviors and the risk of harm to patients.
7. Develop and implement a reporting/surveillance system (possibly anonymous) for detecting unprofessional behavior.
8. Support surveillance with tiered, nonconfrontational interventional strategies, starting with informal "cup of coffee" conversations directly addressing the problem and moving toward detailed action plans and progressive discipline, if patterns persist.
9. Conduct all interventions within the context of an organizational commitment to the health and well-being of all staff, with adequate resources to support individuals whose behavior is caused or influenced by physical or mental health pathologies.
10. Encourage interdisciplinary dialogs across a variety of forums as a proactive way of addressing ongoing conflicts, overcoming them, and moving forward through improved collaboration and communication.
11. Document all attempts to address intimidating and disruptive behaviors.

The Joint Commission (2008). Behaviors that undermine a culture of safety. *Sentinel Event Alert. 40.* Retrieved May 15, 2013, from *www.jointcommission.org/assets/1/18/SEA_40.PDF.*
Reprinted with permission. Copyright © 2009.

BOX 25-6   COMMON SUBTLE BEHAVIORS IN NURSE-NURSE BULLYING

- Giving a nurse "the silent treatment"
- Spreading rumors
- Using humiliation and put-downs, usually regarding a nurse's skills and abilities
- Failing to support a nurse because you do not like him or her
- Excluding a nurse from on-the-job or off-the-job socializing
- Repeating information shared by one nurse out of context so that it reflects badly on him or her
- Sharing confidences you were asked to keep private
- Making fun of another nurse's appearance, demeanor, or another trait
- Refusing to share information with another nurse or otherwise setting him or her up to fail
- Manipulating or intimidating another nurse into doing something for you
- Using body language (e.g., eye rolling or head tossing) to convey an unfavorable opinion of someone
- Saying something unfavorable and then pretending you were joking
- Calling names
- Teasing another nurse about his or her lack of skill or knowledge
- Running a smear campaign or otherwise trying to get others to turn against a nurse

Modified from Dellasega, C. (2009). Bullying among nurses. *American Journal of Nursing, 109*(1), 52-58.

that is based on mutual respect. In the book, *When Nurses Hurt Nurses: Recognizing and Overcoming the Cycle of Bullying*, Dellasega (2011) explores the nature of relational aggression within nursing and provides practical strategies to deal with bullying. The ANA (2010) also has resources, including a pocket card on bullying and lateral violence that gives examples of bullying behavior and possible responses to help nurses identify and deal with bullying (Figure 25-2).

EXERCISE 25-2

Think about your behavior in the workplace. Have you ever acted in a way that might be described as lateral aggression or horizontal violence? How might you guard against such behaviors? Do you think you could confront a co-worker participating in an act of lateral aggression? What would you say?

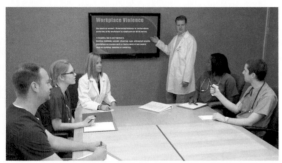

Participating in violence prevention education can prepare staff to deal with situations that contribute to bullying or intimidation.

Education

Education on workplace violence should be provided to all employees but initially to supervisors, whose support is crucial to the success of the program (Papa & Venella, 2013). Interventions aimed at nurse leaders regarding ways to change organizational climates that perpetuate bullying have proved to be a better option than directing education at individual nurses (Johnson, 2009). Education should focus on identifying the potential for violence, managing violent situations, and practicing behavioral and de-escalation techniques. In some settings, more focused training on applying restraints and take-down techniques would be appropriate. This type of training should start in nursing school to prepare those going into the workforce for the realities of their day-to-day work. Training needs to be annual and ongoing and needs to address topics that have been identified through survey, reporting, and data analysis.

Participating in violence prevention education can prepare staff to deal with situations that contribute to bullying or intimidation (Hartley, Ridenour, Craine, & Costa, 2012). In her study, Griffin (2004) used a cognitive behavior technique called *cognitive rehearsal* as an intervention for lateral violence. Cognitive rehearsal involves listening and then holding the information provided in the mind to allow time to process a response in a way the staff have been taught. This change in the way they responded allowed opportunities to change negative perceptions and confront laterally violent

---

Bullying and Lateral Violence

Examples of Bullying Behavior

- Being 'yelled at' or 'screamed at' in front of others
- Being accused of errors made by someone else (Scapegoat)
- Being the subject of gossiping
- Being the topic of rumors
- Being humiliated in front of others
- Being assigned undesirable work
- Being sabotaged

ANA
AMERICAN NURSES ASSOCIATION
8515 Georgia Avenue, Suite 400
Silver Spring, MD 20910
nursingworld.org

- Having key information withheld impacting job performance
- Having thoughts or feelings ignored
- Non-verbal intimidation - stares and glares
- Exclusion from activities or conversations
- Being physically threatened

Possible Responses to Bullying

Verbal Abuse (Yelling in front of others)

"I do not appreciate being yelled at in front of others. It sets a bad example for the staff and does not leave a good impression on the patients and family members. If there is something you need to discuss with me, we can do it in a more private place."

Nonverbal abuse (eye-rolling, making faces)

"I sense that there is something you want to say to me. Do you wish to discuss it?"

Overhearing someone talking about you

"If there is an issue that we need to talk about, please come to me directly so we can discuss it."

Responses When You Witness Bullying

Backstabbing (complaining about a person to someone other than the person)

"I do not know the facts of the situation and do not feel comfortable discussing it."

Lack of Respect

"I do not like to talk about others without their permission."

(Adapted from M. Griffin, 2004; Center for American Nurses, 2007). ANA condemns abuse and harassment of nurses in professional associations and all work environments in which nurses practice, including abuse and harassment, based on age, color, creed, disability, gender, health status, lifestyle, nationality, race, religion, or sexual orientation. ANA is working proactively to reduce the growing problem of workplace abuse, harassment and bullying of nurses and the serious consequences, including serious reprisal and retaliation. Additionally, ANA is exploring collaborative solutions with other disciplines and organizations to leverage resources for research and education. (Adapted from the 2010 House of Delegates Resolution, "Hostility, Abuse and Bullying in the Workplace" and the 2006 House of Delegates Resolution, "Workplace Abuse and Harassment of Nurses.")

FIGURE 25-2 American Nurses Association (2010). Hostility, abuse and bullying the workplace. 2010 House of Delegates Resolution. Bullying and Lateral Violence: Examples of Bullying Behavior Pocket Card. (From http://nursingworld.org/MainMenuCategories/CertificationandAccreditation/Continuing-Professional-Development/NavigateNursing/AboutNN/Tip-Card-Bullying-and-Lateral-Violence-ANA.pdf.)

nurses. This opens the door to better communication and has been shown to help nurses' better cope with potentially violent situations (Dellasega, 2011).

DEVELOPING A SAFETY PLAN

No "one-size-fits-all" strategy exists for an effective safety and violence prevention program or plan. Effective plans may share a number of features, but a good plan must be tailored to the needs, resources, and circumstances of a particular employer and a particular work force. Activities related to developing a good prevention program fall into three domains: administrative, environmental, and interpersonal.

Administrative

To develop an effective workplace violence strategy, support from the top must be present. If an organization's senior executives are not truly committed to a prevention program, it is unlikely to be effectively implemented. Part of the organization's responsibility is to provide a written program for job safety and security. Developing and maintaining a program requires time and resources. Allocations need to be made for a multidisciplinary safety committee, regular worksite analysis, prevention activities, safety and health training, documentation, and evaluation of the overall program. The program should outline the organization's commitment to a safe work environment and the staff's involvement in the plan. The program should be proactive, not reactive, and have clear goals and objectives to prevent workplace violence that is specific to the organization and its characteristics. Personnel, work environments, business conditions, and society all change and evolve. A successful prevention program must change and evolve with them. Policies and practices should not be set in concrete and should be regularly evaluated to determine if they are keeping current with a changing environment. The administration needs to communicate the safety plan effectively and consistently enforce policy to ensure that the staff believes safety is of paramount importance.

A written workplace violence policy sets the standard for acceptable workplace behavior *and* should be available to all employees. The statement should affirm the organization's commitment to a safe workplace, employees' obligation to behave appropriately on the job, and the employer's commitment to take action on any employee's complaint regarding harassing, threatening, and violent behavior. The statement should be in writing and distributed to all employees. In defining acts that will not be tolerated, the statement should make clear that not only physical violence but also threats, bullying, harassment, and weapons possession are against policy and are prohibited.

Plans should consider the workplace culture: work atmosphere, relationships, and management styles. Policies on workplace conduct should be written to clearly state the employer's standards and expectations. Attention should be paid to elements in an organization's culture that foster a toxic work environment, such as the following:

- Tolerance of bullying or intimidation
- Lack of trust among workers
- Lack of trust between workers and management
- High levels of stress, frustration, and anger

The organization should be actively addressing root causes of problems to reduce the potential for frustration to lead to violence. If significant problems are identified, disciplinary actions for violent behavior of any kind must be proportionate, consistent, reasonable, and fair. Erratic or arbitrary discipline, favoritism, and a lack of respect for employees' dignity and rights are likely to undermine an employer's violence prevention efforts. Workers who perceive an employer's practices as unfair or unreasonable will be more unlikely to report problems. Lack of reporting allows unfavorable situations to continue with many negative impacts. When a complaint is made or an incident occurs, an incident response team should conduct or ensure a thorough investigation of the facts and, based on the results, determine appropriate disciplinary measures. Likewise with patients or visitors to a healthcare facility, expectations about acceptable behavior and the consequences of violent behavior should be clearly communicated. Strong administrative commitment to a safety plan serves to reaffirm the employer's commitment to a workplace free from threats and violence.

Environmental

Engineering controls and other environmental adaptations to remove safety hazards can be very effective. Deciding what interventions are needed is the "intelligence" work of organizations. The countermeasures applied can reduce potential risks. The selection of measures to be used is based on the hazards identified in the security risk analysis. Some environmental interventions, such as providing better lighting or restricting access to care areas, can have a significant impact on safety at very low cost. The types of interventions that may be identified by security risk assessment are listed in Box 25-7.

Administrative and work practice controls can also be evaluated to determine the effect on how staff members perform their jobs and how changes in procedures can help reduce the potential for violent incidents. Any process changes that reduce waiting times or improve customer service can help reduce frustration that may lead to violent outburst. Staff training on handling aggressive behavior and how to respond in violent events is discussed in the next section.

Interpersonal

Little research has been done on the effectiveness of training staff to anticipate, recognize, and respond to conflict and potential violence in the workplace. Helping managers to be alert to warning signs of conflict and to know how to respond when indications of a problem arise seems to be beneficial (Johansen, 2012). Training about workplace violence prevention will vary according to different employee groups and issues specific to their work environment. Training should be provided to new and current employees, supervisors, and managers. All training should be conducted on a regular basis and cover a variety of topics, including the following:
- The workplace violence prevention policy, including reporting requirements
- Risk factors that can cause or contribute to threats and violence

---

BOX 25-7   ENVIRONMENTAL SAFETY CONTROLS

- Assess any plans for new construction or physical changes to the facility or workplace to eliminate or reduce security hazards.
- Install and regularly maintain alarm systems and other security devices, panic buttons, handheld alarms or noise devices, cellular phones, and private channel radios where risk is apparent or may be anticipated. Arrange for a reliable response system when an alarm is triggered.
- Provide metal detectors—installed or handheld, where appropriate—to detect guns, knives, or other weapons, according to the recommendations of security consultants.
- Use a closed-circuit video recording for high-risk areas on a 24-hour basis. Public safety is a greater concern than privacy in these situations.
- Create security alert overhead paging protocols and response teams.
- Place curved mirrors at hallway intersections and concealed areas.
- Enclose nurses' stations and install deep service counters or bullet-resistant, shatterproof glass in reception, triage, and admitting areas or patient service rooms.
- Provide employee "safe rooms" for use during emergencies.
- Establish "time-out" or seclusion areas with high ceilings without grids for patients who "act out," and establish separate rooms for criminal patients.
- Provide comfortable client or patient waiting rooms designed to minimize stress.
- Ensure that counseling or patient care rooms have two exits.
- Lock doors to staff counseling rooms and treatment rooms to limit access.
- Arrange furniture to prevent entrapment of staff.
- Use minimal furniture in interview rooms or crisis treatment areas, and ensure that it is lightweight, without sharp corners or edges, and affixed to the floor, if possible. Limit the number of pictures, vases, or other items that can be used as weapons.
- Provide lockable and secure bathrooms for staff members separate from patient/client and visitor facilities.
- Lock all unused doors to limit access, in accordance with local fire codes.
- Install bright, effective lighting, both indoors and outdoors.
- Replace burned-out lights and broken windows and locks.
- Keep automobiles well maintained if they are used in the field.
- Lock automobiles at all times.
- Provide administrative controls such as codes for door access in staff or restricted areas.
- Improve processes to decrease wait times or other activities that create frustration for patients and family members.

Adapted from American Nurses Association: Promoting Safe Work Environments for Nurses, 2002. From Occupational Safety and Health Administration (OSHA). (2004). *Guidelines for preventing workplace violence for health care and social service workers* (OSHA Publication No. 3148-01R). Washington, DC: U.S. Department of Labor (www.osha.gov).

- Early recognition of warning signs of problematic behavior
- Ways of preventing or defusing volatile situations or aggressive behavior, where appropriate
- Information on cultural diversity to develop sensitivity to racial and ethnic issues and differences
- A standard response action plan for violent situations, including availability of assistance, response to alarm systems, and communication procedures
- The location and operation of safety devices such as alarm systems, along with the required maintenance schedules and procedures
- Ways to protect oneself and co-workers, including use of a buddy system
- Policies and procedures for reporting and record-keeping
- Policies and procedures for obtaining medical care, counseling, workers' compensation, or legal assistance after a violent episode or injury

Training employees in nonviolent response and conflict resolution has been suggested to reduce the risk that volatile situations will escalate to physical violence. Training that addresses hazards associated with specific tasks or worksites and relevant prevention strategies is also critical. Training should not be regarded as the sole prevention strategy but, instead, as a component in a comprehensive approach to reducing workplace violence. To increase vigilance and compliance with stated violence prevention policies, training should emphasize the appropriate use and maintenance of protective equipment, adherence to administrative controls, and increased knowledge and awareness of the risk of workplace violence.

No matter how thorough or well-conceived, preparation will not be effective in an emergency if no one remembers or implements the plan. Training exercises should be a regular part of the process. Training must include managers and senior executives who will be making decisions in a real incident. Exercises must be followed by careful evaluation with rapid responses that fix whatever weaknesses have been revealed.

EXERCISE 25-3

Look at an organization's workplace safety plan. Does it have a statement about zero tolerance for violent behaviors? Does it include instructions on how to report violent behavior? Has it been updated recently? Based on what you have read, do you think the plan is comprehensive?

Understanding the Potential for Violence

Though violent incidents can occur seemingly without warning, some theories allow us to assess and predict potential occurrences. Research by John Monahan (1981), a psychologist at the University of Virginia Law School, described basic mental and behavioral cycles and circumstances that can escalate over time into violence. The cycle or spiral has four parts:

- An individual encounters a stressful event.
- The individual reacts to the event with certain types of thoughts that are predisposed based on personality.
- The thoughts lead to emotional responses.
- These responses in turn determine the behavior used to respond to the situation.

Extreme stress may lead to a belief that violence is the only viable way to cope with the situation or to relieve the stress. The responses of the individuals involved can either de-escalate or escalate the situation, influencing the ultimate outcome. Awareness of this basic pattern can help manage the potential for violent situations. Understand that the individual's perception of the stress is what precipitates the spiral. What seems like a minor issue to you may be a huge event for someone else depending on his or her subjective experience. Things as minor as a change in routine or seemingly small annoyances can be a trigger. The stressful event can become magnified when a person is not sure whether he or she has the resources to respond successfully to the stress. It then becomes important to appraise how a person responds to stressors, how he or she views the situation, and what he or she expects to happen.

If the individual is contemplating an assault, anything that can be done to improve communication and decrease frustration can have a significant impact. At this point, the perpetrator may be struggling to overcome internal barriers to lashing out. Taking advantage of this internal struggle and allowing the person a way to back down without embarrassment can de-escalate the situation. This takes good communications skills that can be taught and rehearsed. Another strategy is to not allow an environment that is conducive to a physical assault. In many cases, an assault will not take place in the presence of other staff, in a public area, or where surveillance cameras are present. If an attack is initiated, the goal is minimization of harm and control of the situation or escape.

Physical attacks often occur after several indicators have pointed toward the potential of violence. Case studies of violent behavior are filled with information that show that people felt threatened, intimidated, or unsafe in the presence of the person who later committed an act of violence. In his book, *The Gift of Fear: Survival Signals That Protect Us From Violence*, DeBecker (2000) asserted that fear is an internal warning system, alerting us to potentially threatening situations. In interviews with survivors of violent attacks, they frequently related that they "had a bad feeling" about the situation or that they knew that something was not right. DeBecker postulates that the "gut feeling" or "intuition" is the result of rapid cognitive processing of a complex web of cues or patterns of behavior that the subconscious brain alerts to before the logical part of the brain has the chance to catch up. Learning to use this awareness has formed the basis for many self-defense and workplace violence trainings. Training on subtle clues as well as day-to-day experience in dealing with a variety of people can add to adeptness in reading situations and recognizing danger. Validating that this fear response is useful may help in situations in which that moment of trying to rationalize the fear can give a perpetrator the edge needed to carry out an attack. The trick is not only to listen to your intuition but also to look for behaviors that predict violence or to provide an opportunity for escape. Many overt cues may predict violence. Body language is the most significant of these cues. These are usually easy to identify and may include standing too close, threatening gestures, tense posture, furtive glances, and rapid or repetitive movements. Being aware of your body language can be a critical factor in keeping a situation from escalating. We are generally aware of the body language of others but may not recognize our own body language.

Assessing behaviors that may precede violence and any other clues about a person's history such as mental illness and drug or alcohol abuse may also help predict violent behavior. Luck, Jackson, and Usher (2007) devised a system that helps identify observable behaviors that indicate the potential for violence. Through their research with emergency department personnel, they created five distinctive elements that portend violent behavior. They use the easily remembered acronym *STAMP* to outline cues for an assessment of the behaviors (Box 25-8).

BOX 25-8	STAMP ASSESSMENT COMPONENTS AND CUES	
ASSESSMENT COMPONENT	**ASSESSMENT CUE**
Staring	Prolonged glaring at the nurse while she/he is engaged in nursing practice
Tone and volume of voice	Sharp or caustic retorts
	Sarcasm
	Demeaning inflection
	Increase in volume
Anxiety	Flushed appearance
	Hyperventilation
	Rapid speech
	Dilated pupils
	Physical indicators of pain: grimacing, writhing, clutching body
	Confusion and disorientation
	Expressed lack of understanding about emergency department processes
Mumbling	Talking "under their breath"
	Criticizing staff or the institution just loudly enough to be heard
	Repetition of same or similar questions or requests
	Slurring or incoherent speech
Pacing	Walking around confined areas such as a waiting room or bed space
	Walking back and forth to the nurses' area
	Flailing around in bed
	"Resisting" health care

From Luck, L., Jackson, D., & Usher, K. (2007). STAMP: Components of observable behavior that indicate potential for patient violence in emergency departments. *Journal of Advanced Nursing, 59*(1), 11-19, Blackwell Publishing Ltd.

Often a violent act is preceded by a threat. A threat may be explicit or veiled, spoken or unspoken, specific or vague. It may be an offhanded remark or comments made to people close to the patient or family that may suggest problematic behavior. Detecting threats and/or threatening behavior, evaluating them, and finding a way to address them are important keys to preventing violence. All staff members need to be educated on how to detect threatening behavior and how to report it. All threats should be evaluated to determine when someone is making a threat versus posing a threat. In most cases, a threat will not lead to a violent act, but it still requires a response. The goal of threat assessment is to determine its severity and plan an appropriate intervention.

Personal Safety Training

People are more likely to survive any life-threatening situation when they confront reality and develop a plan. This requires preparation and thinking logically. Frequent training and rehearsal of what to do in a particular situation can help remain clearheaded when fear kicks in. Knowing whom to call, what escape routes are available, and how to defuse violent situations provides readily accessible skills when violent events occur.

Most training on workplace violence prevention is based on basic self-defense techniques that are important for everyone to know. This type of training consists primarily of using common sense and awareness to avoid potentially dangerous situations. Key points are (1) being constantly aware of surroundings and (2) planning ahead or thinking about potential problems and how to respond. Knowing how to call for help or memorizing code names for emergency situations is part of this preparation. Assessing work areas for potential security problems and how to escape if trapped in particular areas is key. Running different scenarios mentally helps create more rapid and safer responses. Assessing how to respond in tense situations can be helpful and provide insight into personal behavior that would escalate a situation. Learning how to project confidence and not being afraid to yell for help are also simple self-defense techniques that everyone can use.

Other conflict-management techniques that can be taught include defusing the aggressive individual. This technique is grounded in basic therapeutic communication theory. The goal is to manage situations in which people experience an escalation of emotion that may lead to violence. De-escalation can reduce the level of tension to the point at which the person under stress can regain control and avoid violence. To defuse situations, remain rational in the face of the irrational. If the affected person senses a prospective victim is losing control, it will increase his or her anxiety and loss of control. Understanding how you handle your own stress can influence your ability to effectively de-escalate others. By practicing therapeutic communication techniques, it is possible to more readily assess the behaviors so that, in a crisis, you can use your skills without freezing. Most important to remember is to look and act calm even if such is not the case. Helping

someone stay calm is often easier if you appear warm and approachable. The person you are de-escalating will notice and take cues from your behaviors, even if he or she is too irrational to hear your words.

People exhibit some identifiable elements of escalation when they become upset. Challenging authority or asking questions that may not seem related to the situation is one common behavior. Another is to refuse or balk when given directions. A person may also temporarily lose some control and use words he or she may not normally use. The agitated person may even become threatening or intimidating. This agitation can rapidly turn life-threatening, so it is important to gain control of the situation quickly. As the situation escalates, you must retain your professionalism. If you become defensive or irrational, the situation only gets worse. It is often easier to react in a professional manner if you are not alone. Using the buddy system can be an easy way to help you retain your professionalism and reduce the chance of injury. Caution must be used when additional people come into an aggressive situation. The aggressor may become more agitated if he or she feels that people are ganging up. On the other hand, a witness may cause the aggressor to reconsider his or her behavior and regain control. One way to help those who are out of control is to validate or empathize with them. When we empathize with others, we are considering their needs and feelings. Expressing empathy helps the other person feel understood. Often, repeating the *feelings* you hear rather than the *content of what was said* is a good strategy. This can highlight the speaker's concerns and fears and may help him or her begin to mentally process what is happening. This validation is powerful in de-escalating a situation. Keeping a calm tone of voice and a relaxed posture can help an agitated person hear the content of your message. Another way to demonstrate we are in control and responsive is to make sure our words and actions are congruent. This means that our words and actions communicate the same thing and form a clear message. For example, nodding and paying attention to the person talking to you is congruent with both sending the message that you would like to hear more and that you are listening. Being incongruent or acting in a way that does not match your words may be interpreted as being untrustworthy or inauthentic. For example, saying "I want to help you" while looking repeatedly at your watch sends a mixed message to the person you are trying to help.

Body language can be used to de-escalate situations. Most communication is nonverbal and involves body language. A basic awareness of body language of people under stress is useful. For example, when someone is upset, his or her personal space tends to increase. The best way to ensure that you are not invading the personal space of others is to stand at an angle to the person, slightly outside his or her personal space (usually about 3 feet or so in the U.S. culture), rather than face to face. Your shoulders should be at about a 90-degree angle to the person to whom you are talking. Keep your arms relaxed and at your sides, and stand with your feet slightly parted. Again, if your body language is aggressive, it may further escalate a situation. You should also be aware of your relationship to an exit. An agitated person may become more aggressive if he or she feels his or her escape from an area is being blocked. You do not want to be the person blocking an exit route if the person does decide to attack. Gender and culture may influence a situation and how you use eye contact, touching, or head movements. It is also important to assess the body language of potentially violent persons, looking for clues as to what they may do next or when they may become violent. Pounding or clenching fists or pointing fingers may indicate the person is about to physically lash out. If these warning signs are present, it may be time to disengage and find help. If you are the one being threatened, any one of these techniques may buy the time needed to get out. The key is to recognize the signs and take action to de-escalate the situation.

EXERCISE 25-4

Have you ever received training from your employer on workplace violence? Would you feel comfortable asking for training from your manager? What type of training would you want?

After a Violent Event

Violence can and will occur despite best efforts at prevention. Like all violent crime, workplace violence creates ripples that go beyond what is done to a particular victim. It damages trust and the sense of security every worker has a right to feel while on the job. In that sense, everyone loses when a violent act takes place. When it does occur, leaders must be prepared to deal with the consequences by providing an environment that fosters honest communication and

support. Lack of commitment in addressing violence can lead to economic loss in the form of high turnover rates, lost work time, damaged employee morale, and reduced productivity. In addition, the organization could face possible legal action from state and federal agencies, increased workers' compensation payments, medical expenses, and possible lawsuits and liability costs. Employees who have been harmed at work in an act of violence should receive assistance with any documentation needed to receive necessary health care. Psychological and other supportive therapies should be offered, and the victims should avail themselves of these services.

When a violent event occurs, the organization should take immediate action to prevent recurrence. An investigation should always follow any violent event to determine if new emergency procedures need to be implemented and if any existing policies or procedures need to be changed to protect staff. Any staff member involved in a violent incident should be supported and offered counseling. Care should be taken to determine if the problem may be related to underreporting of warning signs. Staff of the affected areas should be involved with the investigation and should be given as much information as possible to ensure that they know that the safety issue is being addressed. Additional training should be offered. Existing training should be evaluated to determine if it addresses current situations. Advice from safety experts should be sought to ensure that interventions are addressing any problem areas. This will help the organization keep abreast of new strategies for dealing with workplace violence as they develop.

Finally, the success of safety interventions should be regularly evaluated. An evaluation program should examine the reporting system for incidents to determine whether problems exist with not identifying situations because of underreporting. Data related to the frequency and severity of workplace violence and the subsequent interventions should be examined along

---

EXERCISE 25-5

You have been asked to help an inner-city hospital. The administration staff has advised you that the current safety plan may not be adequate because several incidents have occurred in the hospital in the past year involving violent attacks on staff members. How would you go about conducting an assessment of the facility? What types of things would you look for? What tools would you use to guide your assessment?

---

with the outcomes to determine if changes need to be made. Staff surveys before and after implementing safety interventions should be assessed. The question is do they believe the intervention made a difference?

Employees have the right to expect a safe work environment, but they are also expected to participate in active prevention through gaining knowledge of safety policies, participating in training, and reporting potential problems. Through communication and attention to problems, organizations can foster a climate of trust and respect among workers and between employees and management. This helps reduce the potential for toxic work environments that can allow horizontal violence to flourish.

CONCLUSION

Workplace violence affects us all. Its burden is borne not only by victims of violence but also by their co-workers, their families, their employers, and patients. Although we know that each year workplace violence results nationwide in hundreds of deaths and more than 2 million injuries, it also creates billions of dollars of waste in lost productivity, reduced quality of care, and errors. Our understanding of workplace violence in health care is still in its infancy. Much remains to be done in the area of research, particularly in data collection and interventions for horizontal violence. Without basic information on who is most affected and which prevention measures are effective in what settings, we can expect only limited success in addressing this problem. The first steps have been taken, but a number of key issues have been identified that require future research. All nurses and healthcare leaders need a broader understanding of the scope and impact of workplace violence to reduce the human and financial burden of this significant public health problem.

THE SOLUTION

A team was formed that consisted of the director of security; clinical manager; directors of the emergency department, plant operations safety, and risk management; and numerous other stakeholders. We did an analysis of the event and a comprehensive security assessment. One of our major findings was that there were staff panic buttons in the front treatment areas but not in the back "crash" area where the incident occurred. We also realized that the existing panic buttons were near the heads of the beds but needed to be away from the reach of the patient. We made a lot of changes in the physical layout of the emergency department to enhance security, but we realized this was only part of the solution.

Next we devised a method to identify a potentially violent patient and make sure this information was communicated through each patient hand off. Our existing high alert program indicates previously reported and potential risk behaviors of known patients with different levels. Level 4 indicated no issues. Level 3 indicated patients with suspected narcotic-seeking behavior, previous abusive behavior, or other medical conditions that could increase the potential for violent behavior. Level 2 specified patients who had attempted suicide while hospitalized. Level 1 indicated homicidal behavior such as making threats with a weapon or a history of physical assault. The level is noted in the medical record, indicated on the patient's wristband and on all patient chart labels. Although the emergency department staff was very familiar with the high alert program, we found that this was not the case in the acute care setting.

To ensure that the high alert program was understood throughout the facility, we developed an algorithm that included high alert program levels as well as other prompting questions to identify potential safety threats. If issues are identified, protocols are triggered to ensure appropriate interventions. One intervention is a gray flag, used at the room door to notify staff of the safety risk and to enter only in pairs. The staff knows the meaning of the gray flag; for visitors or others who may ask, the gray flag is to indicate the patient is not to be disturbed. Reduction of disruptions and the pair staff approach decreases the potential for a violent event. The gray flag icon also appears on the bed board in the emergency department with the potentially violent patient's room highlighted in aqua. This alerts security staff to round more frequently in those areas. This also makes everyone in the department aware of the security risks. Security is now part of hand-off communication, notifying staff when at-risk patients are transferred to any other area in the facility.

We also started communicating our zero tolerance for violence with a poster campaign. Around that same time, a bill was moving through the Texas Legislature aimed at increasing the penalty from a misdemeanor to a felony for anyone who injures an emergency services worker. The bill passed at the end of the session, allowing us to strengthen the message that we will not tolerate injury to our staff.

Lastly, we looked at the support available to staff who were victims of violence by patients. We have psychological services available to help them with any issues they may have as the result of an attack or injury.

We are two years into this process. As we go along we are discovering other ways to improve safety and focus on prevention of violent events.

—*The ED Staff and Safety Manager*

Would this be a suitable approach for you? Why?

THE EVIDENCE

Workplace violence is recognized as a significant problem within health care, whether the threat comes from within the organization or from the outside. Reviews of nursing literature indicate that violence and incivility in the workplace is a significant reason why nurses leave their jobs and, in some cases, the profession. With continued concern about a nursing shortage and growing awareness that violence in any form impacts the safety and quality of care, nurse leaders need to implement effective intervention programs to foster a safe and civil workplace. Direct care nurses need to have an awareness of how to identify and prevent bullying or lateral aggression so cultures of incivility can be eradicated. The impact of not taking action will be a higher cost of care, greater risk to patients, and potentially a critical decrease in the nursing workforce.

WHAT NEW GRADUATES SAY

• I was just starting my residency program and was in that place after you get your license where you realize you know just enough to be dangerous. I was feeling insecure and asked my preceptor lots of questions. Each time she rolled her eyes at me and asked "What <u>do</u> you know?" It made me not want to ask her any questions. I kept wondering what I would do if I really needed help. I made a pledge to always be a friend and support to the new graduates.

• As a new grad I felt I had to prove myself to fit into the unit where I was first hired. I took on the harder patients and I had to be there earlier and stay later than everyone else. I got really burned out that year. During the course of the year I floated to a different unit and experienced a totally different environment. The nurses were supportive of one another, the manager responded to conflicts and mediated solutions. There was a real sense of teamwork. I am glad to say that is now where I work; I am back to loving my job!

• I started my healthcare career as an RN in the emergency department. As a new nurse, I observed great differences in how the experienced nursing staff managed difficult patients. Some nurses seemed to be able to manage hostile patients with patience, calmness, and sometimes humor. Other nurses seemed to have great difficulty with patients that would escalate to the point where security needed to be called. I am trying to learn from the seasoned nurses who handle these situations with skill. They used communication and body language to keep the situation under control. The best protection is prevention, or stopping the situation from getting out of control.

CHAPTER CHECKLIST

This chapter focused on two kinds of workplace violence: physical attacks and bullying. Nursing research indicates violence in any form can drain nurses of their enthusiasm for their work and undermines efforts to create a satisfied workforce. It also impacts the quality of care and patient safety. At a time when we are facing a nursing shortage and skyrocketing healthcare costs, preventing or eliminating violence is paramount. All nurses—leaders, managers, and followers—must be aware of the potential for all forms of violence and strive to not participate in horizontal violence, which weakens us as a profession. The key to preventing violence is to understand the potential and implement interventions to minimize that potential.

• Defining workplace violence and incivility
• Scope of the problem
• The cost of workplace violence
• Ensuring a safe workplace
• Making a difference
• Prevention strategies
  • Types of violence
  • Risk assessment
  • Firing right
• Horizontal violence: The threat from within
  • Increasing awareness of horizontal violence
  • Education

- Developing a safety plan
  - Administrative
  - Environmental
  - Interpersonal

- Understanding the potential for violence
- Personal safety training
- After a violent event

▌ TIPS FOR PREVENTING WORKPLACE VIOLENCE

- Take a self-defense course to help you develop other skills to keep you safe at work and elsewhere.
- Take advantage of training offered on workplace violence. If training is not offered, ask your employer to consider providing it.

- Make a personal commitment to not participate in any behaviors that perpetuate horizontal violence.
- Practice precautionary strategies such as the STAMP assessment.
- Analyze workplaces for safety risk factors using the checklists provided by OSHA.

REFERENCES

Agarwal, R., Sands, D. Z., & Diaz-Schneider, J. (2008). *Quantifying the economic impact of communication inefficiencies in US Hospitals.* Winter College Park, MD: University of Maryland Center for Health Information and Decision Systems, CHIDS Research Briefing, 3(18).

American Nurses Association. (2002). *Promoting safe work environments for nurses.* From Occupational Safety and Health Administration (OSHA). (2004). Guidelines for preventing workplace violence for health care and social service workers (OSHA Publication No. 3148-01R) Washington, DC: U.S. Department of Labor. www.osha.gov.

American Nurses Association. (2010). *Hostility, abuse and bullying in the workplace. 2010 House of delegates resolution. Bullying and lateral violence examples of bullying behavior pocket card.* Retrieved February 15, 2013, from http://nursingworld. org/MainMenuCategories/CertificationandAccreditation/ Continuing-Professional-Development/NavigateNursing/ AboutNN/Tip-Card-Bullying-and-Lateral-Violence-ANA.pdf.

American Nurses Association. (2012). *Nationwide state legislative Agenda: Workplace violence map.* Retrieved February 15, 2013 from, http://nursingworld.org/MainMenuCategories/ Policy-Advocacy/State/Legislative-Agenda-Reports/ State-WorkplaceViolence.

Bureau of Labor Statistics, U.S. Department of Labor. (2012a). *Census of fatal occupational injuries.* USDL 12-1888. Retrieved May 15, 2013, from www.bls.gov/iif/oshcfoi1.htm.

Bureau of Labor Statistics, U.S. Department of Labor. (2012b). *Nonfatal occupational injuries and illnesses requiring days away from work, 2011.* USDL 12-2204 . Retrieved May 15, 2013, from www.bls.gov/news.release/pdf/osh2.pdf.

DeBecker, G. (2000). *The gift of fear: Survival signals that protect us from violence.* New York: Little, Brown and Co.

Dellasega, C. (2009). Bullying among nurses. *American Journal of Nursing, 109*(1), 52–58.

Dellasega, C. (2011). *When nurses hurt nurses: Recognizing and overcoming the cycle of bullying.* Indiana: Sigma Theta Tau International.

DeVito, J. A. (2008). *Essentials of human communication* (6th ed.). Boston, MA: Pearson, Allyn and Bacon.

Farrell, G. (2001). From tall poppies to squashed weeds: Why don't nurses pull together more? *Journal of Advanced Nursing, 35*(1), 26–33.

Freire, P. (2003). *Pedaogogy of the oppressed* (30th ed.). New York, NY: International Publishing Group.

Gacki-Smith, J., Juarez, A. M., & Boyett, L. (2009). Violence against nurses working in U.S. emergency departments. *The Journal of Nursing Administration, 39*(7/8), 340–349.

Gates, D. M., Gillespie, G. L., & Succop, P. (2011). Violence against nurses and its impact on stress and productivity. *Nursing Economics, 29*(2), 59–67.

Gallant-Roman, M. (2008). Strategies and tools to reduce workplace violence. *American Association of Occupational Health Nurses, 56*(11), 449–454.

Griffin, M. (2004). Teaching cognitive rehearsal as a shield for lateral violence: An intervention for newly licensed nurses. *Journal of Continuing Education in Nursing, 35*(6), 257–263.

Hartley, D., & Ridenour, M. (2011, September 13). *Workplace violence in the healthcare setting.* Medscape. Retrieved February 15, 2013 from www.medscape.com/viewarticle/749441_print.

Hartley, D., Ridenour, M., Craine, J., & Costa, B. (2012). Workplace violence prevention for healthcare workers: An online course. *Rehabilitation Nursing, 37*(4), 202–206.

Holloway, L. E., & Kusy, M. E. (2010, May/June). Disruptive and toxic behaviors in healthcare: Zero tolerance, the bottom line, and what to do about it. *Medical Practice Management, 25*(6), 335–340.

Hutchinson, M., Vickers, M., Jackson, D., & Wilkes, L. (2006). Workplace bullying in nursing: Towards a more critical organizational perspective. *Nursing Inquiry, 15*, 118–126.

Iowa Injury Prevention Research Center (IIPRC). (February 2001). *Workplace violence: A report to the nation.* University of Iowa— Iowa City. Retrieved May 15, 2013, from www.public-health. uiowa.edu/iprc/resources/workplace-violence-report.pdf.

Johansen, M.L. (2012). Keeping the peace: Conflict management strategies for nurse managers. *Nursing Management, 43*(2), 50–54.

Johnson, S. (2009). Workplace bullying: Concerns for nurse leaders. *Journal of Nursing Administration, 39*(2), 84–90.

Lewis, P. S., & Malecha, A. (2011). The impact of workplace incivility on the work environment, manager skill and productivity. *The Journal of Nursing Administration, 41*(1), 41–47.

Longo, J. (2007). Leveling horizontal violence. *Nursing Management, 38*(3), 34–37, 50–51.

Luck, L., Jackson, D., & Usher, K. (March 2007). STAMP: Components of observable behavior that indicate potential for patient violence in emergency departments. *Journal of Advanced Nursing, 59*(1), 11–19.

Maslow, A. H. (1943). A theory of human motivation. *Psychological Review, 50*(4), 370–396.

Monahan, J. (1981). *Predicting violent behavior: An assessment of clinical techniques.* Beverly Hills, CA: Sage.

Occupational Safety and Health Administration (OSHA). (2004). *Guidelines for preventing workplace violence for health care and social service workers.* (OSHA Publication No. 3148-01R) Washington, DC: U.S. Department of Labor.

Occupational Safety & Health Act (OSH Act). (1970). *Public Law 91-596, 84 STAT. 1590, Section 5. 91st Congress, S.2193, December 29, 1970.* as amended through January 1, 2004 .

Occupational Safety and Health Administration (OSHA). (2013). *Workplace violence.* Retrieved from www.osha.gov/SLTC/workplaceviolence/.

Paludi, M., Nydegger, R., & Paludi, C. (2006). *Understanding workplace violence: A guide for managers and employees.* Westport, Connecticut: Praeger.

Papa, A., & Venella, J. (2013). Workplace violence in healthcare: Strategies for advocacy. *The Online Journal of Issues in Nursing, 18*(1), 1–10.

Pearson, C., & Porath, C. (2009). *The cost of bad behavior: How incivility is damaging your business and what to do about it.* London: Portfolio.

Porto, G., & Lauve, R. (2006, July/August). *Disruptive clinical behavior: A persistent threat to patient safety.* Patient Safety and Quality Healthcare. Retrieved February 15, 2013, from www.psqh.com/julaug06/disruptive.html.

Purpora, C., & Blegen, M. A. (2012). Horizontal violence and the quality and safety of patient care: A conceptual model. *Nursing Research and Practice,* 2012:306948.

Reason, J. (2000). Human error: Models and management. *British Medical Journal, 320*(7237), 768–770.

Roberts, S. J., Demarco, R., & Griffin, M. (2009). The effect of oppressed group behaviors on the culture of the nursing workplace: A review of the evidence and interventions for change. *Journal of Nursing Management, 17,* 288–293.

Rosenstein, A. H. (2010). Measuring and managing the economic impact of disruptive behaviors in the hospital. *Journal of Healthcare Risk Management, 30*(2), 20–26.

Shields, M., & Wilkins, K. (2009). Factors related to on-the-job abuse of nurses by patients. *Health Report, 20*(7), 7–19.

Stokowski, L. A. (2010, August 23). *Violence: Not in my job description.* Medscape. Retrieved February 15, 2013, from www.medscape.com/viewarticle/727144/print.

The Joint Commission (TJC). (2008). Behaviors that undermine a culture of safety. *Sentinel Event Alert,* (40). Retrieved May 15, 2013, from www.jointcommission.org/assets/1/18/SEA_40.PDF.

The Joint Commission (TJC). (2010). Preventing violence in the health care setting. *Sentinel Event Alert,* (45). Retrieved May 15, 2013, from www.jointcommission.org/assets/1/18/sea_45.pdf.

Winfeld, L. (2001). *Training tough topics.* New York: American Management Association.

Woelfle, C., & McCaffrey, R. (2007). Nurse on nurse. *Nursing Forum, 42*(3), 123–131.

SUGGESTED READINGS

Colling, R. L., & York, T. W. (2010). *Hospital and healthcare security* (5th ed). Burlington, Massachusetts: Elsevier.

Dellasega, C. (2011). *When nurses hurt nurses: Recognizing and overcoming the cycle of bullying.* Indianapolis: Sigma Theta Tau International.

Holloway, E. L., & Kusy, M. E. (2009). *Toxic workplace! Managing toxic personalities and their systems of power.* San Francisco: Jossey-Bass.

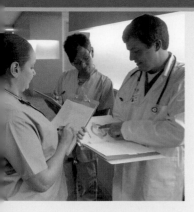

Delegation: An Art of Professional Nursing Practice

Maureen Murphy-Ruocco

Delegation, a multifaceted decision-making process, is a learned leadership behavior acquired by understanding the art of delegation, developing critical judgment skills, and applying delegation decisions in clinical nursing practice. The overall purpose of delegation is to achieve nursing goals and improve patient care outcomes. Registered nurses accountable for other staff members work must learn how to master the art of delegation. This chapter discusses different aspects of delegation, describes the implementation of effective delegation decisions, and explores the legal parameters of delegation in professional nursing practice. The chapter's emphasis is on the role of registered nurses as delegators, regardless of the formal position they hold in the healthcare organization.

LEARNING OUTCOMES

- Define delegation.
- Understand the five rights of delegation.
- Explain the different components of delegation.
- Understand the role of unlicensed nursing personnel/unlicensed assistive personnel (UNP/UAP) in the delivery of health care.
- Differentiate between assignments and tasks in the delegation process.
- Evaluate how tasks and relationships influence the process of delegation.
- Examine the role of the registered professional nurse in delivering high-quality health care.
- Discuss the complexity of delegation decisions for registered nurses.
- Comprehend the legal authority of the registered nurse in delegation.

KEY TERMS

Accountability
Active delegation
Authority
Delegatee
Delegation
Delegator

Individual Accountability
Licensed practical nurse (LPN)/
   licensed vocational nurse
   (LVN)
Organizational accountability
Patient care associate (PCA)

Passive delegation
Responsibility
Supervision
Unlicensed nursing personnel
   (UNP)/unlicensed assistive
   personnel (UAP)

THE CHALLENGE

Kathryn King-Dyker, RN, MSN, CSN
Former Emergency Trauma Nurse, Hackensack University
Medical Center, Hackensack, New Jersey

Not all emergency trauma care centers are created equally. Trauma centers are classified from Level 1 to 5, with Level 1 being the most equipped to meet the needs of critically ill patients. Emergency medical technicians (EMTs) often transport patients to hospital emergency trauma centers by ambulance, or patients are transported by a family member or friend.

Hospital emergency trauma centers are staffed by physicians, registered professional nurses, radiology technicians, respiratory therapists, emergency technicians, transportation aides, clerks, and secretaries. When a patient arrives at a hospital emergency trauma center, critically injured patients should be immediately triaged by a registered nurse to determine the nature and acuity of their illness/injury. The challenge is to assess the patient's condition and provide

emergency health care. If necessary, they must stabilize and transfer the patient to the most appropriate facility.

Recently, the emergency trauma department has been expanded and needs to accommodate 15 more patients. To support patient care, the hospital administration hired additional staff, unlicensed nursing personnel (UNP), whose positions were being phased out in their free standing urgent care center, and employed them as emergency room technicians. The next emergency technician training program will not begin for 2 months. Therefore the new UNPs will be working as emergency room technicians in the emergency department before they are trained.

The emergency department received a call that an explosion at a local chemical plant just occurred. The emergency medical services will be arriving with multiple patients injured in the accident.

What do you think you would do if you were this nurse?

INTRODUCTION

Delegation, an art and skill of professional nursing, is a complex decision-making strategy implemented to improve the work-related performance of the staff employed in health care organizations. Learning how to distribute work appropriately builds the staff members' confidence about caring for groups of patients safely and effectively. Conversely, inappropriate delegation of tasks creates apprehension in staff members' about caring for the same group of patients. Therefore delegation used effectively improves patient care outcomes; used ineffectively it can produce negative effects on patient care delivery. The development of delegation skills and strategies often improve as the registered nurse gains more clinical experience and transitions from novice, advanced beginner, competent, proficient, to expert (Benner & Benner, 1984). Delegation is the most effective professional management strategy registered nurses (RNs) implement in clinical practice to improve the safety and quality of patient care.

HISTORICAL PERSPECTIVE

Until the early 1970s, registered nurses were somewhat familiar with the concept of delegation. At that time, the majority of patient care delivery occurred in acute care hospitals, which were staffed by registered nurses (primarily diploma nursing graduates prepared in

hospital-based nursing programs), licensed practical nurses/licensed vocational nurses (LPNs/LVNs) and nurses' aides (commonly known today as unlicensed assistive personnel [UAP], unlicensed nursing personnel [UNP], or patient care associate [PCA]). UNPs provide direct patient care under the supervision of the registered nurse who retains accountability for patient care outcomes.

Historically, concepts such as "team nursing" and "staffing ratios" permitted LPNs/LVNs and nurses' aides to function as part of a staff on nursing units, limiting the number of registered nurses employed on the unit. This allowed a large portion of direct patient care to be provided by LPNs/LVNs, and nurses' aides. During that time, direct patient care included providing physical comforts and basic treatments to patients. As health care advanced, patient care and treatments became more complex.

As the complexities of patient care delivery increased, the work demands and expectations of registered nurses became more challenging and created the need to provide a higher staff ratio of registered nurses to UNPs to support patient care. During the 1970s and 1980s, many nurses entered the profession with relatively limited content knowledge and/or clinical experience about how, what, and when to delegate to others.

In the mid-1990s, a dramatic shift from a model of primary nursing (an all professional nursing concept), to a multilevel nursing model (registered nurses mixed with LPNs/LVNs, and UNP) occurred. Fiscal constraints and the new complexities in health care created an urgent need for nurses to learn more about how to use effective delegation skills to deliver safe and effective nursing care. As the healthcare industry emphasized community-based care, delegation and supervision of staff became even more challenging. Today, a comprehensive knowledge base in delegation, and diagnostic reasoning and decision-making skills in clinical practice are required to provide expert nursing care.

During the early part of the twenty-first century, the American Nurses Association (ANA) and the National Council of State Boards of Nursing (NCSBN) became increasingly concerned about the quality of the delegation decisions. The NCSBN stated that the "State Boards of Nursing should regulate nursing assistive personnel across multiple settings" (NCSBN, 2005, p. 160). It became evident that the approach in many states to regulate and certify nursing assistants in hospitals and/or health care facilities no longer met the needs of nursing. In addition, the NCSBN added an expectation that the basic education for nursing assistive personnel include an emphasis on how to receive delegation from nurses (NCSBN, 2005). The ANA (2005) outlined the principles of delegation for registered nurses. The ANA and the NCSBN (2006) collaboratively published a joint statement that serves as general guidelines for delegation decisions for registered nurse practice. The joint statement explains that the authority for delegation resides within the Nurse Practice Act of each state, examines the value of unlicensed personnel in patient care delivery, and declares that the importance of delegation decisions is safety and welfare of the public. The joint statement acknowledged that the decision to delegate should be based on multiple factors such as the patient's condition, complexity of the task to be performed, and predictability of outcomes. Nurses need to understand that the "pervasive functions of assessment, planning, evaluation and nursing judgment cannot be delegated" (NCSBN, 2005 p. 1). Principles of Delegation (ANA, 2012) outline what nurses need to know and do in relation to this complex task.

In the past, nursing content knowledge related to the principles of delegation, and successful strategies on how to delegate had not been a major focus in schools of nursing, especially as it related to nursing delegation in the community health setting. Nursing leaders also acknowledged that new nurses were not adequately prepared to master delegation decisions. Because of the changing healthcare delivery system, faculty in schools of nursing must teach, mentor, and develop students' competencies in delegation. These competencies can be developed through different teaching learning strategies, such as didactic content, case studies, simulated experiences, online learning, and clinical nursing practica. Students' proficiency in delegation is "greatly improved by pairing the active learning didactics from education and the clinical experience from the healthcare practice site" (Powell, 2011, p. 10). The nursing practicum experiences foster the application of theory to practice, the development of clinical judgment, and the ability to comprehend the legal authority of delegation decisions. Early in the nurse's career, high-quality clinical delegation experiences and engagement with a nursing mentor foster professional self-confidence. These experiences advance the nurse's ability to become a successful delegator and broker of patient care resources (Weydt, 2010). Delegation knowledge should also be reinforced in nursing continuing education programs. (Kaernested & Bragadóttir, 2012). These educational opportunities are essential to further develop "delegation and supervisory strategies to adapt to the RNs changing role" (Saccomano & Pinto-Zipp, 2011, p. 532).

Delegation can be further complicated by other factors such as age, gender, and ethnicity. Younger generations, for instance, have a different view of the world and are often more open and flexible regarding change than older generations. Gender may play a role in learning delegation skills. The women's movement and feminism have assisted female nurses in becoming "assertive and autonomous" (Harmer, 2010, p. 298). However, it appears that the "minority gender achieves a proportionally better and higher status than the traditional female nurse" (Harmer, 2010, p. 297). Ethnicity also plays a role in the process of delegation because individuals from diverse cultures perceive information and their ability to direct others to perform tasks differently.

The need to increase the number of staff, especially UNPs, was usually directly related to the shortage of nurses. Today, with 50% of registered nurses near retirement age, an increase in medical and healthcare needs of individuals approaching 65 years of age, a greater emphasis on preventive health care, advances in medical technology, and recent healthcare reform that provides millions of individuals access to health care, another shortage of nurses and other healthcare professionals is predicted (ANA, 2013). Because of the potential challenges related to the supply of RNs and cost-effectiveness in health care, the role of RNs must change to meet the growing demands for patient care delivery. A nursing shortage is a "global challenge affecting every country in the world" (Littlejohn, Campbell, Collins-McNeil, & Khayile, 2012). The shortage will grow to one million nurses in the United States by 2020, and employment of RNs is expected to grow 26% from 2010 to 2020, faster than average for most occupations (U.S. Bureau of Labor Statistics, 2012). The registered nurses' ability to delegate, assign, supervise and be ultimately accountable for providing safe, competent, and effective patient care are critical competencies for the twenty-first century nurse. Nursing's ability to acclimate to new advances in health care will allow us to survive, often thrive, and be more effective as a profession.

DEFINITIONS

Delegation, a multifaceted decision-making process, has multiple definitions; however, all definitions have some consistent elements. The principles of effective delegation are derived from the corresponding states' nurse practice act and through an understanding of the key concepts of responsibility, authority, and accountability (Weydt, 2010). *Delegation* is defined as the "transfer of responsibility for the performance of a task from one individual to another while retaining the accountability for the outcome" (ANA, 2012, p. 6). The NCSBN defines delegation as an "act of transferring to a competent individual the authority to perform a selected nursing task in a selected situation" (NCSBN, 2005, p. 1). ANA and NCSBN collaboratively define delegation as the "process for the nurse to direct another person to perform nursing tasks and activities" (ANA & NCSBN, 2006, p. 1). Delegation always involves at least two individuals (delegator and delegatee) who engage in open communication to achieve a goal. The terms delegator and delegatee represent the two key roles enacted in

the process of delegation. Delegators are registered nurses who allocate a portion of work related to patient care to another individual. Delegatees are often comprised of UNPs, often called assistants, technicians, patient care associates, or aides. Although registered nurses do not supervise all unlicensed assistive personnel (e.g., physical therapy technicians), they have exchanges regarding patient care with UNPs and LPNs/LVNs. Some states have different delegation standards depending on the type of healthcare facility. For example, a long-term care facility may have an LPN/LVN responsible for a nursing unit with a registered nurse supervising the patient care. Nurses need to understand the nurse practice acts of their states, understand the delegation standard related to individual job descriptions, and function within their states' regulatory guidelines.

Responsibility refers to the reliability, dependability and obligation to accomplish work. It is a "two way process that is allocated and accepted" (Weydt, 2010, p. 3). Authority is the ability to perform duties in a specific role. Each individual is obligated to perform to the best of his or her ability and at a quality level. These individuals are also responsible for informing the delegator about any limitations that may prevent the accomplishment of the task or fulfillment of the expected outcome. In contrast, accountability determines if the actions were appropriate and provides a detailed explanation of what occurred (ANA, 2012; Weydt, 2010). The delegator discusses with the delegatee what tasks must be completed and transfers the responsibility and authority for those tasks to the delegatee. Even though the delegatee performs a task related to patient care, the registered nurse does not abandon the patient or the accountability for patient care. It is essential that the registered nurse complete a critical analysis, using the nursing process, to determine if the actions taken in a situation were appropriate, and if not, what occurred and why.

In contrast, *legal authority*, by virtue of the professional nursing license, is the ability to transfer selected nursing activities in a given situation to a competent individual (Anthony & Vidal, 2010). When a nurse gives the delegatee the responsibility and authority for completing a task, the nurse retains accountability for ensuring that the task is completed by the right person and that person is supervised appropriately. Supervision is defined as the "provision of guidance and oversight of a delegated nursing task" (ANA & NCSBN, 2006, p. 1). Open lines of communication must occur between the delegator and delegatee to eliminate any misunderstanding about delegated tasks. The application of essential delegation skills is necessary for effective nursing management and high quality patient care outcomes.

Figure 26-1 describes how delegated work is transferred along with the responsibility and authority to the delegatee; however, the nurses' accountability remains constant. Communication must be clear, concise, timely, and reliable to produce safe and successful patient care outcomes. For example, when Hurricane Irene damaged much of the Caribbean and East Coast of the United States in 2011, and Hurricane Sandy damaged parts of the Caribbean, Mid-Atlantic and Northeastern United States in 2012, important lessons emerged about providing health care in a natural disaster. Communication, between and among healthcare professions and among state and national agencies, was the most critical factor in determining when and how to evacuate safely and effectively (U.S. Bureau of Labor Statistics, 2012).

Delegation

The ANA and NCSBN (2006) joint statement illustrates the process of delegation and describes how registered nurses must learn to delegate the right task, under the right circumstances, to the right person, with the right direction and communication, and under the right supervision and evaluation. Table 26-1 describes the Five Rights of Delegation, specific questions to ascertain before delegating, and a "yes" response if the delegation is appropriate.

Delegation is achieving performance of care outcomes by sharing activities with others who have the appropriate authority to accomplish the work. In this process, acceptance of the delegated work must occur either actively (i.e., communication indicates acceptance) or passively (i.e., no protest occurs). Delegation occurs only when two people are involved in a mutual work situation and one of the individuals has accountability and the other has some authority to perform the specific tasks.

Delegation to UNPs can be challenging. Today, UNPs are educated in a formal program of study; however, the programs still vary in length from 1 week to several weeks. The position descriptions of UNPs define the authority for the specific position. The educational preparation and job description of UNPs are not consistent and remain a concern. NCSBN (2005) has expressed concern about the inconsistencies in the educational preparation of UNP and recommends that these educational programs have greater public accountability. A critical component of delegation is authority, and the delegated task must comply with the law, such as the state nurse practice act, and/or comply with the educational preparation and certification of the individual.

Improper follow-through is another concern with delegation. An example of improper follow-through is when the delegator does not provide clear and concise directions to the delegatee. An example of improper follow-through on the part of a delegatee is failure to report results and findings. The nurse's prior knowledge of the delegatee's qualifications and experience related to the task is crucial for safe and successful delegation decisions.

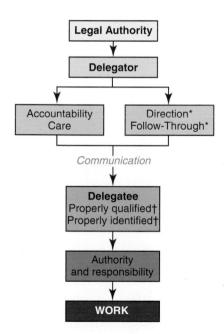

*Two common failures identified by Standing, Anthony, and Hertz (2001).
†Two key recommendations by Fagin (2001).

FIGURE 26-1 A delegation framework: delegation to achieve care outcomes.

TABLE 26-1   THE FIVE RIGHTS OF DELEGATION

DELEGATION RIGHTS	THE RIGHT QUESTIONS (ANSWER THE FOLLOWING QUESTIONS)	YES RESPONSES
Task	• Is the task appropriate to delegate based on institutional policies and procedures? • Is the task legally appropriate to delegate?	The right task
Circumstance	• Is the delegation process appropriate to the situation? • Is the environment conducive to completing the task safely? • Are the equipment and resources available to complete the task? • Do staffing ratios demand the use of high-level delegation strategies? • Does the delegatee have appropriate supervision to complete the task?	The right circumstances
Person	• Is the prospective delegatee a willing and able employee? • Does the delegatee have the knowledge and experience to perform the specific task safely? • Does the delegatee have the expertise to complete the task safely and effectively in relation to the acuity of the patient?	The right person
Direction/communication	• Do the delegator and delegatee understand a common work-related language? (Do terms such as *time frame, patient needs,* and *critical* mean the same to each of them?) • Does the delegator provide clear and concise directions for the task? • Does the delegatee understand the assignment, directions, limitations, and expected results as they relate to the task? • Do the delegator and delegatee know how to maintain open lines of communication for the purpose of questions and feedback? • Does the delegatee understand how, what, and when to report to the delegator?	The right direction/communication
Supervision	• Is it clear that the delegatee will provide feedback related to the task, when appropriate? • Is the delegator able to monitor and evaluate the patient appropriately?	The right supervision

Adopted from American Nurses Association and National Council of State Boards of Nursing. (2006). Joint Statement on delegation. https://www.ncsbn.org/.Jointstatement.pdf and American Nurses Association. (2012). *ANA's principles for delegation by registered nurses to unlicensed assistive personnel.* Silver Spring, Maryland. © 2013 M. Murphy-Ruocco.

Achieving Optimum Outcomes

Achieving optimum performance outcomes is the driving force of all health care. Thus all patient care is based on attaining expected outcomes, whether that care is provided directly by an individual or group of professionals, or shared between professionals and assistants. The communication style of the nurse influences how delegatees respond to assigned tasks and "influences teamwork and relationships" (Weydt, 2010, p. 3).

Anthony and Vidal (2010) explore the effects of mindful communication as an approach to improving delegation and increasing patient safety. They explore "information quality, mindful communication (mindfulness) and mutual trust within the relational context of the delegation … improving the effectiveness of the delegation" (p. 1) Regarding the Five Rights of Delegation, the "right communication and direction" is the cornerstone of delegation and may arguably be the most instrumental in shaping quality and safety outcomes" (Anthony and Vidal, 2010, p. 3). The quality of the communication must be timely, meaningful, understood, and effective. Nurses who provide high quality information in a timely manner in the right context and consider cultural competencies of the delegatee enhance the safety and quality of patient care.

Anthony and Vidal (2010) also describe characteristics of communication that interfere with the delegation process, such as "information decay," that can occur when the patient's health status changes rapidly and specific information loses its value or becomes irrelevant to the patient's condition. An example is a rapid change in one or more of the patient's vital signs: temperature, blood pressure, heart rate, respiratory rate, and pain. When the reported information is decayed or incomplete, it leads to poor clinical judgments that may have adverse effects on patient care. Another characteristic of communication is "information salience," which assesses the quality, meaning, and clarity of the information. Diverse cultural, educational, and experiential backgrounds shape the meaning of information, and therefore, when delegating, the salience of the information that is shared between the delegator and the delegatee must be clearly understood (Anthony & Vidal, 2010).

Healthy work relationships among all personnel, including registered nurses and unlicensed assistive personnel, promote a "synergy between team members, enabling them to work together more effectively" (Weydt, 2010, p. 3). Understanding another individual and developing a trusting relationship are critical components to successful delegation. Trust is developed through gaining "knowledge of one another's capabilities and confidence in their abilities" (Weydt, 2010, p. 5). Delegating with confidence requires considerable trust between two or more individuals to create an effective team. Effective teams agree on specific times to meet to ensure that task achievement occurs within the agreed upon time frame.

Specific time frames may include, but are not limited to, before and after breaks and meals as well as any time when the UNP has any questions or concerns. When working with UNPs, the "delegation potentials are significantly higher when caregivers are paired or partnered, with partnered scenario generally having the highest delegation potential" (Weydt, 2010, p. 6).

Nurses with limited delegation experiences and UNPs with limited clinical experience can misuse valuable resources and diminish patient care outcomes. Nurses who do not trust other individuals and/or are unable to delegate appropriately because they choose to perform the tasks themselves, compromise efficient health care and limit their career opportunities. In the ever-changing healthcare setting, knowing and valuing how to be a successful delegator achieves optimum outcomes.

Individual and Organizational Accountability

Individual accountability is a component of delegation. The term refers to the individuals' ability to explain their actions and results. The Code of Ethics for Nurses, Provision 4 (ANA, 2011), identifies the expectation of accountability and responsibility and specifically references delegation. Legally, the registered nurse has accountability for nursing care. For example, even when some portion of patient care is delegated to someone else, each individual nurse is accountable and responsible for his or her nursing practice, including the decision to delegate and the outcome of the delegated task.

Organizational accountability is another component of delegation. The NCSBN concurs with ANA that the driving principle in decision making is patient (public) safety. Making appropriate decisions depends on how well the organization provides adequate resources, including an appropriate ratio of registered nurses to LPNs/LVNs and UNPs. Successful organizations that have achieved Magnet™ status, through an extensive evaluation process, usually have supportive work environments and assist teams to function effectively. Chief nursing officers (CNOs) are accountable for establishing systems to assess, monitor, verify, and communicate competency requirements related to delegation (NCSBN, 2005).

Sharing Activities with Unlicensed Personnel (UAP/UNP)

During the delegation process, the delegator allocates work to other unlicensed staff and gives them the responsibility to perform the work. When the registered nurse delegates work, he or she is merely sharing a set of functions to ensure quality patient care outcomes. In essence, sharing work does not negate the registered nurse's accountability for the total patient care. The definition of delegation emphasizes that patient care itself is not delegated; only a group of tasks/functions/activities are delegated. Thus the final accountability remains with the delegator. Requesting UNPs to perform a specific task or activity within their scope of function or asking them to perform the same tasks as the previous day can be expected. For delegation to be effective, the nurse must understand that sharing activities is essential to benefit patient care. Professional aspects of care may never be delegated—only basic skills, such as activities of daily living and personal hygiene. In addition, some monitoring and technical skills may be delegated. Some organizations have UNPs with a two-level or three-level designation system, with the higher level designations indicating the ability to perform more skills. As advances in health care continue, more tasks and activities may need to be delegated to assist registered nurses in the delivery of quality patient care.

Span of Control

The registered nurse, the leader of the team, has responsibility for a group of individuals who work on the team. These individuals may include those with no formal preparation or legal recognition (e.g., unit secretary) and those with dependent status (e.g., UNP and LPNs/LVNs who function under the direction of a registered nurse or physician), or those who are designated as being answerable to the delegator (e.g., other RNs or healthcare providers who report to a designated delegator, such as a nurse manager).

Span of control, the number of individuals you are ultimately responsible for, is an important concept to master as you interact with others to achieve optimum patient care. For example, if a nurse has responsibility for 5 staff members, each of whom cares for 10 patients, the registered nurse, in effect, has responsibility for 5 staff members and 50 patients. At first, this may seem overwhelming; however, if patients are in stable condition and the nursing care is somewhat predictable, it may be manageable. When nursing staff are well-prepared providers of routine care and the care environment is limited to a designated area, it makes patient care responsibilities less challenging. If these factors are not consistent, the responsibility for this number of patients may become overwhelming. When nursing staff render a portion of the care, these factors need to be assessed to determine the appropriateness of the patient care workload and whether it can be managed safely and effectively in each clinical situation.

Appropriate Authority

Appropriate authority to perform certain functions comes from various sources. Registered nurses have the appropriate authority to perform certain functions as healthcare providers. This authority is derived from state nurse practice acts and institutional policies. For example, the practice of LPNs/LVNs is defined by state titling or practice acts, as well as by institutional policies. UNPs are prepared to meet a specific set of tasks and the educational preparation of UNPs varies considerably. The education of the UNP, coupled with institutional policies, defines how the UNP may or may not function. Position descriptions should provide more specific details about the level of authority within each role. These elements—the titling or practice acts, position descriptions, and policies—form the expectations for what individuals in certain positions are expected to be able to accomplish safely.

All organizations have descriptors of what tasks may be performed by an individual in a particular position. When a position description contains functions that are normally performed or are an essential part of the practice of a licensed individual (e.g., physician, nurse, pharmacist), the individual functioning in this role performs these functions through passive delegation. Therefore no active delegation decision is made by the registered nurse. In active delegation, the registered nurse assesses the situation, determines what is appropriate for patient care, directs a UNP to perform certain tasks and holds the individual accountable. Even when protocols/policies within organizations indicate that an individual may perform a task on behalf of a registered nurse, the delegatee must be competent to perform the task. This expectation suggests that the delegator makes an initial and ongoing assessment of the delegatee performance as well as an assessment of patient care needs. Furthermore, state laws governing professional nursing practice define what the registered nurse must do when another individual assumes certain tasks.

A FRAMEWORK FOR DELEGATION

Hersey's (2006) Situational Leadership® Model, even though not originally designed for the process of delegation, provides a solid foundation for delegation decisions. The "core competencies of a situational leader are the ability to diagnose the performance, competence and commitment of others, to be flexible and to partner for performance" (Lynch et al., 2011, p. 3). Multiple factors influence the effectiveness of the leader, including an assessment of personality characteristics, and readiness level of the individual as it relates to the type of task and goals to be attained, and specific environmental conditions. Hersey's model (Figure 26-2) describes two factors that need to be assessed to determine the level of the followers' readiness: ability and willingness. How these factors interact with each other also needs to be considered. Ability relates to knowledge and skills in a specific situation (job readiness). An individual's ability does not change from one moment to the next (Hersey, Blanchard, & Johnson, 2013). Willingness relates to the individual's attitude, confidence, and commitment toward the specific situation (psychological readiness). Willingness, however, can fluctuate from one moment to another (Hersey, Blanchard, & Johnson, 2013). If a delegatee indicates reluctance to perform some work, the delegator must evaluate the situation to determine if there is a knowledge deficit, if there is a psychomotor deficit that interferes with performing the work, or if the delegatee is bored, anxious, upset, or just unwilling to meet the expectations. Thus if the delegatee is less able or unwilling to perform in a specific situation, the delegator must be more actively engaged in the situation. In theory, the greater the ability and willingness of the delegatee, the more likely it is that the delegator can implement delegation strategies while interacting with individuals in a specific situation. The model also describes the style of the leadership required of an effective leader and its relationship between task behavior (the amount of guidance) and relationship behavior (the amount of support) needed in the given situation. In the Situational Leadership® Model (Figure 26-2), if

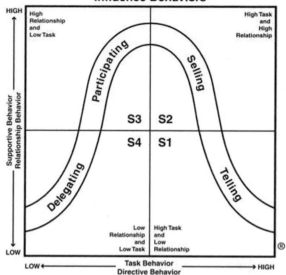

FIGURE 26-2 Situational Leadership® Model. © 2006 Reprinted with permission of the Center for Leadership Studies. Escondido, CA 92025 www.situational.com All Rights Reserved.

you insert a vertical line from the follower performance readiness box to intersect with the bell-shaped curve for a given situation, you will determine the most effective leadership strategy.

In Figure 26-2, situation one, if the delegatee has limited knowledge and ability to perform a task, the delegator needs to provide more guidance. However, if the relationship is limited (when two or individuals are unlikely to work together again), the delegator simply "tells" the individual what to do and how to perform. Hersey's Model (2006) describes the leader's behavior as guiding or directing, which is characterized as "telling." In situation two, if a situation involves a new task and the relationship is ongoing (two individuals who will usually continue to work together), the delegator explains what to do and how to do it. Hersey's Model (2006) describes the leader's behavior as explaining or persuading, which is characterized as "selling." Logically, if producing outcomes in a given situation is the driving force, the delegators are much less likely to spend the time and effort investing in limited relationships than in established relationships. In situation three, if the delegatee has the ability and willingness, but the relationship between the delegator and delegatee is relatively new, they need to establish mutual expectations and conditions of performance. Hersey's model (2006) describes the leader's behavior as encouraging or problem solving, which is characterized as "participating." Finally, in the last situation, if the delegatee has the ability and willingness, the expertise to accomplish the work, and an established relationship, Hersey's Model (2006) describes the leader's behavior as observing or monitoring, which is characterized as "delegating."

Situational Leadership® styles can be observed in real work-related situations. For example, when a new team begins to work together to build a trusting relationship, the delegator must evaluate the ability and willingness of the delegatee. If the ability and willingness is low, the delegator should use the leadership style of telling or selling. If the nature of the relationship is limited, such as a when someone is only going to work for half a day on the unit, the leadership style should be telling because it provides a fair amount of guidance but limits the time spent on the interactions. Additionally, if the relationship is developing or ongoing, the delegator needs to understand the delegatee's motivation related to the situation and the leader's style should be selling, which takes more time, but leads to a supportive relationship. If the relationship is new or developing, more support is needed and the delegator and delegatee need to inter-

act in a participatory manner. When a delegatee has a high degree of ability and willingness and is familiar with the expected task, little guidance is required. In theory, the greater the ability and willingness of the delegatee, the more likely the delegator can implement delegation strategies while interacting with that individual in a specific situation. In other words, both the amount of guidance (task behavior) and the amount of support (relationship behavior) would be relatively low, which works well for established work relationships. However, delegation can be viewed as a spectrum of behaviors based on the context and needs in a specific situation. To achieve effective outcomes, knowing how to interact with a given delegatee is one of the key challenges for the delegator. The Theory Box illustrates how Hersey's Model applies to nursing. Table 26-2 presents the delegatee condition, relevance to the delegator, the original terminology, and a clinical exemplar on how to structure communication with the delegatee to achieve a goal.

> **EXERCISE 26-1**
> Interview three RNs employed as direct care nurses, and ask them the following questions:
> 1. What factors need to be assessed before delegation?
> 2. What strategies are used by the delegator to interact with a delegatee?

Figure 26-3 integrates the various considerations for delegation. Each registered nurse has assistants available during a designated shift. Mutual trust and shared responsibility must exist between the registered nurse and the assistants, and the focus is on the patients, the center of the model. The registered nurse retains accountability for the patient and considers

THEORY BOX

Situational Leadership® Model

THEORY	KEY IDEAS	APPLICATION TO PRACTICE
Hersey's model contends that leaders/managers need to behave differently in specific situations.	Registered nurses must analyze an individual's knowledge and the work-related task before delegating. Registered nurses make decisions based on this analysis.	Before delegating, the registered nurse must understand the kind of support an individual needs to successfully accomplish the work related task. Each staff member may need a different level of support for different tasks.

TABLE 26-2 COMMUNICATING WITH A DELEGATEE

DELEGATEE CONDITION	DELEGATOR RELEVANCE	TERMINOLOGY	CLINICAL EXEMPLAR
Has limited knowledge and ability to perform the task	Requires more guidance	Tell (if the relationship is not going to be ongoing)	"It is important that you take his blood pressure every 15 minutes."
Has ongoing relationship, however a new task is delegated	Requires explanation	Sell	"This is what you need to accomplish; in fact, let me show you what is necessary."
Has willingness and ability, but the relationship is new	Requires that both individuals create mutual expectations and conditions for performance	Participate	"Please tell me how you go about performing this procedure, and I will share with you my expectations about how frequently and under what conditions we need to communicate/report to each other."
Has established relationship and expertise	Little guidance is needed	Delegate	"I know you know what you are doing and when to report. Just remember that I am available to you at any time if an issue or concern arises. Thank you for being part of the team."

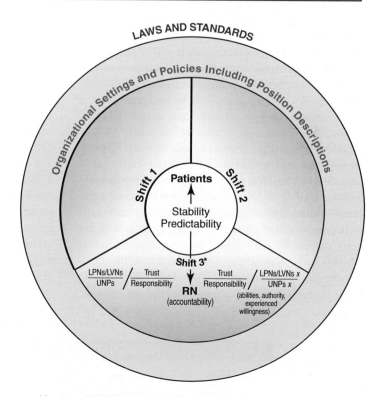

FIGURE 26-3 Delegation framework.

x = Number of LPN/LVNs and UNPs working with a specific RN.

*Repeated for other shifts.

each nursing assistant's abilities, authority, experiences, and willingness before delegating tasks to meet the needs of the patient. This decision-making process occurs in view of the organizational settings and policies, and in relation to laws and standards.

EXERCISE 26-2

Select three experienced unlicensed nursing personnel (UNP) who work on a specific nursing unit and ask them what they expect from their interactions with the registered nurse delegator. Using the information you ascertained, consider the model in Table 26-1, Figure 26-2, and Figure 26-3 to determine what type of relationship the delegator has with each delegatee as it relates to specific tasks.

ASSIGNMENT VERSUS DELEGATION

Assignment has two different meanings. It refers to the work every individual is responsible to accomplish in a designated work period. This assignment consists of patient care expectations and unit-related tasks, which may include, but are not limited to, learning activities, regulation activities, and unit management activities. The second meaning of assignment relates to the transference of both responsibility and accountability among RNs. Whereas registered nurses can be assigned patients, UNPs receive delegated tasks. Delegation is "task based rather then judgment based" (Weydt, 2010, p. 4). Thus, when a registered nurse assigns a patient to another registered nurse, both responsibility and accountability are transferred. When a registered nurse delegates care to a UNP, responsibility is transferred, however, accountability for patient care is not transferred and remains constant with the registered nurse. Thus, "accountability rests within the decision to delegate while responsibility rests within the performance of the task" (Anthony and Vidal, 2010, p. 3). Table 26-3 depicts the difference between assignment and delegation.

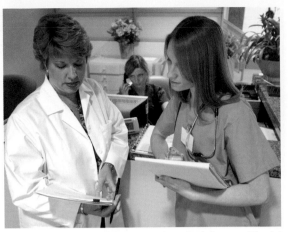

Nursing managers face complex decisions with delegation involving patients and staff.

IMPORTANCE OF DELEGATING

Delegation, a critical leadership skill, must be learned and implemented to accomplish patient care in a timely and cost-effective manner. A common misconception about the nursing profession is that nursing care is a series of psychomotor tasks. Therefore professional nurses must convey the consistent message that performing a task is only one component of patient care. Although the performance of a psychomotor task is essential to providing patient care, it is the second component, the critical analysis, performed by the registered nurse that is clearly the determining factor for nursing action. To perform a critical analysis, the nurse uses the nursing process as a guide for delegation. The nurse assesses the situation to determine what is legally appropriate to delegate, plans an intervention and determines whether the delegatee is competent to perform the task safely, implements the plan including an observation of the delegatee (directly or by general supervision), and evaluates whether the delegation process was completed safely and effectively

TABLE 26-3 ASSIGNMENT VERSUS DELEGATION		
CONCEPT	**RESPONSIBILITY**	**ACCOUNTABILITY**
Assignment (RN)	Yes	Yes
Delegation (UNP)	Yes	No

(Neumann, 2010). Critical thinking, diagnostic reasoning, and the ability to synthesize information from various sources are what characterize the nurse as a licensed professional who plans effective nursing care. The role of the registered nurse in providing safe effective patient care is critical, whether patient care is performed by an individual registered nurse or by other members of the team through the process of delegation. Delegation has direct patient care and professional practice benefits. One benefit is that delegation allows more staff availability to assist with activities of daily living (ADLs). Another benefit is that an effective team utilizes members of the team to conserve time; however, decisions to delegate should never be solely based on time-saving considerations.

EXERCISE 26-3

Interview a nurse manager, a direct care nurse, and a UNP about their perspective on the pros and cons of delegation. Compare and contrast the similarities and differences in the three perspectives and roles.

Delegation is more challenging when the geographic area is greater, when other resources are limited, or when vulnerable populations are receiving care. The Literature Perspective illustrates delegation in a school setting.

LEGAL AUTHORITY TO DELEGATE

Most state nurse practice acts address the concept of delegation; including some rules and regulations governing when and what tasks can be delegated. State boards of nursing are vested in protecting the public; therefore they regulate the educational preparation and practice of professional nursing. Legally, delegation is also a complex process. First, the delegator is personally responsible for prudent action. If the delegation task is not performed within acceptable standards, a potential for nursing malpractice emerges. Failure to delegate and supervise within acceptable standards may extend to direct corporate liability for the institution. Whenever care is provided by other staff rather than a registered nurse, the accountability for care remains with the delegator even though others provide various aspects of care. This view of professional liability is consistent with the concept that licensure conveys both privileges and expectations.

Specific knowledge about nursing and delegation is necessary to make appropriate nursing judgments. The nurse is legally accountable and thus liable for his or her actions and those of the delegatee. Because the role of the nurse has evolved over time, maintaining current and accurate knowledge about the scope of liability of nurses is essential.

 LITERATURE PERSPECTIVE

Resource: Resha, C. (May 31, 2010). Delegation in the school setting: Is it a safe practice? OJIN: The Online Journal of Issues in Nursing, Vol. 15, No. 2, Manuscript 5.

Delegation in the K-12 school setting has become a necessity because of the limited number of qualified school nurses, expanded responsibilities of school nursing practice, increased complexities of healthcare needs of children and adolescents, and limited resources. The appropriate school nurse-to-student ratio recommendation is 1 nurse to 750 students; however, in reality many school nurses provide coverage for more than one school building and the nurse-to-student ratios are extremely high and not conducive to providing high quality health care. UAPs can be a valuable asset to the school nurse when they understand the legal parameters of their role. School nurses must develop effective delegation skills to properly train and safely supervise UAPs.

A challenge regarding delegation for school nurses is when other non-nurse employees of the school do not realize the legal regulatory mechanisms that guide nursing delegation. They do not understand the necessity for medical orders for healthcare procedures performed in the school setting as opposed to those performed at home by the parent. Some administrators view nursing as a set of "tasks" rather than a "process" that assists in making nursing judgments that lead to high-quality nursing care. School administrators and others who delegate nursing tasks to non-nurse employees create litigious situations for themselves, the school nurse, and the school district.

Implications for Practice

The responsibility of a school nurse is to supervise UAPs and develop effective delegation skills to maintain a safe school health practice. School nurses also educate school employees (administrators, principals, teachers, psychologists, social workers, and other staff members) about the legal accountability of delivering nursing care. Therefore only nurses should delegate nursing care. The development of policies and procedures regarding delegation and open lines of communication with school employees prevent inappropriate delegation of nursing care and protect the employees, school nurse, administrators, and school district from any unnecessary liability.

EXERCISE 26-4

Review your state's nurse practice act, rules, and regulations. Discuss with two or more colleagues what your state identifies as delegation. Create a written summary related to your conclusions.

SELECTING THE DELEGATEE

The selection of an assistant is extremely important as their work impacts patient care outcomes. In many settings, even though the registered nurse has the authority to delegate, he or she may not be able to select the nursing assistants with whom he or she works. However, at other times, the nurse will have the ability to select his or her own nursing assistants. For example, an LPN/LVN who has functioned in a physician's office for a long time and is not familiar with working under the direction of a registered nurse may be concerned about being supervised by a registered nurse. Initiating a conversation about that person's new role and function in the organization can open lines of communication to explain why supervision is necessary and can eliminate or diminish any negative feelings about being supervised. Thus the registered nurse's ability to assess and communicate effectively is essential.

Improving lines of communication can also occur by appreciating and valuing each other's cultural perspectives. For example, a nursing assistant who does not concur with the philosophy of the organization, such as the goals of hospice care, might have a negative influence on patients. In addition, nursing assistants who have similar strengths as the delegator might want to perform the same tasks as the delegator, thus creating a gap in the delivery of patient care. However, experienced nursing assistants are more likely to adapt to changing situations. Therefore selecting an individual who has different strengths from the nurse enhances the work both can accomplish together. Building on the strengths and minimizing the challenges of the team prove to be an effective strategy. Realistically, balancing strengths through the deliberate selection of a delegatee may be almost impossible. However, it is even more important to consider all aspects of patient care to ensure that all of the patient care needs are addressed.

SUPERVISING THE DELEGATEE

Because registered nurses are always accountable for the assessment, diagnosis, planning, nursing judgment, and evaluation of patient care, UNPs must understand what elements of implementation they may complete and what elements must be completed by the registered nurse, such as the analyses of data. Both elements must be understood to ensure effectiveness in entrusting an element of care to another individual. Registered nurses are accountable for an initial assessment and the ongoing evaluation of patient care.

When delegators decrease the amount of direct patient care they perform, they automatically increase their supervisory work. The importance of

LITERATURE PERSPECTIVE

Nursing Delegation and Consumer-Directed Patient Care

Resource: Reinhard, S. (2011). A case for nurse delegation explores a new frontier in consumer-direct patient care, *Journal of American Society of Aging, Winter 2010-2011*, 75-81.

This article addresses older adults and younger individuals with disabilities and how delegating health maintenance tasks to unlicensed assistive personnel (UAP) can make a valuable contribution in assisting these individuals to manage their long-term health conditions at home. A major New Jersey pilot project, supported by the Robert Wood Johnson Foundation and the Office of the Assistant Secretary for Planning and Evaluation, was developed by the New Jersey Department of Human Services Division of Developmental Disabilities, and the Rutgers Center for State Health Policy to investigate how collaboration among nursing and consumer advocacy organizations can improve consumer choice and the quality of care. Because the health requirements of these individuals living in the community can be complex, some states have been discussing supporting safe delegation (or exemptions) for delegating health maintenance tasks to UAPs. Reinhard reports that barriers to delegation remain, even when states have broad regulatory guidelines that permit this type of delegation in these settings.

Implications for Practice

With a predicted shortage of nurses and a growing population of consumers living at home with chronic health needs, nurses must examine their norms and attitudes regarding delegation, eliminate any unnecessary barriers to health maintenance tasks being provided by UAPs, and educate themselves on how to delegate effectively. Training of UAPs in how to receive and implement delegated tasks is crucial for positive patient care outcomes. Consumers, nurses, and unlicensed assistant personnel must work collaboratively to improve the quality of community living for older adults and younger individuals with disabilities within a broad regulatory framework.

giving clear directions, asking and receiving quality feedback regarding tasks, and having an agreed upon schedule for checkpoints are essential for a well-executed plan. This evaluation plan is influenced by factors such as knowledge of and experience with the delegatee, the number of delegatees and patients for whom the delegator is accountable, the geographic design of the unit, the stability of the patients, and the resources available to staff. Evaluating how the delegatee and patients are doing throughout the work period is also critical to work performance and patient care outcomes. The Literature Perspective on p. 498 presents a delegation situation related to home care.

DELEGATION DECISION MAKING

Figure 26-4 illustrates the delegation process, which begins with assessing the health needs of the patient and the skills of the UNP. Key elements must be considered while assessing the UNP's abilities to perform the work; they include, safety, critical thinking, stability, and time. Safety is a basic physiological need, and when a patient is unsafe for any reason, delegation may not be appropriate. Exceptions to this rule are usually related to monitoring behaviors of patients (e.g., when patients are placed on suicide precautions). Critical thinking, the intensity and complexity of nurses' decision-making process, is vital to patient care decisions. For example, simple (straightforward) teaching, such as washing hands, can be performed by a UNP; however, complex (multifaceted) teaching, such as care required by diabetic patients, cannot be delegated. Stability, the patient's level of strength or steadiness, is also a major factor in making patient care decisions. The greater the stability of a patient, the more likely a UNP can provide safe patient care. Time, the intensity and length of the interactions with the patient, is also a significant factor to consider in planning patient care. For example, emergency departments usually employ relatively few UNPs because patients are less stable; however, in extended-care and long-term care facilities where patients are more stable, a higher number of UNPs are employed. In these facilities, "delegation is the primary mechanism ... for ensuring that professional nursing standards of care reach the bedside" (Corazzini et al., 2010, p. 1).

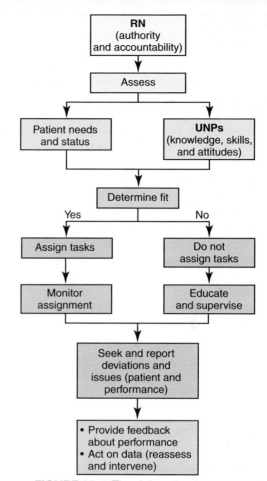

FIGURE 26-4 The delegation process.

Assuming that it is appropriate for a UNP to assist with patient care, the registered nurse must first assess the ability of the UNP. When the delegatee has the appropriate work and performance abilities, tasks can be delegated. When a delegatee has limited work and performance abilities, tasks can still be delegated, but the delegator must educate, monitor, and evaluate care very closely to ensure quality patient care. In this case, the UNP is performing tasks (their responsibility); the registered nurse is monitoring care and outcomes (accountability). The nurse should maintain open lines of communication and seek information, and the UNP should know how, when, and what to report. This two-way communication and follow-through allows patient care to be altered, if necessary, in a timely manner. At times, especially as new skills are acquired or new relationships are forged; the registered nurse should provide feedback to the UNP during the process of providing patient care. In all situations, the registered nurse needs to provide feedback about performance at the end of the activity. Furthermore, the UNP needs to understand that he or she is receiving support and direct feedback and is being monitored for professional growth and development to improve patient care outcomes.

Failure to delegate to others is also an issue of concern. Some registered nurses believe delegation is too time-consuming or that it requires more energy to delegate to others. Others believe that they can do a better job themselves or want the recognition for providing total patient care. However, when we delegate we maximize our contributions to patient care.

EXERCISE 26-5

Select three patient records from a clinical setting that involve delegation decisions. Based only on written documentation, evaluate any indications and assumptions about safety, critical thinking, stability, and time.

Using Figure 26-3, identify how you would work with a prospective delegatee to accomplish patient care goals. State the rationale for your delegation decisions.

Integrating Elements

Applying the four elements of safety, critical thinking, stability, and time into decision making creates an integrative process that fosters effective delegation decisions. However, one of the elements may play a more important role than the other in different patient care situations. For example, when critical-thinking skills are of utmost importance in the patient care situation, other elements may be relatively less important in the delegation decision. Therefore making decisions about to whom to delegate, what to delegate, and when to delegate is a complex process.

Creating a work environment where specific feedback about performance is ongoing is the best strategy for shaping the future behavior of individuals. A statement such as "You performed that procedure safely and professionally" is more effective than the statement "Nice job." The first statement clearly identifies what the individual did well, whereas, the second statement is vague and not specific to the behavior. Equally important is the feedback from the individual performing the tasks. To elicit feedback a series of questions should be asked by the registered nurse, such as, "Has the work/task been completed?", "What changes were observed with the patient?", and "How did the patient respond?" Open-ended questions allow the registered nurse to gain pertinent information from the individuals delegated a portion of patient care. The experienced registered nurse also identifies verbal or nonverbal clues about the UNP's perception of patient care interactions, and allows that information to continue to build a trusting relationship.

The delegator should provide constructive feedback to the delegatee regarding his/her work-related performance whenever possible. However, to convey satisfaction with an individual's performance that is less than satisfactory diminishes the credibility of the registered nurse. A verbal attack on an individual does not produce effective change, and potentially undermines any long-term working relationship, such as "What is wrong with you today?" The best strategy is to provide open, honest, and constructive feedback, such as "Let me demonstrate a more effective way to perform the task." Honest feedback about work-related performance and specific strategies for change provide the delegatee a quality improvement plan. Table 26-1 (p. 490) poses some appropriate questions for making delegation decisions.

Another concern regarding delegation is that some individuals are not competent to hold their current position. One strategy for managing this issue is to temporarily lower expectations and provide additional support. This strategy allows individuals to build on their strengths, minimize their weaknesses, and gain confidence. However, it is essential to examine the effect the strategy of lowering expectations for an individual has on other members of the team. Many questions need to be considered in the decision, such as, Why is one employee held to a standard and another is not? Who becomes responsible for the work that one individual cannot accomplish? Is it fair to compensate an individual for work that does not meet performance expectations? What are the potential liabilities of altering the standards of performance? Because delegation decisions are a complex process, registered nurses must understand that having individuals assigned to work that they are not capable of performing safely and effectively, and then not intervening creates a high risk for legal liability.

"No one should delegate work unless they are certain the person expected to perform the task is competent to perform it" (Kline, 2013, p. 19). In addition to the legal ramifications of poor delegation decisions, ethical considerations should also influence the registered nurse's decisions.

CHALLENGES RELATED TO THE DELEGATION PROCESS

Delegation, a complex decision making process, is successful when effective delegation strategies are utilized by the registered nurse. Understanding the specific skill set and capabilities of the delegatee are crucial elements to the delegation process. For example, selecting a delegatee who has the specific skill set for the particular task is a more productive strategy than just selecting a competent individual. In large organizations, registered nurses usually are afforded more opportunities to select their delegatee than in smaller facilities with fewer employees. In rural settings, the choice of the delegatee is usually more predictable because of the longevity of the employees; thus the delegation process may be easier because the delegator is more familiar with the skills and abilities of the various delegatees.

When the registered nurse has limited clinical experience, whether in a career or a particular workplace, the nurse's ability to make delegation decisions, especially during complex situations, can be difficult. In those situations, working together with the delegatee, as a team, to deliver patient care allows time to assess willingness and ability. Maintaining open lines of communication with the delegatee, without any derogatory or offensive comments, creates a collaborative and productive work environment. Providing constructive feedback allows the delegatee to be more receptive to and understand feedback. However, the ultimate goal of delegation remains the same: maximizing patient care outcomes.

Another challenge related to delegation occurs when a registered nurse does not provide clear direction to the delegatee about the task and the delegatee implements the task based on their own decisions. It is important to have the delegatee understand how and when you want the task accomplished. Sometimes, when the delegator intervenes, the delegatee may lose confidence or become frustrated, and the delegator losses the benefit of effective delegation. However,

assuming that no safety or ethical concern exists, the delegation process should continue to improve communication and build trust between the delegator and the delegatee.

During delegation, the delegator must make sure two essential factors occur in the delegation process. First, the delegatee must be able to recall and understand what is expected, and second is that appropriate resources are available to accomplish the work. Deadlines for completing tasks keep the delegatees on target without having them feel they are being micromanaged. Clear expectations about task accomplishments provide a structure for ongoing evaluation of a delegatee. In settings outside hospitals, (long-term care facilities, clinics, school nurse offices) one of the greatest challenges of delegation relates to supervision. In these situations, it is especially important to be clear about what is expected of the delegatee. Box 26-1 presents a communication template used for the delegation of tasks. When there is a clear understanding between the delegator and the delegatee about a particular delegation situation, the greater the chance it will produce a positive outcome.

EXERCISE 26-6

Develop a case study in which you must make a delegation decision. Use the delegation communication template found in Box 26-1 to practice with a classmate how to transfer the specific responsibilities for patient care.

BOX 26-1   DELEGATION COMMUNICATION TEMPLATE

- State exactly what is being delegated and the expected outcome.
- Convey the authority to perform what is expected.
- Identify priorities.
- Acknowledge monitoring activities that may be performed.
- Specify any performance limitations.
- Specify deadlines, including the exact times if appropriate.
- Specify report time frames and data expected.
- Specify deviations, including when immediate action must be taken.
- Identify appropriate resources, including individual consultants.
- Emphasize what may not be delegated.
- Ask the delegatee to provide examples of each.

In other instances, a problem or issue related to delegation arises, and the nurse observes it but has no authority specific to the situation. If there are no safety issues, urgency to intervene, or potential negative patient outcome, the nurse can assist other registered nurses with delegation decisions by using three strategies: "asking," "offering," and "doing." The first strategy, asking, begins with questions related to the problem or issue regarding patient care. Often, asking questions provides an opportunity to open lines of communication between delegator and the delegatee. It also allows the delegator to examine the situation differently and allows the nurse to reassess. The second strategy, offering, involves making a suggestion to facilitate the achievement of a desirable patient care outcome. The third strategy, doing, occurs by demonstrating the specific task or behavior to improve patient care. Briefly, the approach is described in Box 26-2.

EXERCISE 26-7

Review a delegation decision made by a nurse manager or charge nurse related to a clinical experience. After reviewing the nurse practice act and professional standards, provide answers with an evidence-based rationale to the following questions:
1. Did the nurse manager or charge nurse make clear what was delegated? Why or why not?
2. Were the delegation decisions logical? Why or why not?
3. Were the delegation decisions made within legal and ethical parameters?

BOX 26-2 CRITICAL COMMUNICATION

1. Challenge (use his or her first name and a qualifier [e.g., "Susan, isn't this a sterile procedure?"]).
2. Perhaps you can use the gloves from the sterile kit you have.
3. Would you go check with the unit clerk to see if any of my lab results are back? I'll take care of this procedure.

CHARGE NURSES

Charge nurses frequently emerge as the delegator because they have demonstrated their knowledge and expertise in the clinical setting. When registered nurses do not delegate (usually because of the limited numbers of LPNs/LVNs or UNPs), the charge nurse usually delegates. Thus a charge nurse usually has acquired a sophisticated level of competency skills in critical thinking, clinical practice, organization, leadership, communication, and time management.

CONCLUSION

Delegation is a multifaceted decision-making process necessary to achieve nursing goals and improve patient care outcomes. Regardless of the method of nursing care delivery, the registered nurse must master the art of delegation, develop critical judgment skills, and apply delegation decisions in nursing practice to provide safe, high-quality health care.

THE SOLUTION

In a Level I emergency trauma department, the patient acuity is serious and is often changing. EMS is arriving with multiple patients injured in an accident at the chemical plant.

The registered professional nurse managing the trauma center must understand the qualifications, experience, and abilities of the nurses assigned patients. The nurses also need to understand the qualifications, experience, and abilities of the emergency technicians to whom they delegate tasks.

The emergency technicians who have been working in the center for a minimum of 1 year can be delegated tasks by the registered nurse. However, the qualifications and experience of the newly employed emergency technicians (UNP) were unknown. Since they would not begin the emergency technician training program for another 2 months, one experienced technician and a newly employed emergency technician worked with each registered nurse accountable for patient care. Each technician was directly supervised, observed, and evaluated by their registered nurse.

Each staff member needed to understand what tasks can be delegated and what tasks cannot be delegated.

—*Kathryn King-Dyker*

Would this be a suitable approach for you? Why?

THE EVIDENCE

Effective delegation skills are essential competencies necessary to practice as a registered professional nurse in the 21st century. Multiple factors play a role in the ability of the registered nurse to delegate effectively. These factors include, but are not limited to, the nurses' educational preparation, demographic area, state practice acts, leadership style, employment area, clinical experience, and the individual's self-confidence. When nurses are engaged in a work environment that utilizes an RN/UNP care model, they gain the clinical experience to effectively utilize delegation skills. Today, this type of care model supports nurses in providing high quality cost effective health care.

Implications for Practice

Nursing research, an instrument to support evidence based practice, should be utilized to manage patient care delivery. Nursing internships, offered in school, that provide delegation and supervisory experience of UNPs can enhance an individual's clinical experience and confidence, allowing them to learn how to delegate safely and effectively. As registered nurses adapt to the rapidly changing healthcare environment, nurse managers must continue to support nurses with clinical experiences and continued professional education that enhances their leadership skills, allowing them to effectively delegate and supervise others.

WHAT NEW GRADS SAY

- The hardest part is "being in charge" of someone much older than me.
- I love knowing I can count on _____ [name of nursing assistant]. I appreciate the delegated tasks UNPs perform in providing safe and effective patient care.

CHAPTER CHECKLIST

Delegation, a decision-making process, needs to be learned in order to make appropriate nursing judgments and achieve maximum patient care outcomes. One of the critical roles of registered nurses is maintaining the cohesiveness of the team by coordinating care across the spectrum of providers and improving the quality of care. Important concepts in this chapter include the following:
- Historical perspective
- Definitions
  - Delegation
  - Achieving optimal outcomes
  - Individual and organizational accountability
  - Sharing activities with unlicensed personnel (UAP/UNP)
- Span of control
- Appropriate authority
- A framework for delegation
- Assignment versus delegation
- Importance of delegating
- Legal authority to delegate
- Selecting the delegatee
- Supervising the delegatee
- Delegation decision making
  - Integrating elements
- Challenges related to the delegation process
- Charge nurses

TIPS FOR DELEGATING

- Understand the organizational structure, policies, and culture of the institution to make delegation decisions.
- Comprehend the job description of individuals before delegating tasks.
- Assess the knowledge, skills, and attitudes of the individual staff members before delegating tasks.
- Use your nurse practice act and standards for clinical practice to determine how to appropriately delegate tasks.

- Use communication strategies to develop successful delegating skills.
- Apply a decision-making framework or model to determine the type of work-related tasks that can be successfully delegated.

- Implement decision-making strategies based on the individual's work-related performance regarding delegated tasks.
- Evaluate the effectiveness of delegating tasks to others on a regular basis.

REFERENCES

American Nurses Association. (2012). *ANA's principles for delegation by registered nurses to unlicensed assistive personnel.* Retrieved from, www.nursesbooks.org/Homepage/Hot-off-the-Press/eBook-Principles-Delegation.aspx.

American Nurses Association. (2013). Nursing shortage. *In Nursing World.* Retrieved from http://www.nursingworld.org/MainMenuCategories/ThePracticeofProfessionalNursing/workforce/IOM-Future-of-Nursing-Report-1.

American Nurses Association (ANA). (2005). *Principles for delegation.* Silver Spring, MD: Author.

American Nurses Association (ANA). (2011). *Code of ethics for nurses with interpretive statements.* Washington, DC: Author.

American Nurses Association and National Council of State Boards of Nursing. (2006). *Joint Statement on delegation.* https://www.ncsbn.org/.Jointstatement.pdf.

Anthony, M. K., & Vidal, K. (2010). Mindful communication: A new approach to improving delegation and increasing patient safety. *The Online Journal of Issues in Nursing, 15*(2), 2.

Benner, P., & Benner, R. (1984). *From novice to expert: Excellence and power in clinical nursing practice.* Menlo Park, CA: Addison-Wesley.

Corazzini, K. N., Anderson, R. A., Rapp, C., Mueller, C., McConnell, E. S., & Lekan, D. (2010). Delegation in long-term care: Scope of practice or job description? *Online Journal of Issues in Nursing, 15*(2), 4.

Harmer, V. (2010). Are nurses blurring their identity by extending or delegating roles? *British Journal of Nursing, 19*(5), 295–299.

Hersey, P. (2006). *Situational leadership® model.* Escondido, CA: The Center for Leadership Studies, Inc. http://www.situational.com .

Hersey, P., Blanchard, K. H., & Johnson, D. E. (2013). *Management of organizational behavior: leading human resources* (10th ed.). Upper Saddle River, NJ: Pearson.

Kaernested, B., & Bragadóttir, H. (2012). Delegation of registered nurses revisited: Attitudes towards delegation and preparedness to delegate effectively. *Nordic Journal of Nursing Research & Clinical Studies / Vård I Norden, 32*(1), 10–15.

Kline, R. 2013a. Safe to delegate. *Nursing Standard, 27*(26), 19.

Littlejohn, L., Campbell, J., Collins-McNeil, J., & Khayile, T. (2012). Nursing shortage: A comparative analysis. *International Journal of Nursing, 1*(1), 22–27.

Lynch, B. M., McCormack, B., & McCance, T. (2011). Development of a model of situational leadership in residential care for older people. *Journal of Nursing Management, 19*(8), 1058–1069.

National Council of State Boards of Nursing. (2005). *Working with others: A position paper.* https://www.ncsbn.org//Working with Others.pdf.

Neumann, T. A. (2010). Delegation: Better safe than sorry. *AAOHN Journal, 58*(10), 321–322.

Powell, R. M. (2011). Improving students' delegations skills. *Nurse Educator, 36*(1), 9–10.

Reinhard, S. C. (2011). A case for nurse delegation explores a new frontier in consumer-directed patient care. *Generations, 34*(4), 75–81.

Resha, C. (2010). Delegation in the school setting: Is it safe practice? *Online Journal of Issues in Nursing, 15*(2), 5.

Saccomano, S. J., & Pinto-Zipp, G. (2011). Registered nurse leadership style and confidence in delegation. *Journal of Nursing Management, 19*(4), 522–533.

U.S. Bureau of Labor Statistics. (2012, November). *Hurricane Sandy: A pre-storm look at affected areas.* Retrieved from www.bls.gov/spotlight/2012/sandy/.

Weydt, A. (2010). Developing delegation skills. *The Online Journal of Issues in Nursing, 15*(2), 1.

SUGGESTED READINGS

Athlin, E., Hov, R., Petzäll, K., & Hedelin, B. (2013). Being a nurse leader in bedside nursing in hospital and community care contexts in Norway and Sweden. *Journal of Nursing Education and Practice, 4*(3).

Bain, H., & Baguley, F. (2012). The management of caseloads in district nursing services. *Primary Health Care, 22*(4), 31–38.

Barra, M. (2011). Nurse delegation of medication pass in assisted living facilities: Not all medication assistant technicians are equal. *Journal of Nursing Law, 14*(1), 3–10.

Brunero, S., & Stein-Parbury, J. (2008). The effectiveness of clinical supervision in nursing: An evidenced based literature review. *Australian Journal of Advanced Nursing, 25*(3), 86–94.

Buchan, J., & Aiken, L. (2008). Solving nursing shortages: A common priority. *Journal of Clinical Nursing, 17*, 3262–3268.

Chabot, G., Gagnon, M., & Godin, G. (2012). Redefining the school nurse role: An organizational perspective. *Journal of Health Organization and Management, 26*(4), 444–466.

Clark, R., & Allison-Jones, L. (2011). Investing in human capital: An academic-service partnership to address the nursing shortage. *Nursing Education Perspectives, 32*(1), 18–21.

Cohen, S. (2014). Braving the new manager world. *Nursing Management (Springhouse), 45*(1), 8–9.

Dayer-Berenson, L. (2014). *Cultural Competencies for Nurses, Impact on Health and Illness* (2nd ed). Sudbury, Massachusetts: Jones & Bartlett Learning.

Gillen, P., & Graffin, S. (2010). Nursing delegation in the United Kingdom. *The Online Journal of Issues in Nursing, 15*(2), 6.

Hand, T. (2012). The developing role of the HCA in general practice. *Practice Nurse, 42*(19), 14–17.

Harrington, C., & Estes, C. (2013). *Health policy, crisis and reform in the U.S. health care delivery system* (6th ed.). Burlington, Massachusetts: Jones & Bartlett Learning.

Haugen, N., Galura, S., & Ulrich, S. P. (2011). *Ulrich & Canale's nursing care planning guides: Prioritization, delegation, and critical thinking.* Maryland Heights, MO: Saunders/Elsevier.

Hasson, F., Mckenna, H. P., & Keeney, S. (2013). Delegating and supervising unregistered professionals: The student nurse experience. *Nurse Education Today, 33*(3), 229–235.

Hopkins, U., Itty, A. S., Nazario, H., Pinon, M., Slyer, J., & Singleton, J. (2012). The effectiveness of delegation interventions by the registered nurse to the unlicensed assistive personnel and their impact quality of care, patient satisfaction, and RN staff satisfaction: A systematic review. *JBI Library of Systematic Reviews, 10*(15), 894–934.

Institute of Medicine. (2011). *The future of nursing: Leading change, advancing health.* Washington, D.C.: National Academies Press.

Jennifer, M. (2010). When does delegating make you a supervisor? *The Online Journal of Issues in Nursing, 15*(2), 3.

Jennifer, M. (2010). When does delegating make you a supervisor? *The Online Journal of Issues in Nursing, 15*(2), 3.

Josephsen, J. (2013). Teaching nursing delegation: An on-line case study. *Teaching and Learning in Nursing, 8*(3), 83–87.

Kendall-Raynor, P. (2012). New delegation standards could strengthen nurses' accountability. *Nursing Standard, 26*(5), 5.

Kline, R. 2013b. Safe to delegate? *Nursing Standard, 27*(26), 19.

Lightfoot, R. J. (2011). Nurse delegation in LTC and assisted living. *Long-Term Living: For the Continuing Care Professional, 60*(11), 42–44.

Masters, K. (2014). *Role development in professional nursing practice* (3rd ed.). Burlington, Massachusetts: Jones & Bartlett Learning.

Matthews, J. (2010). When does delegating make you a supervisor? *The Online Journal of Issues in Nursing, 15*(2), 3.

McCarty, M. N. (2012). The lawful scope of practice of medical assistants – 2012 update. *AMT Events, 29*(2), 110–119.

Motacki, K., & Burke, K. (2011). *Nursing delegation and management of patient care.* St. Louis, MO: Mosby/Elsevier.

Mueller, C., & Vogelsmeier, A. (2013). Effective delegation: Understanding responsibility, authority, and accountability. *Journal of Nursing Regulation, 4*(3), 20–27.

Persily, C. A. (2013). *Team leadership and partnering in nursing and health care.* New York: Springer Publishing Company.

Plawecki, L. H., & Amrhein, D. W. (2012). Legal issues. A question of delegation: Unlicensed assistive personnel and the professional nurse. *Journal of Gerontological Nursing, 36*(8), 18–21.

Randolph, P. K., Hinton, J. E., Hagler, D., Mays, M. Z., Kastenbaum, B., Brooks, R., et al. (2012). Measuring competence: Collaboration for safety. *Journal of Continuing Education in Nursing, 43*(12), 541–547.

Randolph, P. K., & Scott-Cawiezell, J. (2010). Developing a statewide medication technician pilot program in nursing homes. *Journal of Gerontological Nursing, 36*(9), 36–44.

Schluter, J., Seaton, P., & Chaboyer, W. (2011). Understanding nursing scope of practice: A qualitative study. *International Journal of Nursing Studies, 48*(10), 1211–1222.

Selekman, J. (2013). *School nursing: A comprehensive text.* Philadelphia: F.A. Davis.

Shannon, R. A., & Kubelka, S. (2013). Reducing the risks of Delegation: Use of Procedure Skills Checklists for Unlicensed Assistive Personnel in Schools, Part 1. *NASN School Nurse, 28*(4), 178–181.

Siegel, E. O., & Young, H. M. (2010). Communication between nurses and unlicensed assistive personnel in nursing homes: Explicit expectations. *Journal of Gerontological Nursing, 36*(12), 32–37.

Spriggle, M. (2009). Developing a policy for delegation of nursing care in the school setting. *The Journal of School Nursing, 25*(2), 98–107.

U.S. Bureau of Labor Statistics. (2009, November). *Health care.* Retrieved from www.bls.gov/spotlight/2009/health_care/.

United Nations. (2011). *The Millennium Development Goals Report 2011.* New York: United Nations.

White, M. J., Gutierrez, A., Davis, K., Olson, R., & McLaughlin, C. (2011). Delegation knowledge and practice among rehabilitation nurses. *Rehabilitation Nursing, 36*(1), 16–24.

Whiting, M., & O'Loughlin, J. (2012). Training high: A clinical skills initiative for families and staff. *Nursing Children and Young People, 24*(7), 30–33.

Role Transition

Diane M. Twedell

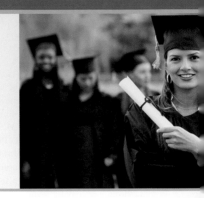

This chapter provides information about role transition—the process of moving from a clinically focused position to a supervisory position with increased responsibility. The basic overview of management roles illustrates the complexity of managing work done by others and provides a foundation for understanding role transition. The exercises offer opportunities to recognize one's own expectations, resources, and management potential.

LEARNING OUTCOMES

- Construct the full scope of a manager role by outlining Responsibilities, Opportunities, Lines of communication, Expectations, and Support (ROLES).
- Analyze specific examples of role transitions as a direct care nurse and a nurse manager.
- Describe the phases of role transition by using a life experience.
- Construct a response to an unexpected role transition.
- Compare strategies to facilitate a successful role transition.

KEY TERMS

mentor	role internalization	role transition
role development	role negotiation	roles
role discrepancy	role strain	
role expectations	role stress	

THE CHALLENGE

Melissa J. Bertelson, RN, BSN
Nurse Manager, Mayo Clinic Health System – Albert Lea
and Austin, Albert Lea, Minnesota

Transitioning from house supervisor registered nurse (RN) position to that of a nurse manager was more complex of a change than I had anticipated! I had to transition from being a peer in the supervisor group to being their new manager. Suddenly I was privy to all issues and concerns within the supervisor group that were occurring and being addressed by the two hospital managers. The harder aspect of this for me was participating in bi-weekly meetings that are held one-on-one with just a small group of the supervisors.

These meetings were held to address any immediate concerns or complaints that occurred as part of ongoing performance. The transition into participating and then conducting these meetings, sometimes on my own, was not comfortable. I also was now in charge of two departments, bringing with them employee concerns, operating budgets, audits, and equipment. I had to make sense of the issues that people brought to me rather than depending on a nurse manager to address it. I was now the nurse manager!

What do you think you would do if you were this nurse?

INTRODUCTION

Role transition involves transforming one's professional identity. A new graduate makes a transition from the student role to the nurse role. Expectations of students are clearly specified in course and clinical objectives. Expectations for a new nurse as an employee may not be so clear. The new graduate nurse faces the first of several professional transitions. These transitions will continue with career growth and development.

Consider the direct care nurse who becomes a nurse manager. The direct care nurse performs tasks related to the care of patients. As a follower, the direct care nurse has accountability and responsibility for the work that is accomplished. A direct care nurse who becomes a nurse manager must transition into the new role as a generalist, orchestrating diverse tasks and getting work done through others.

A direct care nurse who moves from an acute care setting to a home health agency must also undergo a role transition. Instead of balancing the needs of multiple patients, the home health nurse can focus on one patient at a time. Yet when a collegial opinion is needed during a visit, there are no peers there to consult with. Registered nurses who transition to nurse practitioner roles and other advanced practice roles experience this same type of role transition.

Organizations play a key role in assisting employees through role transitions. Changes in roles can be either painful or exciting and depend largely on the work culture and support provided. According to Chari (2008), "Transitions are critical times and are extremely challenging as modern organizations are of bewildering complexity and do business at a rapid pace" (p. 111).

Knowing what to expect during this transformation can reduce the stress of accepting and transitioning into a new role and result in quality outcomes. After an overview of the roles of leader, manager, and follower, this chapter describes the process of role transition, with an emphasis on strategies that can be used to ease the transition.

TYPES OF ROLES

Accepting a management or formal leadership position dictates accepting three roles that involve complex processes. The roles of leader, manager, and follower are complex because they involve working through and with unique individuals in a rapidly changing environment. Examples of the people with whom you interact and the processes involved in each role are shown in Table 27-1. In nursing, each of these roles relates to patients and clients.

The transition from a direct care nurse role to a nurse manager/leader role can occur overnight. The nurse moves from the clinical work of patient care to lead a group of employees.

LEADERSHIP

The role of follower involves respecting the authority of others and working within the system to contribute to the organizational outcomes. Managers as followers recognize their accountability to the persons above them on the organizational chart. Within a team, the manager recognizes the leadership being provided by others and supports decisions made by the group. Weinstock (2011) notes, "Every new role creates a

TABLE 27-1 LEADER, MANAGER, AND FOLLOWER ROLES: PEOPLE WITH WHOM YOU INTERACT AND PROCESSES INVOLVED IN EACH ROLE

ROLE	PEOPLE WITH WHOM INTERACTIONS OCCUR	PROCESSES INVOLVED IN THE ROLE
Leader	Persons being led Peers	Listening Encouraging Motivating Organizing Problem solving (high level) Developing Supporting
Manager	Persons being supervised Administrators Supervisors Regulating agencies	Organizing Budgeting Hiring Evaluating Reporting Disseminating Listening Problem solving (unit level)
Follower	Supervisor Peers	Conforming Implementing Contributing Completing assignments Alerting Listening Problem solving (patient and team level)

change in work tasks, leadership hierarchy, productivity demands, and shifts in all relationships, including one's relationship with oneself" (p. 211).

In the evolving healthcare environment, the nurse leader providing direct patient care also must function as a leader, manager, and follower. As *leader,* the nurse leader recognizes the uniqueness of each patient and provides feedback on clinical progress. As *manager,* the nurse leader links the patient to the resources to achieve clinical outcomes. Medical information is translated into a format that the patient can use to make informed decisions about treatment and self-care. Through referrals, the nurse leader facilitates

continuity of care within the larger system. As *follower,* the nurse leader is accountable to the team and the supervisor for completing the work that is assigned. The nurse leader as a follower practices within the policies and procedures of the organization and the standards of the profession.

Learning the leader, manager, and follower aspects of any new role can be overwhelming. Another approach to the complexity of role transition is the acronym ROLES, in which each letter represents a component common to all roles.

ROLES: THE ABCs OF UNDERSTANDING ROLES

Acronyms help us retain and organize information. ROLES (Box 27-1) is an acronym that is useful in role transition.

R stands for responsibilities. What are the specified duties in the position description for the new position? What tasks are to be completed? What decisions must the person in this position make? For example, the job for a nurse manager might include 24-hour accountability, whereas a job description for a nurse practitioner may involve direct care in a primary care setting. Every position has specific tasks for which the position holder is responsible.

O stands for opportunities, which are untapped aspects of the position. In the employment interview, the nurse executive may have said that the previous manager did not encourage the direct care nurses to participate in continuing education. Or, while touring the unit, a manager observes that the report room lacks amenities. Maybe there is a new method of delivering patient care that is appropriate for the unit. These possibilities represent opportunities for a manager to influence organizational and unit goals.

L represents lines of communication, which are at the heart of every leadership role. No matter what role an individual is in, multiple relationships

---

BOX 27-1   ROLES ACRONYM

Responsibilities
Opportunities
Lines of communication
Expectations
Support

exist with individuals including supervisors and peers. Roles incorporate patterns of structured interactions between the manager and people in these groups. The nurse manager receives and sends messages. Being a skillful listener can be more important than being skillful in sending messages. Skill is required to communicate both the content and the intent of the message effectively. Only through practice can one develop skill. In Chapter 18, techniques of effective communication are described that are extremely important to a new manager in building the team.

_E_ stands for expectations. Expectations vary depending on your goals. Colleagues may expect a new nurse anesthetist to be on call every weekend. Direct care nurses have specific expectations of their managers and particularly want the manager to be a facilitator and a leader. The nursing executive or administrator will likely have expectations about how managers spend their time on the job—even about how much time they spend at work. Nurse executives' expectations evolve from their perspectives of the manager's accountability and duties.

Finding out in advance what the explicit and implicit expectations are of the people involved can facilitate a smoother role transition by decreasing role ambiguity (Hardy, 1978). Hardy's work with role theory suggests a strong relationship between role ambiguity (one type of role stress) and role strain.

The major concepts of role theory are presented in the Theory Box.

Personal expectations related to performance as a manager is another factor to consider. You have a mental image of the role of a manager or person in this position. The process of role transition unfolds as a new manager identifies expectations, recognizes the similarities and differences, and develops the roles of leader, manager, and follower.

_S_ stands for support, which is closely tied to expectations about performance. All roles are shaped to some degree by the support and services others provide. The acute care nurse has peers readily available when a second opinion is needed. The same nurse may feel lost when confronted with questionable findings during a home visit. The nurse manager who must develop the unit's budget in a skilled care facility may have no accounting department to provide services, such as a detailed analysis of the facility's expenditures. Each role has some support available. When a new position is being considered, it is important to evaluate whether support is available in areas in which a manager may lack knowledge or skill. When implementing changes in roles, the organization needs to develop support services to facilitate role transition.

ROLE TRANSITION PROCESS

One way to think about the way in which someone transitions to a new role is illustrated in Box 27-2 and Table 27-2. Thinking about transitions in terms of a common social perspective may be helpful for some.

THEORY BOX

Hardy's Role Theory

THEORY/CONTRIBUTOR	KEY IDEAS	APPLICATION TO PRACTICE
Hardy (1978) is credited with applying role theory to healthcare professionals. Role is the expected and actual behaviors associated with a position. **Role expectations** are the attitudes and behaviors others anticipate that a person in the role will possess or demonstrate. **Role stress** is a social condition in which role demands are conflicting, irritating, difficult, or impossible to fulfill. **Role strain** is the subjective feeling of discomfort experienced as the result of role stress.	Role stress is a precursor to role strain. Role stress is associated with low productivity and performance. Role stress and role strain can lead a person to withdraw psychologically from the role. Clear, realistic role expectations can decrease the role stress for a new nurse manager.	Clear, realistic role expectations can increase productivity.

Data from Hardy, M.E. (1978). Role stress and role strain. In M.E. Hardy & M.E. Conway (Eds.), _Role theory: Perspectives for health professionals_. New York: Appleton-Century-Crofts.

BOX 27-2   ROLE TRANSITION PROCESS

Unlearning old roles while learning new roles requires an identity adjustment over time. The persons involved must invest themselves in the process. In this way, role transition can be compared to developing a relationship. The process of developing an intimate relationship with another person provides a familiar framework for considering role transition. Relationships typically move through the phases of dating, commitment, honeymoon, disillusionment, resolution, and maturity.

Role Preview

During the dating phase, the interested persons spend structured time together. Both parties present their best characteristics and dedicate much energy to developing the relationship. Although both parties present their best characteristics, both also are alert to clues that the other party cannot meet their expectations. For example, one may consider the financial and emotional resources that the other person would bring to the relationship. The individuals might spend time with each other's families to get a feel for the emotional climate in which the other person grew up.

Interviewing for a management position is similar to dating. An interview involves touring the unit, visiting with people, and attempting to make a good impression. The potential employer is also attempting to make a favorable impression. The interviewee wants to find out whether this is an organization that will support his or her growth as he or she supports the growth of the organization. Questions are asked about the role of the manager, and the potential manager mentally evaluates whether the described role matches personal expectations about management. Both of these examples represent the phase "role preview."

Role Acceptance

Through the dating process, two people may decide that they want to spend the rest of their lives together and commit to the relationship. Sometimes, one or both of the people decide that they do not want to establish a long-term relationship. In a similar way, following the role preview of the interview process, both parties may agree to establish a relationship as employee and employer. Or one or both of the parties may decide not to establish the relationship. In dating, the public decision to leave other similar relationships and establish this new relationship represents a formal commitment. In role transition, the formal commitment of the employment contract implies acceptance of the management role, or "role acceptance."

Role Exploration

In new relationships, a time of dating and commitment is usually followed by a honeymoon. More than a trip to a vacation spot, the honeymoon has become synonymous with excitement, happiness, and confidence. In a new work role, people also experience a honeymoon phase. The new graduate may be relieved that the educational program was successfully completed and now a salary can be earned. When a new manager is hired, the employer is excited that the search is over. The staff is happy to have a leader, especially if staff members had input into the hiring decision. The new manager

is happy, excited, and, most of all, confident in exploring the new roles involved in the management position.

Role Discrepancy

Whether by a gradual process or as the result of a particular event that serves as the turning point, eventually the honeymoon is over and disillusionment about the relationship occurs. For example, one person may make an expensive purchase without consulting the partner. An argument is followed by a period of painful silence. Similarly, the honeymoon phase in a new employment position can be followed by a period of disillusionment.

Role discrepancy, a gap between role expectations and role performance, causes discomfort and frustration. Role discrepancy can be resolved by either dissolving the relationship or by changing expectations and performance. The importance of the relationship and the perceived differences between performance and expectations, the basis of role discrepancy, must be considered in light of personal values. When the relationship is valued and the differences are seen as correctable, the decision is made to stay in the relationship. This decision requires the couple or the manager to develop the role.

Role Development

Choosing to change either role expectations or role performance or to change both is the process of role development. In an intimate relationship, open communication can clarify expectations. Negotiation may result in reasonable expectations. Certain behaviors may be changed to improve role performance. For example, one person in the relationship learns to call home to let the other know about the possibility of being late.

To reduce role discrepancy in a new management position, the same open communication and negotiation must occur. Expectations need to be clarified and stipulated by both parties. New managers evaluate management styles and techniques to determine which ones best fit them and the situation. The personal management style evolves as the individuals develop the management roles in their own unique ways. If role discrepancy can be reduced and the role developed to be satisfactory to both parties, the new manager can focus on developing the roles of the position and proceed to the phase of role internalization.

Role Internalization

Role internalization occurs in relationships as they mature. No longer do the persons in the relationship consciously consider their roles. They have learned the behaviors that maintain and nurture the relationship. The behaviors become second nature. The energy spent on establishing and developing the relationship can be redirected toward achieving mutual goals. In the same way, managers who have been in management positions for several years have internalized their roles. Usually they do not consciously consider their roles. Managers know they have reached the stage of role internalization when they focus on accomplishing mutual goals instead of contemplating whether their role performance matches their role expectations. Managers who have internalized their roles have developed their own unique

BOX 27-2 ROLE TRANSITION PROCESS—cont'd

personal style of management. Table 27-2 summarizes the comparison between the phases of developing an intimate relationship and the phases of role transition to a nurse manager.

Unexpected Role Transition

Not every relationship is successful. Some relationships end in an argument, divorce, or death. When a relationship ends unexpectedly, a person goes through a grieving process. In a similar way, when a person is fired, a position is eliminated, or a job description changes dramatically, the person may have to grieve before being able to engage in role transition. Health care is in a tumultuous state. Mergers, acquisitions, and reductions in force are commonplace. To be successful, workplace restructuring must be undertaken with the same sensitivity afforded a person who has lost a relationship through death or divorce. Role transition takes time, even in reverse.

The initial response to a change in role can be shock and disbelief. The person may feel numb and unable to function. As the numbness wears off, the person may become angry. The anger fuels resistance to the change and may be directed toward those who initiated the role change. The anger may be directed internally, leading to depression. If the person is unable to acknowledge and talk about the loss, the period of grief may be extended or emotional baggage may be created that is carried into the next role. Grieving can eventually resolve in acceptance. Lessons learned from the experience are identified and internalized. A new role is sought, and the "dating" begins again.

When a relationship is dissolved in the case of death or divorce, a legal document is prepared to formally dissolve the financial and social obligations between the persons involved. The loss of a position as a result of restructuring or a buyout should involve a similar process. The employer may offer the nurse a severance package that includes financial compensation and outplacement services. If the employer does not offer a written agreement, the nurse should formally request and negotiate reasonable compensation and assistance. Similar to signing a prenuptial agreement, a nurse may have signed a contract with the employer when hired. The terms of that agreement may require the employer to buy out (pay the salary and benefits) for the time remaining on the contract.

Written by Jennifer Jackson Gray.

TABLE 27-2 COMPARISON OF PHASES IN DEVELOPING AN INTIMATE RELATIONSHIP AND IN UNDERGOING ROLE TRANSITION AS A NURSE MANAGER

PHASE IN DEVELOPING AN INTIMATE RELATIONSHIP	PHASE IN ROLE TRANSITION AS A NURSE MANAGER	CHARACTERISTICS OF PHASE
Dating	Role preview	Presentation of best characteristics to make favorable impression; both parties evaluate each other to determine likelihood of the other being able to fulfill one's expectations
Commitment to relationship	Role acceptance	Public announcement of mutual decision to initiate contract
Honeymoon	Role exploration	Experience of excitement, confidence, and mutual appreciation
Disillusionment	Role discrepancy	Awareness of difference between role expectations and role performance; reconsideration of whether to continue with contract
Resolution	Role development	Negotiation of role expectations; adjustment of role performance to approximate expectations and to find own unique style
Maturation of relationship	Role internalization	Performance of role congruent with own beliefs and individual style; achievement of mutual goals

STRATEGIES TO PROMOTE ROLE TRANSITION

Becoming a manager or assuming a new role requires a transformation—a profound change in identity. Such a transformation invokes stress as the person unlearns old roles and learns the management role. Several strategies can be helpful in easing the strain and speeding the process of role transition (Box 27-3).

BOX 27-3 STRATEGIES TO PROMOTE ROLE TRANSITION

- Strengthen internal resources
- Assess the organization's resources, culture, and group dynamics
- Negotiate the role
- Grow with a mentor
- Develop management knowledge and skills

Internal Resources

A key strategy in promoting role transition is to recognize, use, and strengthen one's values and beliefs. Behavior is influenced by values and beliefs. It is important that new leaders do not lose sight of their own values and beliefs. The role of manager is not for everyone. One must consider whether personal goals and professional fulfillment can best be achieved through management. One's commitment to the challenges of managing can provide the desire to persevere during the process of role transition.

If an individual in transition understands his or her own personal values, these will help the person respond to situations and relationships. A person's value does not depend on the quality or quickness of the adjustment to the management role. An exercise such as writing down short statements of belief or self-affirmations and posting this information may be helpful as a visual reminder.

Changing circumstances in health care raise the need for flexibility. The effective leader must be able to learn and master new skills, translate information for staff, and adapt behavior to the situation. It is also important for the new leader to not expect too much of oneself all at once; understanding that this transition takes time will help with flexibility. Weinstock (2011) states that new leaders often take a year to understand their role, system, and boundaries.

Organizational Assessment

A new manager is much like an immigrant in a new country. An immigrant learns how to access the available resources to acclimate to the new environment. Cultural practices of the new country may seem strange or odd. Such differences can be analyzed and decisions made about which aspects to incorporate into one's own culture. More subtle differences in communication patterns or group dynamics can also be identified. Understanding the nuances of social interactions is often the most difficult aspect of acclimating to a new country. The transition is smoother for the immigrant who understands himself or herself, assesses the new environment, and learns how to communicate within groups.

The new manager must also learn how to access resources in the organization. Approaching the organization as a foreign culture, the new manager can keenly observe the rituals, accepted practices, and patterns of communication within the organization. This ongoing assessment promotes a speedier transition into the role of manager. The immigrant who spends energy bemoaning the difficulties of the new country may fail to enjoy the advantages that drew him or her to the country in the first place. In the same way, the manager who focuses on the weaknesses of the organization may lack the energy to internalize the new role, a step that is critical to being an effective leader.

Role Negotiation

A strategy that is helpful during conflicting role expectations is **role negotiation.** The ROLES assessment (see Exercise 27-1) may have identified areas of significant conflict. Writing down the expectations is the first step in resolving areas of conflict. It is important to review the expectations listed to determine whether they are realistic. Unrealistic expectations strongly held by others may require diplomatic reeducation so that their expectations can become more realistic.

The priority of different role expectations may also require role negotiation with the person above you in the line of command. Ask for input as to which expectations have the highest priorities. Explain personal and family expectations and clearly state the priority that meeting those expectations has. The process may have to be repeated several times before agreement on the expectations related to roles and the priority of each expectation is found. Rewriting the unrealistic expectations to be achievable can reduce three common sources of role stress—ambiguity, overload, and conflict. Each person's role contributes to the end result. All individuals must understand their roles, or the team may fail.

EXERCISE 27-1

ROLES Assessment

Answer these questions for a position in management that you would consider.

Responsibilities

1. From the position description, what are the responsibilities?
2. For what decisions are you responsible?
3. Consider information about the management position that you learned during the interview (this may be role-played). Also consider the responsibilities of managers you have observed. Are there other responsibilities to add to your list?

Opportunities

4. What would you like to do differently from the previous manager?
5. How could your strengths or expertise benefit the people or nursing unit you would manage?
6. Dream a little (or a lot). If a person who had been a patient on the unit were describing the nursing care to another potential patient, what would you want the first patient to say? Describe the unit as you want it to be known.

Lines of Communication

7. Draw yourself in the middle of a separate piece of paper. Now fill in the people above you and below you with whom you would communicate. Draw lines from you to each person or group. On the line, identify the form of communication. For example, if you communicate with the director of nursing through a weekly report, write on the line, "Written report."

Expectations

8. This may be the most difficult part to assess. List in short sentences or phrases the expectations each person or group may have for you in relation to your management position.

SELF   FAMILY
ADMINISTRATION   IMMEDIATE SUPERVISOR
PEOPLE YOU WILL MANAGE

Support

9. What people do you know in the organization who could provide information that you will need to do your job?
10. What departments provide services that you could access for assistance?

Next Steps

Now compare the lists.

Place a star next to those expectations that are held by more than one person or group. For example, you want to handle the budget of the unit efficiently, an expectation shared with nursing administration.

Circle those items that could cause conflicts.

Refer to the Strategies to promote role transition section in this chapter on how to resolve these conflicts.

Save your responses to these questions to review in 3 months. You may be surprised how your own perception of your ROLES may change over time.

Mentors

The process of mentoring is not a new concept. This concept has been alive since Homer's *Odyssey*. Odysseus leaves Ithaca to fight in the Trojan War. Before leaving, he entrusts his son to Mentor. Mentor was to develop and prepare him for his life and duties. Race and Skees (2010) note "a **mentor** has the job of helping others learn. The goal of the mentor-mentee or protégé relationship is to promote a mentee's career development" (p. 164).

The Literature Perspective provides insight into the need for mentors throughout one's professional career.

LITERATURE PERSPECTIVE

Resource: Race, T.K. & Skees, J. (2010). Changing tides: Improving outcomes through mentorship on all levels of nursing. *Critical Care Nurse Quarterly, 33*(2), 165-174.

This article focuses on the need for mentoring in all levels of nursing careers from nursing student to new graduate to seasoned nurse to nurse faculty. The authors' lived experiences in the transition from critical care practice to faculty in an academic nursing program serve as the basis for the call for mentoring.

Nursing has a history of being unsupportive of new nurses. The importance of a formal mentoring program for nurses is critical in recruiting and retaining new graduate nurses. Nurse leaders play a pivotal role in promotion of a mentoring culture. Nurse leaders must be visible and perceptive, and acknowledge, value, and recognize staff achievements.

The authors' strategies for successful role transitions include a collegial mentoring model, formal or informal mentoring programs, learning needs assessments, careful mentoring, and reward mechanisms for nurses transitioning into new roles.

Implications for Practice

Formal or informal mentoring is a critical success factor in transitioning nurses into new roles. Nurse leaders must embrace a mentoring environment and be open and responsive to new nursing staff. Satisfied nursing staff promote satisfied patients, which is a key focus in the transparent healthcare environment.

Mentors can be a tremendous source of guidance and support for direct care nurses and managers, serving both career functions and psychosocial functions. Career functions are possible because the mentor has sufficient professional experience and organizational authority to facilitate the career of the "mentee." Box 27-4 highlights some key functions of mentors.

Sponsorship involves volunteering or nominating the mentee for additional responsibilities. A mentor can be a sponsor by creating opportunities for individual achievement and providing encouragement. The mentor may suggest the mentee be appointed to a key nursing committee or volunteer for a special assignment. Sponsorship leads to exposure or opportunities for the mentee to build a reputation of competence. With exposure, the mentor provides protection by absorbing negative feedback, sharing responsibility for controversial decisions, and teaching the unwritten rules about "how things are done around here." These unwritten rules may be more important to job success than the written rules.

Coaches provide information about how to improve performance, including feedback on current performance. *Coaching* requires frequent contact and willingness on the part of the mentee to accept feedback. Challenging assignments are given to the mentee that will stretch the limits of knowledge and skill. The mentor helps the mentee learn the technical and management skills necessary to accomplish the task, such as which numbers on the budget printout are added to achieve the total expenditures.

The interpersonal relationship between the mentor and the mentee involves mutual positive regard. Because the mentee respects the career accomplishments of the mentor, the mentee identifies with the mentor's example. This role modeling is both conscious and unconscious. The mentee with character and self-respect will evaluate the behaviors of the mentor and select those behaviors worthy of being emulated.

Counseling, as another psychosocial function of the mentor, allows the mentee to explore personal concerns. Confidentiality is a prerequisite to sharing personal information. Because the opinion of the mentor is respected, the mentor may provide guidance to the mentee. The best mentors can provide guidance while recognizing that the mentee may choose to disregard the advice.

Being mentored is a learning process. Admiration for a mentor and recognition of the mentor's commitment to self-success can provide an environment of trust in which a mentor-mentee relationship begins. Both persons develop positive expectations of the relationship, and both take the initiative to nurture the new relationship. As more of the mentor functions are experienced, the bond between the mentor and mentee grows stronger.

Relationships between mentors and mentees vary because of individual characteristics and the career phase of each. During the early phases of a career, a nurse manager is concerned about competence and a mentor can provide valuable coaching. As the nurse manager develops, sponsorship by a mentor can prepare the manager for a promotion. A mentor nearing the end of the work career can find fulfillment in sharing knowledge with new managers and at the same time benefit from the counsel of a recently retired colleague.

BOX 27-4	**BENEFITS OF MENTORING**
MENTOR	**MENTEE**
Role model	Develop career goals
Nurturer	Recognize strengths and weaknesses
Caregiver	One to one relationship with mentor
Develop larger network	

Modified from Funderburk, A. (2008). Mentoring: The retention factor in the acute care setting. *Journal for Nurses in Staff Development, 24*(3), E1-E5.

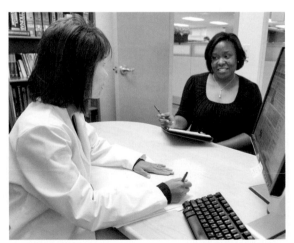

Keeping up with current research is an effective management and education strategy.

Management Education

Management performance can be hindered by a specific knowledge deficit. For example, the manager may lack business skills or knowledge about legal aspects of supervision. Cathcart, Greenspan, and Quin (2010) share that "the nurse manager now has tremendous responsibility to sustain quality, safety, innovation, efficiency and financial performance at the unit level" (p. 441). In addition, the authors note, "Nurse managers require ongoing support and development by senior nursing leadership to sustain the complex and demanding relational work of practice development" (p. 447).

Ongoing professional development is needed at all levels of leadership. The Research Perspective illustrates the importance of education for charge nurses.

 RESEARCH PERSPECTIVE

Resource: Patrician, P.A., Oliver, D.O., Miltner, R.S., Dawson, M., & Ladner, K.A. (2012). Nurturing charge nurses for future leadership roles. *Journal of Nursing Administration, 42*(10), 461-466.

Charge nurses are key to running a busy inpatient or ambulatory nursing setting. Charge nurses run the unit in the absence of the nurse manager or in conjunction with the nurse manager. Charge nurses serve as resource people for the staff and keep the day-to-day operations of the unit flowing. This role is often learned on the job, and many organizations offer no specific educational curriculum.

This qualitative descriptive study used focus groups of charge nurses to determine what the professional educational development needs were to prepare for the role. Charge nurse challenges identified were categorized into four themes: managing staff performance, clarifying the role, feeling powerless in the face of system complexities, and lacking support of leadership.

Recommendations for nursing leaders included formal education and orientation to the role, managing performance and development of staff, and developing communication skills. Additional education should be focused on unit finances and patient relations. Leadership support was found to be pivotal for charge nurses to feel successful or hinder their work.

Implications for Practice

Charge nurses need to have formal preparation and mentoring to be successful in their roles. The role of the charge nurse has often been discounted and yet it needs to be elevated to prominence. A focus on this role can form an effective succession planning model for other nursing leadership roles.

Experience and education provide a firm basis for seeking additional credentials. A nurse holding an administrative position at the nurse executive level with a baccalaureate preparation and 24 months of experience can take an examination to become a certified nursing executive. Nursing administrators with master's degrees and experience at the executive level can take an examination to become a certified nurse executive, advanced. The Website of the American Nurses Credentialing Center (ANCC, 2013) has more detailed information about certification examinations (*www.nursecredentialing.org*). A certification credential also was developed by the American Organization of Nurse Executives (AONE, 2013) exclusively for the nurse executive and the certified nurse manager leader—the Certification in Executive Nursing Practice (CENP) and Certified Nurse Manager Leader (CNML) (*www.aone.org/certification*).

FROM ROLE TRANSITION TO ROLE TRIUMPH

Developing an intimate relationship can be a difficult process, but most people still value relationships enough to make the effort. Making the transition and transformation into a management role is also worth the effort. Leading lives of integrity and commitment, nurse managers set examples, bringing out the best in direct care nurses and thereby multiplying their influence on quality patient care.

CONCLUSION

Transitions from a direct care nurse position to charge nurse or nurse manager pose new challenges. Nurses who make these transitions with minimal discomfort are reflective of role theory in action. Although nurses today are better prepared to take on more formal leadership roles, the roles themselves are more challenging. Charge nurses and managers are responsible for mentoring and coaching new staff as they transition to their new roles. These transition activities take time and effort to achieve the best results possible.

THE SOLUTION

Transitioning from a member of the supervisor group to the manager of the supervisor group has been a balancing act. My approach to the role transition was to be well-informed and to be very mindful in all communication with the supervisor group. I took the time to review each performance situation that had occurred and gather insight from all points of contact. I made sure I addressed the nursing supervisors with the utmost respect and listened actively. Overall, my relationships with the nursing supervisors have been positive; however there are several formal colleagues who are still adjusting to the change.

I also focused on learning my resources as a major strategy. Learning who and where the appropriate resources resided was more difficult than I had thought because our medical center was being integrated with a similarly sized medical center. I have tried to adjust my work style to meet the demands of my position through project management tools including electronic and paper methodology. Organization of my thoughts and schedule has been very important to accomplish all that I need to do on a daily basis.

—*Melissa J. Bertelson*

Would this be a suitable approach for you? Why?

THE EVIDENCE

Role transition occurs throughout a nurse's career both personally and professionally. Successful role transition takes time and requires support by preceptors, mentors, managers, and colleagues. A pivotal relationship to cultivate early in one's career is that of a mentor as one's professional nursing career develops. The relationship between mentor and mentee is positive for both individuals. Leadership coaching is a critical component of developing oneself as a follower and a leader. Nurse residency programs provide an avenue to assist with role transition for new graduates, and leadership development programs assist with providing new leaders with a supportive environment.

WHAT NEW GRADS SAY

- I was worried that I would be viewed as incompetent by seasoned nurses; however my preceptors assured me it would take up to a year to feel confident in my new clinical role.

- I was surprised at how tired I was during my first 6 months. My sleep was consumed by dreams about work and what would happen.

CHAPTER CHECKLIST

Role transition is a process that takes time and energy—two scarce resources for nurse managers. Knowing what to expect and how to facilitate the process can speed role transition and minimize the expenditure of energy as the nurse manager negotiates new roles.
- Types of roles
- Leadership
- Roles: The ABCs of understanding roles
- Role transition process
- Strategies to promote role transition
  - Internal resources
  - Organizational assessment
  - Role negotiation
  - Mentors
  - Management education
- From role transition to role triumph

TIPS FOR ROLE TRANSITIONING

- Role transition is a normal process. Anticipate and prepare for role changes.
- Identify the responsibilities, opportunities, lines of communication, expectations, and support for the role.

- Use your internal resources to negotiate a role that is consistent with your values and life commitments.

REFERENCES

American Nurses Credentialing Center (ANCC). (2013). *Certification eligibility criteria.* Retrieved June 7, 2013, from www.nursecredentialing.org/NurseExecutive.

American Organization of Nurse Executives (AONE). (2013). *AONE credentialing center.* Retrieved June 7, 2013, from www.aone.org.

Cathcart, E. B., Greenspan, M., & Quin, M. (2010). *Journal of Nursing Management, 18,* 440–447.

Chari, S. (2008). Handling career role transitions with confidence. *The International Journal of Clinical Leadership, 16,* 109–114.

Hardy, M. E. (1978). Role stress and role strain. In M. E. Hardy &

M. E. Conway (Eds.), *Role theory: Perspectives for health professionals.* New York: Appleton-Century-Crofts.

Patrician, P. A., Oliver, D. O., Miltner, R. S., Dawson, M., & Ladner, K. A. (2012). Nurturing charge nurses for future leadership roles. *Journal of Nursing Administration, 42*(10), 461–466.

Race, T. K., & Skees, J. (2010). Changing tides: Improving outcomes through mentorship on all levels of nursing. *Critical Care Nurse Quarterly, 33*(2), 165–174.

Weinstock, B. (2011). The hidden challenges in role transitions and how leadership coaching can help new leaders find solid ground. *Holistic Nursing Practice, 25*(4), 211–214.

SUGGESTED READINGS

Batson, V., & Yoder, L. H. (2012). Managerial coaching: A concept analysis. *Journal of Advanced Nursing, 68*(7), 1658–1669.

Kuthy, J. E., Ostmann, J. O., Gonzales, R., & Biddle, D. A. (2013). Predicting successful nursing performance. *Nursing Management, 44*(1), 42–52.

28

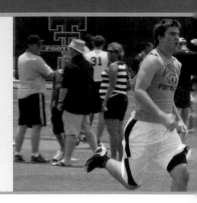

Self-Management: Stress and Time

Mary Ann T. Donohue, Jeannette T. Crenshaw

This chapter examines the concept of self-management—developing self-expression and behaviors that complement rather than duplicate organizational cultures, social contexts, and occupational expectations as a professional nurse. Positive outcomes include effective organization of your day, higher degree of engagement, and enjoyment of daily renewal. Three components of self-management are explored: time management, meeting management, and overall stress management. Methods for managing stress and organizing your time are introduced. Practical exercises and suggestions for stress management and day-to-day time management are presented so they may be used in personal and professional situations and thereby enhance one's personal and professional growth.

LEARNING OUTCOMES

- Define self-management.
- Explore personal and professional stressors.
- Analyze selected strategies to decrease stress.
- Assess the manager's role in helping team members manage stress.
- Evaluate common barriers to effective time management.
- Critique the strengths and weaknesses of selected time management strategies.
- Evaluate selected strategies to manage time more effectively.

KEY TERMS

agenda	fatigue	procrastination
burnout	general adaptation syndrome	role stress
coping	(GAS)	self-management
delegation	information overload	self-reflection
depersonalization	overwork	time management
employee assistance program	perfectionism	

THE CHALLENGE

Mariebelle del Mundo, RN-BC
Nurse Manager Jersey Shore University Medical Center

I had been a nurse manager for a very long time—over 23 years—and was very proud that my dedication to my team had brought my unit to success. We were truly a family; we had barbecues and parties together and celebrated births, graduations, and other important milestones. I supported them and they supported me through the death of my father and throughout his very long illness. My unit was Booker 2, a unit that cared primarily for women's health surgical patients, and

we always scored tops in patient satisfaction as well as team member employee satisfaction. My scores were always the best in the hospital! Unfortunately, the unit census kept dropping, as more surgeries were scheduled on an outpatient basis. Finally, my Vice President/ Chief Nursing Officer (VP/CNO) told me that my unit would close. I was devastated, as were all the members of my team. We were truly in a state of grieving. We would never be together as a "family" again.

What do you think you would do if you were this nurse?

INTRODUCTION

What should you do when you have tried your best in a given situation, but things are still not going well? What needs changing? Where do you begin? Emotional intelligence, a critical leadership competency, involves four skills. Personal competence includes the skills of self-awareness and self-management (TalentSmart®, 2011). Social competence involves the skills of social awareness and relationship management. The good news is that emotional intelligence can be learned. Emotional intelligence is linked to improved self performance, employee performance, and organizational performance (TalentSmart®, 2011; Ingram & Cangemi, 2012). Emotionally intelligent leaders create leadership opportunities that inspires, to transform themselves and others within organizations (Ingram & Cangemi, 2012). As a nurse leader, your goals will include growth and self-knowledge, learning to balance new as well as formerly held personal and professional objectives, and reorganizing your time and activities to reach these goals. The literature suggests that nurse leaders cope with the stresses and crises of everyday life in a variety of ways (Hirokawa, Taniguchi, Tsuchiya, & Kawakami, 2012). The so-called stress hardiness of nurses and leaders is thought to be essential to safe, high-quality patient care (Halm et al., 2005), as well as staff recruitment and retention (Bailey, 2009). In the past, seasoned nurses would pride themselves on being able to "take it," meaning silently work without openly challenging certain unfavorable aspects of the workplace, however unacceptable they might be. Those who left nursing, unable or unwilling to tolerate difficult conditions in the practice setting, were labeled as "weak," "bad nurses," or simply,

"not a good fit" for the organization. Historically, research on stress in the nursing workplace focused on the individual's acceptance of demanding work environments, complex role requirements, and recurring staff shortages instead of proactive problem solving (Shirey, 2006). However, true hardiness, as described in the seminal work by Lambert and Lambert (1987), incorporates control, commitment, and challenge as tools in one's personal repertoire to better deal with what cannot easily be changed. In fact, investing in leadership development was found to provide healthcare leaders with opportunities to connect, strengthen social support networks, and mitigate against the toxic effects of burnout (Lee et al., 2010). Leaders in progressive and innovative thinking, called "thought leaders," reflected in the meta-analysis of Zangaro & Soeken (2007), suggested that cultivating stress hardiness produces nurse managers with a leadership style and resilience that actually improves overall working conditions. Fortunately, stress management can be taught and personal hardiness can be acquired, yet interventions at all organizational levels must be tested for their value in reducing caregiver burnout and stress (Judkins, Reid, & Furlow, 2006; Epp, 2012).

To develop stress hardiness, we must actively improve our skills related to stress management, adaptive coping, healthy communication, and problem solving. The three key strategies introduced in this chapter—stress management, time management, and meeting management—are important ways to do more with fewer resources. Time and stress are somewhat of a chicken-and-egg phenomenon—running out of time contributes to stress, and stress may further erode efficiency and thus decrease time on task. The key lies in our ability to "take charge," and strive to manage both time and stress, personally and professionally. Over time, the outcome of skillful self-management is hardiness and an improved ability to accomplish worthwhile goals.

UNDERSTANDING STRESS

Nurses have learned about the effect of stress on patients and how to teach them to manage its consequences. However, only one third of nurse managers have any sort of formal leadership or managerial training (Bailey, 2009) that would prepare them for dealing with competing needs and priorities; that is, being able to skillfully manage multiple sources of stress at the same time. Nurses need to recognize the unique stressors in their professional and personal lives. The ubiquitous use of the Holmes-Rahe Stress Scale reinforces that everyone experiences stress—the exhilaration of a joyous event, as well as the negative feelings and unpleasant physical symptoms that may be associated with a difficult life situation or even the anticipation of a specific difficulty, such as meeting the new girlfriend's parents or taking an exam in a tough subject area. Stress is defined as the uncomfortable gap between how we would like our life to be and how it actually is. Nurses are not immune to the effects of stress and, in fact, modern nursing is a very stressful occupation, with fewer nurses taking care of more and more critically ill patients (Chen, Davis, Davis, Pan, & Daraiseh, 2010). Learning what stress is, its dynamics, and some strategies to manage stress is a part of the personal and professional maturation of all individuals. Because nurses tend to work in areas and in situations that are stressful, it is very important that stress management skills continuously improve over time.

Definition

In this chapter, *stress* and *distress* (Selye, 1965) are used interchangeably, although some writers regard stress as neutral and refer to positive attributes or preceptions of stress as *eustress* and negative attributes or perceptions of stress as *distress*. Stress is a consequence or response to an event or stimulus. Stress is not inherently bad. It is each individual's interpretation that determines whether the event is viewed as positive or threatening. In addition, stress management does not necessarily mean stress reduction or elimination. More than

30 years ago, Kobasa, Maddi, and Kahn (1982) characterized successful stress management as emotional and behavioral control, perseverance, and a sense of challenge in the face of stressful events. Stress management is a nurse manager competency (Jennings, Scalzi, & Rodgers, 2007) and how leaders incorporate ways to mitigate stress in one's leadership style is tied to employee stress (Lopez, Green, Carmody-Bubb, & Kodatt, 2011). Stress management has important implications for the workplace because of its link to low absenteeism rates, improved quality, and increased productivity (Judkins, Reid, & Furlow, 2006).

SOURCES OF JOB STRESS

Job stress can be defined as the physical and emotional responses that arise when the job requirements do not match the abilities, resources, or needs of the worker. Work-related stress can lead to poor physical and emotional health and injury. Job-related challenges (eustress), which motivate us to learn new skills, master our jobs, and manage new situations, differs from distress, which can lead to symptoms in a range from fatigue to exhaustion, feelings of inadequacy, and failure, or even, complete burnout. If you are involved in an oral interview for a job, you will benefit from a certain amount of stress (eustress). It is stress that provides you with determination and gives you the "edge" we all need to help us think quickly and clearly and express our thoughts in ways that will benefit the interview process. On the way to the interview, however, having the car break down or missing the bus or train connection certainly creates stress (distress) as you realize that you will most certainly be late for the anticipated appointment. However, as more is learned about the relationship of stress to physiologic changes, stressors will become even easier to identify. When one looks at job-related stressors, the stressors fall into one of two categories: external (working conditions) and internal (worker characteristics).

External Sources

Nursing is a very stressful occupation (Dickerson, 2013). Work-related stressors, such as an ever-increasing workload, rotating shifts, high patient acuity, inadequate staffing, ethical conflicts, dealing with acute illness and death, role ambiguity, the multiple, complex, and continually growing number of responsibilities, constant multitasking, work relationships, and job insecurity have all been associated with increased stress, possibly culminating in complete exhaustion and burnout (Rudan, 2002; Krichbaum et al., 2007). Nurses spend more and more time at work, and nurse managers report 12- to 14-hour days with accountability 24 hours a day, 7 days per week, tied to a cellphone or other electronic device that is never completely "powered down." Nurse leaders, managers, and charge nurses often supervise direct-care workers who are unlicensed. Unlicensed direct care workers also have jobs that are fraught with ethical conflicts, require complex decision making, and are physically taxing (Seavey, 2010).

Change

Although the distress that results from change takes many forms, two underlying patterns appear to be constant. Often, nurses feel trapped by conflicting expectations. They expect to furnish evidence-based clinical care, to meet all their patients' and families' emotional needs, and to be warm, friendly, and nurturing to their co-workers. Ultimately, organizations also require nurses to be knowledgeable about their business unit and have a financial awareness about how they contribute to overall efficiency and cost-effectiveness and receive high marks on their patient satisfaction scores. Because individuals—frontline direct care nurses, nurse managers, and chief nursing executives alike—cannot easily balance caring and clinical expectations with business and administrative demands, it is completely normal to sometimes experience considerable role overload, frustration, and distress.

Social

Interpersonal relations can buffer stressors or can in themselves become stressors. Outside the work setting, home may represent a refuge for harried nurses; however, stressors at home, when severe, can impair work performance and relationships among staff or even include violent patterns that may invade the workplace and create an unhealthy work environment. When one parent in the home works hours other than daytime hours, significant behavior problems may occur in infants during the first 2 years of life as compared to children in families where both parents work standard day shifts (Rosenbaum &

Morett, 2009). Therefore the cycle of work pressure and home pressure can at times seem insurmountable, especially to the younger nurse who may be caring for an elderly parent, sick partner, or child. Added to the mix may be attending school to attain a university degree and studying for a national board certification, all common requirements of the contemporary work setting.

Changes in healthcare delivery systems, as well as the cycles in the nursing workforce supply and demand, have impacted professional nursing in many ways. Some work settings may have a disproportionate representation of *Gen X or Y* or perhaps a larger percentage of older nurses, the *Baby Boomer Generation*. In situations where the values of one generation of workers clash with that of another, conflict occurs unless the manager becomes aware of how to best maximize the positive behaviors of each generation (Thomas, 2010).

In geographic areas suffering from staffing shortages, inpatient settings may have minimally safe levels of professional caregivers. Because of the economy, and changes in federal financial reimbursement in the form of greatly reduced Medicare payments to U.S. hospitals, overly strict adherence to unit budgets may result in rigid staffing patterns that are not realistically flexed to actual patient acuity. Consequently, layoffs or buyouts may occur and with it, the struggle to maintain supportive, collegial relationships that were established over many years. Still other institutions have turned to supplemental staffing with agency or "traveling" nurses, thus creating a very transient nursing staff. When nurses are reassigned or "float" to unaccustomed patient care units, they often work with unfamiliar staff. Thus they may feel isolated or become unwillingly involved in dysfunctional politics on the unit. Floating, by definition, means that nurses work with patients whose requirements for care may be unfamiliar, resulting in further stress related to patient safety concerns.

Persons in management level positions may also become stressors. Communication may come from the top down, with little opportunity for nurses to participate in decisions that affect them directly or that they may need to implement without proper training or support. On units or in hospitals without a viable shared governance system of shared decision making, nurses may experience distress from feelings of frustration and helplessness without an opportunity for input to improve the clinical care and work environment of the frontline direct care nurse.

In addition, disruptive behavior from members of the healthcare team in itself, poses considerable work stress (see Chapter 25). Although healthy workplaces include freedom from such behavior, too many instances of disruptive behavior occur in healthcare settings. In addition to being stressful for nurses, such behavior can disrupt patient safety efforts (see the Research Perspective).

The Position

Upon entering nursing school, most students expect that caring for patients who are chronically or critically ill and for families who have experienced tragedy will be stressful. The current environment in many healthcare agencies, however, is even more complex than ever before and is often characterized by **overwork,** as well as by the stresses inherent in contemporary nursing practice. In some settings, direct care nurses have been expected to stay beyond the designated assignment period, constituting mandatory overtime, often with little or no notice. Owing

 RESEARCH PERSPECTIVE

Resource: Johnson, S. & King, D. (2012). Nurses' perceptions of nurse-physician relationships: Medical-surgical vs. intensive care. *MEDSURG Nursing, 21*(6), 343-347.

This study was based upon the premise that positive relationships between nurses and physicians promote improved patient-centered outcomes, particularly in the area of preventable "never events" and in patient safety. Medical/surgical nurses were less likely to participate in interdisciplinary rounds compared to ICU nurses; ICU nurses were more likely to report that their physician colleagues treated them like handmaidens. The researchers' conclusion was that no specialty within nursing practice is immune to issues related to the RN–MD relationship, that all nurse leaders should promote activities designed to raise awareness of the impact of unhealthy RN–MD relationships and report disruptive behaviors at every level.

Implications for Practice
Disruptive behaviors in the work environment must be reported. Because disruptions negatively impact patient care, organizational support must exist for a zero tolerance environment, and a mechanism for reporting disruptive behaviors must be endorsed by executive, administrative, and professional leaders.

to the nature of stress and crisis, some patients and families may escalate in their own threatening behaviors and verbally or physically attack their own caregivers. Several states, in response to legislative efforts and pressure from their constituents, have enacted criminal laws to protect healthcare workers from such violence. Many healthcare institutions have established relationships with local police departments in order to convey a zero tolerance policy to those who are violent toward their team members (see *www.nursingworld.org/WorkplaceViolence.aspx*). A zero tolerance workplace means that acts of violence toward staff are not acceptable and will, in most cases, be prosecuted to the full extent of the law.

Another common stressor for nurses is the paradox of the presence and/or the lack of technology in the workplace. Often, nurses face stress as they attempt to learn and then integrate multiple systems that may lack sufficient interface, which often leads to frustration when they must toggle between multiple screens to complete necessary patient documentation. When healthcare software is not designed well, the user can get stuck in a cycle when there is no logical or correct answer in a mandatory field. Many times, nurses experience this as a burden because they are, so to speak, feeding *data hungry systems* that were created and put into a production workflow to solve individually focused tasks, such as entering a patient's blood pressure or blood glucose levels, without regard to the comprehensive effect upon workflow (see *http://ncbi.nlm.nih.gov/pubmed/10730596* and *http://ncbi.nlm.nih.gov/pmc/articles/PMC61466*). Or some areas within the same facility may still use paper documentation. Nurses may need to bridge the gap to safely communicate with their internal and external colleagues whose workplaces are more technologically advanced.

Role stress is an additional stressor for nurses. Viewed as the incongruence between perceived role expectations and achievement (Chang & Hancock, 2003), role stress for new graduates is related to role ambiguity and role overload. Role stress is particularly acute for new graduates, whose lack of clinical experience and organizational skills, combined with new situations and procedures, may increase feelings of overwhelming stress. Conflict between what was learned in the classroom and actual practice compounds the situation and increases stress. This concept has been so historically common in nursing that the phenomenon gave rise to the term "reality shock," in Dr. Marlene Kramer's (1974) seminal work. Unfortunately, transition to practice issues have endured to present day because academic and practice leaders have not yet managed to completely eradicate its unfortunate effects upon ensuing generations of nurses.

Gender Roles

Approximately 9.4% of the nation's 3.1 million licensed registered nurses working in the United States are men (Health Resources and Services Administration, 2013), and so most nurses are women and go home at the end of their shift to traditional responsibilities, including managing the household and caring for young children and aging parents with healthcare demands of their own. When added to the already stressful workday of the nurse, the additional responsibilities often contribute to the level of distress that is experienced. Male nurses may experience these same challenges. Thanks to Generation Y's (those born in the 1980s) entry into the workforce, the importance of work-life balance has become increasingly emphasized but has not yet entirely translated into improvements in the American workplace. Owing to the economy, spouses or partners may be unemployed or experience sharply reduced work hours with poor or nonexistent health benefits. Children or even grandchildren may have returned to live at home. Therefore many nurses are shouldering the burden of another full- or part-time job and increasing their requests for overtime so they can add additional income to already overstretched household budgets. Lack of financial security means that in times of severe economic hardships, such as in a national economic recession or perhaps regional threats to the local economy, such as in a severe hurricane, living from paycheck to paycheck sharply reduces one's options to improve oneself through career advancement. Financial insecurity may actually curtail career opportunity. For example, some nurses may be too afraid to seek a better position because of concern for not succeeding in a new position, not liking a new job, losing health benefits, or experiencing layoffs in an uncertain economy.

Evans and Steptoe (2002) examined the associations of work stress and gender-role orientation to psychological well-being and sickness-related work absences in male-dominated (accounting) and female-dominated (nursing) occupations in England. They concluded that when men and women are occupationally engaged in gender-dominated occupations in which they are in the gender minority, the men and women perceived more work-related hassles and exhibited gender-specific health effects. Therefore special consideration must be recognized in males; gay, lesbian, and transgender (GLTG) individuals; and members of minority racial and ethnic groups, who may experience stress or forms of bias or prejudice in the workplace.

Internal Sources

Personal stress "triggers" are events or situations that have an effect on specific individuals. A personal trigger might be a specific event such as the death of a loved one, an automobile accident, losing a job, or getting married or divorced. These events are in addition to daily personal stressors such as working in a noisy environment, experiencing job dissatisfaction, or having a long or difficult daily commute to work. Negative self-talk, pessimistic thinking, self-criticism, and overanalyzing situations can be significant ongoing stressors. These internal sources of stress usually stem from unrealistic self-beliefs (unrealistic expectations, taking things personally, all-or-nothing thinking, exaggerating, or rigid thinking), perfectionism, or the type A personality.

An individual's ability to deal with stress may be moderated by psychological hardiness. According to Lambert, Lambert, and Yamase (2003), psychological hardiness is a composite of commitment, control, and challenge. These form a constellation that (1) dampers the effects of stress by challenging the perception of the situation and (2) decreases the negative impact of a situation by moderating both cognitive appraisal and coping. Maddi (2002), in a 12-year longitudinal study, found that individuals thriving in a stressful work environment displayed the same psychological hardiness. The *commitment attitude* led the individuals to be actively involved in the changes that decreased isolation. The *control attitude* led them to try to influence outcomes rather than sink into powerlessness and passivity. The *challenge attitude* led them to believe that the stressful events were opportunities for new learning.

Poor and unhealthy lifestyle choices, such as the use of caffeine, lack of exercise, a fat-ridden diet, inadequate sleep and leisure time, and cigarette smoking, have a direct effect on the amount of one's stress and create a vicious lose-lose cycle. Nurses attending a 2012 House of Delegates and Healthy Nurse Conference participated in a survey. Only 30 reported being at a healthy weight (not overweight or obese; exercised the recommended four to five times a week); 78% drank one or less sugary drink per day; and only 40% ate the suggested four or more servings of fruits and vegetables a day (*Georgia Nursing* 2012-2013). The recent ANA campaign, *The Healthy Nurse,* which promotes healthy and safe work environments as well as healthy personal choices and behaviors, underscores the need for us to improve our overall health in order to safely care for others and live longer, more satisfied lives (*www.nursingworld.org/MainMenuCategories/WorkplaceSafety/Healthy-Nurse*).

Dynamics of Stress

Stress may result from unrealistic or conflicting expectations originating from oneself or others, the pace and magnitude of change, human behavior, individual personality characteristics, the characteristics of the position itself, or the culture of the organization. Other stressors may be unique to certain environments, situations, and persons or groups. Initially, increased stress produces increased performance. However, when stress continues to increase or remains intense, performance decreases. Hans Selye's midcentury investigations to decode the nature of and reactions to stress (Selye, 1956) have been very influential. In his classic theory, Selye (1991) described the concept of stress, identified the **general adaptation syndrome (GAS),** and detailed a predictable pattern of response (see the Theory Box on p. 525 and Figure 28-1).

More recent investigations of the relationship among the brain, the immune system, and health (psychoneuroimmunology) have generated models that challenge Selye's (1956) general adaptation syndrome. Although Selye states that all people respond with a similar set of hormonal and immune responses to any stress, Kemeny (2003) has since proposed that there are two stress responses: (1) the classic GAS and (2) a withdrawing reaction, in which the person pulls back to conserve energy. Kemeny hypothesized that people respond to the same psychological event in different ways, depending on their independent appraisal of the situation (DeAngelis, 2002).

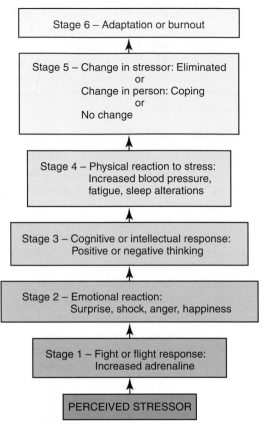

FIGURE 28-1 The stress diagram.

Critical of stress research using predominately (87%) male subjects, Taylor et al. (2000) proposed a model of the female stress response, the "tend and befriend," as opposed to the male's "fight or flight" model. The "tend and befriend" response is an estrogen and oxytocin–mediated stress response that is characterized by caring for offspring and befriending those around in times of stress to increase chances of survival.

Most nurses can easily recognize the origins of stress and its symptoms. For example, a healthcare agency may make demands on nurses, such as excessive work, that the nurses regard as beyond their capacity to perform. When they are unable to resolve the problem through overwork, with more staff, or by looking at the situation in another way, nurses may feel threatened or depressed and increase the number of callouts on the job. They may also experience headaches, fatigue, inability to concentrate, or other physical symptoms. If the stress persists, such symptoms

THEORY BOX

Theories Applicable to Self-Management

KEY CONTRIBUTORS	KEY IDEAS	APPLICATION TO PRACTICE
Maslow's Hierarchy of Needs: Maslow (1943) identified five need levels of every human.	Although recent research shows the five levels are not always present or in order, it is reasonable that unmet needs motivate most employees most of the time.	Nurse wages should be sufficient to provide shelter and food. Job security and a social environment that rewards and recognizes nurse performance are important.
General Adaptation Syndrome: Selye (1956) is credited with developing this theory.	The "stress response" is an adrenocortical reaction to stressors that is accompanied by psychological changes and physiologic alterations that follow a pattern of fight or flight. The general adaptation syndrome includes an alarm, resistance, and adaptation or exhaustion.	Change, lack of control, and excessive workload are common stressors that evoke psychological and physiologic distress among nurses.
Complex Adaptive Systems: Plsek and Greenhalgh (2001).	This theory of unpredictable interactions between interdependent people and activities emphasizes the importance of innovation and rapid information sharing to improve performance.	Nurse engagement in self-managed groups and teams allows organizations to shape their environment through controlled "experimentation" using the rapid-cycle plan-do-study-act improvement method.
The Pareto Principle: Hafner (2001).	The "Pareto Principle" refers to a universal observation of "vital few, trivial many." Pareto (1848-1923) studied distribution of personal incomes in Italy and observed that 80% of the wealth was controlled by 20% of the population. This concept of disproportion often holds in many areas. Although the exact values of 20% and 80% are not significant, the observation of considerable disproportion is important to remember.	The 80-20 rule can be applied to many aspects of health care today. For example, 80% of healthcare expenditures are on 20% of the population, and 80% of personnel problems come from 20% of the staff. In quality improvement, 80% of improvement can be expected by removing 20% of the causes of unacceptable quality or performance. A nurse can also expect that 80% of patient-care time will be spent working with 20% of his or her patient assignment.

may increase and manifest themselves in negative outcomes such as medication errors or musculoskeletal or needle-stick injuries. Nurses may attempt to cope by becoming completely apathetic or by resigning their positions. These are signs of **burnout.** Table 28-1 gives physical, mental, and spiritual/emotional signs of overstress in individuals.

In 2004, Segerstrom and Miller published a meta-analysis of research on the relationship between stress and the human immune system. They found that acute stressors (very short-term) "revved up" the immune system, preparing for infection or injury. Short-term stressors, such as difficult exams, tended to suppress cellular immunity while preserving humoral immunity. The immune systems of those who are older or already sick are more prone to stress-related immune system changes.

Physical illnesses linked to stress include visceral adiposity (body fat), type II diabetes, cardiovascular disease (hypertension, heart attack, stroke), musculoskeletal disorders, psychological disorders (anxiety, depression), workplace injury, neuromuscular disorders (multiple sclerosis), suicide, cancer, ulcers, asthma, and rheumatoid arthritis. Stress can even cause life-threatening sympathetic stimulation.

MANAGEMENT OF STRESS

Individuals respond to stress by eliciting coping strategies that are a means of dealing with stress to maintain or achieve an improved sense of well-being or work-life balance. Certain strategies may be ineffective because of their reliance on methods such as

TABLE 28-1   SIGNS OF OVERSTRESS IN INDIVIDUALS

PHYSICAL	MENTAL	SPIRITUAL/EMOTIONAL
Physical signs of ill health: • Increase in flu, colds, accidents • Change in sleeping habits • Fatigue **Chronic signs of decreased ability to manage stress:** • Headaches • Hypertension • Backaches • Gastrointestinal problems **Unhealthy coping activities:** • Increased use of drugs and alcohol • Increased weight • Smoking • Crying, yelling, blaming	• Dread going to work every day • Rigid thinking and a desire to go by all the rules in all cases; inability to tolerate any changes • Forgetfulness and anxiety about work to be done; more frequent errors and incidents • Returning home exhausted and unable to participate in enjoyable activities • Confusion about duties and roles • Generalized anxiety • Decrease in concentration • Depression • Anger, irritability, impatience	• Sense of being a failure; disappointed in work performance • Anger and resentment toward patients, colleagues, and managers; overall irritable attitude • Lack of positive feelings toward others • Cynicism toward patients, blaming them for their problems • Excessive worry, insecurity, lowered self-esteem • Increased family and friend conflict

excessive alcohol or prescription drug or substance abuse. Other methods, such as exercise, meditation, or professional counseling, may be quite effective in helping to restore a greater sense of well-being and effectiveness. More examples of effective strategies are discussed here.

Stress Prevention

One effective way to deal with stress is to determine and manage its source. Discovering the origin of stress in patient care may be difficult because some environments have changed so rapidly that the nursing staff is overwhelmed trying to balance bureaucratic rules and limited resources with the demands of vulnerable human beings. *Complexity compression* is the name given to conditions in which change occurs with great intensity (Krichbaum et al., 2007). When in distress, nurses may need to step back and look at the big picture. By identifying daily stressors, the nurse can then develop a plan of action for management of the stress. This plan may include eliminating the stressor, modifying the stressor, or changing the perception of the stressor (e.g., viewing mistakes as opportunities for new learning) by the use of the reframing technique.

Many of the day-to-day activities of nursing can create workplace stress. Consider the nature of acute care nursing and the potential for serious injury to others. Staffing shortages create situations of caring for more patients with less help while pulling, moving or pushing equipment. Nurses may have inadequate rest because of rotating shifts or irregular schedules or because they may come to work already tired from caring for other family members or working additional jobs *and* going to school. Nurses are subject to significant occupational hazards such as musculoskeletal stress caused by lifting, pulling, and turning patients. Nurses give physical care to those who have potentially communicable diseases or may become verbally or physically abusive or assaultive. Nurses are highly engaged with patients and their families who suffer with acute pain and grief associated with either chronic or acute illness. Of course, such on-the-job stressors are often counterbalanced by the rewards of patient appreciation, the joy of seeing a healthy baby born, or seeing firsthand, the relief brought by a nursing intervention such as appropriate pain medication or repositioning of an uncomfortable limb. However, given the nature of nursing practice, it is wise for the nurse to be alert to his or her own signs of stress and to be able to develop self-awareness about work-life balance. Each of us has to understand how many hours in a day, how many shifts in a row, and how many hours or days between shifts is sufficient so that one may become comfortable with saying "no" to an unreasonable workload rather than risk personal health and patient safety. It is important to cultivate healthy lifestyle habits to help reduce stress. Adequate sleep, a balanced diet, regular exercise, and frequent interactions with friends are excellent stress-buffering habits to develop.

According to Stöppler (2005), the top five stress-management mistakes are poor calendar habits, clutter, perfectionism, self-treatment, and following others' expectations. These may be high on your list of stress experiences. Analyze your stress experiences by completing Exercise 28-1.

EXERCISE 28-1

Identify what stress you experience and how you usually manage it. Create and complete the following log at the end of every day for 1 week. Review the log and note what situations (e.g., people, technology, values conflict) were the most common. Also identify how you most often react to stress: physically, mentally, and emotionally/spiritually. Keeping this diary for a week is helpful to determine what you respond to with stress and learn about your reactions. Enter a date, and describe a situation and your response. Ask yourself if the stress was good stress (eustress) or bad stress (distress). Then, with a trusted colleague, conduct a peer review about what more-positive strategies could be used to deal with a similar situation.

Date_____

Situation_____

Your response_____

Good stress or bad_____

Action (how you dealt with your response)

_____

Evaluation_____

Look over your week of stressors. Are there some that you encounter on a regular basis? If so, try to formulate a plan to conquer the problems. You may need to role-play or get continuing education to improve a specific skill. You may need to simply break a task down into smaller pieces or to eliminate interruptions.

Symptom Management

Unpredictable and uncontrollable change, coupled with immense responsibility and little control over the work environment, produces stress for nurses and other healthcare professionals. Consequently, nurses may develop emotional symptoms such as anxiety, depression, or anger; physical alterations such as fatigue, headache, and insomnia; mental changes such as a decrease in concentration and memory; and behavioral changes such as smoking, drinking, crying, and swearing. The important factor is not the stressor but, rather, how the individual perceives the stressor and what coping mechanisms are available to mediate the hormonal response to the stressor.

Multiple stress-buffering behaviors can be used to reduce the detrimental effects of stress. The stressor-induced changes in the hormonal and immune systems can be modulated by an individual's behavioral coping responses. These coping responses include spending time developing a particular interest such as dancing or playing an instrument, leisure activities with friends and family, and taking time for self, decreasing or discontinuing the use of caffeine, positive social support, a strong belief system, a sense of humor, developing realistic expectations, reframing events, regular aerobic exercise, meditation, and use of the relaxation response.

Everyone needs to balance work and leisure in his or her life. Leisure time and stress are inversely proportional. If time for work is more than 60% of awake time or if self-time is less than 10% of awake time, stress levels will increase. Changes should be made to relieve stress, such as decreasing the number of work hours or finding more time for leisure activities. Caffeine is a strong stimulant and, in itself, a stressor. Slowly weaning off caffeine should result in better sleep and more energy. Positive social support can offer validation, encouragement, or advice. By discussing situations with others, one can reduce stress. A great deal of stress comes from our belief systems, which cause stress in two ways. First, behaviors result from them, such as placing work before rest or pleasure. Second, beliefs may also conflict with those of other people, as may happen with patients from different cultures. Articulating beliefs and finding common ground will help reduce anger and stress. Humor is a great stress reducer and laughter a great tension reducer. Other activities may include self-reflection in the form of guided imagery, journaling, or debriefing with a mentor or peer.

A common source of stress is unrealistic expectations. Realistic expectations can make life feel more predictable and more manageable. *Reframing* is changing the way you look at things to make you feel better about them or to obtain a different perspective. A situation can be seen in multiple ways, so taking the positive view is less stressful. Regular aerobic exercise is a logical method of dissipating the excess energy generated by the stress response.

Meditation to elicit the relaxation response can be beneficial. The benefits of practicing relaxation techniques for 20 minutes daily include a feeling of well-being, the ability to learn how tension makes the body feel, and the sense that tension can be controlled. In cases of some stress-related disorders (e.g., hypertension), biofeedback may be used to monitor physiologic relaxation processes. Exercise 28-2 outlines one systematic relaxation technique.

EXERCISE 28-2

This exercise can be used in the middle of a working day, the last thing at night, or at any time you feel tense or anxious. Review the information and strategies at the Mayo Clinic Website: *www.mayoclinic.com/health/meditation/HQ01070*. Make a short list of steps to take, and put it in your smartphone, personal digital assistant (PDA), or notepad.

- Use meditation DVDs or audio products readily available for any smartphone or portable electronic device. These applications can be downloaded for repeat viewing or listening, such as in the car going back and forth to work.
- Purchase and learn how to operate a portable, electronic listening device and listen to audio books while working at home or walking in the neighborhood or in the car.

Social support in the form of positive work relationships, as well as nurturing family and friends, may be an important way to buffer the negative effects of a stressful work environment. Although friendships may be formed with colleagues, the workload and the shifting of staff from one unit to another make it difficult sometimes to establish and maintain close relationships with peers. For many people at work, the time spent with their managers and co-workers represent one of the strongest sources of community in their lives. Sherman (2013) advises leaders to invest in team building activities to strengthen the sense of camaraderie. The Gallup Organization, in its study of more than 80,000 managers to better understand the relationship of great managers to a quality workplace, created the Q-12 survey question; *I have a best friend at work.* Employees who believe they have formed strong friendships with co-workers who will help them get through rough spots positively correlates with employee retention, customer metrics, productivity, and profitability (*http://businessjournal.gallup.com/content/511/item-10-best-friend-work.aspx*). Leaders who provide regular recognition feedback, in the form of personal notes that are mailed to their team members' homes; annual Nurses' Week celebrations, or through participation in the DAISY Foundation, a not-for-profit organization that formally recognizes the extraordinary contributions of nurses help to shape the organization's culture in a way that patients, families, and nurses value (Lefton, 2012).

Young nurses in their first position, those who find themselves in an unfamiliar geographic area, or nurses who switch employers after long tenure at another hospital—all want to anticipate that they will be part of a work group that will furnish emotional support and a sense of belonging to an endeavor that is greater than themselves. Too often, nurses overlook the benefits of active membership in their professional association or specialty associations. Connections established at the beginning of one's career will serve the nurse with an unending lifelong source of enthusiastic colleagues who are as passionate about their individual professional careers as they are about serving their profession. Opportunities to become active members help nurses discover and refine brand-new leadership skills in a warm, comfortable setting. Ongoing mentorship, by seasoned nursing leaders from academia, private practice, and organizational settings, are often free for the taking and add dimension and perspective to nurses at every level. Such efforts may help nurses cope with workplace demands that seem to exceed their capabilities. Positive coping strategies may make nurses less likely to adopt negative coping strategies such as withdrawing, lowering their standards of care, abusing alcohol or prescription or illegal drugs, and leaving nursing entirely.

Stress applies to all positions. Direct care nurses may experience stress from a patient's deteriorating condition or lack of ability to function autonomously. A nurse manager may experience role conflict between being an administrative representative and being a nurse. A leader may be more stressed about potentials for downsizing or planning a new service. The stress (distress) experienced by one group can affect another. The challenge is how to manage individual reactions to stress so that it results in growth rather than inhibiting it, and how to manage the effects of stress on others (see the Research Perspective).

RESEARCH PERSPECTIVE

Resource: Kath, L.M., Stichler, J.F., Ehrhart, M.G., & Schultze, T.A. (2012). Predictors and outcomes of nurse leader job stress experienced by AWHONN members. *Journal of Obstetrical, Gynecological and Neonatal Nurses, 42*(1), 12-25.

This study's objectives were to measure relationships between typical life stressors (work, home, and personal factors) experienced by nurse leaders and investigate the relationship between autonomy, leadership style, and stress. Role overload, constraints imposed by the organization, and role ambiguity represented the most significant areas of stress. These factors affected patient outcomes, personal health, and job satisfaction, and also increased the intent to quit. The recommendations from this study endorsed activities designed to raise the leader's level of personal autonomy and to create opportunities for stress reduction and stress management.

Implications for Practice

Given the geographic and cyclic nursing oversupply and shortages, nurse job satisfaction and employee retention are very important to current healthcare industry demands for safe, effective, patient-centered, timely, efficient, and equitable care. Nurses and nurse managers in all settings are faced with resource constraints. Identifying and validating nurse perceptions about stress, collaboration, and autonomy facilitate accurate assessment and effective management of staff, turnover rates, and performance.

Burnout

Sometimes individuals cannot manage stress successfully through their own efforts and require assistance. Examples of behavior related to stress that feels overwhelming are found in Table 28-1 on p. 526. Coping strategies, such as those described previously, may furnish temporary relief or none at all. With this level of distress, one can feel overwhelmed or helpless and may be at greater risk for mental or physical illness. This constellation of emotions is commonly called *burnout.*

Burnout is a psychological term to describe the effects of prolonged emotional and physical exhaustion and diminished interest caused by an unrelenting workload, without relief (Maslach & Leiter, 1997). The sources of the stressors may exist in the environment, in the individual, or in the interaction between the individual and the environment. Some stressors, such as employment termination, death in the family, or the breakup of a relationship appear to be universal, whereas other stressors, such as meeting deadlines, are more personal. For example, some nurses thrive on goals and timetables, whereas others feel constrained

and frustrated and experience distress. Sometimes, stress is experienced when others around the individual have a dominant personality style and few possess characteristics that are not complementary. Burnout is not an objective phenomenon as if it were the accumulation of a certain number and type of stressors. It is more important how the stressors are perceived and how they are mediated by an individual's ability to adapt that are crucial variables in determining one's levels of distress.

Nurses who are burned out feel as though their resources are depleted to the point that their well-being is at risk. A self-analysis usually uncovers the characteristics of burnout. First, a feeling of physical, mental, and emotional exhaustion can be recognized. Historically, Greenglass, Burke, and Fiksenbaum (2001) found that emotional exhaustion was directly related to workload. For example, recent graduates may value total, detailed care for individuals and may have little experience in caring for more than two patients simultaneously. When confronted with the responsibility of caring for a group of six to eight acutely ill patients, they may have difficulty adapting to the realities of the workplace, and emotional exhaustion ensues. Emotional exhaustion in turn has a direct effect on levels of cynicism and somatization. A second characteristic of burnout is **depersonalization,** a state characterized by distancing oneself from the work itself and developing negative attitudes toward work in general (Greenglass et al., 2001). Depersonalization is commonly described as a feeling of being outside one's body, feeling as if one is a machine or robot, an "unreal" feeling that one is in a dream or that one "is on automatic pilot." Generally, subjective symptoms of unreality make the nurse uneasy and anxious. Others may view this as callousness. Nurses pushed to do too much in too little time may distance themselves from patients as a means of dealing with emotional exhaustion. Also, nurses' personality characteristics may lean too heavily on the caregiving dimension, which often carries over into one's personal life. For example, caregiving individuals may be further challenged by life partners who demand a disproportionate amount of time and energy, either because of physical disabilities or because of latent personality disorders or, even, alcoholism. There is little chance for renewal and a safe haven at home in such cases.

A decreased sense of professional accomplishment and competence is the third hallmark of burnout. Low professional efficacy has been found to be a function of higher levels of cynicism (Greenglass et al., 2001). *Efficacy* is one's belief in his or her capabilities to organize and execute goal-oriented activities. Nurses are more inclined to take on a task if they believe they can succeed. Low efficacy can lead nurses to believe tasks are harder than they actually are. This can lead to a sense of failure, perceived helplessness, and finally crisis. Bolton, Harvey, Grawitch, and Barber (2012) studied counterproductive work behaviors in response to burnout and found that depersonalization and becoming completely oppositional to the organization were indirect predictors of active (harming elders or deliberately bypassing handwashing) or passive (taking longer breaks off the unit, or calling in sick on a busy weekend) counterproductive work behaviors. At this point, one's coping skills are no longer effective. Immediate referral to mandated employee assistance program (EAP) counseling, and perhaps a medical leave of absence may be recommended. At its best, a healthy peer discussion, whether it is formal or informal, can help to identify when a nurse is troubled. However, it is often the task of the assistant nurse managers, nurse managers, or nursing supervisors to address and refer nurses to seek help for themselves, before the stress escalates to a state of crisis.

RESOLUTION OF STRESS

Resolution of stress in its early stages can be accomplished through a variety of techniques. Nurses must be able to reach a balance of caring for others and caring for self. Table 28-2 summarizes physical, mental, and emotional/spiritual strategies.

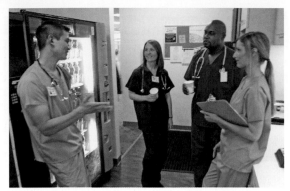

Peers and followers can be supportive and help reduce stress.

When stress rises to unacceptable or even dangerous levels, colleagues can be supportive and perhaps even point out the stress level or recommend appropriate help.

Social Support

Peers and followers can be supportive and help reduce stress by assisting with problem solving and by presenting different perspectives. Family and friends can provide an affirming, loving perspective and much-needed respite from stress in the form of celebrations around birthdays, graduations, and seasonal holidays. Social isolation increases stress. When nurses find themselves in a never-ending cycle of work, sleep, school, and conflicting calendars with escalating pressures at home, relief must be actively sought. True social support allows us to relax, be playful, have fun, laugh, vent emotions, and enjoy life to the fullest.

TABLE 28-2 STRESS-MANAGEMENT STRATEGIES		
PHYSICAL	**MENTAL**	**EMOTIONAL/SPIRITUAL**
• Accept physical limitations • Modify nutrition: moderate carbohydrate, moderate protein, high in fruits and vegetables, low caffeine, low sugar • Exercise: participate in an enjoyable activity five times a week for 30 minutes • Make your physical health a priority • Nurture yourself by taking time for breaks and lunch • Sleep: get enough in quantity and quality • Relax: use meditation, massage, yoga, or biofeedback	• Learn to say "no"! • Use cognitive restructuring and self-talk • Use imagery • Develop hobbies or activities • Plan vacations • Learn about the system and how problems are handled • Learn communication, conflict resolution, and time-management skills • Take continuing education courses	• Use meditation • Seek solace in prayer • Seek professional counseling • Participate in support groups • Participate in networking • Communicate feelings • Identify and acquire a mentor • Ask for feedback and clarification

Counseling

Persistent, unpleasant feelings; problem behavior; helplessness; and withdrawal during prolonged stress may suggest the need for assistance from a mental health professional. Examples of problem behaviors include tearfulness or angry outbursts over seemingly minor incidents, traffic violations, major or subtle changes in eating and/or sleeping patterns, frequent unwillingness or lack of desire to go to work, and even substance abuse. In such cases, the aforementioned coping strategies afford only temporary relief; nurses with this level of distress feel overwhelmed and believe that they simply cannot go on this way. In these stressful situations, individuals may feel helpless and see no way out. They may require professional assistance from an advanced practice psychiatric nurse, clinical psychologist, psychiatrist, or another mental health worker.

In some organizations, leaders may refer their peers or subordinates to employee assistance programs (EAPs). They are a source of free, voluntary, confidential, short-term professional counseling, and other services for employees either via in-house staff or through a contract with a separate mental health agency. This type of counseling can be effective because the counselors are usually already well aware of organizational issues and stressors in the workplace. Some nurses may have confidentiality concerns when using employer-recommended or employer-provided counseling services. However, mental health professionals are bound by their professional standards of confidentiality. Additionally, sometimes it is in the nurse's best interest to sign a release of information, such as when seeking employer accommodation for a certain physical or emotional problem.

Those who seek counseling outside of the workplace may be guided in their selection of mental health professionals by a personal provider (physician or nurse practitioner), a knowledgeable colleague in the human resources department, or such online publications as the most recent edition of their health insurance referral book. A phone call to the state nurses' association and an inquiry for lists of advance practice nurses in adult psychiatric–mental health practice in your region will often yield significant results. When the problem underlying the distress is ethical or moral, a trained pastoral counselor or spiritual director may be very helpful. Some clergy and mental health professionals are certified in pastoral care or have earned a degree in another discipline such as psychology or spiritual direction counseling. Referrals can be obtained from hospital pastoral care departments or places of worship that affiliate with regional centers where certified counselors are available. When private counseling is being arranged, the health insurance contract should be checked to determine mental health benefits and the payment limitations and types of providers eligible for reimbursement.

Leadership and Management

Although social support and counseling can alter how stressors are perceived, effective leadership that is shared and time management that supports involvement at the level of direct care nurse in the unit can certainly modify or remove stressors. Historically, nurses have had limited formal authority as individuals in most organizations. Shared governance, defined by Tim Porter-O'Grady describing the pioneer efforts of Vanderbilt University Medical Center in the 1980s, "is a professional practice model, founded on the cornerstone principles of partnership, equity, accountability and ownership" (Porter-O'Grady, 2013). Organizations that implement shared governance systems are either "on the bus or off the bus," according to Dr. Robert Hess (2013), creator of the only measurement tool designed to analyze organizational readiness and level of participation in shared governance activities. In Hess's study (2011), Magnet™ hospitals reported 37%, non-Magnet hospitals reported 16%, and hospitals pursuing Magnet™ designation reported 32% of involvement in shared governance activities that bring policy-making to the nurses whose job it is to implement them. Chief nursing executives and the managerial and administrative groups at which tables they sit continually advocate for nursing resources, and certainly influence policy and resource allocation. Nurse managers can and must continue to articulate clinical and workplace issues as they work to control existing environmental stressors on their own units. In addition, managers ought to examine their own behavior as a source of their subordinates' stress via peer review, coaching, and regularly scheduled leadership rounds.

In some cases, a controlling or autocratic style of management is appropriate, such as in emergency situations and when working with a large percentage of new and inexperienced team members. For the most part, however, professional nurses need, want, and deserve the latitude to direct their activities within their sphere of competence. "Letting go," or delegating, means that the nurse leader trusts the personal integrity and professional competence of the team. It does not mean abdicating accountability for achieving accepted standards of patient care and agreed-upon outcomes. Such an attitude provides ample opportunity to provide invaluable coaching that has the potential to teach, motivate and guide others toward reaching their full potential.

Assistance with problem solving is another way to reduce environmental stressors. Nurse leaders may provide technical advice, refer staff to appropriate resources, or mediate conflicts. Often, nurse leaders enable staff to meet the demands of their work more independently by providing time for continuing education and professional meetings to enhance their clinical competence and exert control over their own workplace.

Another way in which nurse leaders can reduce stress is to be supportive of staff. Support is not equated with being a friend but, rather, with helping one's peers accomplish good care, develop professionally, and feel valued personally. Leaders can ensure that the expected workload is in line with the nurses' capabilities and resources. They can work to ensure meaningfulness, stimulation, and opportunities for nurses to use their skills. Nurses' roles and responsibilities need to be clearly and publicly defined. Work schedules should be posted as far in advance as possible and should be compatible with what is known about patient safety and respect for their team members' private lives and school schedules. Encouraging innovation and experimentation, as in self-scheduling for example, can motivate staff and give them a sense of greater control over their environment. Affirming a good idea, finding resources for further study, or implementing a promising new procedure or proposal by a direct care nurse are all characteristic of supportive leadership. It is possible to be supportive even when things are not necessarily going well. For example, when staff members struggle with their methods of coping with overwork and other stressors, supportive leadership behaviors include helping staff members recognize the need to avoid passive coping strategies

that fuel helplessness and lower the standards of care. Nurse leaders must be sensitive to the distress of the nursing staff and acknowledge it without themselves becoming therapists or counselors, which would present a role conflict. Support may involve raising the staff's knowledge of counseling resources.

Nurse leaders also must be careful to avoid diagnostic labels and to maintain strict confidentiality. This is difficult to do, for example, when a nurse's practice is impaired by alcohol or drug use. Sometimes the staff on the entire unit and even staff on other units may already be aware of the impairment. When distress relates to the personal life of subordinates, managers should focus on the effect of such situations on workplace performance and ask for outside assistance, if necessary, to help the members of the team work through the events. The individual who has produced the stress can then be welcomed back to the job following recovery in a program designed to aid the person in appropriate coping approaches.

In addition, leaders can enhance the workplace by dealing effectively with their own stressors. Maintaining a sense of perspective as well as a sense of humor is important. Some stressors, in fact, can be ignored or minimized by posing three questions:

1. Is this event or situation important? Stressors are not all equally significant. Do not waste energy on little stressors.
2. Does this stressor affect me or my unit? Although some situations that produce distress are institution-wide and need group action, others target specific units or activities. Do not borrow stressors from another unit. Individuals can "cross-pollinate" stressors by spreading gossip about the misfortunes of other units' team members.
3. Can I change this situation? If not, then find a way to cope with it, or if the situation is intolerable, make plans to change positions or employers. This decision may require gaining added credentials that may produce long-term career benefits or contacting a search firm to simply discover "what's out there."

Keeping stressful situations in perspective can enable nurses to conserve their energies to cope with stressful situations that are important, that are within their domain, or that can be changed or modified.

MANAGEMENT OF TIME

A very close relationship exists between stress management and time management. Time management is one method of stress prevention or reduction. Stress can decrease productivity and lead to poor use of time. Time management can be considered a preventive action to help reduce the elements of stress in a nurse's life.

Everyone has two choices when managing time: organize or "go with the flow." Everyone has only 24 hours in every day, and it is clear that some people make better use of time than others do. *How* people use time makes some people more successful than others. The effective use of time-management skills thus becomes an even more important tool to achieve personal and professional goals. Time management is the appropriate use of tools, techniques, and principles to control time spent on low-priority needs and to ensure that time is invested in activities leading toward achieving desired, high-priority goals. More simply, time management is the ability to spend your time on the things that matter to you and your organization. However, it does take time to plan daily time-management strategies! By setting goals and actively working to reduce time stealers, you will have the extra time to accomplish them.

Where Does Your Time—and the Day—Go?

Have you ever wasted time? Time, although a cheap commodity, is our most valuable resource. There are some commonly identified time stealers, and individuals must recognize them to guard against them. At the heart of time management is an important shift in focus. Concentrate on results, not on being busy.

Doing Too Much

Do you try to do too much at once? At work, do you have three or four major projects going simultaneously? Are you a member of more than one organizational committee? Do you have to worry about what will be on the table for dinner or who will get your child to soccer while you are hanging an IV and planning a staff meeting? Have you ever completed a nursing intervention and realized that your mind was really somewhere else and you had ignored the patient? If you *think* you have too much to do, you probably do! Learn to have fewer projects running simultaneously and to concentrate your efforts on one thing at a time. The first step is to be realistic and limit

major commitments, and then give each activity your full and undivided attention. Sometimes completing one task before starting another is the most efficient method for getting everything done. Prioritization of goals and activities each day is very helpful.

In the nursing profession, however, limiting commitments is not always possible. When you are feeling overwhelmed by the sheer volume of tasks to be completed, take the time to establish priorities for the day. Decide what must be done versus what would be nice to do. Do not let yourself get distracted from your priority tasks. Nursing is a balancing act; priorities are always changing.

Inability to Say "No" or "Not Now"

Sometimes the smallest and simplest words are the most difficult to learn. If you are suffering from overload, you probably have gotten there by not being able to say "no," or not being able to prioritize the "yes." Learning to say "no" to requests is difficult, and in the process, others may be displeased. If you do not say "no," however, you may end up spending much time on projects that are uninteresting or have no relationship to your personal goals and priorities. When someone asks you to do something, you need to stop and consider the request. Do you want to do the task now or sometime in the future? If not, then say so. If you wish to do the task but simply do not have the time, consider delegation. However, be honest with the requester. If you simply do not have the time, say so as politely as possible. If you wish to take on the task but at a later date, negotiate. Remember, accepting an assignment you will never be able to complete sheds an unfavorable light on you.

Procrastination

Do you put off important tasks because they are not enjoyable or because they may be difficult? Do you find excuses for not starting or completing tasks? Are you a procrastinator? By engaging in procrastination, or doing one thing when you should be doing something else, you give up time to complete your task and therefore limit the quality of the work you produce. Specific techniques can help deal with procrastination. First, identify the reason for procrastinating. Then make that task your highest priority the next day. Reward yourself after you finish the task. Another technique is to select the least attractive element of the task to do first, and the rest will seem easy.

Some people find that they procrastinate when the task ahead is very large. The solution is to break the task down into manageable pieces and plan rewards for accomplishing each of the smaller tasks. Developing a program evaluation and review technique (PERT) chart or a Gantt chart may help in this process. PERT charts were originally developed as tools to assist in complex projects that require a series of activities, some of which must be performed sequentially and others that can be performed in parallel with other activities. Envisioned as a network diagram, a PERT chart indicates dependent activities that must be completed before a new activity is undertaken. A Gantt chart (Table 28-3) consists of a table of project task information and a bar chart that graphically displays the project schedule. This method of tracking project activities in relation to time is often used in planning and project management. Both chart techniques can be used to outline how you will approach a large project.

Technology can be a "time waster" or it can be a tool that benefits the nurse leader. How often have you looked at the clock and been startled to see how much time has passed? To learn from time stealers such as answering copious amounts of e-mail from friends, family and work colleagues, it is helpful to organize folders to which e-mails automatically are sent. Stay away from social networking sites and instead, register for a class on how to use technology to your advantage. These are available in the community adult education sector, at colleges and universities and in the health education departments, common in most facilities.

Complaining

Complaining is the act of expressing dissatisfaction or annoyance with persons, places, things, and situations (Merriam-Webster Online, 2013). Often, the time people spend complaining about a task or a particular situation is greater than the time needed to complete the task or to deal with the issue. If you find yourself complaining repeatedly or justifying complaining by saying you are only venting about something, stop and ask yourself what would be the ideal solution and then take the risk to act on it. If the complaint is related to another person, either take the time to talk with the person and get the problem out in the open or write a letter or an e-mail to the person discussing your point of view (stop short of pushing "send," because this is an effective technique even if you do not mail it). If you find yourself complaining about something within the workplace, rethink the problem, generate some possible solutions, and then talk to your manager. Look for solutions that are very simple or "outside the box." Talk to your manager and be prepared to discuss solutions, not just your dissatisfaction or annoyance. In this way, your manager will see you as interested and capable in contributing to the goals of the organization.

Perfectionism

Perfectionism is the tendency to never finish anything because it is not yet perfect. This approach tends to consume much time when your expected outcome is not attainable. Overcoming perfectionism takes considerable effort. However, this does not mean that you should do less than your best. Being aware of perfectionism means that you occasionally need to give yourself permission to do slightly less than a perfect job, such as buying a carryout dinner rather than preparing a home-cooked meal after a hard day at work.

TABLE 28-3 SAMPLE GANTT CHART

TASK	ACCOUNTABILITY	JAN	FEB	MAR	APR	MAY	JUNE
1. Conduct literature search	Unit clinical nurse specialist	⟶					
2. Hold nursing practice committee meeting to review material	Chair, nursing practice committee		X				
3. Create a report for the medical staff	Chair, nursing practice committee		⟶		⟶		
4. Disseminate findings to nursing and medical staff	Chair, nursing practice committee				⟶		⟶

Interruptions

One common distraction from priority activities is interruptions. Most interruptions are integral to the positions that you hold, but others can be controlled. A home care nurse with a large caseload can expect to be paged at any time. More commonly, however, are the numerous small interruptions by individuals who want just a "minute of your time" and take much longer than that getting to the point! Box 28-1 identifies some specific strategies to prevent and control interruptions. The two keys to dealing with interruptions are to resume "doing it now" so that an interruption does not destroy your schedule and to maintain the attitude that whatever the interruption, it is a part of your responsibility. When you make a conscious decision not to worry about the things you cannot

control, you have more energy to maintain a positive perspective and to move projects forward.

Disorganization

One of the most serious time wasters of all is disorganization. How many times have you had to spend 5 minutes trying to find something you have misplaced or misfiled? Organization can be a great time saver. Remember that the guiding principle is that organization is a process rather than the product. You can spend so much time organizing that you will never get to the task at hand (procrastination). Simple organizing guidelines include eliminating clutter, keeping everything in its place, and doing similar tasks together. In contrast, Abrahamson and Freedman (2008) make the case that disorder has benefits because disorder often is more efficient and may produce better outcomes. For example, ideas that seem to happen spontaneously in the middle of the night or in the car on the way home from work are seemingly not borne of ritualistic adherence to meticulous filing or rigidly documented note-taking systems. Everyone creates and enjoys creating in many diverse ways, the key is learning by mistakes and seeing the patterns that emerge as potentially useful elements in problem solving.

Too Much Information

The newest time waster to evolve is data proliferation. The technology within our workplace forces us to receive huge amounts of data and to transform these data into useful information. The computer workstation, once touted as a time-saving device, has become the driving force behind care delivery. Patients even complain that they may feel at times that the nurse is busy nursing the computer instead of them! Nurses, depending on where they are according to their specific generational differences, can view the computer either as an inescapable stress-producing slave driver or as a useful tool to assist them in their daily activities.

Information overload, or "data smog," occurs when you are overwhelmed by too much information, too fast, and too often and do not have the skills to interpret the data as useful information. Developing data and information gathering, receiving, and sending skills (known as *information literacy*) can greatly reduce stress and improve efficiency and productivity

---

BOX 28-1 TIPS TO PREVENT INTERRUPTIONS AND WORK MORE EFFECTIVELY

- Ask people to put their comments in writing in an e-mail—do not let them catch you "on the run." On the same note, do not use others as you would a Post-it note!
- Let the office/unit secretary know what information you need immediately.
- Conduct a conversation in the hall to help keep it short or in a separate room to keep from being interrupted.
- Be comfortable saying "no" and "not yet."
- When involved in a long procedure or home visit, ask someone else to cover your other responsibilities.
- Break projects into small, manageable pieces.
- Get yourself organized.
- Minimize interruptions—for example, allow voice mail to pick up the phone; shut the door.
- Keep your work surface clear. Have available only those documents needed for the task at hand.
- Keep your manager informed of your goals.
- Plan to accomplish high-priority or difficult tasks early in the day.
- Develop a plan for the day and stick to it. Remember to schedule in some time for interruptions.
- Schedule time to meet regularly throughout the shift with staff members for whom you are responsible.
- Make an effort to round with the night and weekend team; conduct early morning breakfasts so that night staff can meet with you away from their unit.
- Recognize that crises and interruptions are part of the position.
- Be cognizant of your personal time-wasting habits, and try to avoid them.

(Englebardt & Nelson, 2002). Gaining a new appreciation for how to manage the flow of information, called knowledge management (McDermott, 2000) is important. Information is simply a tool for planning action or making decisions. By forming or joining knowledge communities, such information can be condensed and shared over every imaginable medium, inclusive of podcasts, e-mail synopses of weekly healthcare news items, Twitter and Facebook notifications, and many more.

Time-Management Concepts

Table 28-4 presents a classification scheme for time-management techniques. The unifying theme is that each activity undertaken should lead to goal attainment and that goal should be the number one priority at that time.

Goal Setting

The first steps in time management are goal setting and developing a plan to reach the goals. Set goals that are reasonable and achievable. Do not expect to reach long-term goals overnight—*long-term* means just that. Give yourself time to meet the goals. Determine many short-term goals to reach the long-term goal, giving you a frequent sense of goal achievement. Give yourself flexibility. If the path you chose last year is no longer appropriate, change it. Write your goals, date the entry, keep it handy, and refer to it often to give yourself a progress report. Very often, goals are an important discussion point of the annual performance evaluation process. Unfortunately, the time for reviewing goals ought not to be the period immediately preceding this year's discussion, yet too often this is the case. The savvy nurse leader will refer to goals mutually set by his or her direct report frequently throughout the year and address progress toward achievement during monthly meetings.

Setting Priorities

Once goals are known, priorities are set. They may, however, shift throughout a given period in terms of goal attainment. For example, working on a budget may take precedence at certain times of the year, whereas new staff orientation is a high priority at other times. Knowing what your goals and priorities are helps shape the "to do" list. On a nursing unit or as you work in a community setting, you must know your personal goals and current priorities. How you organize work may depend on geographic considerations, patient acuity, or some other schema.

A particular strategy to assist in prioritization suggests that people generally focus on those things that are important and urgent. By placing the elements of importance and urgency in a grid (Figure 28-2), all activities can be classified as shown (Covey, Merrill, & Merrill, 1996).

Typically, we tend to focus on those items in cell A because they are both important and urgent and therefore command our attention. Making shift assignments is an A task because it is both important to the work to be accomplished and commonly urgent because a time frame is specified during which data about patients and qualifications of staff can be matched. Conversely, if something is neither

		IMPORTANT	
		yes	no
URGENT	yes	A	C
	no	B	D

FIGURE 28-2 Classification of priorities.

TABLE 28-4	CLASSIFICATION OF TIME-MANAGEMENT TECHNIQUES	
TECHNIQUE	**PURPOSE**	**ACTIONS**
Organization	Designed to promote efficiency and productivity	Organize and systematize things, tasks, and people. Use basic time-management skills.
Keep focused on goals	Focuses on goal achievement	Assemble a prioritized "to do" list daily, based on goals.
Tool usage	Uses the right tool for planning and preparation	Use tools such as a smartphone.
Time-management plan	Helps to refocus, to gain control, and to use information	Develop a personal time-management plan appropriately.

important nor urgent (cell D), it may be considered a waste of time, at least in terms of personal goals. An example of a D activity might be reading "junk" e-mail. Even if something is urgent but not important (cell C), it contributes minimally to productivity and goal achievement. An example of a C activity might be responding to a memo that has a specific time line but is not important to goal attainment. The real key to setting priorities is to attend to the B tasks, those that are important but not urgent. Examples of B activities are reviewing the organization's strategic plan or participating on organizational committees.

Organization

A number of simple routines for organization can save many minutes over a day and enhance your efficiency. Keeping a workspace neat or arranging things in an orderly fashion may be a powerful time-management tool. Rather than a system of "pile management," use "file management." The following are a few hints:

- Plan where things should go: your desk or your disk
- Keep a clean workspace
- Create a "to do" folder
- Create a "to be filed" folder for any papers
- Schedule time to work your way through the folders

If you don't have a physical desk at work, you typically use something—a designated space, a tablet, a clipboard, or your phone. Consider how to translate the above into a nondesk format.

Determine your priority goals for the next day, and have the materials ready to work on when you start the next day. If you are fortunate to have the resources of a secretary or administrative assistant, even for very limited periods of the day, be sure to discuss with this individual how creative scheduling has the power to either maximize your day or sap your energy and strength to deal with your obligations.

Time Tools

Sometimes, the real problem is that the events of the day become the driving force, rather than a planned schedule. Days may become so tightly scheduled that any little interruption can become a crisis. If you do not plan the day, you may be responding to events rather than prioritized goals. If you think you are a reactor rather than a proactive time user, use a time log to list work-related activities for several days. You

may not be able to plan well because you really do not have a good estimate of how long a particular activity actually takes or you do not know how many activities can be accomplished in a given time frame. Ask others around you if *your* lack of planning has a negative impact upon *their* work day. The answer may be as unsettling as it is startling: Your work habits may be impacting *their* lives.

As the nurse's role in care management becomes more complex, the need for organizational tools increases. Tracking the care of groups of patients, either as the member of a care team or in a leadership capacity, can be overwhelming. Each nurse must devise a method for tracking care and organizing time, as well as delegating and monitoring care provided by others. Although some nurses depend on a shift flowsheet, many more now have the benefit of computerized information tracking systems. Handheld computer devices such as PDAs provided by the hospital or bar-code scanners for medication administration are other methods to track information and increase safety and efficiency. The issue of patient confidentiality and organizational privacy cannot be ignored when entering data into any device. Check with your organization's privacy officer and appropriate policies to verify that you are on the right side of managing paper and electronic information.

Managing Information

The first step in managing information is to assess the source. Once you have identified the sources of your data, you have a better idea of how to deal with the information. Track incoming information for a few days. Patterns will begin to emerge and will give clues as to how to deal with it. You can generally predict that, using the Pareto principle, 80% of your incoming data comes from approximately 20% of your sources, and that 80% of useful information comes from 20% of information received (see the Theory Box on p. 525).

By developing information-receiving skills, you can quickly interpret the data and convert them to useful information, discarding unneeded data. Initially, you should reduce or eliminate that which is useless. Label files and folders to which e-mail messages can be directed. Delete e-mails, or encourage administrative leaders to endorse systems that automatically archive older messages. Toss the memo in the trash. Next, monitor the information flow and decide what to do with incoming data. Find and focus on the most important pieces, and then quickly narrow down the specific details you need. Identify resources that are most helpful, and have them readily available. Be able to build the big picture from the masses of data you receive. Finally, recognize when you have enough information to act.

Once you have mastered the receiving end of information, concentrate on information-sending skills. Remember, your information is simply another person's data! Try to keep your outflow short; make it a synthesis of the information. Remember, if your e-mail message is more than a few sentences in length, your message probably warrants a phone call instead. Finally, select the most appropriate mode of communication for your message from the technology available. You may be sending your information in written (memo or report) or verbal (face-to-face or presentation) form or via telephone, voice mail, e-mail, text, Twitter, or fax. Remember, the most important skill is to know when you have said enough. Exercise 28-3 will help you consider how you have dealt with information.

EXERCISE 28-3

Think of the last time you were in the clinical area. How often did you record the same piece of data (e.g., a finding in your assessment of the patient)? Remember to include all steps, from your jotting down notes on a piece of paper or entering data into the computer to the final report of the day. What information processing tools could decrease the number of steps?

MEETING MANAGEMENT

Two key time-management strategies that are critical to success are managing meetings and delegating, which are discussed in the next two sections of this chapter. Even nurses who may not have extensive management responsibilities usually are in the position of delegating tasks to less-skilled workers and can benefit from learning to make the most of meetings, either as the leader or as a group member.

Managing Meetings

Meetings serve various purposes, ranging from creating social networks to setting formal policy. In Lencioni's (2004) book, *Death by Meeting*, defines four types of meetings, as follows:

- The first meeting type is the daily check-in, which takes about 5 minutes and is the opportunity to check schedules and activities. This might be analogous to a "touch base" or huddle meeting to ensure that everyone is progressing as planned and that no patient care issues are unattended.
- The second meeting type is the daily or weekly tactical meeting, which is used to resolve issues. This type would be reflective of what the unit staff needs to address to ensure that it has the resources to achieve what it needs to do for patients.
- The third meeting type, the monthly strategic meeting, is used to address big issues that have longer-term implications. These meetings are frequently standing committees of the organization on which staff serve and include reports from subgroups. An example of this meeting can be illustrated by unit based councils, often found in Magnet™ organizations where shared governance provides opportunities for staff decision making at the unit level.
- The fourth meeting type is the quarterly off-site review, which is designed to analyze progress and to develop the team. It is uncommon to find that many organizations provide this frequency and intensity except at higher levels in the organization. Lencioni (2004) suggests this type of meeting should be 1 to 2 days.

Meetings may be designed to solve problems, disseminate information, seek input, inspire the group, delegate work or authority, or create or maintain a formal power base. Unless the purpose of a meeting is to socialize, the meeting is unlikely to be effective if it is poorly managed.

Tips for Managing Meetings Effectively

Consider if this meeting is necessary. For example, a conference call, Skype, posted notice, e-mail, or brief huddle (a short, check-in meeting) might suffice. If the right people are not available, rescheduling may be a good option.

Schedule meetings right before lunch or at the end of the day. Participants will have an incentive to stick to the schedule. Set a start time and a stop time, and reward prompt members by starting on schedule and closing the door. Avoid holding meetings that will last longer than 2 hours. Select an appropriate setting in which the participants are not readily accessible to interruptions. If necessary, plan the seating arrangement to prevent inappropriate behaviors such as whispering or other interruptions such as managers who answer their phones in the meeting. Place such individuals near the door, so they can easily slip out of earshot and handle emergencies as needed. If the group meets over a period of time, have group members set group expectations, such as setting devices on vibrate and requesting a "no texting while meeting" agreement. Create agreements about how the group will interact. These agreements need to be created mutually by the group because the group will be implementing them (see Chapter 18).

Distribute an agenda. Whenever possible, provide a written agenda to each member in advance of the meeting. Establish and make known the goal of the meeting. Be mindful of the time allotted to each topic and prioritize issues in order of importance. Review the agenda at the onset of the meeting so there is general buy-in about it. Attach all needed preparation reading to the agenda. The more advanced the reading or preparation that is required, the earlier members should receive agendas.

Different types of agendas can be used for different purposes:

- *Structured agendas:* If a topic is particularly controversial, consider the expectation that requires any negative comment to be preceded by a positive one.
- *Timed agendas:* Consider setting a specific amount of time to be dedicated to each item on the agenda. If you stick to the schedule, discussion will stay focused and you will be more likely to make it through the agenda. However, setting realistic times is critical to the success of this strategy.
- *Action agendas:* Consider submitting an agenda with a description of the needed/desired action, such as review proposals, approve minutes, or establish outcomes.

Keep the group on task. Use rules of order to facilitate meetings. Robert's Rules of Order (Robert, Honemann, & Balch, 2011) may seem overly structured; however, Robert's Rules are well known and are particularly helpful when diversity of opinion is likely or important. Specifically, these rules help the chairperson set time limits on discussion and provide a specific order of priorities to deal with concerns.

Keep minutes and distribute them to participants. The minutes provide a record for reference if needed and convey content to persons unable to attend.

Planning for the meeting is a group leader's best strategy for a satisfactory experience. Participants must also prepare for meetings. Reviewing the agenda (or requesting one in advance if not provided), reviewing preparatory materials, and thinking through agenda items are ways that group members may assist in accomplishing the meeting goals. Meeting participants should be on time for all meetings or communicate that they will be late or unable to attend. Participants should be prepared to leave on time as well. When a meeting is poorly chaired, a committee member could volunteer to ensure that the meeting agendas and minutes are distributed. Some people deliberately avoid preparing agendas and distributing minutes in an attempt to control the meeting. Exercise 28-4 will help you understand the importance of well-run meetings.

> **EXERCISE 28-4**
> Have you ever sat in a meeting and wondered why you were there? Perhaps the purpose of the meeting, where the meeting was heading, or even who was supposed to be in charge was unclear to you! Write down the three things about that type of meeting that were most annoying, and then analyze how the situation could have been handled better.

DELEGATING

Delegation is a critical component of self-management for nurse managers and care managers. Appropriate delegation not only increases time efficiency but also serves as a means of reducing stress. Delegation is discussed in depth in Chapter 26, but it is also appropriate to discuss briefly as a time-management strategy. Delegation works only when the delegator trusts the delegatee to accomplish the task and to report findings back to the delegator. The delegator wastes time if he or she checks and redoes everything someone else has done. Delegation requires empowerment of the delegatee to accomplish the task. If the nurse does not delegate appropriately, with clear expectations, the delegatee will constantly be asking for assistance or direction. Delegation can also be a means of reducing stress if used appropriately. If the nurse does not understand delegation and does not use it appropriately, it can be a major source of stress as the nurse assumes accountability and responsibility for care administered by others.

CONCLUSION

Self-management is a means to achieve a balance between work and personal life, as well as a way of life to achieve personal goals within self-imposed priorities and deadlines. Time management is clock-oriented; stress management is the control of external and internal stressors.

To achieve a balance in life and minimize stressors, nurses must learn to sit back and see their own personal big picture and examine their personal and professional goals. Personal priorities also must be established. Stressors and coping strategies need to be identified and used. By developing these techniques, nurses can gain a sense of control and become far better nurses in the process.

THE SOLUTION

Since the unit was closing, I accepted a nurse manager role in another unit at the hospital. However, this unit was the complete opposite of the one I had led to success. It was way at the bottom in every single metric you could think of! I became focused trying to help my old team during the anticipated closure as best as I knew how: I invited the VP/CNO to come to breakfast frequently on the unit, along with the bargaining unit and human resources leadership. I constantly checked in with them to help them apply for posted positions and help some of them transition to new roles in other units. On my new unit, I brought in seasoned assistant nurse managers and encouraged the high performing staff to apply for the vacancies that were created when the low-performers either resigned or were disciplined. In terms of my own stress, I definitely felt I had to get better at taking care of myself. My VP/CNO encouraged me to take days off and I went on a cruise for a family vacation and celebration. Considering the increased load, I guess I had to! I try to get enough sleep; I try to eat a balanced diet; I take a vitamin daily; I exercise by doing the weighted hula hoop and by enjoying dancing; and I am a spiritual person so I pray and attend religious services.

My family and my nurse leaders are really supportive, and I feel lucky to have people like that around me! I really love my job, and although I miss and mourn for my old unit, I know I can turn this unit around so it can be successful.

—*Mariebelle del Mundo*

Would this be a suitable approach for you? Why?

THE EVIDENCE

Sayre, McNeese-Smith, Philips, and Leach (2012) studied effective leadership styles and the phenomenon of "speak up," that is the degree of comfort and ease with which team members advocate for the perspective of the patient. This study was designed to investigate whether an education module could lead to an increase in advocacy behaviors and included nurse support groups following five actual patient care scenarios by the hospital risk manager, where the end result could have been prevented had the nurse voiced his or her actual care concerns. The participants also heard or read affirmations of support from their medical and nursing administrative leaders. A personal action plan incorporated self-identified barriers to their advocacy role with recognition of past, present, and future behaviors. Finally, a commitment to implement the plan was endorsed by the participants. Following the intervention, three questionnaires were administered, which included baseline demographic data, the Speaking Up Measurement Tool, and the Collaborative Practice Scale (CPS). The results showed a statistically significant difference for the intervention group for speaking up and for collaborative practice. Several months postintervention, anecdotal reports demonstrated that nurses perceived that they had more options than previously thought in conflict-laden situations.

WHAT NEW GRADUATES SAY

- I thought my faculty were weird when they talked about caring for myself. Now I see what they meant. I am proactive so I can continue in an emotionally challenging profession—one I love.

- The first meeting I attended used several of the strategies I had learned. I was impressed with how much we accomplished in a short time! Organization is important!

CHAPTER CHECKLIST

Stress management and time management are two strategies for self-management. Balancing stress means caring for your emotional, physical, and mental needs. Delegating effectively, using schedules and calendars and other planners, using time-management principles, and managing meetings are key strategies to be integrated into the nurse leader role. By developing self-management skills, managers, leaders, and followers will find themselves in control of work time and stressors, and they will become more skilled at achieving both personal and work-related goals.

Stress and overwork are inherent in the nursing profession, and nurses can adapt and cope with stress and time pressures by learning effective ways to care for themselves and to manage time. By assessing and reducing specific stressors and time wasters, nurses can thrive within the healthcare challenges before them. Increasing skills in coping, organization, delegation, and effective time management is vital for effective leadership. A nurse manager who can be a role model and support his or her staff in turbulent times is a true leader.

- Understanding stress
  - Definition
- Sources of job stress
  - External sources
    - Change
    - Social
    - The position
    - Gender roles
  - Internal sources
  - Dynamics of stress
- Management of stress
  - Stress prevention
  - Symptom management
  - Burnout
- Resolution of stress
  - Social support
  - Counseling
  - Leadership and management
- Management of time
  - Where does your time—and the day—go?
    - Doing too much
    - Inability to say "no" or "not now"
    - Procrastination
    - Complaining
    - Perfectionism
    - Interruptions
    - Disorganization
    - Too much information
  - Time-management concepts
    - Goal setting
    - Setting priorities
    - Organization
    - Time tools
    - Managing information
- Meeting management
  - Managing meetings
  - Tips for managing meetings effectively
- Delegating

TIPS FOR SELF-MANAGEMENT

- Make your health a priority and use strategies that keep yourself feeling cared for and in control.
- Make and keep personal physical and mental health appointments.
- Know your personal response to stress and self-evaluate frequently.
- Know what your high-priority goals are and use them to filter decisions.
- Refocus on your priorities whenever you begin to feel overwhelmed.
- Use organizational systems that meet your needs; the simpler, the better.
- Simplify.

REFERENCES

Abrahamson, E., & Freedman, D. H. (2008). *A perfect mess: The hidden benefits of disorder.* New York: Little, Brown and Co.

Bailey, J. (2009). The challenge for today's nurse managers: How to be fiscally competent & efficient while nurturing the workforce and sustaining self. *Spinal Cord Injury, 29*(1), 25–28.

Bolton, L. R., Harvey, R. D., Grawitch, M. J., & Barber, L. K. (2012). Counterproductive work behaviours in response to emotional exhaustion: A moderated meditational approach. *Stress and Health, 28*, 222–233.

Chang, E., & Hancock, K. (2003). Role stress and role ambiguity in new nursing graduates in Australia. *Nursing and Health Sciences, 5*, 155–163.

Chen, J., Davis, L. S., Davis, K. G., Pan, W., & Daraiseh, N. M. (2010). Physiological and behavioural response patterns at work among hospital nurses. *Journal of Nursing Management, 19*, 57–68.

Covey, S. R., Merrill, A. R., & Merrill, R. R. (1996). *First things first: To love, to learn, to leave a legacy.* New York: Simon & Schuster.

DeAngelis, T. (2002). A bright future for PNI. *Monitor on Psychology, 33*(6), 46. Retrieved March 10, 2014, from www.apa.org/monitor/jun02/brightfuture.html.

Dickerson, P. (2013). An algorithm to help you manage your stress. *American Nurse Today, 8*(3), 28–31.

Englebardt, S. P., & Nelson, R. (2002). *Health care informatics: An interdisciplinary approach.* St. Louis: Mosby.

Epp, K. (2012). Burnout in critical care nurses: A literature review. *Canadian Association of Critical Care Nurses, 23*(4), 25–31.

Erdwins, C. J., Buffardi, L. C., Casper, W. J., & O'Brien, A. S. (2001). The relationship of women's role strain to social support, role satisfaction, and self-efficacy. *Family Relations, 50*(3), 230–238.

Evans, O., & Steptoe, A. (2002). The contribution of gender-role orientation, work factors, and home stressors to psychological well-being and sickness absence in male- and female-dominated occupational groups. *Social Science and Medicine, 54*(4), 481–492.

Gallup Business Journal. (1999). *Item 10 I have a best friend at work.* Retrieved on March 20, 2014, from http://businessjournal.gallup.com/content/511/item-10-best-friend-work.aspx.

Georgia Nurses Association (2012–2013). Results from ANA's 2012 health risk assessment are in! *Georgia Nursing, 9.*

Greenglass, E., Burke, R., & Fiksenbaum, L. (2001). Workload and burnout in nurses. *Journal of Community and Applied Social Psychology, 11*, 211–215.

Hafner, A. W. (2001). *Pareto's Principle: The 80-20 rule.* Retrieved May 25, 2010, from www.bsu.edu/libraries/ahafner/awh-th-math-pareto.html.

Halm, M., Peterson, M., Kandels, M., Sabo, J., Blalock, M., Branden, R., et al. (2005). Hospital nurse staffing and patient mortality, emotional exhaustion, and job dissatisfaction. *Clinical Nurse Specialist, 19*(5), 241–251.

Health Resources and Services Administration, Bureau of Health Professionals, National Center for Health Workforce. (2013). *The U.S. nursing workforce: Trends in supply and education.* Retrieved March 20, 2014, from http://bhpr.hrsa.gov/healthworkforce/reports/nursingworkforce/nursingworkforcefullreport.pdf.

Hess, R., DesRoches, C., Donelan, K., Norman, L., & Buerhaus, P. (2011). Perceptions of nurses in Magnet® hospitals, non-Magnet hospitals, and hospitals pursuing Magnet status. *Journal of Nursing Administration, 41*(7/8), 315–323.

Hirokawa, K., Taniguchi, T., Tsuchiya, M., & Kawakami, N. (2012). Effects of a stress management program for hospital staffs on their coping strategies and interpersonal behaviors. *Industrial Health, 50*, 487–498.

Ingram, J., & Cangemi, J. (2012). Emotions, emotional intelligence and leadership: A brief, pragmatic perspective. *Education, 132*(4), 771–778.

Jennings, J. M., Scalzi, C. C., & Rodgers, J. D. (2007). Differentiating nursing leadership and management competencies. *Nursing Outlook, 55*(4), 169–175.

Johnson, S., & King, D. (2012). Nurses' perceptions of nurse-physician relationships: Medical-surgical vs. intensive care. *MEDSURG Nursing, 21*(6), 343–347.

Judkins, S., Reid, B., & Furlow, L. (2006). Hardiness training among nurse managers: Building a healthy workplace. *Journal of Continuing Education in Nursing, 37*(5), 202–207.

Kath, L. M., Strichler, J. F., Ehrhart, M. G., & Schultze, T. A. (2012). Predictors and outcomes of nurse leader job stress experienced by AWHONN members. *Journal of Obstetrical, Gynecological and Neonatal Nurses, 42*(1), 12–25.

Kemeny, M. (2003). The psychobiology of stress. *Current Directions in Psychobiological Science, 12*, 124–129.

Kobasa, S. C., Maddi, S. R., & Kahn, S. (1982). Hardiness and health: A perspective study. *Journal of Personality and Social Psychology, 42*(1), 168–177.

Kramer, M. (1974). *Reality shock: Why nurses leave nursing.* St. Louis, MO: Mosby.

Krichbaum, K., Diemert, C., Jacox, L., Jones, A., Koenig, P., Mueller, C., et al. (2007). Complexity compression: Nurses under fire. *Nursing Forum, 42*(2), 86–94.

Lambert, C. E., & Lambert, V. A. (1987). Hardiness: Its development and relevance to nursing. *Journal of Nursing Scholarship, 19*(2), 92–95.

Lambert, V., Lambert, C., & Yamase, H. (2003). Psychological hardiness, workplace stress and related stress reduction strategies. *Nursing and Health Sciences, 5*, 181–184.

Lee, H., Spiers, J. A., Yurtseven, O., Cummings, G. G., Sharlow, J., Bhatti, A., et al. (2010). Impact of leadership development on emotional health in healthcare managers. *Journal of Nursing Management, 18*, 1027–1039.

Lefton, C. (2012). Strengthening the workforce through meaningful recognition. *Nursing Economics, 30*(6), 331–338.

Lencioni, P. (2004). *Death by meeting.* San Francisco: Jossey-Bass.

Lopez, D., Green, M., Carmody-Bubb, M., & Kodatt, S. (2011). The relationship between leadership style and employee stress: An empirical study. *The International Journal of Interdisciplinary Social Sciences, 6*(3), 169–180.

Maddi, S. R. (2002). The story of hardiness: Twenty years of theorizing, research and practice. *Consulting Psychology Journal, 54*, 173–185.

Maslach, C., & Leiter, M. P. (1997). *The truth about burnout: How organizations cause personal stress and what to do about it.* San Francisco: Jossey Bass.

Maslow, A. H. (1943). A theory of human motivation. *Psychological Review, 50,* 370–396.

McDermott, R. (2000). Why information technology inspired but did not deliver knowledge maintenance. In E. L. Lesser, M. A. Fontaine, & J. A. Slisher (Eds.), *Knowledge and communication.* Butterworth Heine: Worburn, MA.

Merriam-Webster Online. (2013). *Complain.* Retrieved October 21, 2009, from www.merriam-webster.com/dictionary/complain.

Plsek, P. E., & Greenhalgh, T. (2001). The challenge of complexity in health care. *British Medical Journal, 323*(7313), 625–628.

Porter-O'Grady, T. (2013). Retrieved on March 23, 2013. www.mc.vanderbilt.edu/root/vumc.php?site=Shared%20Governance&doc=23733.

Robert, H., Honemann, D. H., & Balch, J. (Eds.) (2011). *Robert's rules of order newly revised* (11th ed.). Cambridge, MA: Perseus Book Group.

Rosenbaum, E., & Morett, C. R. (2009). The effect of parents' joint work schedules on infants' behavior over the first two years of life: Evidence from the ECLSB (early childhood longitudinal surrey, birth cohort). *Maternal and Child Health Journal, 13,* 732–744.

Rudan, V. T. (2002). Where have all the nursing administration students gone? *Journal of Nursing Administration, 32,* 185–188.

Sayre, M., McNeese-Smith, D., Philips, L., & Leach, L. S. (2012). A strategy to improve nurses speaking up and collaborating for patient safety. *Journal of Nursing Administration, 42*(10), 458–460.

Seavey, D. (2010). Caregivers on the front line: Building a better direct-care workforce. *Journal of the American Society on Aging, 34*(4), 27–35.

Segerstrom, S., & Miller, G. (2004). Psychological stress and the human immune system: A meta-analytic study of 30 years of inquiry. *Psychological Bulletin, 130*(4), 601–630.

Selye, H. (1956). *The stress of life.* New York: McGraw-Hill.

Selye, H. (1965). The stress syndrome. *American Journal of Nursing, 65,* 97–99.

Selye, H. (1991). History and present status of the stress concept. In A. Monat, & R. Lazarus (Eds.), *Stress and coping: An anthology* (pp. 21–36) (3rd ed.). New York: Columbia University Press.

Sherman, R. O. (2013). Building a sense of community on nursing units. *American Nurse Today, 8*(3), 32–33.

Shirey, M. (2006). Stress and coping in nurse managers: Two decades of research. *Nursing Economic$, 24*(4), 193–211.

Stöppler, M. (2005). *Top five stress management mistakes. Your guide to stress management.* Retrieved October 21, 2009, from http://stress.about.com/cs/copingskills/a/mistakes_p.htm.

TalentSmart®. (2011). *About emotional intelligence.* Retrieved from, www.talentsmart.com/about/emotional-intelligence.php.

Taylor, S. E., Klein, L. C., Lewis, B. P., Gruenewald, T. L., Gurung, R. A., & Updegraff, J. A. (2000). Biobehavioral responses to stress in females: Tend-and-befriend, not fight-or-flight. *Psychological Review, 107,* 411–429.

Thomas, E. (2010). Generational differences and the healthy work environment. *Med/Surg Matters! 21*(6), 20–21.

Zangaro, G. A., & Soeken, K. L. (2007). A meta-analysis of studies of nurse's job satisfaction. *Research in Nursing & Health, 30,* 445–458.

SUGGESTED READINGS

Centers for Disease Control and Prevention. (2013). *Stress and work.* Retrieved on March 23, 2013, from www.cdc.gov/niosh/docs/99-101/.

Collins, J., & Hansen, M. T. (2011). *Great by choice.* New York: Harper Collins.

Covey, S. R. (2011). *The seven habits of highly effective people.* 15th anniversary edition, New York: Simon & Schuster.

Lenson, B. (2002). *Good stress, bad stress.* Cambridge, MA: De Capo Press.

McKenna, E. P. (1998). *When work doesn't work anymore: Women, work and identity.* New York: Dell Publishing.

Oncken, W., & Wass, D. (November/December, 1999). Management time: Who's got the monkey? *Harvard Business Review,* reprint 99609.

Tracy, B. (2004). *Time power.* New York: AMACOM.

29

Managing Your Career

Debra Hagler

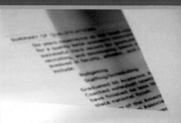

Successful people actively manage their careers rather than wait for "lucky breaks." Although trusted others may guide or influence career development, individuals manage their own reputations and careers. Continuous lifelong learning and the ability to demonstrate and document competence are critical elements in effective career management. This chapter includes tools to document accomplishments and ways to extend career development beyond the work setting.

LEARNING OUTCOMES

- Differentiate among career styles and describe how career styles influence career options.
- Develop a cover letter and résumé targeted for a specific position.
- Analyze critical elements of an interview.
- Describe a variety of professional development activities, including academic and continuing education programs.
- Identify contributions you could make and benefits you could derive from active involvement in professional organizations.

KEY TERMS

career	curriculum vitae	professional association
certification	licensure	(organization)
continuing education	portfolio	résumé

Daniel Weberg, RN, PhD, MHI
Director of Nursing Innovation, Kaiser Permanente

When I graduated with a BSN, I knew that I wanted to work in the emergency department right away. I was surprised at the opposition from most faculty and friends who told me, "You have to get at least a year of experience in med-surg first." Another challenge for me early on was the drive I felt to expand my skills in different directions, not only in direct bedside care. During my undergraduate nursing courses, I taught myself how to run the human patient simulators used in the learning laboratory, and I thought there might be a market for those skills. My struggle during this time was finding the direction to get to an objective that I could not clearly express and find a unique type of job that had not been created yet.

What do you think you would do if you were this nurse?

INTRODUCTION

The number of career options and paths within nursing is remarkable. Some of these options are the "traditional" roles nurses have performed for centuries—providing direct care to patients, leading teams or organizations, teaching, providing public health or school health services, or working in an occupational field. Yet new roles continue to emerge. Serving healthcare consumers as a legislative aide, for example, is not a common role, but it is one that helps shape the state's or nation's view of health care. Coordinating preventive care and health coaching are becoming more common health promotion roles. However, having these numerous options creates challenges in determining how to build a career, which educational path best serves the role, which experiences best prepare nurses for a specific field or role, who might be a willing and helpful mentor, and what new activities and roles need to be developed. Some options build primarily on experience and others on education and experience; all, however, require that a nurse engage in professional development and continue to advanced expertise to meet the evolving challenges in health care. How nurses reach their career goals depends on the goals they set and how they manage their career development.

A FRAMEWORK

A career, defined as progress throughout an individual's professional life, is developed by selecting positions that contribute to professional goals. A relationship exists between an individual and a position, and that same relational fit is exhibited in a career path. A good fit is built on strong, similar goals and tolerable (or growth-producing) differences. The whole of any work situation is composed of the two elements—person and position—interacting in a complex environment. Analyzing positions and the required skills in light of individual talents can help applicants determine positions that fit with their strengths. When gaps occur between the requirements of a "dream" position and the person's skills, applicants can consider whether professional development activities might help improve the match between their current and desired future qualifications.

Consideration of a career path, such as practitioner or administrator or educator, includes reflection on the most rewarding aspects of prior work. As an example, a nurse who determined that teaching patients, families, and students was the most personally rewarding aspect of practice might plan to develop a career as an educator. Whatever career is pursued, one key strategy is planning to obtain the right education and experience to meet future goals.

Broscio and O'Brien (2011) described a range of attitudes toward career development. Some individuals, although satisfied with their roles, are intent on continued improvement and seek continued development opportunities. Others may see the current role as a springboard to a future desired role or position, are uncertain about what they want, or are unhappy in their positions and don't know what to do about it. In each of these cases, clarifying future goals is an early step to finding the right new role or continuing a role that is meaningful and satisfying. It is in the best interest of both organizations and individuals to seek a good fit between the position and person. See Box 29-1 for elements to achieving career success that depend on both the individual and collaboration with the organization.

BOX 29-1   ELEMENTS IN CAREER SUCCESS

1. **Taking ownership:** Own the process and take responsibility for your career.
2. **Taking risks:** Don't be afraid to try something new. Adjust course and challenge yourself.
3. **Seeking to learn:** Be inquisitive. Ask questions. Listen. Be open to feedback.
4. **Choosing to engage:** Take the initiative and inspire yourself.
5. **Setting a goal and making a plan:** Know what you want and create the path forward.
6. **Striving to align:** Connect with your current or future organization's priorities.

From Broscio, M., & B O'Brien, M. K. (2011). Taking charge of your career: Good career management results in "shared success" between individuals, organizations. *Healthcare Executive, 26*(6), 64-66.

Another way to think about career development is to consider the work of Citrin and Smith (2003), who studied "extraordinary" careers. Their identification of three broad phases—*promise, momentum,* and *harvest*—suggest movement from early to late career. Thus, early in one's career, the focus is on developing skills, establishing credentials, and socializing into the role. Mid-career, the focus often shifts to honing specific areas of expertise (the things by which we will be known) and being more aware of the fit of positions within the broad array of opportunities that will enhance some goal. Finally, in a later career stage, many individuals focus on strengthening the profession (the broad view of the work). This movement through nursing life is predicated on having a vision of a career as opposed to a series of jobs.

Being a professional includes both privileges and obligations. The legal privileges and expectations are codified in the state nursing practice acts, rules, and regulations. Because **licensure** is designed to provide the baseline (i.e., the minimum expectation), it does not identify or obligate any practitioner to function in a professional manner as defined by the profession itself. For example, no practice act identifies membership in a professional association or providing community/professional service as an expectation. Yet the profession, through various professional organizations, embraces the expectation that nurses will belong to professional associations and provide leadership in improving communities. For example, the Forces of Magnetism (*www.nursecredentialing.org/ForcesofMagnetism.aspx*) include the expectation that nurses are involved in their community. The challenge, of course, is how to incorporate these activities into a busy, committed life! It often is those "additional" activities and interests that enrich a career and provide for invaluable insight into clinical and professional issues.

Knowing Yourself

The best opportunity for nurses to manage their careers and for a manager to help nurses gain important experiences is for the individuals to know themselves.

Knowing what is important, what is valued, and the commitment needed forms the basis for understanding one's self. Whether positions are plentiful or scarce, knowing one's self can focus the available work or selection process toward capitalizing on one's strengths. Even assessing one's strengths through a formal avenue (e.g., StrengthsFinder 2.0 at *www.strengthsfinder.com/home.aspx*) can provide insight. Therefore the beginning of creating a person/position fit is in understanding the person involved. Throughout school and initial experiences in nursing, insight begins to evolve that helps each of us determine our preferences for our life work. Some positions add more to what we want to be able to achieve in the long term than other positions. As an example, a position that offers educational compensation or flexible scheduling might be preferable when the goal is to return to school and complete advanced education for a specialized role.

Being able to describe yourself from various perspectives is useful. First, knowing your strengths tells you what you bring to a position and what you can rely on. When you know your strengths, you can say what they are in a succinct manner and use them as a filter in reading position descriptions to find your fit in an organizational. An analysis of your current competencies allows you to see what work needs to be done to meet required or desired standards and competencies. Finally, entering into such analyses can help you see the bigger picture of your career and how what you can learn from a particular position might contribute to your overall goals. The career styles described in Table 29-1 include the motivation and characteristics of each style. Seeing how your self-analysis fits with the descriptors in the third column may suggest how you see yourself approaching your career. The goal of all this work is to know yourself well so that your pursuit of a position or career path fits you and your strengths.

TABLE 29-1   CAREER STYLES

	EXAMPLE	DESCRIPTION	MOTIVATION AND CHARACTERISTICS	MANAGERIAL CONSIDERATIONS
Steady State	Direct care nurses	Constancy in position with increasing professional skill	Increasing expertise High professional identity Obligation to serve Maintenance of standards Autonomy in performance of care Preference for action Personal accountability The work itself Stability	Hold work in high esteem Decentralize Use and recognize abilities Provide feedback about patient outcomes Reward competence and tenure Provide continuing education Provide permanent assignment
Linear	Nursing service administrator	Hierarchical orientation with steady climb	Requisite authority and power Had a challenging first job Guided by internalized norms Money Recognition Opportunities for self-development	Provide management development Reward and value both education and competence Modify management selection and development systems Provide decreasing supervision
Entrepreneurial and Transient	Nurses in private practice; temporary assignments	Desire to create new service; meeting own priorities	Limited organizational commitment Opportunists Novelty/creativity Other people Achievement	Use flexibility to organization's benefit Avoid burdening them with organizational and practice decisions Provide immediate feedback
Spiral	Nurse who returns after raising a family	Rational, independent responsibility for shaping career	Novelty Prestige Intense period of employment followed by non-employment or a different employment Care for others Opportunities for self-development Typically well paid, service-oriented Recognition	Configure specific job that needs doing Be flexible about terms and length of commitment Find challenging initial assignment Negotiate Encourage creativity

Data from Friss, L. (1989). *Strategic management of nurses: A policy oriented approach.* Owings Mills, MD: AUPHA Press.

Knowing the Position

Few people, including nurses, hold the same position forever. Thus most nurses hold more than one position throughout their work life. Rapid changes in health care require an evaluation of each employment opportunity through a series of questions. Can a position contribute to increased skills and competencies? Does a position have the potential to recast one's professional profile so that others see the potential for greater contributions? Are the benefits of the position so enticing that they offset limitations of the position itself? Is the professional practice environment in that organization a safe and collaborative setting for healthcare professionals and patients (AACN, n.d.)?

Position assessment begins with understanding the vision and mission of the organization. Assessment also requires finding out specifics of the position, which may be available only through an interview. Bolles (2012) pointed out that although most often people apply for a similar position at several organizations, most managers look first within the organization to hire by transferring someone from a different position. So one key strategy to use is selecting an organization where you want to work, even if the position is not exactly the right one. The potential for inside connections and networking, in addition to knowledge about management styles in the organization and future position openings, can lead you to the position that is the right fit for you.

CAREER DEVELOPMENT

A career extends beyond employment positions. A career includes the various ways in which an individual engages in activities that provide care to patients, support that care, educate for that care, support the providers of that care, study the ways in which to deliver the care, and engage in the broader perspective of professional and community service. Thinking broadly about a career in a rapidly changing field such as health care is critical to remaining competent and relevant. Licensure carries certain expectations about maintaining competence and reflecting professional standards. Legislators enact legislation based on the needs of the citizens and in response to political pressures. When a profession is protected by legislation, others, such as consumers, insurers, regulatory agencies, and employers, expect that professional standards have been and will continue to be met. Continuing competence is a focal professional issue, but nursing has not identified a unified standard for maintaining competence, so requirements for demonstrating continued competency vary by state (Watson & Hillman, 2011). Changing geographic locations during a career may entail meeting different regulatory requirements for continuing professional development.

Over the course of a career, a position that was once a good fit may no longer work. The position may have evolved as much as the person did. If the movement was in harmony, the fit remains, but if the position changes one way and the person another, the fit devolves.

Bolles (2012) also suggested that some positions are life-changing. These can best be described as changing positions and fields simultaneously (such as may occur with a spiral career style). For example, when a charge nurse in a critical care unit assumes the role of a chief nursing officer in a rural community hospital, a major shift has occurred. Nurses who follow a spiral career path, especially if they were second-degree students (meaning they have a degree in another field and then entered nursing), may also experience this phenomenon. These individuals may have worked in another field and now are pursuing their hearts. They may have become bored with a career that had few interactions with people, or they may have studied in fields such as science and realized that the best application of knowledge could occur in patient care. Because of prior career successes, these individuals may craft career patterns that appear very different from the majority of the profession: they are using talents from two or more fields and are trying to capitalize on both.

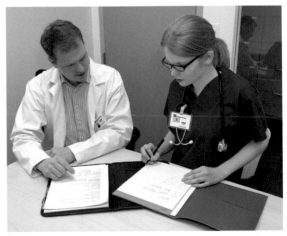

A mentor can inspire new thinking and new opportunities and steer you toward various roles and clinical areas.

Core career development strategies are important to success. Selecting professional peers and mentors to share in your development is crucial to gaining good, ongoing advice. Having a few well-chosen peers, mentors, and role models who respond openly from various perspectives can enrich career planning

LITERATURE PERSPECTIVE

Resource: Zachary, L. & Fischler, L. (2011). Begin with the end in mind: The goal-driven mentoring relationship. *T+D, (65)1*:50-53.

Most mentees do not come to a mentoring relationship with well-defined goals. A mentor can help mentees express their general ideas about future hopes and dreams as well as guide them to articulate and prioritize specific goals and timelines. Both "do goals" and "be goals" are important for career development. Do goals involve short-term measurable changes in knowledge, skills, or behavior. Be goals involve more nebulous areas, such as character and personal development. Mentors are especially helpful in planning a balance of one or two quick goal successes that will increase mentee confidence along with a longer-term, more challenging goal to make career impact.

Implications for Practice
- Choose a mentor with whom you feel comfortable sharing your career dreams.
- Match your mentor choice to the type of guidance you hope to receive.
- Like other types of relationships, a strong mentoring relationship takes an investment of time and effort to develop.

and development. A mentor can inspire new thinking and new opportunities and steer you toward various roles and clinical areas. That person can also create connections for you and help guide decisions related to timing and context. Mentors might even be able to create opportunities for you to test new approaches to clinical care or to new aspects of a position. See the Literature Perspective above.

EXERCISE 29-1
Think about an experienced nurse who serves as a role model to you. Would you want that person as a mentor? If so, consider how you would enlist that person's assistance in molding your career.

Through its Career Center (www.nursingsociety.org/Career), Sigma Theta Tau International (STTI) actively supports nursing professionals in identifying life-long learning for career enhancement, and in attaining their career goals. The STTI Career Center offers access to expert advisors, books, continuing education courses and nursing career opportunities. Resources to help you make the right career choices and transition into new roles, work life harmony, dealing with difficult people, succeeding in a multigenerational work force, and information specifically for new graduates are all examples of topics in which the STTI Career Center can assist fellow nurses. The STTI Career Center provides the opportunity to pose real time, personal career questions and receive responses from experienced expert professionals.

CAREER MARKETING STRATEGIES

Even the steady-state or experienced nurse who is not seeking a new position needs to have a curriculum vitae (CV) or résumé that can document continued development of expertise. Interviewing, which is a two-way process, also contributes to successful position choices and career development.

Although professional data can be recorded in numerous ways, most people do not do so in a systematic manner. Therefore, when information is needed quickly, it is difficult to recall and then to hone the most pertinent information for a position. A goal of this chapter is to develop a systematic strategy for creating marketing documents that you can use throughout your professional career. Some organizations use an electronic form of professional records so that an individual can readily access and convert the information into various documents. As an example, the National Student Nurses Association; the American Nurses Credentialing Center; and the Honor Society of Nursing, Sigma Theta Tau International, provide access to such an electronic approach. Portability of information is an important consideration so that information moves with an individual throughout a career.

Many position searches, even those internal to an organization, begin with a résumé. The key is to make information distinctive in telling your professional story and in establishing the appearance of a competent professional.

Data Collection

Depending on your unique background, the extent of data collection varies considerably. The first step is to collect all your professional career information. If you are fairly new in the profession, analyze anything special you did in school, such as electives, offices held, and special assignments, honors, and recognitions. If you are a second-career nurse, consider your previous work and how it relates to your profession now. If you have an employment history, start with your nursing positions. Include relevant information from volunteer roles, which can illustrate skills such as in leadership, ability to balance budgets, communication, and political astuteness, as well as indicate professional commitment.

To begin data collection, begin with where you are and think back. If you have short experience or no difficulty recalling details, you are in great shape to start a systematic plan. If, however, you have a long history as a nurse or a prior relevant career, your task is more challenging because you have to actively think about what you did in the past and, for a prior career, determine how to translate those experiences into relevance for nursing. The important aspect of this phase is to begin the process and to save it electronically so that you can shape information for specific reasons using a cut-and-paste technique rather than creating an original document each time you need to provide information about yourself.

Compile as many facts as possible for each of the ten categories identified in Table 29-2. Even if you have no entry for a specific category, retain the heading as a reminder and think about what you would like to be able to list there in the future. This is your private data bank for information to list on a curriculum vitae or to select for a résumé.

Curriculum Vitae

A curriculum vitae (or CV) is the documentation of one's professional life. It is designed to be all-inclusive but not detailed. A curriculum vitae follows some designated flow of information reflective of the ten categories identified in Table 29-2, however, empty categories are not listed on a CV.

Typically, a CV begins with your name and contact information. Your name should be most prominent (e.g., larger type size, bolded) and should be followed with contact information listed on separate lines. Your contact information should include address with zip code; phone numbers, designated by work, home, and cell; fax number; e-mail address; and, a Website address. If you include a Website address, use an e-mail account with a professional name; avoid usernames that are overly casual or personal such as "*sweetiepie@ domain.com*". Center the contact information on the CV or place a dividing line under it to help a prospective employer quickly locate that information. Information in the body of the CV should be presented in reverse chronological order. This approach allows a prospective employer to find the most recent information quickly and gain a sense of where you are in your career.

TABLE 29-2 DATA COLLECTION

TOPICS	FACTS NEEDED
1. Education	Name of school, address, phone numbers, Website address, years of attendance, date of graduation, name of degree(s) received, minor earned, honors received (e.g., Dean's List)
2. Continuing education	Dates attended, places, topics and any special outcomes, type and amount of credit earned
3. Experience	Dates of employment, title of position, name of employing agency, location and phone numbers, Website address, name of chief executive officer, chief nursing officer, immediate supervisor, salary range, typical duties (role description)
4. Community/institutional service	Dates of service, name of committee/task force and the parent organization (e.g., name of hospital or professional organization), your role on the committee (e.g., chairperson, secretary, member), general description of committee's functions, any distinctive accomplishments
5. Publications	Articles: author(s) name(s), year of publication, title, journal, volume, issue, pages; books: author(s), year of publication, title, location and name of publisher
6. Honors	Date, description of award, special factors related to award (e.g., competitive, community-wide, national)
7. Research	Date, title of research, role in research (e.g., principal investigator, co-investigator, team member), funded/unfunded
8. Speeches/presentations given	Date, title of speech presented, place, name of sponsoring organization, nature of the presentation (e.g., keynote, concurrent session)
9. Workshops/conferences presented	Date, title of workshop/conference presented, place, name of sponsoring group and nature of the presentation, brief description of the activity
10. Certification	Initial date of certification, expiration date, certifying body, area/type of certification

EXERCISE 29-2

Create a CV from your data. Define a plan to keep your CV current, such as copying data facts from your collection system onto the CV each time you enter data into your files.

Resumé

Resumés are customized documents that relate to the qualifications of a specific organizational position and help create an image of you serving in that position. Unlike the CV, a resumé provides details. It is presented in sentences or phrases (not both) to share the value of the information. For example, rather than listing years of service in a position by title and organization, a resumé might include information that you served as the only nurse to provide some distinctive service. For the experienced nurse, a resumé could be used to reflect increasing skills and abilities; for the new nurse, it could focus on specific "extra" abilities (e.g., competencies) that are not normally expected of a new graduate.

The resumé is a better choice than a CV for advertising your skills and talents to a prospective employer. Because a resumé is brief (typically no more than two pages) and tailored to the position being sought, the information is pointed toward specific position requirements. Details and action words help the reader view you as accomplishing important work. Verbs that relate to outcomes (produced, created) are the most powerful in conveying your achievements.

Basically, resumés can be produced in two ways. One is *conventional,* and it provides chronological information about positions and activities. The other approach, called *functional,* may combine multiple positions into role areas you are trying to highlight. So, rather than using experience as a heading (as in a conventional resumé), the functional resumé heading may relate to writing or client education and describe how you achieved results across several positions. A functional approach is best if you are planning a sharp departure from your present position or if you have considerable experience before entering nursing. The focus is on experience in diverse roles/positions rather than the specific positions held.

As with the CV, your resumé should be error-free, grammatically correct, accurate, and logical. Both of these documents should be printed on high-quality paper. Electronic resumés are best sent as a pdf or image file so that no distortion in the design or layout can occur. This is also a universally accepted electronic format, so recipients should have no difficulty opening the attachment. Bringing a resumé to an interview is especially useful if you were asked previously to provide a CV. This additional work of applying your talents to the specific position in the resumé helps the interviewer see you as fitting in the organization.

EXERCISE 29-3

Draft statements you could use in a resumé (conventional or functional, whichever would best serve your purpose) to describe one of your strengths or best outcomes.

Professional Letters

During your career, you will need to communicate effectively through letters. Every well-designed letter markets you as a professional. The commonly used letters are a cover letter, a thank-you letter, and a resignation letter. You may also write letters declining positions that you have been offered or recommending others for positions.

All of these types of letters include your name and contact information and should match the comparable contact information on your resumé and CV. This is especially important for the cover letter because it accompanies another document. The same quality paper should be used for letters as is used for the CV and resumé. If any of these documents are sent by e-mail or fax, you may still choose to send a hard copy.

These letters should be no longer than one page. The date and an inside address with the name (and credentials) of the addressee, the person's title, the name of the organization, street address, city, state, and zip code should be included. The next area of the letter is the greeting. The typical salutation (greeting) (e.g., "Dear Ms. Smith") is followed by a colon or comma. The end of the letter (closing) allows several line spaces between the word (e.g., *Sincerely*) and your printed name followed by credentials. If your address did not appear at the top of the letter, it should appear below your typed name. The space between the closing and your name should allow enough room for your signature. Between the greeting and the closing are paragraphs conveying the letter's main message. As with all formal documents, the letters should be proofread for layout, typographical errors, spelling, and content. E-mail communication contains essentially the same information, although no inside address is used. A discussion of each of the major types of letter follows.

Cover Letter

The cover letter is the key to getting your CV read and reiterates or supplements a résumé. A cover letter is a brief and carefully written document that includes why you are writing, why you "fit" the position, and how you will follow up.

Numerous positions may be advertised by an organization simultaneously. Thus immediately stating which position interests you and how you learned of it is helpful. Once you have stated your reason for writing, you should address the issue of "why you."

The second paragraph should indicate why someone should take time to read your attached résumé or CV. This section should state how you see yourself fitting with the organization (by experience, by philosophy, by clinical focus, and so forth). Two or three examples are helpful to provide the details of any general statements. It is also appropriate to refer to the attachment (your CV or résumé, whichever the organization requested).

The final paragraph should convey your optimism—you anticipate being interviewed. If you want to ensure that you have an additional opportunity to market yourself, you should indicate when you will follow up with a phone call.

EXERCISE 29-4

Write a cover letter that highlights information from at least two items from your data bank. Select items that best market you and that will entice the reader to call you for an interview.

Thank-You Letter

The business format described earlier can be used also for a formal thank-you letter, expressing appreciation for the opportunity that you had to interview. A more personal approach is to handwrite a thank-you note. Either way, the thank-you letter is your last chance to provide information about your communication skills, and values at this point in the process. A quick e-mail message to acknowledge the interview is not sufficient; if you send an immediate e-mail, a formal note should follow.

The lead paragraph of the thank-you letter may help the interviewer recall your interview. Identify which position you are seeking and perhaps a key statement that you discussed during the interview. If you discussed multiple positions, you should identify which of those positions most interested you. The next paragraph should reiterate one of your strengths and what you found most interesting in the interview. This paragraph could also answer any question that was left unanswered during the interview.

The closing paragraph should reference specific times when you expect to hear about the interview outcomes and when you will follow up. If you decided the position was not a fit, you should thank the person for the time devoted to the interview and wish him or her success in seeking the best candidate. Even the worst interview should be followed by a thank-you letter expressing your appreciation for the interviewer's taking time to talk with you and sending the organization your best wishes for the future. These actions create a positive impression both for the present and for future interactions. Finally, if the position is offered to you, another thank-you letter is appropriate and might include a statement related to your excitement about joining the organization, the date you expect to transition, and any key agreements that were made verbally but that are not yet in writing.

Resignation Letter

When you secure a new position, it is essential to resign effectively from your current position. Occasionally this is not applicable—for example, if you are transitioning from a student or military role or if you were terminated or laid off. Otherwise, being polite and diplomatic in your resignation process keeps communications open with your current agency so that you could return or seek support from the colleagues you left behind. The best approach to resigning is having a personal meeting with your manager and indicating that you will provide a formal letter of resignation. Your resignation should be given with adequate notice, which depends on your conditions of employment. Being flexible in your resignation date and negotiating that date with your manager create a positive exit strategy.

The letter of resignation follows the format guidelines described for other professional letters and begins with an acknowledgment of your intent to resign. Your date of resignation should be stated, and you might include whether this date is negotiable. This first paragraph should also reference the oral discussion you had with your manager.

The second paragraph highlights aspects of the employment experience that enhanced your career development. Identifying any major contribution you made to the organization is also appropriate. The worst thing to do would be to offload any negative feelings you have for the organization, manager, or co-workers in writing. Always say something positive about the position you have held.

The closing paragraph concludes by asking for a copy of your exit evaluation. It is important to learn your final standing as you leave an organization, and this appraisal for your own records may be valuable to you in the future.

Data Assembly for Professional Portfolios

The checklist in Box 29-2 will help you assemble your data attractively. Inclusion of these elements ensures a comprehensive view of your professional contributions and makes up a **portfolio.** Creating a professional portfolio, the basics of which are found in the citations made in your CV, can help organize one element of your professional life. Keeping notes of recognition, copies of evaluations, and pictures of your successes are examples that help round out the resource documents behind the CV data. Although a portfolio takes time to develop and to maintain, that work pays off at evaluation, promotion, and position-seeking times. Consider organizing your data in an electronic portfolio format. Some employers prefer receiving portfolio application materials in electronic form rather than large

---

BOX 29-2 CHECKLIST FOR CONSTRUCTING MARKETING DOCUMENTS

Data Assembly
_____ 1. Discrete categories are used.
_____ 2. Assembly addresses specific position.
_____ 3. Current name, address, phone numbers, e-mail address, and Web address are prominent (use as many as are appropriate for you).
_____ 4. Career summary (if used) (or cover letter) is prominent.
_____ 5. Key points about positions/experiences are evident.
_____ 6. A logical flow is evident.
_____ 7. Grammar, spelling, and syntax are correct.
_____ 8. Writing style is positive and direct, but not terse.
_____ 9. Action verbs are evident.
_____10. If writing in full sentences, third person and passive voice are avoided (i.e., write in the active voice).
_____11. "Canned" résumé language is avoided (e.g., "distinguished" and "all phases of ...").
_____12. Emphasis is on competence, not years (cover letter).
_____13. Specific examples of key competencies are cited (cover letter).
_____14. The format is consistent throughout.
_____15. Personal information (e.g., health, marital status) is absent.

Appearance and Format
_____ 1. There are no typographic errors.
_____ 2. The product is "clean" (e.g., no smudges, no discrepant margins).
_____ 3. The product is readable (e.g., layout design is pleasing: white space, capitalization).
_____ 4. The paper is high-quality bond (100% cotton), white or cream.
_____ 5. The type is businesslike (no script); text is at least 10 to 12 point, and fonts are limited to one or two.
_____ 6. Emphasis is evident (e.g., centering and bold print or underlining).
_____ 7. The product is only one or two pages in length (not applicable for a curriculum vitae [CV]).

Overview
_____ 1. It is attractive, interesting, quick-reading, and competency-based.
_____ 2. The package sells you.
_____ 3. You are pleased to have it precede you.
_____ 4. Additional items are enclosed, or they are assembled for personal handling at an interview.
_____ 5. If you were receiving this CV or résumé, you would want to interview this person.

collections of paper. The electronic format allows for easy customization based on a specific position. In other words, this system of maintaining professional information provides a resource to respond promptly to new or emerging opportunities.

The Interview

After your letters and résumé are effective in career marketing, the next step is participating in an interview. Interviewing is a two-way proposition; the interviewee should be gathering as much information as the interviewer is. Both should be making judgments throughout the process so that if a position is offered, the interviewee will be prepared to accept, decline, or explore further. Interviews may take place with one or more individuals and may include a range of activities. To be at ease, the interviewee should wear professional and comfortable clothing. Rehearse specific questions to ask and points to make so that you can feel more at ease during the interview. Be prepared to cite how you have faced challenges and dilemmas, because those types of questions are likely to be asked (see The Evidence, p. 563).

Even in times of a nursing shortage, employers are using behavioral interviewing techniques to identify the most appropriate applicant for the vacant position. Rather than being asked, "What are your weaknesses?" you may be asked, "Tell me how you handled the last mistake you made" or "How did your educational program prepare you for critical care nursing?" Applicants in some organizations are screened and interviewed by a panel and then asked to participate in a series of interviews to allow fellow employees more say in the hiring process. In business and healthcare settings, many prospective employers administer basic skills tests. Researching the organization in advance can help prepare you for the interview.

Interview Topics and Questions of Concern

During interviews, employers should ask all applicants for a given position the same questions. In addition to providing comparable information as the basis for a decision, the applicant's expectation for equal treatment is upheld. Only questions related to the position and its description are legitimate. Employers should not ask other questions (Table 29-3), and applicants should decline to answer if asked such inappropriate questions.

If the interviewer asks an inappropriate question, the applicant can choose not to answer the direct question by addressing the content area. For example, if asked about your spouse's employment, you might say, "I believe what you are asking is how long I will be able to be in this position. Let me assure you that I intend to be here for at least 2 years."

Each of the content areas identified in Table 29-3 may be acceptable, but the initial question is phrased inappropriately. The second column identifies approaches that are both appropriate and legal. The key to ensuring a fair interviewing process is being prepared, knowing what can be asked legitimately, and knowing how to respond to inappropriate questions.

TABLE 29-3   INAPPROPRIATE AND APPROPRIATE QUESTIONS

SAMPLE OF INAPPROPRIATE QUESTIONS	SAMPLE OF APPROPRIATE AND LEGAL QUESTIONS
1. How old are you?	1. Do you know that this position requires someone at least 21 years old?
2. What does your husband (wife) do?	2. This position requires that no one in your immediate family be in the healthcare field or own interests/shares in any healthcare facility. Does this pose a problem?
3. Who takes care of your children?	3. Attendance is important. Are you able to meet this expectation?
4. Are you working "just to help out"?	4. What are your short-term and long-term goals?
5. Do you have any disabilities?	5. Is there anything that would prevent you from performing this work as described?
6. Where were you born?	6. This position requires U.S. citizenship. May I assume you meet this criterion?
7. What are the names of all of the organizations to which you belong?	7. To which professional organizations do you belong?
8. What is your religious preference?	8. We subscribe to a specific religious philosophy and mission. Do you understand that all employees are expected to promote this philosophy?

If you have prepared well, you will know what the organization's stated beliefs are and whether they are compatible with yours. The challenge in an interview is to determine whether those stated beliefs are lived or are merely printed words. If numerous people can relate how the mission is translated into a specific role, the beliefs are likely lived ones.

Plank (2010), in an article in *The Wall Street Journal*, identified the five must-ask questions, and therefore the five must-be-prepared-to-answer questions:

1. In what ways will this role help you stretch your professional capabilities? (This is designed to provide clues about weaknesses.)
2. What have been your greatest areas of improvement in your career? (This identifies weaknesses again and this time identifies what action you took; just knowing one's weaknesses is not good enough.)
3. What's the toughest feedback you've ever received and how did you learn from it? (This question is designed to identify candidates who can be forthright and who are learners.)
4. What are people likely to misunderstand about you? (This question is all about how the candidate "reads" others.)
5. If you were giving your new staff a "user's manual" to you, what would you include in it to accelerate their "getting to know you" process? (This reveals information about how the person will function in the team.)

This chapter includes two tools designed to be used in preparing for an interview: "Checklist for Interviewing" (Box 29-3), and "Interview Goals and Content" (Table 29-4). Using the thank-you letter described earlier in this chapter is an additional opportunity to market yourself, especially if you wish to correct or expand on an answer you provided during the interview.

BOX 29-3 CHECKLIST FOR INTERVIEWING

1. Check interviewing guides, such as *What Color Is Your Parachute?*
2. Check out the new organization:
   a. Review the organization's mission, vision, and values statements before the interview (via the Web or hard copy).
   b. Obtain statistics and facts.
   c. Ask about new program directions.
3. Recheck your résumé or curriculum vitae for the following:
   a. Emphasis
   b. New information
4. Practice using "action" words.
5. Decide about the following:
   a. Appearance
   b. Key points:
      i. To make
      ii. To learn
   c. Tool for quick check (e.g., a file card with key points)
6. Arrive on time and alone.
7. Make a memorable entrance:
   a. Make eye contact.
   b. Shake hands.
   c. Smile.
   d. Say, "Hello, I'm [name]."
8. Position yourself with the interviewer (e.g., decide to sit at an angle).
9. Keep in mind your key points.
10. Appear interested—project competence, confidence, and energy.
11. Accentuate the positive!
12. Answer questions directly but know when not to.
13. Ask for more information.
14. Say only positive and honest things about your present employer.
15. Secure a time frame for notification of a position offer.
16. Thank interviewer personally.
17. Write a thank-you letter.
18. Let interviewer know your decision.
19. Put commitments in writing.

EXERCISE 29-5

Select a partner and role-play an interview for a professional nursing position. The potential employer (manager) should focus on competencies of the prospective employee. Include questions and scenarios about common conflicts and challenges seen in the clinical setting. The interviewee (prospective employee) should highlight competencies, decision-making abilities, and critical-thinking abilities when responding to the situation-based questions. Reflect on the process and discuss what you learned that you can apply to future interviews.

PROFESSIONAL DEVELOPMENT

A key message from the Institute of Medicine (IOM, 2011) report, *The Future of Nursing: Leading Change, Advancing Health,* is that "Nurses should achieve higher levels of education and training through an improved education system that promotes seamless academic progression." Although there is hope that such a seamless system will exist in the future, nurses most often have to forge their own paths to academic and career progression.

TABLE 29-4	INTERVIEW GOALS AND CONTENT
INTERVIEW GOALS	**CONTENT**
1. Personal characteristics	Describe the type of person you are, including personality traits. Be expected to cite examples of when these traits helped or hindered you in previous situations.
	List situations that characterize your energy, initiative, drive, ambition, and enthusiasm.
	Clarify your professional values.
	Have a story ready that illustrates how you see yourself.
2. The work itself	Emphasize what makes you distinctive. Describe how your education and experience prepared you for this position.
	Describe your skills as a member of a team and a leader of a team.
	Prepare to address hypothetical situations that display your problem solving, reasoning, self-confidence, knowledge, and critical thinking. (Creates opportunity to evaluate you in action and under some stress.)
	Ask intelligent questions that suggest you have prepared for this interview and know something about this organization.
3. The organizational fit	Be clear about what you believe to be distinctive about this organization and how it meets your expectations for a position.
	Articulate your "fit" with the organization's philosophy, mission, and vision.
4. The professional opportunities	Be clear about what you expect to obtain from any position you consider. Include advancement opportunities, educational support, and work/life balance.

Active involvement in education, service, and scholarship opportunities can help prepare you to deal with new roles and challenges in your employment setting and the larger scope of nursing and health care. Engaging in service activities (both community and professional organizations) and sharing your knowledge through research, writing, and speaking (scholarship) allow you to influence others in the profession and through the profession. When positions are scarce or when you are competing for a very desirable position, community and professional service experience and scholarly contributions to nursing may give you the advantage over other candidates.

One of the keys to maintaining competence and versatility is continued learning. "Nursing professional development is a vital phase of lifelong learning in which nurses engage to develop and maintain competence, enhance professional nursing practice, and support achievement of career goals" (American Nurses Association [ANA] and National Nursing Staff Development Organization [NNSDO], 2010b, p. 1). Learning can occur also through informal means: in a conversation with colleagues, by observing leaders in the workplace, reading an article in the general literature, or sometimes in an "ah ha" reflective thought that provides sudden enlightenment.

ACADEMIC AND CONTINUING EDUCATION

A graduate degree opens the door to numerous career opportunities. Graduate education consists of either master's-level or doctorate-level study in a clinical specialty area, in preparation for a specific role, or a combination of both.

Some employment situations or career specialties require advanced education. As health care has become more complex, nurses recognized as independent practitioners need more education to meet healthcare demands. For example, nurse practitioner preparation requires graduate-level degree preparation as opposed to the earlier certificate programs. If you dream of conducting clinical research, earning a PhD is likely to be the best preparation for the role. If you want to teach future healthcare professionals, you may be able to prepare for that role in a variety of ways: a master's degree or doctoral degree in nursing or education, or a graduate degree in a related field such as public health, sociology, genetics, or informatics. Choose a graduate program based on your future career plans.

Admission to graduate programs may require taking a test (often the Graduate Record Examination

[GRE]), having an above-average grade point average (GPA), and graduating from a professionally accredited school of nursing.

Deciding to pursue graduate education may be very simple. Some applicants to associate degree and baccalaureate programs already have a specific career focus requiring graduate preparation in mind. In the past, new graduates were often encouraged (or even required) to gain work experience before seeking a master's degree or doctorate. Although experience can enrich the learning process, the philosophy of delaying entry into graduate education is changing as nurse leaders have identified the profession's need for nurses who have completed graduate degrees earlier in their careers. In addition, the increasing complexity of health care leads to a need for nurses who are simultaneously experts in areas outside nursing. Earning a graduate degree in another field may put you in the position of translating advanced knowledge from other disciplines to improve health care. Working while attending a graduate program may be difficult, but it is common among graduate students in nursing. Box 29-4 lists some factors to consider in selecting a graduate program.

Consider the following example of seeking out a graduate program that fits:

> You know you want to work with elderly patients. Your library subscribes to the *Journal of Gerontological Nursing* and *Geriatric Nursing.* You review the most recent year's issues of both. You scan the page with the editors and board members. Where are these individuals affiliated? Now you scan the articles. Are there some that are particularly intriguing? Where are the authors affiliated? Finally, look back over the lists. Are there any places emerging where the leaders in the field may be? What centers of excellence in geriatrics have related graduate programs? This is a good starting place.

Distance education online provides an additional option for earning an advanced degree. Flexible scheduling and the convenience of online courses permit many individuals to participate who would not be able to attend traditional programs because of class times or geographic distance.

BOX 29-4   FACTORS TO CONSIDER IN SELECTING A GRADUATE PROGRAM

Accreditation	• Does the program have national nursing accreditation (master's/doctoral level)?
	• Is the institution regionally accredited (e.g., North Central Association of Colleges and Schools)?
Clinical/functional role	• How closely do the descriptions of clinical/functional courses of study meet career goals?
Credits	• How many graduate credits are required to complete the degree?
	• How many are devoted to clinical or practicum experiences?
	• How many relate to classroom experiences?
Thesis/research	• Is a thesis/dissertation/capstone project required?
	• If not, what opportunities exist for research development?
	• What support is available for graduate students?
Faculty	• What credentials do faculty members hold?
	• Are they in leadership positions in the state/national/international scenes?
	• Are they competent in your field of interest?
	• What is their reputation?
Current research	• What are the current research strengths of the institution?
Flexibility	• Do these strengths fit with your interests, or is there flexibility to create your own direction?
	• Is flexibility present in scheduling and progress through the program?
	• Is consistent classroom attendance required or is online/blended attendance an option?
Admission	• What is required?
	• Is the GRE used?
	• What is the minimum undergraduate GPA expected?
	• Is experience required? What kind? How much?
Costs	• What are the total projected costs?
	• What financial aid is available?

GPA, Grade point average; *GRE,* Graduate Record Examination.

EXERCISE 29-6

Assume you are interested in graduate education.

- Use the Internet or the library to locate information about graduate education and financial assistance.
- Determine what specialties exist at the master's/doctoral level.
- Determine the location of programs nearby and access to distance programs.
- Evaluate the clinical interest of the programs of study.
- Decide if the diverse roles of the advanced practice registered nurse appeal.
- Consider doctoral programs, including those permitting entrance from the baccalaureate level.

EXERCISE 29-7

Imagine you have decided to earn a master's or doctoral degree in nursing. Develop a strategic plan for your graduate education.

- What values do you have that influence your plan?
- Are your interests in primary care, administration, or education?
- What is your target date for completion of the program?
- What other factors would interfere with your strategic plan?
- Do you have specific short-term goals or operational plans that must be attained before enrollment?

Continuing education also contributes to professional growth. **Continuing education** is defined as "systematic professional learning experiences designed to augment the knowledge, skill, and attitudes of nurses, thereby enriching the nurses' contributions to quality health care and their pursuit of professional career goals" (ANA, 2010b, p. 6).

Numerous opportunities for continuing education exist at local, state, regional, and broader levels. Selecting among the numerous opportunities to pursue may be difficult. Box 29-5 lists factors to consider in selecting any offering, but depending on your particular goal, certain factors may be more influential than others. For example, if cost is a major factor, length and speaker may be less influential factors.

In addition to increasing your knowledge base, continuing education provides professional networking opportunities, contributes to meeting certification and licensure requirements, and documents additional pursuits in maintaining or developing clinical expertise. Sponsors of continuing education include employers, professional associations, schools, and private entrepreneurial groups.

BOX 29-5	FACTORS TO CONSIDER IN SELECTING A CONTINUING EDUCATION COURSE
Accreditation/approval	• Is the course accredited/approved? If so, by whom? • Is that recognition accepted by a certification entity and by the board of nursing (if continuing education is required for re-registration of licensure)?
Credit	• Is the amount of credit appropriate in terms of the expected outcomes?
Course title	• Does it suggest the type of learner to be involved (e.g., advanced)? • Does it reflect the expected outcomes?
Speaker(s)	• Is the instructor known as an expert in the field? • Is the instructor experienced in the field?
Objectives	• Are the objectives logical and attainable? • Do they reflect knowledge, skills, attitudes, or a combination of these? • Do they fit a learner's needs?
Content	• Is the content reflective of the objectives? • Is the content at an appropriate level?
Audience	• Is the audience designed as a general or target one (e.g., all registered nurses or experienced nurses in state health positions)?
Cost	• Is the cost equitable with that of similar nursing conferences? • Is travel required? • What is the actual direct expense for an individual to attend? Is it affordable?
Length	• Is the total time frame logical in terms of objectives, personal needs, and time away from work? • Does the time frame permit breaks from intense learning?
Provider	• Does the provider have an established reputation?

Both types of formal professional development (i.e., graduate education and continuing education) are valuable, and both can contribute to a specific area of career development—certification.

CERTIFICATION

Certification signifies completion of requirements in a particular field beyond basic nursing educational preparation for licensure. Nurses can be certified as recognition of competence in a number of different specialty areas. Certification is an expectation in some employment settings for career advancement; in the field of advanced practice nursing, it is a requirement for practice and reimbursement. In many states, certification in advanced practice is the mechanism to achieve recognition as an advanced practice registered nurse from the board of nursing. Consumers, nurses, managers, and administrators value certification. See the Research Perspective on this page.

Obtaining certification may require testing, continued education, and documented time in practice in a specific practice area. Recertification is a process of continued recognition of competence within a defined practice area and may require participation in continuing education. Certification plays an important part in the advancement of a career and the profession. In some fields, more than one examination exists; in others, there is an examination in the broad field and numerous options for defined subspecialties. The American Nurses Credentialing Center (ANCC) (*www.nursecredentialing.org*) offers numerous certification examinations for nurse generalists, nurse practitioners, clinical specialists, nurse administrators, nurse case managers, ambulatory nurses, and informatics nurses. In addition, other certifications are offered by nursing specialty organizations. The Websites of these specialty organizations (or their credentialing organizations) provide specific certification requirements.

 RESEARCH PERSPECTIVE

Resource: Kendall-Gallagher, D., Aiken, L.H., Sloane, D.M., & Cimiotti, J.P. (2011). Nursing specialty certification, inpatient mortality, and failure to rescue. *Journal of Nursing Scholarship, 43*(2), 188-194.

In order to establish the possible value of certification to improving health care, researchers analyzed data from 1,283,241 surgical patients in 652 hospitals. They used patient outcome data, administrative staffing data, and nurse characteristics such as education completed and certifications achieved to estimate the effect of specialty certification on patient mortality and failure to rescue. Each 10% increase in a hospital's proportion of baccalaureate nurses decreased the likelihood of inpatient mortality and failure to rescue by 6%, and every 10% increase in the proportion of those baccalaureate staff certified in a nursing specialty decreased the likelihood of inpatient mortality and failure to rescue by an additional 2%. Overall, nursing specialty certification had a higher correlation with better patient outcomes than baccalaureate or other graduate preparation alone.

Implications for Practice
Consider preparing for specialty certification as a direct contribution to improved patient outcomes. Some organizations actively support certification activities. If yours does not, ask administrators to support certification efforts at your workplace through sponsoring attendance at certification preparation courses or holding courses on site. Point out the value of nurses' certifications for the organization from the perspective of patient safety and outcomes. Having support from the organizations might require you to encourage colleagues in the workplace to share efforts for future certification by organizing study plans and groups. Finally, ask nurse leaders and staff about characteristics of nursing staff such as percentage of certified nurses in workplaces where you seek employment. Working in settings striving for better patient outcomes may contribute to your satisfaction with your nursing career. If you are interviewing in a Magnet™ organization, this information will be readily available.

PROFESSIONAL ASSOCIATIONS

Belonging to a professional association not only demonstrates leadership but also provides numerous opportunities to meet other leaders, participate in policy formation, continue specialized education, and shape the future of the profession. Professional associations (organizations) are groups of people who share a set of professional values and who decide to join their colleagues to effect change. Many nursing associations set standards and objectives to guide the profession and specialty practice. Standards can also serve as critical measurements for the profession and its practitioners. In today's changing healthcare environment, increasing numbers of associations are serving unique healthcare interests in society. Although associations have very different agendas and goals, many nursing organizations share the same motivation and long-term goal of uniting and advancing the profession.

More than 75 specialty nursing organizations represent nurses in particular areas of the profession. Some are clinically focused, such as the American Association of Critical-Care Nurses, the Oncology Nurses Association, and the American Association of Neuroscience Nurses. Others are role focused, such as the American Organization of Nurse Executives and the National League for Nursing. Still others represent specific groups in nursing, such as the American Assembly for Men in Nursing and the National Black Nurses Association. To attract future members, many specialty organizations offer reduced membership rates to students and new graduates, which include discounted meeting and convention rates, discounts on insurance, networking opportunities, and informative publications and mailings about the association. Go to the *Evolve* Website (*http://evolve.elsevier. com/Yoder-Wise*) to see a listing of nursing specialty organizations.

The "umbrella organization" that represents all nurses is the American Nurses Association (ANA), which comprises registered nurses throughout the United States and its territories and various organizational affiliate members (*www.ana.org*). The ANA advances the nursing profession by fostering high standards of nursing practice. Some functions of the ANA include projecting a positive and realistic view of nursing, promoting the economic and general welfare of nurses in the workplace, and lobbying Congress and regulatory agencies on healthcare issues affecting nurses and the public (ANA, 2010a). When the ANA was formed in 1897 and officially founded in 1901, its purpose was to protect the public from unsafe nursing care and to set standards for practice and education that could be changed and adapted over the years (Joel, 2003). Today, the ANA continues to speak for nursing. Policymakers look to the ANA for guidance on nursing and health policy issues.

Unlike most professional associations that are open memberships (i.e., if you meet the basic criteria, you are eligible to be a member), Sigma Theta Tau International is an invitational association. Established in 1922, membership is available to nurses enrolled in baccalaureate, masters, and doctoral education programs and community leaders through a nomination process. Its mission is to create a global community of nurses who lead in using scholarship, knowledge, and technology to improve the health of the world's people (*www.nursingsociety.org*). This organization is one of the primary sources for small grants to aid in beginning research and disseminates research and leadership information through various publications and international meetings.

A MODEL FOR INVOLVEMENT

Upon graduation, nurses often are focused on key aspects of professional life, such as learning basic policies and the organizational culture, evaluating peers to determine who to trust and who to avoid, and resolving numerous transitional issues, such as where to live, how to afford housing, how to manage payment of student loans, how to network with old and new friends, and how to be safe practitioners. Few new graduates think about how they can benefit from professional organizational membership, and unfortunately, many nurses never pursue membership in any professional organization. Many others participate only through a financial contribution, by paying the membership dues.

Connecting with an Organization

The size of an organization is not as important as how the group is organized and who is leading it. Therefore it is extremely important to do some online reading about the officers and membership composition of the organization before making a commitment through membership. Most associations have a Website that lists information regarding leader contact and biographical information, locations of their next meetings or activities, current policy issues and their positions, election information, and other valuable resource links. Some organizations permit e-mail subscriptions so that you are notified on a regular basis about events.

> **EXERCISE 29-8**
> Research the ANA and your state nursing organization on the Internet (*www.nursingworld.org*). Find the mission of the organization and the legislative issues of interest. Obtain/download association brochures or further information.

Expectations of Membership

Upon joining a nursing organization, you may receive information on the history of the organization, future meetings and current activities, officer contact information, and local contacts. One of the most important things that you can do is connect with your local organization so that you can immediately begin networking. Decide how much time you can allocate to the organization. Multiple ways to be involved carry different time commitments. Do not assume that a certain role or committee position entails a set amount of time. The fact remains that most associations are composed of volunteers, all of whom have very busy schedules and different motivations for becoming involved. Taking time to talk to an officer or attend a local meeting and observe the group and the dynamics before deciding to make commitments will help ensure that you make an informed decision. Some members enter into the organizational experience with unreal expectations and quickly become disenchanted and disappointed with the organization, which results in completely pulling away from the organization. To maximize your experience, you owe it to yourself to do your homework, research the organization, talk to the members, determine the sense of the group dynamics, and assess what you want to derive from the experience and how you can contribute to the organization. Look at your strengths and talents to determine if there is a need or a fit within the organization. Finally, remember that the organization is composed of humans who are volunteering their time; therefore you should not expect a "perfect" organization. Every organization has its struggles, but you can gain tremendous personal and professional benefits from your involvement. Examples of tangible benefits of membership can be found in Box 29-6.

BOX 29-6   TANGIBLE BENEFITS FROM ORGANIZATIONAL INVOLVEMENT

- Substantial discounts on continuing education and professional journals
- Promote professional standards beyond the individual's workplace
- Certification
- Quick access to staff experts
- News on legal, legislative, and educational issues
- Group insurance plans for professional liability, health care, and disability
- Travel services, such as auto rentals, hotel stays, and restaurant visits
- Discounted retail services

Joining/Reasons for Involvement

Nurses may hold membership in a variety of social and professional organizations, devoting more time to particular areas of interest. Nurses who define themselves as leaders and who want to have influence beyond their workplaces should join at least one professional association. Some reasons for joining organizations include feeling a sense of responsibility to the profession, contributing to the greater good of the profession, enhancing your résumé and marketability, supporting particular legislative interests, and social networking. A common belief among nurses is that their organization of choice can help improve conditions and care for their patients. In addition, some choose to be active participants by joining committee work, running for office, or taking on other leadership roles. Organizations need all types of members, both active and passive participants, so that they can carry out their missions and conduct activities and business. Organizational involvement is a socialization process that can improve morale—being around others who take pride in and celebrate the nursing profession is contagious. Whatever your preferred level of involvement, you can contribute greatly to your profession by simply becoming a member of a professional association, and progressing to active involvement guarantees a world of opportunities.

Some nurses choose to belong to their state nurses' association because they want to improve health care through influencing legislation. Others choose to belong because of specific benefits such as liability insurance and education. Some individuals belong to professional organizations because they are required to do so; employment contracts in some states can make it mandatory for the nurse to join a union and pay dues in order to receive a paycheck.

Personal and Professional Benefits

Some associations offer substantial scholarships for nurses who are pursuing higher education and certifications. They might also offer scholarships to attend policy meetings, such as the Nurse in Washington Internship (organized by the Nursing Organizations Alliance) or the Annual Health Policy Institute, conducted by the Center for Health Policy, Research, and Ethics of George Mason University. These two internships are examples of opportunities through which nurses can learn about legislative issues, the political process, healthcare advocacy, and how to be more effective on local, state, and national levels. Another potential benefit of membership is the opportunity to travel for conventions and meetings. Most organizations rotate their regular convention meeting sites so that members throughout the country will have an opportunity to attend.

Networking and exposure to different opportunities within the nursing profession are two of the most valuable benefits of belonging to an organization. Some nurses may stop working for a time because of family or educational priorities. Organizational membership can help these nurses stay connected to professional issues and colleagues through meetings and publications and smooth the transition back into practice.

Membership in nursing organizations can provide a continuous source of professional colleagues for today's nurse to draw upon for advice and support. All nurses encounter ethical dilemmas and professional challenges. Members of a nurses' professional association can be nonbiased, safe colleagues to ask for advice about your situation, especially when you may not want to discuss it with co-workers who could be directly involved. They also may be connected to the experts in the field.

With abundant opportunities in nursing, chances are that most nurses will work in a variety of settings over the course of their career. Therefore today's nurse needs to socialize with nurses in different professional career paths. This socialization can take place through local meetings, state or national conventions, or online. For example, conferences might feature a nurse panel representing a variety of innovative positions within the field, which will introduce the member to networking contacts in those emerging fields. In addition to networking, the professional organization can serve as a training ground through which nurses can build skills and gain wonderful experiences. Examples of these skills can be found in Box 29-7. They also provide opportunities for leadership development through committees or in officer positions, which can provide invaluable skills training.

Professional organization members can influence healthcare policy through opportunities to influence and educate policymakers. Members of nursing associations learn firsthand about diversity among

---

BOX 29-7 SKILLS DEVELOPED THROUGH ORGANIZATIONAL INVOLVEMENT

- Conflict management
- Interpersonal communication
- Public speaking
- Mentoring
- Meeting management
- Agenda development
- Facilitation
- Delegation
- Consensus-building
- Strategic-thinking
- Team-building
- Political advocacy
- Legislative work/lobbying
- Problem solving

---

the patient populations and clinical issues of fellow members, as well as diversity within the profession. On the most basic level, nurses can influence legislation for health and the profession by simply becoming a member and adding political strength through numbers. Further, nurses can participate on a legislative committee and become involved in their local grassroots politics. Nurses' ability to advocate for their patients is not confined to the bedside; nurses must learn to use advocacy skills in the political arena as well. By being acquainted with the key political figures in their area, nurses can ensure that they are at the table for discussions on healthcare and policymaking decisions. Consistently, the Gallup poll reports that the public trusts information about health care

---

EXERCISE 29-9

Attend a local meeting of a professional association, observe the dynamics, and network with the members. Challenge yourself to speak to at least two members to learn about their work setting and their nursing role. Make sure to get contact information or a business card from at least two individuals whom you can call in the near future. On the back of the business card, write something about that person that will help you remember him or her for the future (e.g., long black hair, nurse manager on the neurology unit at General Hospital). It is also helpful to have a date and the name of the meeting so you can "place" the person in your mind. You may use these cards in the future when you are looking for a job or need a specific question answered.

provided by registered nurses. This powerful influence of the nursing profession on public trust reinforces that nurses must be involved in healthcare discussions and decision-making policies.

EXERCISE 29-10

Make a list of your strengths (communication, organization, budgeting, legislative interests) and connect them to positions within the nurses' organization that interests you. On a separate list, write out reasons why you would want to be a part of the association.

CONCLUSION

A wise mentor can provide a safe learning environment for honest reflection and discussion about challenging issues while acting as a sounding board, an advisor, a role model, a bridge to connections with new colleagues, and a support structure for new responsibilities. Working with a helpful mentor provides support for career development through facilitating learning new roles and leadership skills. In addition to the benefits for those who work with a mentor, the mentoring relationship can benefit the mentor and the organization in improving organizational commitment. Organizations need to have future leaders prepared at every level to progress into positions of more responsibility as other formal leaders retire or move within the organization. Some organizations offer structured mentoring programs as a path to leadership development.

THE SOLUTION

I started by volunteering in the emergency department (ED) before I graduated, which gave me the firsthand view that this chaotic environment was the right place for me to start. I was confident that I knew myself and my passions, so I was willing to challenge the tradition of working in medical-surgical units before the ED. I had to work hard to convince my friends, my faculty, and myself that I could work in the ED directly out of nursing school. I wrote down the pros and cons, created my résumé, and made phone calls to a nurse I knew who worked at the medical center and could introduce me to the ED manager there. I was hired, so I worked in the ED as a new graduate, and before my first year, I had earned my Certification in Emergency Nursing (CEN).

I thought that creating the nontraditional job that I wanted for myself would be easier if I had the credibility of a graduate degree. I began taking graduate courses one at a time to find a good fit and found that I did not want to obtain the traditional MSN degree, so I applied and was accepted into a new master of healthcare innovation (MHI) degree program. I e-mailed some contacts I had met while attending conferences, asking them if they had a human patient simulator and if they needed help learning how to use it, all the while staying in contact with the faculty from my undergraduate program. Within 4 years, I had earned my MHI, started my own patient simulation consulting company, published three peer-reviewed articles in national journals, and started coursework in a PhD program. After I completed my dissertation in nursing and healthcare innovation leadership, my career trajectory shifted to administration: I recently accepted a position as Director of Nursing Innovation at a very large healthcare system in California. My nontraditional path made this dream job possible.

Navigating the traditions and socialization of nursing is tough, but you should not let other people direct or constrain your dreams. I did not know it at the time, but networking, joining professional organizations, and looking for the right fit in my career goals made a huge difference in how these ventures developed. Connections with mentors, colleagues, and friends who agree with me, as well as those that challenge my views, keep me moving forward.

—*Daniel Weberg*

Would this be a suitable approach for you? Why?

THE EVIDENCE

Asbury: Don't wait until you are offered a job interview to clean up your social networking sites. Assume that as soon as potential employers receive your application, they will search the internet for mentions of you. What they find on the internet about your activities may prevent them from calling you for an interview, or you might be asked about what is found.

Be pleasant to everyone you meet in the organization where you are applying for work. Some managers rely on the impressions of secretaries and the other staff with whom you interact with during the application process.

Stafford: Take a copy of your resume along in case you need to refer to dates or titles. Don't take your cell phone along, though, unless you are sure it is turned off. Receiving a phone call during your interview would not reflect a serious attitude about work.

Nutter: The interview is no time to be humble. Be prepared to describe specific accomplishments and ways that you have added value in organizations where you have been employed or volunteered.

Vilorio: Knowing about the organization helps convey a sense of enthusiasm for the position. Study the organization's mission, vision, and expectations through their Website, advertisements, and published news reports before you go to the interview.

Asbury, S. (2011). Just the job. *The Safety & Health Practitioner, 29*(8), 48.

Stafford, D. (2012). Beware of interview landmines. *Women in Business, 64*(1), 14.

Nutter, R.W. (2013). Give yourself an edge during a job search. *Healthcare Executive, 28*(1), 76.

Vilorio, D. (2011). Focused jobseeking: A measured approach to looking for work. *Occupational Outlook Quarterly, 55*(1), 2-11.

WHAT NEW GRADUATES SAY

- I am interviewing the organization where I am applying for a job, just as they are interviewing me.
- It seemed so hard at first to put together my résumé, gathering all the information and organizing it to look nice. But now that I've done it, I feel proud of what my résumé shows.
- As a student, I didn't really think nursing organizations were very important to join. But where I work now, most of the nurses belong to a professional nursing organization. The organization's Website has a lot of information I can use for patient care. Now I'm planning to go to the national conference and attend the educational sessions.

CHAPTER CHECKLIST

Nurses must make decisions about career goals and career development. Managing a career requires a set of planned strategies designed to lead systematically toward the desired goal. The use of each strategy should be geared toward finding a good person-position fit. Career planning and development is a lifelong process focused on continual competence. Continued professional development, whether via graduate education, continuing education, certification, or service in professional associations, is a crucial component of success as a nurse. Involvement in professional associations can open doors to opportunities and skill development that would never have been possible otherwise.

- A framework
  - Knowing yourself
  - Knowing the position
- Career development
- Career marketing strategies
- Data collection
- Curriculum vitae
- Résumé
- Professional letters
  - Cover letter
  - Thank-you letter
  - Resignation letter
- Data assembly for professional portfolios
- The interview
  - Interview topics and questions of concern
- Professional development
- Academic and continuing education
- Certification
- Professional associations
- A model for involvement
  - Connecting with an organization
  - Expectations of membership
  - Joining/reasons for involvement
    - Personal and professional benefits

TIPS FOR A SUCCESSFUL CAREER

- Use an expanding file to organize hard copies of your accomplishments, such as continuing education certificates (by year) so that you can report accurate data for licensure or certification. Keep electronic versions of documents filed together in an electronic folder.
- Update your CV at least once a year (every 6 months is even better) so that you always have an accurate, current set of accomplishments and qualifications to share with should a special opportunity appear.
- Keep connected with people.
- Find a mentor; be a mentor; self-mentor.
- Learn from what you do each day: what to do differently, how to preempt errors, who to seek as a supporter.
- Focus on your strengths and build them into spectacular performances; hone the basics so that you are always prepared.
- Create an individual mission statement.
- Think about the future and what you need to be employable in the face of health system changes.
- Research and create a file of educational programs of interest.
- Join two or more professional organizations: a broad professional group (e.g., the American Nurses Association) and a specialty (e.g., the American Association of Critical-Care Nurses).
- Read professional journals and at least one other general news journal.
- Attend at least one professional meeting each year to network with colleagues. When possible, travel outside of your geographic area.
- Volunteer in your profession and your community.

REFERENCES

American Association of Colleges of Nursing (AACN). What every nursing student should know when seeking employment: An interview tip sheet for baccalaureate and higher degree prepared nurses. Retrieved May 14, 2013 from www.aacn.nche.edu/publications/hallmarks.pdf.

American Nurses Association (ANA). (2010a). *ANA nurse's career center*. Retrieved February 8, 2013 from, www.nursingworld.org/careercenter.

American Nurses Association and National Nursing Staff Development Organization. (2010b). *Nursing professional development: Scope and standards of practice*. Silver Spring, MD: Nursesbooks.org.

Bolles, R. N. (2012). *What color is your parachute? A practical manual for job-seekers and career-changers*. Berkeley, CA: Ten Speed Press.

Broscio, M., & O'Brien, M. K. (2011). Taking charge of your career: Good career management results in "shared success" between individuals, organizations. *Healthcare Executive*, *26*(6), 64–66.

Citrin, J. M., & Smith, R. A. (2003). *The five patterns of extraordinary careers*. New York: Crown Business Books.

Friss, L. (1989). *Strategic management of nurses: A policy oriented approach*. Owings Mills, MD: AUPHA Press.

Institute of Medicine. (2011). *The future of nursing: Leading change, advancing health*. Washington, D.C.: National Academic Press.

Joel, L. (2003). *Kelly's dimensions of professional nursing* (9th ed.). New York: McGraw-Hill.

Plank, W. (2010). *Five must-ask questions*. Retrieved February 9, 2013, from, http://online.wsj.com/article/SB1000142405274870430230457521396279439000.html.

Watson, E., & Hillman, H. (2011). Practice of registered nursing: Are you competent? *Journal of Legal Nurse Consulting*, *22*(2), 27–28.

SUGGESTED READING

Enelow, W. S., & Kursmark, L. M. (2010). *Expert resumes for health care careers* (2nd ed.). Indianapolis, IN: Jist Works.

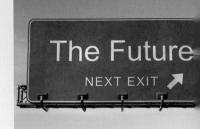

This chapter explores the potential for the future and how the changes we face can be maximized to our benefit—organizationally and personally. The key leadership skills of forecasting and visioning are presented. Projections for the future and their implication for nursing are included.

LEARNING OUTCOMES

- Value the need to think about the future while meeting current expectations.
- Ponder two or three projections for the future and what they mean to the practice of nursing.
- Determine three projections for the future that have implications for individual practice.

KEY TERMS

chaos	shared vision
complexity compression	vision

Sara McCumber, APRN, BC, MSN
Adult/Family Nurse Practitioner, Duluth Clinic, Duluth,
  Minnesota

I had been working for several years and had just accepted a position as a correctional nurse working with high-risk adolescents and adults. I pictured my job of completing physical assessments and managing the medication-delivery system. Over time, I learned that I was working with a population who were poor, had high-risk health behaviors, lacked access to health care, and often had physical and mental health problems. They often were returned to the community with many of the same problems. As the only nurse and health advocate in the facility, I realized that I had to search out and develop innovative solutions to the multitude of unmet health needs. I also knew I didn't have the skills or experiences to develop effective interventions. In addition, I determined that changes in the future that would improve the care for this population were unlikely.

What do you think you would do if you were this nurse?

INTRODUCTION

Leading and managing in nursing constitute a consistent challenge. Even nurses who say they do not want to lead or manage find that new demands call for continuous leadership and increased self-management skills. More important, the increased emphasis on teams will continue, and a strong team does not emerge from members with limited talents. Bringing leadership and management talents to the team strengthens the work of the team. The core point is this: We are all accountable for something, and by virtue of our professional licensure status, we must lead when we have the insight, the ability, or the skill needed to move a situation forward. As stated in Chapter 1, every role has expectations associated with it. Thus every nurse has some leadership role to execute in practice.

Changes affecting health care occur at a rapid clip. Even though healthcare changes have often happened as a result of something, rather than the organizations leading change, thinking proactively will be useful. Just when some stability seems likely, another new project or invention alters the currently established practice. Today, most people accept apps for phones as standard, yet only a few decades ago, a phone was wired and in the house. Two or three generations ago, people received health care (if they sought any) in the home and if they went to the hospital, it was for weeks. Additionally, many people believed that is where people went to die! Today people tend to seek illness care and if they are hospitalized, it is for hours or days. Tomorrow people will be rewarded for seeking wellness care and may receive actual physical care in the home, but this time through remote interactive devices. And, who among us wouldn't think that not having robotics isn't antiquated! Now think what changes have already occurred as a result of the Affordable Care Act and what yet could be! These events illustrate the dichotomous times in which we live and how the future is expected to be.

LEADERSHIP DEMANDS FOR THE FUTURE

Nurse administrators and leaders consistently say that the characteristic they are most seeking in tomorrow's professional nurse is leadership. In probing what that means, we often find themes that relate to our activities that may have serendipitous outcomes. We shape the public's view of the profession, the organization in which we work, and health care in general. We influence interprofessional views of what it is to be a professional, and we create the expectations of the nursing profession's potential. All of those examples form some of the leadership potential that exists for the future.

If we think about the world as a loose web, we know that every element has the potential to influence every other element. This connectivity with each other, whether within our profession or within the team, means that we influence others all of the time just as others influence us. This influence molds our practices and beliefs as we move health care forward and also changes how we influence others subsequently. Thus even positions without formal leadership titles contain expectations for leadership, and we must all be prepared and willing to lead whenever the need arises. This response is exhibited every time a mass casualty occurs. The ability to be bicultural—both leading and following—is crucial to quality care.

EXERCISE 30-1

When a spider is decapitated, it dies. When a starfish is severed in half, each half regenerates to form a new starfish. Using the comparison of a starfish (decentralized) and a spider (centralized), analyze two or three community organizations. If the respective leader left, would the organization diminish or suffer its demise or would the organization thrive? What rationale supports this conclusion?

 LITERATURE PERSPECTIVE

Resource: Crenshaw, J.T. & Yoder-Wise, P.S. (2013). Creating an environment for innovation: The risk-taking leadership competency. *Nurse Leader, 11*(1), 24-27.

Most of the efforts of nurses in practice focus on providing evidence-based care and adopting new practices. A relatively small amount of the time (or of the population) is devoted to considered risk taking. Using Rogers' theory of diffusion of innovation, the authors suggest that little time or talent is spent in being the innovator in the profession. However, being willing to take careful risks (considered risk taking) leads to innovative approaches of practice. The reason this type of work is not evidence-based is because this work is, in essence, creating the innovation. Innovators are at the cutting edge of change and laggards are at the tail end; in between is the majority of the profession: those who practice based on evidence and who do so in a safe and documented manner. The value of innovation is not only creating the next step for new evidence-based research but also disrupting current thinking and practices.

In order to promote innovation in an organization, the culture has to support the idea of considered risk taking. Everyone needs to have protected time to reflect on events to consider how a change might have produced even better outcomes.

Implications for Practice

In order to support innovation in the workplace, nurse leaders must support a culture that allows for diverse viewpoints and reflection about events. Providing support for considered risk taking allows individuals who might not otherwise risk wild thinking to do so in an attempt to find different solutions to ongoing clinical and management concerns.

LEADERSHIP STRENGTHS FOR THE FUTURE

Because so much of nursing's work is accomplished in teams, we have considerable strength in inclusivity (the politics of commonalities). This is in contrast to what many of us face in our everyday work of not capitalizing on thinking long-term and acting short-term. Much of the work of the Institute for Healthcare Improvement (*www.ihi.org*), for example, is built around the fact that change is slow and cumbersome. IHI basically supports small changes and encourages failing fast to determine if a given small change is worthwhile pursuing. It has short-circuited that drawn-out process through its program "Transforming Care at the Bedside." Although this rapid change (known as *rapid cycle change*) has produced positive results, nurses' abilities to embrace this intensity of change may be limited. Yet, almost every healthcare organization is actively engaged in determining best practices and finding or validating evidence. This emphasis is critical for safe patient care. However, what we lack by this intense focus is the passion for innovation (see the following Literature Perspective).

EXERCISE 30-2

Consider a persistent problem in the clinical area. This might relate to the functioning of a team or a clinical care practice. Consider what bothers you about the problem. Then imagine for a moment that you could do something to effect change for this problem. Make a list of "wild" ideas that are not the mainstream responses to such problems.

When we are faced with the pressures of providing care to patients versus changing the system, we often remain focused on the patient, thus losing the opportunity to change an issue for many patients. To be effective in the future, we must embrace the opportunities to think longer term and more broadly so that more people are affected by our actions. Perhaps because of our history of attention to details, we may need to challenge ourselves in developing our ability for leadership. Moving from micromanaging to focusing on setting expectations for those for whom we are accountable may feel uncomfortable. However, that movement reinforces our ability to deal with longer-term issues. In addition, the quest for meaning suggests that our actions today create the foundation on which future leaders will build. Thus if we fail to capitalize on today's opportunities, we are diminishing the place at which future leaders will start their careers. It is incumbent on us to raise expectations about what comprises good, safe, quality care and how nurses contribute to those expectations. This potential is especially critical in times of dramatic changes, such as those that continue to evolve from the Affordable Care Act.

How then do today's practitioners know what is expected in the future? The answer may seem trite: Continue to learn and to practice! Our foundation begins with our concern for and advocacy about patient care. That foundation is fairly well engrained in professional nurses' beliefs. The movement from focusing on the nurse-patient relationship to the big picture of nursing (politics and public or health policy activities) may take several years, but the foundation is there. What we do in our professional lives is the legacy we leave for future generations.

EXERCISE 30-3

Think ahead to the time when you might logically die. Rather than being sad that your life has ended, consider all of the good you have done in life and in nursing. Your next of kin is asked to say what he/she believes your nursing legacy to be. What one or two sentences would you want to have said about your contributions to nursing and the patients for whom we provide care?

Nurses who seek leadership opportunities will find that many are available—in the employment setting, in professional organizations, and in voluntary community organizations. Balancing the multiple demands in an era of rapid changes and the resultant new expectations becomes an even greater challenge. Merely being employed is no longer sufficient; we must be *employable*. This suggests that we must constantly be focused on competence, on learning, on what the future holds, and on what patients want and need. Failure to do so will make us unemployable and will make the profession undesirable. To be valued in the future, we need to know what the future might encompass.

VISIONING

Whether you are a leader, a follower, or a manager, being able to visualize in your mind what the ideal future is becomes a critical strategy. A **vision** can range from that of an individual to that of a group or to a whole organization. No matter how we engage in this visioning activity, we must be open and honest about what we think for the future. Creating our own circle of advisors or brain trusts (those who do not necessarily think as we do, but who are creative thinkers) allows us to test ideas so that we enhance our own thinking and performance to higher levels (see the Literature Perspective).

 LITERATURE PERSPECTIVE

Resource: Batcheller, J. & Yoder-Wise, P.S. (2011). Creating insight when the literature is absent: The circle of advisors. *Nursing Administration Quarterly, 35*(4), 338-343.

Some areas of practice are fairly narrow and few people work in those narrow fields; other areas lag behind the massive push toward safety related issues. Thus, the literature can be limited or absent related to a concern a person might have. Having a circle of advisors is a strategy to overcome merely thinking by yourself. This circle of advisors is not restricted by geographic or cultural constraints. Rather, resourceful nurses can find others with similar interests and filter information based on the area of the country or world or taking into account various values prevalent in a given field or area. Surrounding yourself with others interested in your specific area provides the opportunity to exchange ideas. The process is somewhat analogous to qualitative research in that little appears in the literature and the task at hand is to gain insight, seek a solution, or propose new ideas. Advisors provide diverse views. Surrounding oneself within a circle of advisors provides for diverse viewpoints to be shared.

Implications for Practice

Although this article was geared toward chief nursing executives, this practice works equally well for nurses in other positions. Careful selection of the advisors is critical to having access to successful advice.

In the classic book, *The Fifth Discipline: The Art and Practice of the Learning Organization,* Senge (2006) said that all leadership is really about people working at their best to create the future. And that, in reality, is what we do everyday. One way to capitalize on your "best" is to consider your strengths (*www.strengthsfinder.com*) and what societal changes could capitalize on your strengths to meet the challenges of the future.

This chapter is designed to share some views about the future so that you can think about them in relation to what it means to lead and manage. This "thinking about" the future, like visions, is further enriched through sharing in open dialogs.

EXERCISE 30-4

Select a group of three or four peers and brainstorm about what you think the future of nursing will be. Consider how technology will affect what we do; consider where our primary place of service will be and how we will deliver care. Think about the changes in society and the political pressures for effective health care and what those might mean for nursing. Think about how you would reform health care. Create a list of ideas to share with others.

Although no one knows the future for certain, many entities engage in formal discussions and predictions. These range from structured groups, such as the World Future Society (*www.wfs.org*), to regular reports and books. Although not everyone is a futurist, each of us needs to be aware of trends. We take for granted that certain practices have remained unchanged. Yet, technology *and* creative thinkers and investigators prove us wrong on a regular basis. Our challenge is to think about the future in a way that does not necessarily rely on history and yet builds on today. Converting problems or challenges into opportunities is a skill that opens up opportunities for the future.

THE WISE FORECAST MODEL©

Yoder-Wise (2011) created The Wise Forecast Model©. Although the model is simplistic (three steps), it is useful in any situation where thinking about the future is important. Box 30-1 portrays the three steps.

This three-step model emphasizes what each of us must do proactively to create our own future rather than to passively react to changes as they occur. The first step, learn widely, means that we must extend our sources of knowledge beyond our role and clinical areas of interest. In fact we must extend our learning beyond nursing and health care. Learning widely might encompass another discipline such as architecture or engineering. This extension doesn't mean that someone has to seek a degree in a new field. Learning about the field and how those professionals think might create new ways to think about issues affecting nursing. Just-in-time learning may feel stressful at times, yet it provides new information when it is needed. Thinking about what that learning means beyond its intent can also create new ways of thinking about an issue. Learning widely might also include readings works related to the future or general publications, such as *Fast Company* or *Wired*. Initially, this kind of learning may be deliberate; in other words, you might need to set aside specified times to garner this diverse information. After a few such sessions, however, it is realistic to think that information from other fields will pique your interest to the point that you will create a file of "tidbits" of information.

The second step is to think wildly. In other words, now we are limited only by our imagination. For example, since they were invented, someone wasn't satisfied with what we could do with computers. So computers evolved from one or two room-sized mainframes to something someone could have in a home, to something someone could carry in a backpack, to something someone could carry in a hand. Step two is designed to create connections among disparate thoughts. This thinking might be seen as the start of innovations. As Crenshaw and Yoder-Wise (2013) identified, risk taking was an important competency to develop. Considered risk taking, that which has the potential to produce innovation without unanticipated results, is practiced by a small portion of the population. Yet, others could engage in the practice in order to develop new and improved ways to practice. Thinking wildly includes creating wild questions. Sometimes they are what lead to a wild idea.

Step three, act wisely, is designed to draw us back to the reality of what is possible within the organization in which we work, with the funding we have available, and with the amount of time we have to invest in an activity. Acting wisely is, in a sense, a recovery phase to help us balance the wild thinking with reality.

Because the future is about teams and group work, many implications exist for nursing. Skills related to working with others and facilitating their work and ways to reach decisions about practice and the workplace will be crucial. If the work is team based, how will evaluations and compensation be structured in the future? Will you receive favorable reviews because the team you work with is productive? Will a team receive a bonus or merit salary increase? If you are not a team player, will you be useful to the organization at all? How will the role of the nurse as a frontline leader and the role of the nurse leader change? These are examples of how to rethink the future.

BOX 30-1	THE THREE STEPS TO THE WISE FORECAST MODEL©

1. Learn widely
2. Think wildly
3. Act wisely

Adapted from Yoder-Wise, P.S. (2011). Creating wise forecasts for nursing: The Wise Forecast Model©. *The Journal of Continuing Education in Nursing: Continuing Competence for the Future, 42*(9), 387.

SHARED VISION

The concept of shared vision suggests that several of us buy into a particular view. If we think of a familiar concept, stress, and what Selye (1978) described as *eustress* and *distress,* we have a continuum.

Eustress ←――――――――――――――→ Distress
Stress

Again, if you think about stress, you recall that each of us views an event differently and that having no stress results in death. Comparably, we can think about how society is evolving. Stability and total chaos are the ends of a continuum. Moving in some way between those two ends suggests that we live in a constant state of disequilibrium in which we strive toward stability while recognizing we experience chaos. The figure below suggests that in times of great stability, society makes little progress, so life may seem serene. In times of great chaos, in contrast, society may transform itself, and life may seem uncontrollable. Thus it is even more important to think about the projections for the future. As one example for most of us, think what we were doing, thinking, believing, and valuing on September 10, 2001. Then think about each in relation to September 11, 2001. We moved from some point on that continuum closer to chaos, no matter where we were in the world or what we were doing. Similarly, when the Boston Marathon was disrupted by bombs exploding near the finish line, we moved closer to the side of chaos. Yet, in both circumstances, healthcare professionals responded magnificently and learned from prior, similar events to make their care progressively better.

Stability ←――――――――――――――→ Chaos
Society

As we continue to move from "traditional" practices to evidence-based ones and from a heavy focus on tertiary care to one that values primary care, we can assume that we might experience more chaos. Think what the formation of accountable care organizations means in terms of the delivery of care and how people will move through a care continuum. The comfort of the known is gone; rather, practices are evaluated on a regular basis and changes are incorporated so that we are all doing the latest "best" for patients. In our efforts to do the best we can as soon as we can, we have experienced the phenomenon of complexity compression, a term that means many changes are happening almost simultaneously. Before one practice can be firmly implanted in our minds, we are already addressing some other new change. This compression can be distracting or useful. As we increase the educational preparation of nurses worldwide, we will be better able to function in this evolving environment.

It is our ability to retrieve information and analyze and evaluate it that influences our currency with practice expectations. We seem to value the need for shared vision, which includes the idea of operating from a rich data-based approach. To be able to do so, however, we also need to hone our skills in projecting for the future so we know where practice is headed. We need to consider how we interact with our patients, and we need to consider how quickly we can elevate all nursing practitioners to a satisfactory level of working with an evidence-based practice approach.

PROJECTIONS FOR THE FUTURE

If you watch future reports on television, read *the TREND letter* or *The Futurist* (a publication of the World Future Society), or read books such as *The World is Flat: A Brief History of the Twenty-First Century* or *Hot, Flat and Crowded* by Thomas L. Friedman, you will find comparable themes about the future. The following are some forecasts for the future that will affect nursing; it is possible to ask the "what if" questions with each (e.g., what if this happens?):
- Knowledge will change dramatically, requiring that we all be dedicated learners. With or without state law, continuing education will be mandatory and essential.

- Knowledge will evolve from the intensity of the current information evolution so that we will access content with meaning and applicability for our work.
- A power shift will occur toward health care because of the intensity of the developing knowledge and its use in making cost-effective decisions about care.
- As the healthcare system continues to evolve, and as employers limit healthcare coverage and genetics allows us to know more about how an individual would respond to treatment, a shift toward eliminating the current disparities is more likely. Health care also seems to invade one's rights to privacy and choice because, as an example, everyone will have an electronic health record.
- The world will be seen increasingly as a continuum without borders that prevent trade and inventions, including those related to health care.
- Technology will continue to revolutionize health care.
- Increasing diversity will result in the following:
  - More people who are older
  - More people moving to different parts of the country or the world
  - A greater need for speaking two or three languages
- People will be satisfied with an experience, not simply service.
- There will be increased violence and simultaneously an increased expectation for civility.
- Stores will be either very small or huge.
- Macromarketing (targeting masses) will be out; micromarketing (targeting specific populations) will be in.
- We could become narrower in our views of the world because we can be catered to based on our distinctive interests. As an example, think about micromarketing where retailers know what brands and sizes of clothing you prefer and send you information about those products on a regular basis.
- Job security will be out; career options will be in.
- Competition will be out; cooperation will be in.
- Work will be sporadic.
- More people will be living with chronic diseases.
- A focus on prevention and wellness care will include patient accountability expectations with

higher insurance rates for those who continue to engage in unhealthy behaviors.
- More people will be overweight and consequently experience various related diseases.
- Robotics will change how chronic diseases can be managed.
- Bioengineering will make possible interventions that currently do not exist.
- Emphasis on prevention will redirect care efforts.
- Work will be accomplished by teams.
- Everyone will need to be a leader.

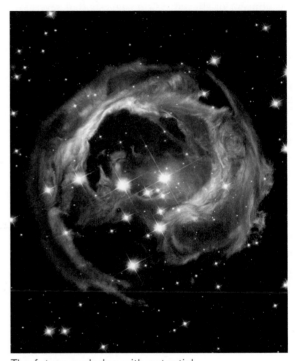

The future explodes with potential.

EXERCISE 30-6

Review the list of projections, and consider how each might affect what you envision as your career. Make a note of one or two phrases that are the top implications. Look at the list again, and evaluate each of the items to determine which ones you believe will be most important to you. Rank in order the top five. Compare your list with two or three colleagues' lists, and offer your rationale for your selection. After you hear other viewpoints, consider if you would change your own rankings.

In nursing, we have issues we can consider in the more narrowed scope of the world, for example:

- How will shared governance continue to enhance the role of direct care nurse?
- How will Magnet™ designations affect where nurses seek employment?
- How will the Pathway to Excellence® Program (ANCC) affect where nurses seek employment?
- Will we have a dramatically richer set of evidence to describe the difference nurses make in patient care and health promotion/disease prevention?
- How will continuing competence be measured in the future?
- How will health care emerge over the next several years as a desirable place to work and as a source of help for health-related needs?
- Will nurses be paid by a classification salary, or will their economic worth be reflected in what they are paid?
- How will the increasing number of men in nursing change the "profile" of the profession?
- What can healthcare organizations learn from business, and vice versa?
- Will increasing concern about terrorism affect the flow of nurses across borders?
- Will educational transition move seamlessly across degrees so that we increase our numbers of highly educated nurses by 2020, as the IOM suggests?

IMPLICATIONS

Should we be concerned with these forecasts? Are they likely to come true? Historically, Cornish (1997) analyzed the predictions from the February 1967 issue of *The Futurist*. Of the 34 forecasts that could be judged, 23 were accurate and 11 were not. However, some of the 11 were accurate trends that did not meet the targeted date, often because of shifting national priorities, such as funding. If this is true historically, we might assume that forecasting, which becomes better refined each year, will continue to be a valuable tool for the future. We can see in the economic downturn starting in 2008 that continued movement occurred, but most time lines for meeting expectations were altered.

CONCLUSION

Numerous changes will occur throughout our lifetimes. It is only a matter of time before we say (if we haven't already), "When I was young…" Our description might be of something that today is considered fairly advanced. For those who want to thrive, the future forecasts are like the gold ring on the merry-go-round. If you risk and reach far enough, you can grasp it! Lead on … ¡Adelánte!

THE SOLUTION

I joined the professional organization for correctional health professionals and reviewed nursing publications to identify some of the possible options that were viewed as currently successful or likely to happen in the near future. I networked with colleagues at local and state meetings and realized that a graduate degree in public health nursing would help me develop the skills to address the health needs of my population. I also decided to pursue the Clinical Nurse Specialist in Community Health Nursing certification. Clearly, society expected more in the future in both education and credentials. I believed that I had the skills to develop community programs and research studies to help me address the high-risk needs of my client population.

—Sara McCumber

Would this be a suitable approach for you? Why?

THE EVIDENCE

Evidence about the future really doesn't exist. That much is obvious. However, people who have been successful in their future lives have done several things, two of which bear mentioning here. Those two items are mindfulness and reflection. Both involve active thinking about what is evolving, what one's performance is like so far, how the person fits within an organization (or not), if the work one is doing contributes to a specific goal, and so forth. Mindfulness requires actively thinking about what you are doing, what choices you make, how you see your career unfolding, and what is missing (if anything) from what you are doing now. To get to a clear picture of where you are in your career requires the strategy of reflection. Proactively thinking about the day, the week, the month, and the year in relation to your career goals creates the op-portunity to be clear about what practices you need to reinforce and which ones would be useful to change. Some authors refer to this synergy between what you see as your desired self and what you are actually engaged in doing as "the zone". That is the focus of getting to the future you desire.

WHAT NEW GRADUATES SAY

- Many other disciplines have a very different perspective of life.
- Learning the concepts in nursing really was important because some of the facts already changed.
- Where you work in your first position can shape what you'll be prepared for in the future.

CHAPTER CHECKLIST

This chapter addresses the need to think about the future and what that means for current practice. Involvement by all nurses is needed to keep the profession relevant to the constantly emerging future.
- Leadership demands for the future
- Leadership strengths for the future
- Visioning
- The Wise Forecast Model©
- Shared vision
- Projections for the future
- Implications

TIPS FOR THE FUTURE

- Scan literature external to nursing and health care.
- Listen to divergent viewpoints about the economy, federal and state policy, and technology.
- Ask yourself "what if" questions.
- Remember what you find disheartening and use that as a filter for what you learn from numerous fields.

REFERENCES

Batcheller, J., & Yoder-Wise, P. S. (2011). Creating insight when the literature is absent: The circle of advisors. *Nursing Administration Quarterly, 35*(4), 338–343.

Cornish, E. (1997). The Futurist forecasts 30 years later. *The Futurist, 31*(January/February), 45–48.

Crenshaw, J. T., & Yoder-Wise, P. S. (2013). Creating an environment for innovation: The risk-taking leadership competency. *Nurse Leader, 11*(1), 24–27.

Selye, H. (1978). *The stress of life.* New York: McGraw-Hill.

Senge, P. (2006). *The fifth discipline: The art and practice of the learning organization.* New York: Doubleday Currency.

Yoder-Wise, P. S. (2011). Creating wise forecasts for nursing: The Wise Forecast Model©. *The Journal of Continuing Education in Nursing: Continuing Competence for the Future, 42*(9), 387.

SUGGESTED READINGS

Auerbach, D. I. (2012). Will the NP workforce grow in the future? New forecasts and implications for healthcare delivery. *Medical Care, 50*(7), 606–610.

Begun, J. W., & White, K. R. (1995). Altering nursing's dominant logic: Guidelines from complex adaptive systems theory. *Complexity and Chaos in Nursing, 2*(1), 5–15.

Dennison Himmelfarb, C. R., & Hayman, L. L. (2012). Heads up: The forecast for cardiovascular health and disease is formidable. *Journal of Cardiovascular Nursing, 27*(6), 461–463.

Institute for Alternative Futures. (2013). What will chiropractic in the U.S. look like in 2025? *Futurist.* www.altfutures.org/chiropracticfutures.

Kowalski, K., Cherry, B., & Yoder-Wise, P. S. (2012). A conversation with Peter Buerhaus: Crucial ideas for the next decade of leadership and administrative research. *Journal of Nursing Administration*, *43*(3), 127–129.

Porter-O'Grady, T., Igein, G., Alexander, D., Blaylock, J., McComb, D., & Williams, S. (2005). Critical thinking for nursing leadership. *Nurse Leader*, *3*(4), 28–31.

Saffo, P. (2009). A looming American diaspora. *Harvard Business Review*, (February), 27.

Scott, E. S., & Yoder-Wise, P. S. (2013). Increasing the intensity of nursing leadership: Graduate preparation for nurse leaders. *Journal of Nursing Administration*, *43*(1), 1–3.

Yoder-Wise, P. S. (2012a). Preparing tomorrow's service leaders: An educational challenge. *Nursing Administration Quarterly*, *36*(2), 169–178.

Yoder-Wise, P. S. (2012b). The complex challenges of administrative research for the future. *Journal of Nursing Administration*, *42*(5), 239–241.

Chapter 2

Unnumbered Figure 2-1: From Lewis, S., Heitkemper, M., Dirksen, S., O'Brien, P., & Bucher, L. (2007). *Medical-surgical nursing* (7th ed.). St. Louis: Mosby.

Unnumbered Figure 2-2: Courtesy Institute of Medicine.

Chapter 3

Figure 3-1: From Fagin, C. (2000). *Essays on nursing leadership.* New York: Springer Publishing.

Unnumbered Figure 3-2: ©2014 Photos.com, a division of Getty Images. All rights reserved.

Chapter 4

Figure 4-1: Reprinted with permission from NMLP Learning Domain Framework. (2011). American Organization of Nurse Executives. Retrieved from www.aone.org/resources/leadership%20tools/NMLPframework.shtml.

Unnumbered Figure 4-2: From Miami Children's Hospital with permission.

Unnumbered Figure 4-3: ©Getty Images, Ablestock.com.

Unnumbered Figure 4-4: From Miami Children's Hospital with permission.

Chapter 5

Unnumbered Figure 5-2: From Leake, P. (2010). *Community/public health nursing online for Stanhope and Lancaster, foundations of nursing in the community.* (3rd ed.). St. Louis: Mosby.

Chapter 6

Figure 6-1: Modified from Sullivan, E.J., & Decker, P.J. (1992). *Effective management in nursing.* Menlo Park, CA: Addison-Wesley.

Chapter 7

Unnumbered Figure 7-1: From Leake, P. (2010). *Community/public health nursing online for Stanhope and Lancaster, foundations of nursing in the community.* (3rd ed.). St. Louis: Mosby.

Unnumbered Figure 7-2: From Leake, P. (2010). *Community/public health nursing online for Stanhope and Lancaster, foundations of nursing in the community.* (3rd ed.). St. Louis: Mosby.

Chapter 12

Figure 12-1: Modified from Ward, W. (1988). *An introduction to health care financial management.* Owings Mills, MD: National Health Publishing.

Chapter 14

Figure 14-1: From Kane, R.L., Shamliyan, T.C., Duval, S., & Wilt, T. (March 2007). *Nursing staffing and quality of patient care: Evidence Report/Technology Assessment No. 151.* (Prepared by the Minnesota Evidence-based Practice Center under Contract N. 290-02-0009.) AHRQ Publication N. 07-E00005. Rockville, MD: Agency for Healthcare Research and Quality.

Chapter 18

Figure 18-1: Adapted from Satir, V. (1988). *The new peoplemaking.* Mountain View, CA: Science & Behavior Books; and Olen, D. (1993). *Communicating: Speaking and listening to end misunderstanding and promote friendship.* Germantown, WI: JODA Communications.

Figure 18-2: Adapted from St. Charles Medical Center. (1993). *People centered teams.* Bend, OR: Author.

Chapter 21

Figure 21-1: From Stetler, C.B. (2001). Updating the Stetler model of research utilization to facilitate evidence-based practice. *Nursing Outlook, 49*(6), 272-279, Figure 3A, p. 276.

Figure 21-2: DiCenso, A., Bayley, L., & Haynes, R. B: Accessing pre-appraised evidence: fine-tuning the 5S model into a 6S model, Evid Based Nurs 2009 Oct;12(4):99-101.

Figure 21-3: CLAHRC for Greater Manchester in collaboration with NHS Manchester. http://clahrc-gm.nihr.ac.uk/heartfailure/about/

Unnumbered Figure 21-2: From Lowdermilk, D., & Perry, S. (2007). *Maternity and women's health care.* (9th ed.). St. Louis: Mosby. Courtesy Cheryl Briggs, RN, Annapolis, MD.

Chapter 22

Figure 22-1: From Leake, P. (2010). *Community/public health nursing online for Stanhope and Lancaster, foundations of nursing in the community* (3rd ed.). St. Louis: Mosby.

Unnumbered Figure 22-2: From Leake, P. (2010). *Community/public health nursing online for Stanhope and Lancaster, foundations of nursing in the community.* (3rd ed.). St. Louis: Mosby.

Chapter 23

Figure 23-2: Almost, J. (2006). Conflict within nursing work environments: Concept analysis. *Journal of Advanced Nursing, 53*(4), 444-453, Blackwell Publishing.

Chapter 25

Figure 25-1: From The American Nurse Association's Nationwide State Legislative Agenda for workplace violence, April 2012. From http://nursingworld.com.

Figure 25-2: From American Nurses Association (2010). Hostility, abuse and bullying in the workplace. 2010 House of Delegates Resolution. Bullying and Lateral Violence: Examples of Bullying Behavior Pocket Card. (From http://nursingworld.org/MainMenuCategories/CertificationandAccreditation/Continuing-Professional-Development/NavigateNursing/AboutNN/Tip-Card-Bullying-and-Lateral-Violence-ANA.pdf.)

Chapter 26

Figure 26-2: © 2006 Reprinted with permission of the Center for Leadership Studies. Escondido, CA 92025 www.situational.com All Rights Reserved.

Chapter 28

Figure 28-1: Adapted from Selye, H. (1991). History and present status of the stress concept. In A. Monat & R. Lazarus (Eds.), *Stress and coping: An anthology* (pp. 21-36). New York: Columbia University Press.

Figure 28-2: Adapted from Covey, S.R., Merrill, A.R., & Merrill, R.R. (1994). *First things first: To love, to learn, to leave a legacy.* New York: Simon & Schuster.

Chapter 29

Unnumbered Figure 29-1: ©José Luis Gutiérrez, iStock Photo.

Chapter 30

Unnumbered Figure 30-1: ©Geoffrey Holman, Zargon Studios Corp.

Unnumbered Figure 30-2: NASA and The Hubble Heritage Team (STScI/AURA), Hubble Space Telescope ACS, STScl-PRC04-10.

A

Absenteeism The rate at which an individual misses work on an unplanned basis. (Ch. 24)

Accommodating An unassertive, cooperative approach to conflict in which the individual neglects personal needs, goals, and concerns in favor of satisfying those of others. (Ch. 23)

Accountability The expectation of explaining actions and results. (Ch. 26)

Accountability measures Quality measures that meet four criteria to produce the greatest positive outcomes for patients. The criteria are (1) scientific evidence about a process, (2) proximity of the process to the desired, intended outcome, (3) accuracy that the process was implemented, and (4) minimal or no adverse effects. (Ch. 20)

Accountable care organization Groups of providers and healthcare organizations that agree to work together to provide coordinated high quality care to patients who receive Medicare. (Chs. 7, 8)

Accreditation Process by which an authoritative body determines that an organization meets certain standards to such a degree that the organization is able to meet the standards as a whole and without ongoing monitoring of each aspect of performance. (Ch. 7)

Acculturation Process by which a person becomes a competent participant in the dominant culture. (Ch. 9)

Acknowledgment Recognition that an employee is valued and respected for what he or she has to offer to the workplace, team, or group; acknowledgments may be verbal or written, public or private. (Ch. 18)

Active delegation Proactively making a decision about tasks and people to accomplish effective work. (Ch. 26)

Active listening Focusing completely on the speaker and listening without judgment to the essence of the conversation; an active listener should be able to repeat accurately at least 95% of the speaker's intended meaning. (Ch. 18)

Advanced generalist Clinical nurse leader, which is a protected title for those who successfully complete the CNL certification examination. (Ch. 13)

Advanced practice registered nurses (APRNs) A group of nurses, prepared at the graduate level, with defined roles and scopes who function in expanded nursing roles. Those roles are: certified registered nurse anesthetists, certified nurse-midwives, clinical nurse specialists, and certified nurse practitioners. (Ch. 1)

Advocate One who proactively speaks for another to ensure certain needs or wishes are met. (Ch. 22)

Agency for Healthcare Research and Quality (AHRQ) The primary federal agency devoted to improving quality, safety, efficiency, and effectiveness of health care. (Ch. 2)

Agenda A written list of items to be covered in a meeting and the related materials that meeting participants should read beforehand or bring along. Types of agendas include structured agendas, timed agendas, and action agendas. (Ch. 28)

American Board of Quality Assurance and Utilization Review Physicians A multidisciplinary professional organization that focuses on those providers in roles related to quality assurance and utilization review. (Ch. 2)

Apparent agency Doctrine whereby a principal becomes accountable for the actions of his or her agent; created when a person holds himself or herself out as acting on behalf of the principal; also known as apparent authority. (Ch. 5)

Associate nurse A licensed nurse in the primary care model who provides care to the patient according to the primary nurse's specification when the primary nurse is not working. (Ch. 13)

At-will employee An individual who works without a contract. (Ch. 19)

Authority The power to make decisions which often derives from policies, laws, and job descriptions. (Ch. 26)

Autocratic An authoritarian style that places control within one person's position. (Ch. 6)

Autonomy Personal freedom and the right to choose what will happen to one's own person. (Ch. 5)

Average daily census (ADC) Average number of patients cared for per day for a reporting period. (Ch. 14)

Average length of stay (ALOS) The number of patient days in a specific time period divided by the number of discharges in that same period. (Ch. 14)

Avoiding An unassertive, uncooperative approach to conflict in which the avoider neither pursues his or her own needs, goals, and concerns nor helps others to do so. (Ch. 23)

B

Bar code technology Systems that encode data electronically into a format of bars and spaces that represents letters or numbers. (Ch. 11)

Barriers Factors, internal or external to the change situation, that interfere with movement toward a desirable outcome. (Ch. 17)

Benchmarking Best practices, processes, or systems identified by a quality improvement team to be compared with the practice, process, or system under review. (Ch. 20)

Beneficence Principle that states that the actions one takes should promote good. (Ch. 5)

Biomedical technology The technological devices and systems that relate to biological and medical sciences. (Ch. 11)

Budget A detailed financial plan, stated in dollars, for carrying out the activities an organization wants to accomplish within a specific period. (Ch. 12)

Budgeting process An ongoing activity of planning and managing revenues and expenses to meet the goals of the organization. (Ch. 12)

Bullying A practice closely related to lateral or horizontal violence, but a real or perceived power differential between the instigator and recipient must be present in bullying. (Chs. 23, 25)

Bureaucracy Characterized by formality, low autonomy, a hierarchy of authority, an environment of rules, division of labor, specialization, centralization, and control. (Ch. 8)

Burnout Disengagement from work characterized by emotional exhaustion, depersonalization, and decreased effectiveness. (Ch. 28)

C

Capital expenditure budget A plan for purchasing major capital items, such as equipment or a physical plant, with a useful life greater than 1 year and exceeding a minimum cost set by the organization. (Ch. 12)

Capitation A reimbursement method in which healthcare providers are paid a per-person-per-year (or per-month) fee for providing specified services over a period of time. (Ch. 12)

Care coordination Organizing patient care activities and sharing information among all of the participants to achieve safe, effective care for patients. (Ch. 22)

Career Progressive achievement through-out a person's professional life. (Ch. 29)

Case management A person-oriented service that reflects multidisciplinary cooperation and coordination. (Ch. 4)

Case-management model A model of delivering patient care based on patient outcomes and cost containment. Components of case management are a case manager, critical paths/critical pathways, and unit-based managed care. (Ch. 13)

Case manager A clinical nurse with a baccalaureate or master's degree who coordinates patient care from preadmission through discharge. (Ch. 13)

Case method A model of care delivery in which one nurse provides total care for a patient during an entire work period. (Ch. 13)

Case mix The volume and type of patients served by a healthcare provider. (Ch. 12)

Cash budget A plan for an organization's cash receipts and disbursements. (Ch. 12)

Certification Designation of special knowledge beyond basic licensure. (Ch. 29)

Chain of command The hierarchy depicted in vertical dimensions of organizational charts. (Ch. 8)

Change agents Individuals with formal or informal legitimate power whose purpose is to initiate, champion, and direct or guide change. (Chs. 4, 17)

Change leaders Those who create the vision and foster major organizational transformation. (Ch.17)

Change management The overall processes and strategies used to moderate and manage the preparation for, effect of, responses to, and outcomes of any condition or circumstance that is new or different from what existed previously. (Ch. 17)

Change process The series of ongoing efforts applied to managing a change. (Ch. 17)

Chaos A condition of disorder or confusion. (Ch. 30)

Chaos theory Theoretical construct defining the random-appearing yet deterministic characteristics of complex organizations (see *Nonlinear change*). (Ch. 17)

Charge nurse A registered nurse responsible for delegating and coordinating patient care and staff on a specific unit. A resource person for all staff; there is usually one charge nurse each shift per unit. (Ch. 13)

Charges The cost of providing a service plus a markup for profit. (Ch. 12)

Chemically dependent A psychophysiological state in which an individual requires a substance, such as drugs or alcohol, to prevent the onset of symptoms of abstinence. (Ch. 24)

Clinical decision support (CDS)/ clinical decision support systems Defined broadly, CDS is a clinical computer system, computer application, or process that helps health professionals make clinical decisions to enhance patient care. (Ch. 11)

Clinical guidelines Statements of practice expectations developed by a group of healthcare practitioners to guide the clinical management of patients. (Ch. 21)

Clinical nurse leader An evolving role of the professional nurse being developed by the American Association of Colleges of Nursing (AACN). (Ch. 13)

Clinical process A defined sequence of steps needed to ensure that basic functions are fulfilled in a standardized manner, ensuring safety and quality, such as medication procurement and administration (Ch. 1)

Coaching The strategy a manager uses to help others learn, think critically, and grow through communications about performance. (Ch. 15)

Coalitions Groups of individuals or organizations that join together temporarily around a common goal. This goal often focuses on an effort to effect change. (Ch. 10)

Collaborating Involves a group of people working together to achieve a common goal. (Ch. 23)

Collective action A mechanism for achieving professional practice through group decision making. (Ch. 19)

Collective bargaining Mechanism for settling labor disputes by negotiation between the employer and representatives of the employees. (Chs. 5, 19)

Commitment A state of being emotionally impelled; feeling passionate about and dedicated to a project or event. (Ch. 18)

Communication technology An extension of wireless (WL) technology that enables hands-free communication among mobile hospital workers. (Ch. 11)

Comparative effectiveness research A form of research that is designed to provide evidence on the effectiveness, benefits, and harms of different treatment options so that best decisions can be made. (Ch. 21)

Competing Assertive, uncooperative approach to conflict in which the individual pursues own needs at the expense of others. (Ch. 23)

Complexity compression The intensity of increasing functions and expectations without a change in resources, including time. (Ch. 30)

Complexity theory Requires leaders to expand and respond to engaging dynamic change and focus on relationships rather than on prescribing and approaching change as a lock-step, pre-prescribed method. Traditional organizational hierarchy plays a less significant role as the "keeper of high level knowledge" and replaces it with the idea that knowledge applied to complex problems is better distributed among the human assets within an organization, without regard to hierarchy. Leaders try less to control the future and spend more time influencing, innovating, and responding to the many factors that influence health care. (Chs. 1, 17)

Compromising Moderately assertive, cooperative approach to conflict in which the individual's ability to negotiate and willingness to give and take result in conflict resolution and fulfillment of priorities for all involved. (Ch. 23)

Computerized provider order entry (CPOE) System that uses computers for creating orders for care to be made electronically and to coordinate with other elements of an individual's care and record so that one entry performs multiple functions. (Ch. 11)

Confidentiality Right of privacy to the medical record of a patient; also, a respect for the privacy of information and the ethical use of information for its original purpose. (Ch. 5)

Conflict A disagreement in values or beliefs within oneself or between people that has the potential to cause harm if unresolved or stimulates change for a more favorable outcome if effectively addressed. (Ch. 23)

Consolidated systems A group of healthcare organizations that are united based on common characteristics of ownership, regional location, or mutual performance objectives for the purpose of optimizing utilization of their resources in achieving their missions. (Ch. 7)

Consumer focus Centering of action or attention on the participant or user as a whole. (Ch. 22)

Continuing education Learning that builds on prior knowledge and experience with the goal of being a more competent professional. (Ch. 29)

Continuous quality improvement (CQI) A comprehensive program designed to continually improve the quality of care. Often used interchangeably with *total quality management, quality management, quality improvement,* and *performance improvement.* (Ch. 20)

Contractual allowance A discount from full charges. (Ch. 12)

Coping The immediate response of a person to a threatening situation. (Ch. 28)

Corporate liability The condition of being responsible for corporate loss related to acts performed and not performed in meeting obligations to operate legally and judiciously. (Ch. 5)

Cost The amount spent on something. The national healthcare costs are a function of the price and utilization of healthcare services; a healthcare provider's costs are the expenses involved in providing goods or services. (Ch. 12)

Cost-based reimbursement A retrospective payment method in which all allowable costs are used as the basis for payment. (Ch. 12)

Cost-based system A cost-based system consists of the cost of providing a service plus a markup for profit. (Ch. 12)

Cost center An organizational unit for which costs can be identified and managed. (Chs. 12, 14)

Creativity Conceptualizing new and innovative approaches to solving problems or making decisions. (Ch. 6)

Critical path/critical pathway A component of a care MAP that is specific to diagnosis-related group reimbursement. The purpose is to ensure patients are discharged before insurance reimbursement is eliminated. (Ch. 13)

Critical thinking A composite of knowledge, attitudes, and skills; an intellectually disciplined process. Also, the ability to assess a situation by asking open-ended questions about the facts and assumptions that underlie it and to use personal judgment and problem-solving ability in deciding how to deal with it. (Ch. 6)

Cross-culturalism Mediating between and among cultures. (Ch. 9)

Cultural competence The process of integrating values, beliefs, and attitudes different from one's own perspective in order to render effective nursing care. (Chs. 9, 22)

Cultural diversity The differences that exist between multiple viewpoints based on ethnicity, gender, religion, socioeconomic status, and other variables. (Ch. 9)

Cultural imposition The condition that exists when one individual or organization attempts to require another individual or group to accept the values, attitudes, and beliefs of the first. (Ch. 9)

Cultural marginality A condition of bordering on one or more cultures and perceiving no membership or affiliation with either. (Ch. 9)

Cultural sensitivity Capacity to feel, convey, and react to ideas, habits, customs, or traditions unique to a group of people. (Ch. 9)

Culture A way of life conveyed strongly enough for a group of people to describe its meaning. It consists of values, beliefs, attitudes, practices, rituals, and traditions. (Chs. 9, 19)

Curriculum vitae A listing of professional life activities. (Ch. 29)

D

Data Discrete entities that describe or measure something without interpretation. (Ch. 11)

Database A collection of data elements organized and stored together. (Ch. 11)

Decision making Purposeful and goal-directed effort using a systematic process to choose among options. (Ch. 6)

Deeming authority A power granted by one with power so that the recipient acts in his or her place. (Ch. 7)

Delegatee The individual who becomes accountable for performing delegated activities. (Ch. 26)

Delegation Achieving performance of care outcomes for which an individual is accountable and responsible by sharing activities with other individuals who have the appropriate authority to accomplish the work. (Chs. 26, 28)

Delegator The individual with authority to share activities with another. (Ch. 26)

Depersonalization Inability to become involved in human relationships and interactions. (Ch. 28)

Det Norske Veritas (DNV) Diagnostic related group (DRG) (Ch. 2)

Diagnosis-related group (DRG) The basis for prospective payment to hospitals that Medicare has used. (Ch. 12)

Differentiated nursing practice A model of care that recognizes the difference in the level of education and competency of each registered nurse. The differentiation is based on education, position, and clinical expertise. (Ch. 13)

Diffusion of innovation Process by which ideas spread through a culture. (Ch. 21)

Direct care hours   The amount of time spent in providing care to patients. (Ch. 14)

DNV (Det Norske Veritas)   A new deeming organization as of 2008 to accredit healthcare organizations. (Ch. 2)

Dualism   An "either/or" way of conceptualizing reality in terms of two opposing sides or parts (right or wrong, yes or no), limiting the broad spectrum of possibilities that exists between. (Ch. 18)

E

Effective communication   A process that leads to positive outcomes for senders and receivers in terms of clarity, usefulness, and efficiency. (Ch. 18)

Electronic health record (EHR)/ electronic medical record (EMR)   Computer-based patient record that capitalizes on the features of electronic processes. (Ch. 11)

Emancipated minor   Person younger than adulthood who is no longer under the control and regulation of parents and who may give valid consent for medical procedures; examples include married teens, underage parents, and teens in the armed services. (Ch. 5)

Emerging workforce   The so-called 20-something generation, who were born between the years of 1965 and 1985. (Ch. 3)

Emotional intelligence   Monitoring emotions in a situation to guide actions and inform thought processes. (Ch. 1)

Employee assistance program   Program designed to provide counseling and other services for employees through either in-house staff or a contracted mental health agency. (Ch. 28)

Empowerment   A sharing of power and control with the expectation that people are responsible for themselves; also, the process by which we facilitate the participation of others in decision making within an environment in which power is equally distributed. (Chs. 10, 15, 19)

Engagement   A workplace approach designed to ensure employees are committed to their organization's goals and values. Intended to motivate and contribute to organizational success and at the same time, enhance an individual's sense of professional satisfaction and personal well-being. (Ch. 19)

Entrenched workforce   Employed persons older than 35 years who are thought of as the *Baby Boomer generation*. (Ch. 3)

Ethics   Science relating to moral actions and moral values; rules of conduct recognized in respect to a particular class of human actions. (Ch. 5)

Ethics committee   Group of persons who provide structure and guidelines for potential healthcare problems, serve as an open forum for discussion, and function as patient advocates. (Ch. 5)

Ethnicity   An affiliation with a group often based on race or language. (Ch. 9)

Ethnocentrism   Viewing the world based on one's own reference group. (Ch. 9)

Evidence-based practice (EBP)   The integration of individual clinical expertise, built from practice, with the best available clinical evidence from systematic research applied to practice. (Ch. 21)

Evidence-based organizational practice   Scientifically derived approaches to delivering care that optimizes professional roles, practices, and coordination of activities. (Ch. 1)

Expected outcomes   The result of patient goals that are achieved through a combination of medical and nursing interventions with patient participation. (Ch. 13)

F

Facilitators   Factors, internal or external to the change situation, that promote movement toward a desired outcome. (Ch. 17)

Factor evaluation system   A patient classification system that incorporates specific elements or critical indicators and rates patients on each of these elements. Each indicator is assigned a weight or numerical value. (Ch. 14)

Failure mode and effects analysis (FMEA)   A method to analyze reliability problems proactively to avoid negative outcomes. (Ch. 20)

Failure to warn   Newer area of potential liability for nurse managers that involves the responsibility to warn subsequent or potential employers of nurses' incompetence or impairment. (Ch. 5)

Fatigue   A physical or emotional exhaustion. (Ch. 28)

Fee-for-service   A system in which patients have the option of consulting any healthcare provider, subject to reasonable requirements that may include utilization review and prior approval for certain services but does not include a requirement to seek approval through a gatekeeper. (Ch. 7)

Fidelity   Keeping one's promises or commitments. (Ch. 5)

First-order change   Evolutionary change that occurs in planned and small steps. (Ch. 17)

Fixed costs   Costs that do not change in total as the volume of patients changes. (Ch. 12)

Fixed full-time equivalents (FTEs)   Full-time equivalent roles that do not fluctuate based on patient care demands. (Ch. 14)

Flat organizational structure   Characterized by decentralization of decision making to the level of personnel carrying out the work. (Ch. 8)

Follower   Person who contributes to a group's outcomes by implementing activities and providing appropriate feedback. (Ch. 4)

Followership   Those with whom a leader interacts; involves assertive use of personal behaviors in contributing toward organizational outcomes while still acquiescing certain tasks to the leader or other team members. (Chs. 1, 19)

Forecast   The process of making decisions about the future based on multiple sources of data. (Ch. 14)

Foreseeability   Concept that certain events may reasonably be expected to cause specific consequences; third element of negligence/malpractice. (Ch. 5)

For-profit organization   An organization, such as a hospital, that is operated to create excess income (profit) for the benefit of owners or stockholders. (Ch. 7)

Full-time equivalent (FTE)   An employee who works full-time, 40 hours per week, 2080 hours per year. (Chs. 12, 14)

Functional model of nursing   A method of providing patient care by which each licensed and unlicensed staff member performs specific tasks for a large group of patients. (Ch. 13)

Functional structure   Arrangement of departments and services by specialties. (Ch. 8)

G

Gatekeeper   Liaison between the consumer and the healthcare market. (Ch. 22)

General adaptation syndrome (GAS)   A set of characteristics first described by Hans Seyle that are identifiable when people experience stress. (Ch. 28)

Governance   System by which an organization controls and directs formulation and administration of policy. (Ch. 19)

Group   A number of individuals assembled together or having a unifying relationship. (Ch. 18)

H

Health Care and Education Reconciliation Act   Federal legislation that amended the Patient Protection and Affordable Care Act to clarify budget resolutions. (Ch. 5)

Health literacy   An individual's capacity to obtain, process, and understand health information needed to make appropriate health decisions. (Chs. 5, 22)

Healthcare consumer   Patient/customer who uses healthcare provider resources. (Ch. 22)

Healthcare providers   Agencies, insurers, physicians, nurses, and allied health people providing health-related business to consumers. (Ch. 22)

Hierarchy   Chain of command that connotes authority and responsibility. (Ch. 8)

High-complexity change   A complicated change situation characterized by the interactions of multiple variables of people, technology, and systems. (Ch. 17)

High tech   Mechanistic perspective that relates to the use of technology in the diagnosis and treatment of disease. (Ch. 22)

High touch   Caring, humanistic perspective that relates to the use of human skills in the care and treatment of patients. (Ch. 22)

Horizontal integration   The condition that results when two (or more) organizations with similar services come together. (Ch. 7)

Horizontal violence   Involves conflictual behaviors among individuals who consider themselves peers with equal power but with little power within the system (Ch. 23). Describes aggressive and destructive behavior of co-workers against each other (Ch. 25).

Hybrid   Possessing characteristics from several types of organizational structures. (Ch. 8)

I

Incivility   The condition of acting in a rude or disruptive manner. (Ch. 25)

Indemnification   Obligation resting on one person to make good any loss or damages another has incurred because of the person's actions or inactions; refers to the total shifting of the economic loss to the party chiefly responsible for that loss. (Ch. 5)

Independent contractor   One who makes an agreement with another to perform a service or piece of work and retains in himself or herself control of the means, method, and manner of producing the result to be accomplished; sometimes called an *independent practitioner*. (Ch. 5)

Indirect care hours   The amount of time spent in activities that support the care of patients but do not involve direct provision of care. (Ch. 14)

Individual accountability   The individuals' ability to explain their actions and results. (Ch. 26)

Influence   The process of using power; may range from the punitive power of coercion to the interactive power of collaboration. (Ch. 10)

Informatics   The use of knowledge technology. (Ch. 11)

Information   Communication of reception of knowledge, consisting of interpreted, organized, or structured data. (Ch. 11)

Information overload   A state of stress brought about by a lack of information-processing skills. (Ch. 28)

Information technology   The use of computer hardware and software to process data into information to solve problems. (Ch. 11)

Informed consent   Authorization by patient or patient's legal representative to do something to the patient. (Ch. 5)

Institute for Healthcare Improvement (IHI)   An independent organization devoted to improving patient safety and health care globally. (Chs. 2, 19)

Institute of Medicine (IOM)   An organization that works outside of the federal government to provide independent, scientific advice. (Ch. 2)

Interest-based problem solving   A method used in collective bargaining that uses structured problem solving techniques to identify mutual interests to achieve mutual goals. Process serves to optimize the potential of mutual or joint gains. Process also known as integrative, win-win, collaborative, or mutual gains problem solving. (Ch. 19)

Interpersonal conflict   Conflict that occurs between or among people. (Chs. 23, 25)

Intrapersonal conflict   Conflict that occurs within an individual. (Ch. 23)

J

Justice   Principle that persons should be treated equally and fairly. (Ch. 5)

K

Knowledge technology   The use of expert and decision support systems to assist in making decisions about patient care delivery. (Ch. 11)

Knowledge worker   An individual who performs nonrepetitive, nonroutine work consuming considerable levels of cognitive activity and judgment. (Ch. 11)

L

Labor cost per unit of service   A comparison of budgeted salary costs per budgeted volume of service with actual salary costs per actual volume of service. (Ch. 14)

Lateral aggression   Aggressive and destructive behavior of co-workers against each other. (Ch. 25)

Lateral violence   Aggressive and destructive behavior or psychological harassment of nurses against each other. (Ch. 23)

Law   Sum total of rules and regulations by which a society is governed; rules and regulations established and enforced by authority or custom within a given community, state, or nation. (Ch. 5)

Leader   Person who demonstrates and exercises influence and power over others. (Ch. 4)

Leadership   The use of personal traits to constructively and ethically influence patients, families, and staff through a process in which clinical and organizational outcomes are achieved through collective efforts. (Chs. 1, 3)

Learning organization   The designation of a type of organization in which continual learning as an expectation permeates all levels to promote adequate responses required by dynamic, accelerated change. (Ch. 17)

Liability   Refers to one's responsibility for his or her own conduct; an obligation or duty to be performed; responsibility for an action or outcome. (Ch. 5)

Liable   Refers to one's responsibility for his or her actions or inactions. (Ch. 5)

Licensed practical nurse (LPN)   Licensed vocational nurse (LVN) (Ch. 26)

Licensure   A right granted that gives the licensee permission to do something that he or she could not legally do absent such permission; the minimum form of credentialing, providing baseline expectations for those in a particular field without identifying or obligating the practitioner to function in a professional manner as defined by the profession itself. (Chs. 5, 29)

Line function   A function that involves direct responsibility for accomplishing the objectives of a nursing department, service, or unit. (Ch. 8)

Low-complexity change   An uncomplicated change situation characterized by the interactions of the limited influences of people, technology, and systems. (Ch. 17)

M

Magnet Recognition Program®   The only national designation built on and evolving through nursing research that is designed to recognize nursing excellence of healthcare organizations through a self-nominating, appraisal process. (Chs.1, 2, 13).

Malpractice   Failure of a professional person to act in accordance with the prevalent professional standards or failure to foresee potential consequences that a professional person, having the necessary skills and expertise to act in a professional manner, should foresee. (Ch. 5)

Managed care   Care purchased through a public or private healthcare organization whose goal is to promote quality healthcare outcomes for patients at the lowest cost possible through planning, directing, and coordinating care delivered by healthcare organizations that it may own, have contractual agreements with, or have authority over by virtue of the fact that it reimburses the organization for services provided its patients. This model rewards providers for low utilization of care that is relatively low in cost; also, a system of care in which a designated person determines the services the patient uses. (Chs. 4, 7, 12)

Management   The activities needed to plan, organize, motivate, and control the human and material resources needed to achieve outcomes consistent with the organization's mission and purpose. (Chs. 1, 3)

Management theory   The theory related to the activities described in *Management*. (Ch. 1)

Manager   The person with accountability for a group of people. (Ch. 4)

Mandatory overtime   The expectation that staff will work beyond the hours assigned, often accompanied by a real or perceived threat. (Ch. 14)

Marketing   Analysis, planning, implementation, and control of programs for meeting organizational objectives. (Ch. 16)

Matrix structure   An organizational structure influenced by dual authority, such as product line and discipline. (Ch. 8)

Meaningful use (MU)   The set of standards defined by the Centers for Medicare & Medicaid Services (CMS) Incentive Programs that governs the use of EHRs and allows eligible providers and hospitals to earn incentive payments by meeting specific criteria. (Ch. 11)

Mediation   A process using a trained third party to assist with conflict resolution. (Ch. 23)

Medical home   Patient-centered, multifaceted source of personal primary health care. (Ch. 22)

Mentor   An experienced person who helps a less experienced person navigate into expertise. (Chs. 3, 19, 27)

Meta-analysis   Statistically combines similar studies on a particular issue to determine if the findings are significant across settings. (Ch. 21)

Mission   The reason for the organization's existence. The purpose it was designed to address. (Ch. 8)

Mission statement   An organization's reason for being. (Ch. 8)

Moral distress   A type of distress that occurs when faced with situations in which two ethical principles compete, such as when the nurse is balancing the patient's autonomy issues with attempting to do what the nurse knows is in the patient's best interest. Moral distress may occur also when the nurse manager is balancing a staff nurse's autonomy with what the nurse manager perceives to be a better solution to an ethical dilemma. (Ch. 5)

Motivation   The instigation of action based on various factors, both intrinsic and extrinsic. (Ch. 1)

Multiculturalism   Maintaining several different cultures. (Ch. 9)

N

National Integrated Accreditation for Healthcare Organization (NIAHO)   Formerly Det Norske Veritas. An internationally based organization that accredits many fields, including health care. (Ch. 2)

National Quality Forum (NQF)   A membership-based organization that sets priorities and goals for performance improvement and endorses standards for measurement. (Ch. 2)

Near miss   A clinical situation that resulted in no injury but that highlights the need for action (e.g., attempted suicide, last minute cancellation of surgery on wrong patient). (Ch. 20)

Negligence   Failure to exercise the degree of care that a person of ordinary prudence, based on the reasonable person standard, would exercise under the same or similar circumstances; also known as *ordinary negligence*. (Ch. 5)

Negotiating Conferring with others to bring about a settlement of differences. (Chs. 10, 23)

Networks Resources of colleagues upon whom you can draw for advice; formal systems to provide services. (Ch. 7)

Never event Error in medical care that is clearly identifiable, preventable, and serious in its consequences for the patient and that indicates a real problem in the safety and credibility of a health care facility. These errors should never occur. Examples of never events include surgery on the wrong body part, foreign body left in a patient after surgery, mismatched blood transfusion, major medication error, severe pressure ulcer acquired in the hospital, and preventable postoperative death. (Ch. 20)

Nonmaleficence Principle that states that one should do no harm. (Ch. 5)

Nonproductive hours See *Nonproductive time.* (Ch. 12)

Nonproductive time Benefit time such as vacation or sick time. (Ch. 14)

Nonpunitive discipline A disciplinary measure, usually verbal, describing existing standards and goals to which the parties agreed; pay is not withheld; employee agrees either to adhere to the standards in the future or to be terminated. (Ch. 24)

Nurse navigator A nurse who helps patients, often in a specific patient population, work through the healthcare system to secure quality, efficient care. (Ch. 13)

Nurse outcomes Typically, a system of classification to evaluate nursing care. (Ch. 14)

Nurse practice act Legal scope of practice allowed by state legislation and authority. (Ch. 5)

Nurse-sensitive data The actual data elements collected that relate to nursing-sensitive outcomes. (Ch. 14)

Nursing care delivery model The method used to provide care to patients. (Ch. 13)

Nursing case management The process of a nurse coordinating health care by planning, facilitating, and evaluating interventions across levels of care to achieve measurable cost and quality outcomes. (Ch. 13)

Nursing productivity The ratio of required staff hours to actual provided staff hours. (Ch. 14)

Nursing-sensitive outcome Patient outcomes that relate to the quality of nursing care provided. (Ch. 20)

O

Operating budget A financial plan for day-to-day activities of an organization. (Ch. 12)

Optimizing A specific decision process that is designed to produce the best (optimal) results. (Ch. 6)

Optimizing decision Selecting the ideal solution or option to achieve goals. (Ch. 6)

Organization A business structure designed to support specific business goals and processes; or a group of individuals working together to achieve a common purpose. (Ch. 8)

Organizational accountability The accountability for the system of operations; the prime accountability of organizations is patient safety. Organizations are accountable for adequate resources to deliver safe care. (Ch. 26)

Organizational chart A chart that defines organizational positions' responsibility for specific functions. (Ch. 8)

Organizational conflict Conflict that occurs when a person confronts an organization's policies and procedures for patient care and personnel and its accepted norms of behavior and communication. (Ch. 23)

Organizational culture The attitudes, behaviors, and policies evident in an organization that create the ambiance and operation of the workplace. (Chs. 4, 8)

Organizational structure A framework that divides work within an organization and delineates points of authority, responsibility, accountability, and non–decision-making support. (Ch. 8)

Organizational theory The systematic analysis of how organizations and their component parts act and interact. (Ch. 8)

Organized delivery system (ODS) Network of healthcare organizations, providers, and payers who provide a comprehensive package of healthcare services at a competitive price. (Ch. 12)

Outcome criteria The result of patient goals that are expected to be achieved through a combination of nursing and medical interventions. (Ch. 13)

Outcomes Anticipated or actual effects of program activities and outputs. (Ch. 21)

Overtime Time in excess of the standard amount per day; often based on an 8-, 10-, or 12-hour shift. (Ch. 14)

Overwork A situation in which employees are expected to become more productive without additional resources. (Ch. 28)

P

Participatory action research A study approach where members of the study population engage in the research design and implementation process. (Ch. 21)

Partnership model A method of providing patient care when an RN is paired with an LPN/LVN or an unlicensed assistive person to provide total care to a number of patients. (Ch. 13)

Passive delegation Delegation that does not require a decision-making process. The decisions derive from job descriptions or policies and thus the tasks are not actively delegated, they are assumed by virtue of the policy or job description. (Ch. 26)

Paternalism Principle that allows one to make decisions for another; often called *parentalism.* (Ch. 5)

Patient activation Patients' willingness and ability to take independent actions to manage their health and care and includes understanding one's role in the process and having the confidence to do so. (Ch. 22)

Patient care associate A title given to individuals who are employed as unlicensed nursing personnel. Formerly nurse aide. (Ch. 26)

Patient-care outcome A measurable end result of patient care. (Ch. 20)

Patient-centered outcomes research Research focused on best evidence in care. (Ch. 21)

Patient-focused care A model in which staff functions become centralized on a unit to reduce the number of staff required; emphasizes quality, cost, and value. (Ch. 13)

Patient outcomes See *Expected outcomes.* (Chs. 13, 14)

Patient Protection and Affordable Care Act (PPACA) Legislation aimed at increasing access to uninsured Americans to quality, affordable care while reducing costs of unnecessary services. The PPACA was upheld as constitutional by the Supreme Court in 2012. (Chs. 1, 5)

Patient satisfaction   Measurement, frequently by an external service, of patient perception about care and services; frequently presented in reports or ratings and often compared with a prior time period and comparable service. (Ch. 22)

Payer mix   The volume and type of reimbursement sources for a healthcare provider. (Ch. 12)

Payers   Sources of healthcare financing or payment for health services; includes government, private insurance, and individuals (self-pay). (Ch. 12)

Percentage of occupancy   The patient census divided by the number of beds on the unit. (Ch. 14)

Perfectionism   The tendency to never finish anything because it is not quite perfect. (Ch. 28)

Performance appraisal   Individual evaluation of work performance. (Ch. 15)

Performance improvement (PI)   The application of quality improvement principles on an ongoing basis. Often used interchangeably with *total quality management, continuous quality management, quality improvement,* and *quality management.* (Ch. 20)

Personal liability   Serves to make each person responsible by law for his or her own actions. (Ch. 5)

Philosophy   Values and beliefs regarding nature of work derived from a mission and the rights/responsibilities of people involved. (Ch. 8)

Planned change   Change expected and deliberately prepared beforehand by using systematic directional processes to develop and carry out activities to accomplish a desired outcome. (Ch. 17)

Policy   A specifically designated statement to guide decisions and actions. (Ch. 10)

Politics   A process of human interaction within organizations. (Ch. 10)

Portfolio   A professional assemblage of materials that represent the work of the professional. These materials include such elements as evaluations, letters of recommendation or appreciation, certificates of accomplishment, copies of articles, documentation of projects (e.g., research, clinical changes, management projects), and additional educational achievements (continuing education and degree achievement). (Ch. 29)

Position description   A general overall description of the duties and responsibilities of the employee. (Ch. 15)

Power   The ability to influence others in the effort to achieve goals. (Ch. 10)

Practice partnership model   A form of primary nursing where an RN is paired with a technical assistant. (Ch. 13)

Practice-based evidence   A research methodology that helps inform practice decisions by examining outcomes in the real world where patients may not be similar and the actual application of an intervention may have multiple variations. (Ch. 21)

Practice-based research network (PBRN)   Originally formed to address research issues in primary care, PBRNs are increasingly being used in large healthcare organizations having the capability of integrating systems across multiple practice sites. Practice-based research networks in nursing exist for primary care, community nursing centers, and school nursing. (Ch. 21)

Preferred provider organizations (PPOs)   Contracts are developed between hospitals and physicians with discounted rates and prompt payment. (Ch. 7)

Price   See *Charges.* (Ch. 12)

Primary care   First access to care. (Ch. 7)

Primary nurse   One who delivers autonomous care. (Ch. 13)

Primary nursing   A model of patient care delivery whereby one registered nurse functions autonomously as the patient's main nurse throughout the entire hospital stay. (Ch. 13)

Privacy   The right to protection against unreasonable and unwarranted interference with one's solitude; the right of an individual to be left alone. (Ch. 5)

Private non-profit (or not-for-profit) organization   Organization that has funds redirected to maintenance and growth rather than as dividends to stockholders. (Ch. 7)

Problem solving   Using a systematic process to solve a problem. (Ch. 6)

Process of care   The desired sequence of steps that have been designed to achieve clinical standardization. (Ch. 1)

Procrastination   Doing one thing when one should be doing something else. (Ch. 28)

Productive hours   Paid time that is worked. (Ch. 12)

Productive time   Time an employee actually works. (Ch. 14)

Productivity   The ratio of outputs to inputs or, in nursing terms, the ratio of services to resources used to provide services. (Ch. 12)

Productivity report   Documentation of the volume of efforts consumed. (Ch. 14)

Professional association (organization)   An alliance of practitioners within a profession that provides opportunities for its members to meet leaders in the field, hone their own leadership skills, participate in policy formation, continue specialized education, and shape the future of the profession. (Ch. 29)

Profit   An excess of revenues over expenses. (Ch. 12)

Progressive discipline   A step-by-step process of increasing disciplinary measures, usually beginning with an oral warning, followed by a written warning, suspension, and termination, if necessary. (Ch. 24)

Prospective payment system   A method in which the third-party payer decides in advance what will be paid for a service or episode of care. (Ch. 12)

Prototype evaluation system   System of classifying in broad categories. (Ch. 14)

Providers   See *Healthcare provider.* (Ch. 12)

Public institution   Providing health services under the support and direction of local, state, or federal government. (Ch. 7)

Q

Quality and Safety Education for Nurses (QSEN)   This acronym refers to the Quality and Safety Education for Nurses, which is an institute devoted to providing resources related to the QSEN Competencies for both undergraduate and graduate practitioners. The knowledge, skills, and attitudes are defined to reflect the necessary abilities one must have to practice safely and to strive for quality. The six competencies are patient-centered care, teamwork and collaboration, evidence-based practice, quality improvement, safety, and informatics. (Ch. 2, 11)

Quality assurance (QA)   A process that focuses on the clinical aspects of a provider's care, often in response to an identified problem. (Ch. 20)

Quality improvement (QI)   An ongoing process of innovation, prevention of error, and staff development used by an organization that has adopted a quality management philosophy. Often used interchangeably with *total quality management*, *continuous quality management*, *quality improvement*, and *quality management*. (Ch. 20)

Quality indicators   Measurable elements of quality that specify the focus of evaluation and documentation. (Chs. 4, 22)

Quality management (QM)   A corporate culture emphasizing customer satisfaction, innovation, and employee involvement in quality improvement activities. Often used interchangeably with *total quality management*, *continuous quality management*, *quality improvement*, and *performance improvement*. (Ch. 20)

Quantum theory   A physics theory stating that energy is not a smooth flowing continuum but, rather, bursts of energy that are related. (Ch. 4)

R

Randomized controlled trial (RCT)   Study in which patients are assigned by chance to one of the groups defined in the study. (Ch. 21)

Redesign   Technique to analyze tasks to improve efficiency. (Ch. 8)

Reengineering   A total reorganization of how an organization will function, with the goal of increased efficiency. (Ch. 8)

Research   A systematic investigation to determine the truth or falsity of a hypothesis. (Ch. 21)

Research utilization   Process of synthesizing, discriminating, and using research-generated knowledge to make an impact or change in existing practices. (Ch. 21)

Respect for others   The highest ethical principle, respect for others acknowledges the right of individuals to make decisions and to live by those decisions. (Ch. 5)

Respondeat superior   A doctrine by which the employer is given accountability and responsibility for an employee's negligent actions incurred during the course and scope of employment. (Ch. 5)

Responsibility   The condition of being reliable and dependable and being obligated to accomplish work. (Ch. 26)

Restructuring   Technique to enhance organizational productivity. (Ch. 8)

Résumé   A summary of professional abilities and facts designed for specific opportunities. (Ch. 29)

Revenue   Money earned by an organization for providing goods or services. (Ch. 12)

Right to work   Statute in the United States that governs the extent to which an established union can require employees' membership, payment of union dues, or fees as a condition of employment, either before or after hiring. Right-to-work laws do not provide a general guarantee of employment, but rather a government regulation of the contractual agreements between unions and employers that prevent the exclusion of non-union workers or to require employee to pay dues prior to representation. (Ch. 19)

Risk management   Integrated into a quality management program as a process of developing and implementing strategies that will minimize risks and mitigate the impact of adverse effects. This includes preventing patient injury, minimizing financial loss after a problem/error occurs, and preserving agency reputation. (Ch. 20)

Role   Expected or actual behavior, determined by a person's position or status in a group. (Ch. 4)

Role ambiguity   A condition in which individuals do not have a clear understanding about performance and evaluation. (Ch. 15)

Role conflict   A condition in which individuals understand the role but are unwilling or unable to meet the requirements. (Ch. 15)

Role development   Choosing to change role expectations and/or role performance. (Ch. 27)

Role discrepancy   A gap between role expectations and role performance. (Ch. 27)

Role expectations   The attitudes and behaviors another anticipates a person in the role will possess or demonstrate. (Ch. 27)

Role internalization   Stage at which a person has learned behaviors that maintain a role so thoroughly that the person performs them without consciously considering them; energy once spent on establishing these behaviors can be redirected to other goals. (Ch. 27)

Role model   A person who enacts a role, typically in a positive way, so that others can follow the example. (Ch. 19)

Role negotiation   Resolving conflicting expectations about personal management performance through communication. (Ch. 27)

Role strain   The subjective feeling of discomfort experienced as a result of role stress; may manifest through increased frustration, heightened emotional awareness, or emotional fragility to situations. (Chs. 24, 27)

Role stress   A social condition in which role demands are conflicting, irritating, or impossible to fulfill. (Chs. 24, 27, 28)

Role theory   A framework used to understand how individuals perform within organizations. (Chs. 4, 15)

Role transition   The process of unlearning an old role and learning a new role. Transforming one's identity from being an individual contributor as a staff nurse to being a leader as a nurse manager. (Ch. 27)

ROLES   An acronym used to identify the components of a role: responsibilities, opportunities, lines of communication, expectations, and support. (Ch. 27)

Root-cause analysis   The process used to identify all possible causes of a sentinel event and all appropriate risk-reduction strategies. (Ch. 20)

S

Satisficing   A decision process where the solution is acceptable (rather than best). (Ch. 6)

Satisficing decision   Selecting an option that is acceptable but not necessarily the best option. (Satisfy + suffice = satisfice.) (Ch. 6)

SBAR   A standard, best practice form of communication between two (or more) healthcare professionals. Situation, Background, Assessment, Recommendation. (Ch. 20)

Scheduling   The implementation of the staffing plan by assigning unit personnel to work specific hours and days. (Ch. 14)

Secondary care   Disease restorative care. (Ch. 7)

Second-order change   Change that is revolutionary, episodic, and that requires radical differences from what exists. (Ch. 17)

Self-management   The ability of individuals to actively gain control of their lives; components include stress management, time management, meeting management, and the ability to delegate. (Ch. 28)

Self-reflection   A process of serious consideration about one's thoughts and actions designed to improve one's performance in the future. (Ch. 28)

Sentinel event   A serious, unexpected occurrence involving death or injury, such as suicide, infant abduction, or wrong-site surgery. (Ch. 20)

Service   In a healthcare context, the interaction between a consumer and the system to the extent needs are addressed. (Ch. 22)

Service-line structures   A type of structure in which the functions necessary to produce a specific service or product are brought together into an integrated organizational unit under the control of a single manager or executive. (Ch. 8)

Service recovery   A strategy for identifying complaints and rectifying service failures to retain or "recover" dissatisfied customers. (Ch. 22)

Shared governance   A flat type of organizational structure with decision making decentralized. (Chs. 8, 19)

Shared vision   Agreement among a team of people working toward a common end; concurrence on what the desired state in the future will be. (Ch. 30)

Smart card   Credit card–like device that stores data. (Ch. 11)

Social networking   The use of technology and other mechanisms to create a web of relationships with common involvement in an area of focus or concern. (Ch. 1)

Span of control   The number of individuals a supervisor manages. For budgetary reasons, span of control is often a major focus for organizational restructuring. (Ch. 8)

Speech recognition (SR)   Electronic devices and programs that permit data entry via oral entry methods. (Ch. 11)

Staff function   Function that assists those in frontline positions in accomplishing primary objectives. (Ch. 8)

Staff mix   The proportion of RNs to LPNs/LVNs to UAPs in a specific setting. (Ch. 13)

Staffing   The function of planning for hiring and deploying qualified personnel to meet the needs of patients for care and services. (Ch. 14)

Staffing plan   The conceptual approach of accomplishing the work to be done on a given unit. (Ch. 14)

Staffing regulations   Licensing regulations required by the state department of health, usually related to the minimum number of professional nurses on a unit at a given time. (Ch. 14)

Standard of care   Level of quality considered adequate by a profession; skills and learning commonly possessed by members of a profession; also written at a minimum level. (Ch. 5)

Statute   Rule/regulation created by elected legislative bodies; also known as *statutory law.* (Ch. 5)

Strategic planning   A process designed to achieve goals through allocation of resources. (Ch. 16)

Strategies   Approaches designed to achieve a specific purpose. (Ch. 17)

Subculture   Element of a main culture that has formed its own culture that differs in some way. (Ch. 19)

Supervision   Provision of guidance and oversight of delegated nursing task (ANA & NCSBN, 2006). (Ch. 26)

Synergy   A phenomenon in which teamwork produces extraordinary results that could not have been achieved by any one individual. (Ch. 18)

Synergy Model   A model of care delivery adopted by the American Association of Critical-Care Nurses that matches the needs and characteristics of the patient with the competencies of the nurse. Seven characteristics are unique to every patient, and each nurse

has varying levels of ability, which are categorized into eight competencies. When the knowledge, skills, and competencies of the nurse are used to meet the complex needs of the patient and family, the care is optimal. (Ch. 13)

System   A group or organization working together as a unified whole. (Ch. 8)

Systems theory   An approach to consider how various independent parts interact to form a unified whole or to disrupt a unified whole; the construct related to the operation of the whole process or entity. (Ch. 8)

T

Tacit knowledge   An implied, unspoken knowledge. (Ch. 1)

Teach-back   A learning evaluation technique where the educator asks the learner to explain the information shared with the learner. (Ch. 20)

Teaching institution   An academic health center and affiliated hospital. (Ch. 7)

Team   A number of people associated together in specific work or activities. (Ch. 18)

Team nursing   A small group of licensed and unlicensed personnel, with a team leader, responsible for providing patient care to a group of patients. (Ch. 13)

TeamSTEPPS   A teamwork system designed to increase patient safety. (Ch. 2)

Telehealth   Use of modern telecommunications and information technologies for provision of health care to individuals at a distance and transmission of information to provide that care; involves use of two-way interactive videoconferencing, high-speed phone lines, fiberoptic cables, and satellite transmissions. (Ch. 11)

Tertiary care   Rehabilitative or long-term care. (Ch. 7)

The Joint Commission   An organization that accredits healthcare organizations and is deemed by the Center for Medicare & Medicaid Services (CMS) as holding healthcare facilities to CMS standards. (Ch. 2)

Third-party payers   Private and public agencies that contract with an individual to assume responsibility to pay under defined conditions for specified healthcare services. (Ch. 7)

Time management The use of tools, techniques, strategies, and follow-up systems to control wasted time and to ensure that the time invested in activities leads toward achieving a desired, high-priority goal. (Ch. 28)

Total patient care See *Case method.* (Ch. 13)

Total quality management (TQM) A comprehensive program designed to achieve perfection in quality of care. Often used interchangeably with *continuous quality management, quality management, quality improvement,* and *performance improvement.* (Ch. 20)

Toxic workplace An organization in which people feel devalued or dehumanized and in which disruptive behavior often flourishes. (Ch. 25)

Transactional leadership The act of using rewards and punishments as part of daily oversight of employees in seeking to get the group to accomplish a task. (Ch. 3)

Transculturalism Bridging significant differences in cultural practices. (Ch. 9)

Transformational leadership An act of encouraging followers to follow the leader's style and change their interests into a group interest with concern for a broader goal. (Ch. 3)

Transforming Care at the Bedside (TCAB) A program of the Institute for Healthcare Improvement designed to improve care of patients. (Ch. 13)

Transitional care models An approach designed by Dr. Mary Naylor to help patients return successfully to their homes (or another facility) after hospitalization. (Ch. 13)

Translating research into practice (TRIP) Approaches that integrate the use of evidence into patient care. (Ch. 21)

Translation science The science of how research is adopted. (Ch. 21)

Triple aim A shortcut for describing contemporary healthcare reform: to improve access, improve quality, and decrease or control healthcare costs. (Ch. 1)

U

Unit of service A measure of the work being produced by the organization, such as patient days, patient or home visits, or procedures. (Chs. 12, 14)

Unlicensed assistive personnel Healthcare workers who are not licensed and who are prepared to provide certain elements of care under the supervision of a registered nurse (e.g., technicians, nurse aides, certified nursing assistants). (Chs. 13, 26)

Unlicensed nursing personnel A term used to distinguish those for whom nurses are accountable as opposed to the numerous unlicensed assistive personnel providing aid in other clinical disciplines. (Ch. 26)

Unplanned change Disconcerting, unanticipated, adaptive change. (Ch. 17)

Utilization The quantity or volume of services provided. (Ch. 12)

V

Value-based purchasing A pay for performance methodology used to reimburse hospitals based on outcomes. (Ch. 12)

Values Inner forces that influence decision making and priority setting. (Ch. 1)

Variable costs Costs that vary in direct proportion to patient volume or acuity. (Ch. 12)

Variable FTEs Those full-time equivalent positions that depend on the demand for care, typically staff positions. (Ch. 14)

Variance Anything that alters a patient's progress through a normal care path. (Chs. 12, 13)

Variance analysis Budget-control process to determine differences between income and expenses, projected and actual costs. (Ch. 12)

Variance report A report defining the difference between the actual and projected staffing or budgeting. (Ch. 14)

Veracity Principle that compels the truth be told completely. (Ch. 5)

Vertical integration Alignment of organizations to provide a full array or continuum of services. (Ch. 7)

Vicarious liability Imputation of accountability upon one person or entity for the actions of another person; substituted liability or imputed liability. (Ch. 5)

Vision The desired future state. (Chs. 1, 8, 30)

W

Whistle blowing The process in which an individual makes public a serious wrongdoing or danger when the organization didn't take action to correct the situation or report the condition. (Ch. 5)

Whistleblower A person who makes public a serious wrongdoing or danger concealed within an organization when internal actions have failed to correct or make public a situation. (Chs. 5, 19)

Workload The amount of work distributed to a person or unit for a given time period. (Ch. 14)

Workplace advocacy Refers to acting on or in behalf of another who is unable to act for himself or herself to effect change about workplace conditions. (Ch. 19)

Note: Page numbers followed by *b* indicate boxes, *f* indicate figures and *t* indicate tables.